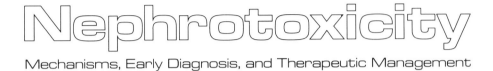

Nephrotoxicity

Mechanisms, Early Diagnosis, and Therapeutic Management

edited by

Peter H. Bach

School of Science
Polytechnic of East London
London, England

Neill J. Gregg

The Boots Company PLC
Thurgarton, Nottingham, England

Martin F. Wilks

ICI Central Toxicology Laboratory
Macclesfield, Cheshire, England

Ligia Delacruz

Robens Institute of Health and Safety
University of Surrey
Guildford, Surrey, England

Marcel Dekker, Inc.   **New York/Basel/Hong Kong**

Library of Congress Cataloging-in-Publication Data

Nephrotoxicity : mechanisms, early diagnosis, and therapeutic
    management / edited by P. H. Bach ... [et al.] .
            p   cm.
        Papers presented, in honor of Karl Ullrich, at the Fourth
    International Symposium on Nephrotoxicity, held at Guildford,
    Surrey, England in 1989.
        Includes bibliographical references and index.
        ISBN 0-8247-8366-2
        1. Nephrotoxicity--Congresses. 2. Ullrich, K. J. (Karl J.)-
    -Congresses. I. Bach, P. H. (Peter H.) II. Ullrich, K. J. (Karl
    J.) III. International Symposium on Nephrotoxicity (4th : 1989 :
    Guildford, England)
    RC918.N45N46   1991
    616.6'1--dc20
                                                    91-6774
                                                      CIP

This book is printed on acid-free paper

MARCEL DEKKER, INC.
270 Madison Avenue, New York, New York 10016

Current printing (last digit):
10 9 8 7 6 5 4 3 2 1

PRINTED IN THE UNITED STATES OF AMERICA

DEDICATION

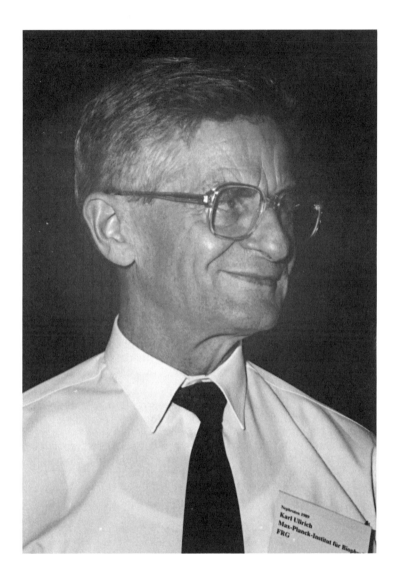

Karl Julius Ullrich

The personality of Karl Julius Ullrich is characterized by his continuous excitement about progression in our knowledge on renal function in particular and science in general. In that respect, he is one of the "youngest" participants.

He graduated with a degree in medicine in 1951, and was much influenced by Homer Smith's book <u>The Kidney in Health and Disease</u>. This stimulated him to switch from clearance experiments in human volunteers to basic studies in renal physiology in Marburg, where Kurt Kramer had founded one of the most successful post-war research groups in that field. Starting from studies on urine concentration in the renal medulla, he found that the solute gradient was composed not only of sodium chloride and urea, but also of organic osmolytes such as glycerophosphorylcholine and inositol, which he described in 1956. Since then, his main interest has focussed on the molecular mechanisms of renal function, applying physical, chemical and biological techniques to the mammalian nephron. Many technical developments carry his experience. The microcatheterization of the collecting duct, microcuvette techniques, the shrinking droplet and microperfusion technique as well as the technique to perfuse peritubular blood capillaries were developed together with Karl Heinz Jarausch, Karl Heinz Gertz, Gundula Pehling, Peter Deetjen and Eberhard Froemter. Using these techniques, he found that the collecting ducts reabsorbed NaCl and urea, and secretes protons and ammonium ions. The recirculation of urea was studied together with Carl Gottschalk and Bodil Schmidt-Nielsen. He was awarded the chair of Physiology at the University of Berlin in 1962 and here and at the Max-Planck Institute for Biophysics in Frankfurt (where he has been since 1967). Karl Ullrich's interest has covered nearly every aspect of kidney function, attracting numerous scientists from all over the world to collaborate with him.

Karl Ullrich has worked with Gerhard Rumrich, Sonia Klsz and Friedron Papavassiliou over the past twenty years to characterise hexose, amino acid, proton, calcium, phosphate, sulphate, monocarboxylate and dicarboxylate transport in proximal tubules. He has recently concentrated his interest on the contraluminal transport steps of the proximal tubule and approached the field of nephrotoxicity by detecting the mechanisms of dicarboxylate, aliphatic monocarboxylate, and para-aminohippurate transport. His systematic study of the role of each moeity of the molecule to its transport has helped further an understanding of the compartmentalisation of xenobiotics in different parts of the kidney. These data are essential for all those studying the many aspects of renal pharmacology and toxicology.

In addition to his scientific activities, Karl J. Ullrich has served many scientific and cultural societies as a continuous supporter and stimulator. His opinion is respected not only by the scientific community, but also by those involved in the general political and cultural life of his country. Supported by his family and friends, Karl J. Ullrich has proved himself a highly engaged representative of the scientific society in defending the principles of openness and truth. His numerous activities have been acknowledged by many honorary medals and prizes. In spite of his full engagement in science, he still finds time for his family, his many friends and the young students whom he encourages to enter the scientific world.

This book is dedicated to Karl J. Ullrich on the occasion of his 65th birthday to acknowledge his important contribution to our understanding of renal transport functions. Young scientists will value the importance of his contribution to the understanding of their experiments in studying the mechanisms of nephrotoxicity. In common with many other scientists, I feel that the many stimulating comments and suggestions from this extraordinary colleague will provide new challenges and understanding that will be significant to all areas of clinical medicine.

Walter G. Guder

Institute for Clinical Chemistry
Munich, Germany

PREFACE

The importance of nephrotoxicity as an aetiological factor in the development of renal disease is now widely appreciated by clinicians, scientists, industry and governmental agencies. The complex structure of the kidney and the processes of renal functional impairment necessitate a multidisciplinary approach to research into the underlying mechanisms and the clinical prevention, diagnosis and treatment of toxic nephropathies.

The aim of the *Fourth International Symposium on Nephrotoxicity* was to provide a forum for life scientists and clinicians to focus on understanding the mechanistic basis of toxic nephropathies as a means for developing new and sensitive markers for the early diagnosis of nephrotoxic damage. The topics included molecular and cellular biology, structure activity relationships, physiology, pathology, in vitro methods, novel techniques of diagnostic imaging and nuclear magnetic resonance, to name but a few. This has moved towards enabling scientists to detect subtle renal damage with unprecedented accuracy in the future, thereby facilitating early therapeutic intervention. Participants from 21 countries presented their findings in 130 oral and poster communications.

A limited number of contributions, representative of the whole symposium, were selected, expanded by the authors and peer-reviewed and have been published in a special issue of *Renal Failure* (Volume 12, Part 3, 1990). This is to widen the clinical awareness of progress being made in nephrotoxicity. Together, both the *Proceedings* and the *Special Issue* form a comprehensive synopsis of the state-of-the-art research in all aspects of toxic nephropathies.

Many people contributed their scientific expertise and organisational skills to the success of the symposium. They include the scientific advisors who provided guidance and suggested **Karl Ullrich** as a luminary whose contributions to nephrotoxicity have been key to its development and should be the opening focus of the symposium. The Proceedings is dedicated to Professor Ullrich on the occasion of his 65th birthday. The scientific advisors also conferred the Young Scientist Award on **Dr Charles Ruegg** for his novel and energetic approach to understanding selective cell injury.

The smooth running of the meeting was ensured by Joanne Thorndike, Sally Nichol, Merce Moret, Yinuo Ding and Cecilia Guastadisegni. The administration of the symposium and the preparation of the proceedings were expertly handled by Lisa Breitner, Gail Sutherland, Monique Rivet and Mimps E. van Ek. Finally, our thanks to the participants, for their scientific contribution, critical appraisal and lively debate.

Peter H. Bach
Neill J. Gregg
Martin F. Wilks
Ligia Delacruz

ACKNOWLEDGEMENTS

The symposium was supported by

Hazleton UK, Harrogate
Upjohn Limited, Crawley
Pfizer Central Research, Sandwich
Ciba-Geigy Pharmaceuticals, Wilmslow
Johnson Matthey Research Centre, Reading
The Procter & Gamble Company, Cincinnati
Roche Products Limited, Welwyn Garden City
ICI Central Toxicology Laboratory, Macclesfield
Esso Exploration and Production UK Limited, London
Smith Kline & French Laboratories Limited, Welwyn

Wellcome Trust, London
Cancer Research Campaign, London
International Programme on Chemical Safety - World Health Organization, Geneva
Commission of the European Communities, Luxembourg

-oOo-

The Young Scientist Award was sponsored by
Smith Kline & French Research Laboratories, Philadelphia

CONTENTS

PART V: ANTIBIOTICS

PART VI: CYCLOSPORINE A

PART VII: RADIOCONTRAST MEDIA

PART VIII: HALOGENATED COMPOUNDS

PART IX: ORGANIC SOLVENTS

PART X: THE MECHANISM OF RENAL CANCER AND ANTI-CANCER THERAPY

PART XI: **HEAVY METALS**

PART XII: **IN VITRO**

PART XIII: MARKERS OF NEPHROTOXICITY

PART I
RENAL PHYSIOLOGY AND FUNCTION

1

RENAL TRANSPORT AND NEPHROTOXICITY

K.J. Ullrich (1), G. Rumrich (1), M.W. Gemborys (2), W. Dekant (3)

Max-Planck-Institut für Biophysik, 6000 Frankfurt/M., Germany (1), McNeil Consumer Products Company, Fort Washington, USA (2), Institut für Pharmakologie u. Toxikologie, Universität Würzburg, 8700 Würzburg, Germany (3)

Many nephrotoxic substances exert their toxic effect preferentially in the kidney because a higher concentration accumulates in proximal tubular cells than in other cells. During net reabsorption or net secretion these nephrotoxic compounds have to cross the two cell membranes of the proximal tubule using specific transport systems which have a broad and overlapping specificity. Thus, a substance may use more than one system at either the apical or basal side of the cell. The direction of net transport depends on the driving forces, which are not only the electrochemical potential differences of the transportees, but also those of their co- or counter-transported partners.

If a substance is freely filtrable, 20% of the total amount in the kidney reaches the luminal cell membrane and 80% the contraluminal membrane. In accordance with this, transport systems at the contraluminal cell side can clear the blood plasma flowing through the kidney completely from organic anions or organic cations. Quite a variety of nephrotoxic substances are organic anions. Others have electronegative groups and are sufficiently hydrophobic to be transported by the organic anion transport system. There are, however, three contraluminal transport systems for organic anions (1,2). Their characteristics are as follows:

1) The transport system for hydrophobic organic anions, i.e. the para-aminohippurate (PAH) transport system, requires molecules with a sufficiently hydrophobic core and one or more electronegative anionic or partially electronegative groups. It is an anion exchange system.

2) The Na^+-dicarboxylate cotransport system accepts molecules with electronegative ionic charges at 50-90nm distance or one ionic and one partial negative group at that distance. Since almost all such molecules are hydrophobic they also fulfil the specificity requirement for the PAH transport system. The Na^+-dicarboxylate transport system is localised to the luminal, as well as the contraluminal cell membrane of proximal tubular cells.

3) The sulphate-oxalate transport system requires an accumulation of electronegative and/or partially electronegative charges (30- 70 nm charge distance). The system also accepts molecules which are hydrophobic and are substrates for the PAH transport system. It also accepts substrates which have some of their anionic charges at 60-70nm distance and are also substrates for the Na^+-dicarboxylate transport system. This means that only small and non-hydrophobic molecules with several electronegative charges are specific substrates for the sulphate-oxalate system.

Unfortunately, there are no specific inhibitors for any of the contraluminal organic anion transport systems. Probenecid has an apparent K_i for the PAH transport system (0.03 mmol/l) which is 4 times higher than the K_m for PAH (0.08). However, it also inhibits the sulphate transport system with an apparent K_i of 7.5 mmol/l which is 6 times higher than the apparent K_m for sulphate (3). Thus, probenecid can be considered as specific inhibitor for the

PAH transport system only with reservation. A second gap in our knowledge is that the effect of overlapping specificities on overall transport and intracellular concentration is not clear. In our studies on contraluminal anion transport we have used the stop-flow capillary perfusion method and have measured the short-term, over 1-4 seconds, influx of ^{3}H-PAH, ^{3}H-succinate and ^{35}S-sulphate in terms of K_m and J_{max}. Furthermore we have measured the apparent K_i of several hundred organic anionic substances carried by these three transport systems. The apparent K_i determines only the interaction of the substance in question with the respective transport system, but it does not give any information about the transport rate of this substance. It is likely that the affinity of a certain substance for the transporter must be high enough to give a reasonable transport rate, but if the affinity is too high, the transport rate of such a substance may become low because of

its low "off" rate. The transport behaviour of toxicologically important substances in terms of apparent K_i values against contraluminal transport of PAH, succinate and sulphate will be discussed below.

Transport of phenolic compounds and their derivatives

The "parent molecule" phenol (Table 1) interacts very weakly with the dicarboxylate system probably because of oligomer formation (4). Benzoate has only a small inhibitory potency against the PAH transporter in common with salicylate, acetylsalicylate (aspirin) and lysyl-acetylsalicylate. This is in agreement with clearance data which indicate filtration, probenecid-sensitive secretion and non-ionic back diffusion (for literature see 5 and 6). The glycine conjugate of salicylate (salicyluric acid), which is the main excretory product of salicylate in urine (up to 70%), potently inhibits contralumi-

Table 1. Effect of salicylate and acetaminobenzene-derived analgesics on contraluminal transport systems of the proximal tubule

	apparent K_i values (mmol/l)		
	PAH	succinate	SO_4^{2-}
phenol	>5 (NS)	9.0±23.3	25 (NS)
benzoate	1.5±0.92	>10 (NS)	>25 (NS)
salicylate	0.93±0.42	>10 (NS)	>25 (NS)
acetylsalicylate (aspirin)	1.1±0.38	>10 (NS)	>25 (NS)
lysyl-acetylsalicylate	2.0±1.0	>10 (NS)	> 25 (NS)
glycine-salicylate (salicyluric acid)	0.03±0.01	>10 (NS)	>25 (NS)
aminobenzene (aniline)	>5 (NS)	>10 (NS)	>25 (NS)
N-phenylhydroxylamine	>5 (NS)	>10 (NS)	>25 (NS)
N-acetaminobenzene(antifebrin)	2.0±1.1	>10 (NS)	>25 (NS)
aminophenol	>5 (NS)	>10 (NS)	>25 (NS)
4-acetaminophenol(paracetamol)	2.8±1.7	>10 (NS)	>25 (NS)
4-ethoxyacetaminobenzene (phenacetin)	1.0±0.4	>10 (NS)	>25 (NS)
4-acetaminoacetophenone	0.75±0.21	>10 (NS)	>25 (NS)
4-ethoxyaminobenzene (phenetidine)	2.2±1.2	>10 (NS)	>25 (NS)

NS = inhibition of transport not significant, compared to controls.

nal PAH transport. In the dog kidney, clearance of salicyluric acid can be 5 x GFR (7), indicating complete excretory clearance as it is the case for PAH which has a $K_{i,PAH}$ value of 0.03 mmol/l. Aniline, N-phenylhydroxylamine and aminophenol do not interact with the PAH transporter, but if the amino group of aniline is acetylated (antifebrin), a moderate inhibition is seen. Further para-hydroxylation to paracetamol or para-ethoxysubstitution to phenacetin gives an inhibitory potency in the same range (8). Interestingly, 4-acetaminoacetophenone (with two C=O groups) has the highest inhibitory potency of this series. The last compound 4-ethoxyaminobenzene (phenetidine) has an inhibitory potency like antifebrin or paracetamol. None of the compounds listed in Table 1 interacts with the dicarboxylate transporter. Clearance data of phenacetin and paracetamol indicate a behaviour similar to that of urea, because of their lipid solubility and therefore good diffusibility (for literature see 8). While there was no indication of secretion in the published literature, such a process is clearly indicated by our data. The conjugates of paracetamol behave quite differently which will be discussed below.

Transport of mercapto compounds and their mercury complexes

The interaction of the thiol-compound dithiothreitol and the mercapto- reagents, 4-chloro-mercuri-benzoate and 4-acetaminophenyl-acetate with the PAH- and the dicarboxylate transporter are as predicted, but the mercuri-compounds behave anomalously with the sulphate transporter. This suggests that the sulphate transporter has reactive SH-groups in the substrate binding site which is supported by the fact that 9 out of 10 mercury complexes tested (data in brackets, Table 2) show an interaction with the sulphate transporter which is not justified by their structure. Thus the sulphate transporter seems to have reactive SH groups in its substrate binding centre in contrast to the other two transporters.

The commercially available mercapto-compounds DL-mercaptosuccinate, meso-2,3-dimercaptosuccinate, 2-mercaptoethane-sulfonate, DL-2,3-dimercapto- propane-sulfonate and N-(2-mercaptopropionyl)-glycine and their respective disulfides, exert a moderate inhibitory potency against the contraluminal PAH transporter ($K_{i\ PAH}$ 0.25 to 1.4 mmol/l). Complexing with Hg does not change this behaviour. Interaction with the dicarboxylate transporter is only seen with the dicarboxylic DL-mercaptosuccinate and meso-2,3-dimercapto-succinate. Here, complexing with Hg diminishes the interaction. A low interaction with the sulphate transporter is seen with the two SH-dicarboxylates and interestingly with DL-2,3-dimercaptopropane sulfonate-disulfide. L-cysteine, N-acetylcysteine, L-cystine, D-penicillamine, N-acetyl-D-penicillamine, and its disulfide, as well as reduced and oxidized L-glutathione do not interact with the PAH transporter, or the dicarboxylate, or with the sulphate transporter. Hg-complexed reduced L-glutathione shows a small, although significant inhibitory potency against dicarboxylate transport.

Of the mercuric-complexes, those of N-acetylcysteine and N-acetyl- penicillamine interacted with the PAH transporter, while the uncomplexed compounds did not. From the data of Table 2 one might hypothesize that only those substances which interact with the transporters will enter the tubular cells, whereby the SH-dicarboxylates might reach higher intracellular concentrations because their Na^+-dependent transporter is located at both cell membranes. N-acetylcysteine and N-acetylpenicillamine do not enter the tubular cells except when they are complexed with Hg. This might have implications for nephrotoxicity. The dicarboxylate transporter may accomplish the uptake of glutathione from the blood into proximal tubular cells and possibly net secretion (9). The mercapto-compounds mentioned in Table 2 serve as complexing agents for toxic metal ions (for literature see 10,20), and at least some of them also act as a reservoir for intracellular SH-groups and scavengers for oxygen radicals (12,22).

Table 2. Effect of mercapto-compounds (and their Hg-complexes, data in brackets) on contraluminal transport systems of the proximal tubule

	apparent K_i values (mmol/l)		
	PAH	succinate	SO_4^{2-}
1,4 dithiothreitol	>5 (NS)	>10 (NS)	>25 (NS)
4-chloromercuri-benzoate	1.2±0.9	>10 (NS)	1.9±0.9
4-aminophenyl-mercuriacetate	>5 (NS)	>10 (NS)	5.7±6.2
DL-mercaptosuccinate	0.77±0.33	0.28±0.07	6.1±6.9
	(0.94±0.28)	(0.73±0.46)	(0.56±0.15)
meso-2,3-dimercapto-	1.4±0.57	2.2±1.6	5.5±5.8
succinate	(>5 (NS))	(5.8±11.5)	(0.7±0.53)
2-mercaptoethane-	1.16±0.62	>10 (NS)	>25 (NS)
sulfonate	(0.62±0.16)	(>10 (NS))	(6.2±8.4)
mercaptoethane-disulfide	0.25±0.08	>10 (NS)	>25 (NS)
DL-2,3-dimercapto-propane-	0.56±0.13	>10 (NS)	>25 (NS)
1-sulfonate	(1.0±0.3)	(>10 (NS))	(2.3±1.4)
DL-2,3-dimercapto-propane-	0.46±0.1	>10 (NS)	1.3±0.52
1-sulfonate-disulfide			
N(-2-mercaptopro-	0.86±0.24	>10 (NS)	>25 (NS)
pionyl)-glycine	(1.21±0.43)	(>10 (NS))	(0.95±0.28)
L-cysteine	>5 (NS)	>10 (NS)	> 25 (NS)
	(>5 (NS))	(>10 (NS))	(>25 (NS))
N-acetyl-	>5 (NS)	>10 (NS)	>25 (NS)
L-cysteine	(1.65±0.75)	(>10 (NS))	(1.6±0.71)
L-cystine	>5 (NS)	>10 (NS)	>25 (NS)
D-(-)-penicillamine	>5 (NS)	>10 (NS)	>25 (NS)
(>5 (NS))	(>10 (NS))	(4.8+5.3)	
N-acetyl-DL	>5 (NS)	>10 (NS)	12.0±25.7
penicillamine	(1.9±0.9)	(>10 (NS))	(7.6±11.1)
D-(-)-penicillamine-disulfide	>5 (NS)	>10 (NS)	>25 (NS)
L-glutathione red.	>5 (NS)	10.6	>25 (NS)
	(>5 (NS))	(18.0)	(1.5±0.65)
L-glutathione ox.	>5 (NS)	>10 (NS)	>25 (NS)

In previous studies it was found that an electronegative ionic charge and a hydrophobic core are the main prerequisites for a molecule to be accepted by the contraluminal PAH transporter (1,2). It seems to be the principle in xenobiotic detoxification to establish both properties, i.e. charge and hydrophobicity. This could best be documented by conjugation of electrophilic xenobiotics with glutathione (13), which is catalysed by glutathione-S-transferases and takes place in the liver. The compounds reach the luminal and contraluminal cell side of renal proximal tubules via the blood stream. As shown in Table 3, hydrophobic glutathione conjugates interact with the contra-luminal PAH transporter and are probably also taken up into the kidney cells by this transporter (14). Alternatively, gamma-glutamyl-transpepti-dase located at the outer surface of the luminal as well as of the contraluminal cell membrane splits off glutamate first. From the resulting S-cysteinyl-glycine conjugate glycine is also removed, catalyzed by cysteinyl-glycine- di-peptidase and aminopeptidase M. The resulting S-cysteinyl-conjugate is much more hydro-phobic than the glutathione conjugate and, as shown in Table 3, in almost every case a good substrate for the contraluminal PAH transpor-ter. Thus, it seems plausible that an electrophilic xenobiotic is taken up from blood into the kidney cell either as glutathione-con-jugate or, more likely as cysteine-conjugate. There is good evidence that S-cysteinyl-con-

jugates are transported into proximal tubular cells by a probenecid inhibitable, i.e. the PAH transport mechanism (for literature see 14). It is, however, debatable whether the cysteine-conjugates can also use amino acid transport systems. N-acetylation of the cysteine con-jugate transforms the zwitterionic molecule into an anionic molecule augmenting the affinity towards the contraluminal PAH transporter (Table 3). Indeed, it was found that N-acetyl-S-cysteine conjugate uptake into proximal tubular cells is inhibited by substrates for the PAH transporter such as PAH itself, probenecid or penicillin G (21). N-acetylation also occurs with-in the kidney cells (15). Finally, the mercapturic acid-conjugates are excreted into the urine.

Several studies have shown that the mercap-turic acid pathway produces toxic compounds from various drugs and xenobiotics (16). Appar-

Table 3. Transport of S-conjugates of glutathione, L-cysteine and N-acetyl- cysteine

| | apparent $K_{I,PAH}$ (mmol/l) | | |
	-L-glutathione	-L-cysteine	-N-acetyl-L-cysteine
S-(2-chloroethyl)-		>5 (NS)	
S-(2-chloro-1,2,2-trifluoroethyl)-		0.66±0.16	
S-(2-chlorovinyl)-		1.10±0.40	
S-(1,2-dichlorovinyl)-	>5 (NS)	0.82±0.24	0.46±0.10
S-(1,2,2-trichlorovinyl)-	1.30±0.48	0.41±0.08	0.22±0.04
S-(3-chloropropenyl)-		1.60±0.70	0.70±0.18
S-(1,2,3,3-pentachloropropenyl)-		0.11±0.02	
S-(1,2,3,4-tetrachlorobutadienyl) -bis-1.4-	>5 (NS)		
S-(1,2,3,4,4-pentachlorobutadienyl)	0.47±0.11	0.16±0.03	0.07±0.01
S-(n-decyl)-	0.35±0.10		
S-(benzyl)-		1.60±0.65	0.32±0.06
S-(pentachlorophenyl		>5 (NS)	
S-(4-nitrophenyl)	>5 (NS)		
S-(2-bromo-hydrochinone)-5-		0.34±0.07	
S-(2-bromo-hydrochinone)-bis-3.5-		0.93±0.28	
S-(4-azidophenacyl)-	2.90±2.00		
S-(4-chlorophenacyl)-	2.25±1.30		
S-(benzthiazolyl)-		0.30±0.06	

Table 4. Effect of 4- acetaminophenol and metabolites on the contraluminal anion transport systems.

	PAH	apparent K_i values (mmol/l) Succinate	SO_4^{2-}
4-acetamino-phenol (APAP)	2.8±1.7	>10 (NS)	>25 (NS)
N-acetyl-4-benzoquinoneimine	>5 (NS)	>10 (NS)	>25 (NS)
3-glutathione-APAP	>5 (NS)	>10 (NS)	>25 (NS)
3-cysteine-APAP	0.67±0.2	>10 (NS)	3.6±2.9
3-N-acetylcysteine-APAP	0.58±0.14	>10 (NS)	4.6±4.4
3-thiomethyl-APAP	1.4±0.6	>10 (NS)	>25 (NS)
3-methyl-sulfone-APAP	1.1±0.4	>10 (NS)	>25 (NS)
3-hydroxy-APAP	1.3±0.6	>10 (NS)	>25 (NS)
3-methoxy-APAP	1.8±1.0	>10 (NS)	>25 (NS)
3-cysteamine-APAP	>5 (NS)	>10 (NS)	>25 (NS)
3-glucuronide-APAP	>5 (NS)	>10 (NS)	>25 (NS)
3-sulphate-APAP	1.7±0.8	>10 (NS)	5.4±5.9

ently cysteine-conjugates are changed to toxic species by cysteine conjugate beta-lyase, a pyridoxal phosphate-dependent enzyme (17). The most sensitive is the S3-segment of the proximal tubule, the pars recta, where the highest rate of PAH transport occurs (18). Thus, the data from the literature provide evidence for the role of the PAH transporter in uptake of xenobiotic-S-glutathione, -S-cysteine and -S-acetyl-cysteine-conjugates into the proximal tubular cells, while the data presented in Table 3 allow quantitative predictions of the affinity of the different conjugates to the PAH transporter.

Transport of paracetamol and its metabolites

Paracetamol (acetaminophen-APAP) is hepatotoxic, when given as massive overdose, and possibly responsible for chronic nephrotoxicity (for literature see 19). APAP itself shows only a small inhibitory potency against contraluminal PAH transport. The reactive species N-acetyl-4- benzoquinoneimine, the 3-glutathione the 3-glucuronide- and the 3-cysteamine conjugate of APAP show no interaction at all because they have no proper electronegative group and/or a hydrophobicity which is too small. 3-cysteamine APAP, however, interacts with the contraluminal organic cation (NMN) transport

system with a $K_{i,NMN}$ value of 1.1 ± 0.3 mmol/l. The 3-cysteine-, 3-thiomethyl-, 3-methyl-sulfone-, 3-hydroxy- and 3-methoxy- and 3-sulphate conjugates of APAP exert a moderate inhibitory potency against the PAH transporter and are probably transported by that transport system. 3-Sulphate APAP interacts, as expected, with the sulphate transporter, as does 3-cysteine and 3-N-acetylcysteine-APAP. It would be interesting to know whether the intracellular concentration for the latter two substances which interact with two contraluminal anion systems is different from those substances which interact only with the PAH transport system.

Summary and Conclusion

The potential nephrotoxicity of a xenobiotic, as well as the efficiency of an anti-nephrotoxic agent (complexer of heavy metals, scavenger of oxygen radicals) depends on their concentrations within renal tubular cells. Anti-nephrotoxic effects are, in addition, exerted by substances which prevent the uptake of nephrotoxic agents into tubular cells. In this paper an overview is given of the characteristics of anion transport mechanisms, responsible for the uptake of xenobiotics from the blood into proximal tubular cells. The interaction of 1. salicylate- and acetaminobenzene-derived analgesics (aspirin, paracetamol, antifebrin, phenacetin, phenetidine); 2. mercaptocompounds and their Hg-complexes; 3. haloalkene conjugates with glutathione, cysteine, N-acetyl-cysteine; and 4. paracetamol metabolites with the contraluminal anion transporters can be explained by the specificity requirements of the transporters as previously established (1,2).

REFERENCES

1. Ullrich KJ, Rumrich G: Contraluminal transport systems in the proximal renal tubule involved in secretion of organic anions. Am J Physiol 245:F453-462, 1988.

2. Fritzsch G, Rumrich G, Ullrich KJ: Anion transport through the contraluminal cell membrane of renal proximal tubule. The influence of hydrophobicity and molecular charge distribution on the inhibitory activity of organic anions. Biochim Biophys Acta 978:249-256, 1989.

3. Ullrich KJ, Rumrich G, Klöss S: Contraluminal organic anion and cation transport in the proximal renal tubule: V. Interaction with sulfamoyl- and phenoxy diuretics, and with beta-lactam antibiotics. Kidney Int 36:78-88, 1989.

4. Ullrich KJ, Rumrich G, Klöss S: Contraluminal para-aminohippurate (PAH) transport in the proximal tubule of the rat kidney. IV. Specificity: mono- and polysubstituted benzene analogs. Pflügers Archiv 413:134-146, 1988.

5. Russel FGM, Wouterse AC, van Ginneken CAM: Physiologically based pharmacokinetic model for the renal clearance of salicyluric acid and the interaction with phenolsulfonphthalein in the dog. Drug Metab Dispos 15:695-701, 1987.

6. Ferrier B, Martin M, Roch-Ramel F: Effects of p-aminohippurate and pyrazinoate on the renal excretion of salicylate in the rat: a micropuncture study. J Pharmacol Exp Ther 224:451-458, 1983.

7. Weiner IM, Washington JA, Mudge GH: Studies on the renal excretion of salicylate in the dog. Bull Johns Hopkins Hosp 105:284-297, 1959.

8. Duggin GG: Mechanisms in the development of analgesic nephropathy. Kidney Int 18:553-561, 1980.

9. Heuner A, Schwegler JS, Silbernagl S: Renal tubular transport of glutathione in rat kidney. Pflügers Archiv 414:551-557, 1989.

10. Aposhian HV: DMSA and DMPS - Water soluble antidotes for heavy metal poisoning. Ann Rev Pharmacol Toxicol 23:193-215, 1983.

11. Ziegler DM: Role of reversible oxydation-reduction of enzyme thiols- disulfides in metabolic regulation. Ann Rev Biochem 54:305-329, 1985.

12. Kato M, Kako KJ: Effects of N-(2-mercaptopropionyl)glycine on ischemic reperfused dog kidney in vivo and membrane preparation in vitro. Mol Cell Biochem 78:151-159, 1987.

13. Habig WH, Pabst MJ, Jakoby WB: Glutathione S-transferases. J Biol Chem 249:7130-7139, 1974.

14. Ullrich KJ, Rumrich G, Wieland T, Dekant W: Contraluminal para- aminohippurate (PAH) transport in the proximal tubule of the rat kidney. VI. Specificity: Amino acids, their N-methyl-, N-acetyl- and N-benzoyl- derivatives; glutathione- and cysteine conjugates, di- and oligopeptides. Pflügers Archiv 415:342-350, 1989.

15. Schrenk D, Dekant W, Henschler D: Metabolism and excretion of S-conjugates derived from hexachlorobutadiene in the isolated perfused rat kidney. Mol Pharmacol 34:407-412, 1988

16. Dekant W, Vamvakas S, Anders MW: Bioactivation of nephrotoxic haloalkenes by glutathione conjugation: Formation of toxic and mutagenic intermediates by cysteine conjugate beta-lyase. Drug Metab Rev 20:43-83, 1989.

17. Stevens JL, Jacoby WB: Cysteine conjugate beta-lyase. Mol Pharmacol 23:761-765, 1983.

18. Nash JA, King LJ, Lock EA, Green T: The metabolism and disposition of hexachloro-1,3 butadiene in the rat and its relevance to nephrotoxicity. Toxicol Appl Pharmacol 73:124-137, 1984.

19. Gemborys MW, Mudge GH: Formation and disposition of the minor metabolites of acetaminophen in the hamster. Drug Metabol Dispos 9:340-351, 1981.

20. Murakami M, Sano K, Webb M: The effect of L-cysteine on the portion- selective uptake of cadmium in the renal proximal tubule. Arch Toxicol 60:365-369, 1987.

21. Lock EA, Odum J, Ormond P: Transport of N-acetyl-S-pentachloro-1,3- butadienyl cysteine in rat renal cortex. Arch Toxicol 59:12-15, 1986.

22. Fuchs J, Mainka L, Zimmer G: 2-Mercaptoproionylglycine and related compounds in treatment of mitochondrial dysfunction and postischemic myocardial damage. Arzneim-Forsch/Drug Res 35:1394-1402, 1985.

2

EFFECT OF AMPHOTERICIN B ON PAH TRANSPORT OF RAT RENAL CORTICAL SLICES IN VITRO AND EX VIVO

G. Inselmann, A. Kutzschbach, J. Heydemann and H. Th. Heidemann

1. Med. Clinic, Christian-Albrechts-University Kiel, D-2300 Kiel, FRG

INTRODUCTION

The therapeutic use of the antifungal drug amphotericin B is limited due to its nephrotoxic side effects. The incidence of this adverse effect is high and may reach 80% (1,2). Amphotericin B-induced impairment of kidney function is characterized by a reduction of renal blood flow with a concomitant decrease in glomerular filtration rate (3), most likely due to an activation of the tubular glomerular feedback (4). The tubular glomerular feedback is an intrarenal mechanism to regulate renal blood flow and glomerular filtration rate (5). Evidence has been accumulated that amphotericin B-induced renal vasoconstriction is one mechanism which may contribute to its nephrotoxicity (6). Little information exists as to what extent amphotericin B has a direct toxic effect on tubular function.

The purpose of this study was to evaluate whether amphotericin B and its vehicle sodium deoxycholate directly influence the PAH transport of rat renal cortical slices. PAH transport by renal cortical cells was studied in vitro after pre-incubation with amphotericin B and its vehicle. In addition, PAH transport of rat renal cortical cells was measured ex vivo after a 3 day treatment with amphotericin B or with the vehicle respectively.

MATERIALS AND METHODS

Male Sprague Dawley rats (200-250 g) were kept on a standard diet and received water ad libitum. Cortical slices were prepared free hand

from kidneys, about 100 mg tissue was used for each sample.

In vitro experiments:

The prepared renal slices were incubated for 60 min., 37°C, pH 7.4 in a sample volume of 4 ml under an oxygen (95%) carbon dioxide (5%) atmosphere. The following final amphotericin B concentrations were tested: 2, 5, 10, 30, 60μg/ml. The basic incubation medium consisted of: 96.7 mM NaCl, 7.4 mM sodium phosphate buffer, 40 mM KCl and 0.74 mM $CaCl_2$ as described (7). The medium was supplemented with 10 mM lactic acid. Since for clinical application amphotericin B is dissolved in sodium deoxycholate, ratio 1:0.82, additional incubations with the vehicle - final concentrations: 1.64, 4.1, 8.2, 24.6, 49.2 μg/ml were performed. Control samples were free of both the drug and the vehicle.

Ex vivo experiments:

Sprague Dawley rats (200-250 g) were treated for 3 days with amphotericin B (3 mg/kg b.w.) by intravenous administration or with sodium deoxycholate (2.46 mg/kg b.w.) respectively. Control animals received glucose 5% in an equal volume only. After in vitro or in vivo exposure to amphotericin B or sodium deoxycholate the renal cortical slices of all series were incubated in a medium as described which contained 0.74 mM para-aminohippuric acid (PAH). Incubations were carried out at 25°C, pH 7.4 in a metabolic shaker for 90 min. Immediately after the incubations were finished, the slices were blotted, weighed and homogenized in 10ml 3% (w/v) trichloroacetic acid. After centrifugation for 10 min at 1000 x g the amount of PAH in the resulted supernatant was measured as described (8). Two ml of the corresponding medium was treated similarly. The accumulation of PAH was expressed as a slice to medium concentration ratio (S:M).

Statistics

Mean values and standard deviation (x ± SD) were calculated followed by ANOV. A p-value of less than 0.05 was considered being significant.

RESULTS

After 1 hr incubation both amphotericin B and the vehicle sodium deoxycholate decreased PAH accumulation in a dose dependent manner (Fig. 1). At the highest amphotericin B concentration of 60 µg/ml a decrease of PAH transport to 17.6% was observed, sodium deoxycholate caused at the corresponding concentration a decrease to 33.3% (Fig. 1). After 3 days of treatment with amphotericin B (3 mg/kg b.w., i.v.) a reduction of PAH transport to 80% resulted (Fig. 2). At the analogous concentration sodium deoxycholate decreased PAH transport to 77% (Fig. 2).

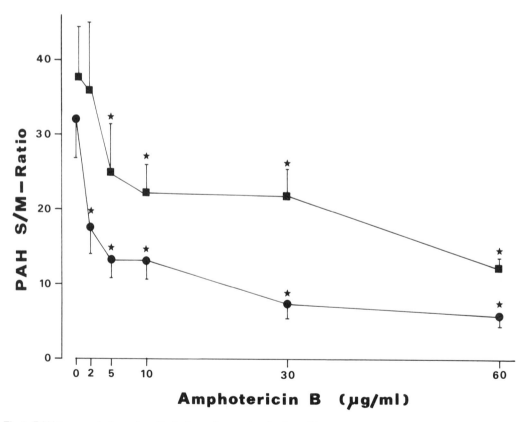

Fig.1. PAH transport of renal cortical slices after preincubation with: amphtotericin B (circle) or sodium deoxycholate (square) for 1hr. Symbols represent mean value ± SD of at least 6 rats. * Significantly different from controls. PAH: slice to medium ratio (S/M).

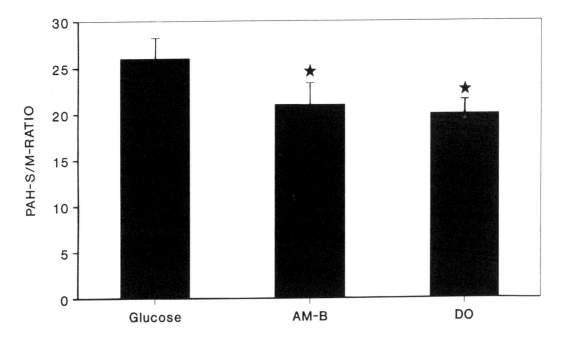

Fig.2. PAH transport of renal cortical slices from rats which were treated for 3 days with amphotericin B (3 mg/kg bw., i.v.) or with the vehicle sodium deoxycholate (DO; 2.41 mg/kg b.w.,i.v.). All being significantly different from controls(glucose 5%). Each symbol represents the mean value ± SD from at least 5 rats. PAH: slice to medium ratio (S/M).

DISCUSSION

The results of this study show that amphotericin B and its vehicle sodium deoxycholate induce impairment of PAH transport in renal cortical cells in vitro and ex vivo. Since a decrease of PAH transport also occurred under the influence of the vehicle it is concluded that the vehicle may participate in the nephrotoxicity of amphotericin B.

It was realized from earlier studies that amphotericin B reduces renal blood flow and glomerular filtration rate (3). It has been suggested that the amphotericin B-induced nephrotoxicity might be due to an activation of the tubular glomerular feedback mechanism (4). This intra-renal mechanism is assumed to be activated by an increased sodium chloride absorption at the macular densa. An activation of this feedback mechanism is considered to be a protective mechanism against volume losses

in the development of tubular dysfunction (5). A possible direct interference of the drug with the proximal renal transport system could result in a decrease of anionic transport and reabsorption and in turn could lead to an activation of the tubular glomerular feedback mechanism. The reduction in glomerular filtration rate might be the consequence of tubular failure which occurred under the influence of amphotericin B. This possibility is favoured by the data presented which shows a direct effect of amphotericin B on the PAH transport of renal cortical cells. The observed depression of tubular function can be explained in two ways. In addition to the possible direct interaction between amphotericin B and the active PAH transport system, the drug could also increase cell membrane permeability with a higher efflux rate of PAH from the cells. However, the latter possibility is excluded, since it has been shown that the drug does not increase the leakage rate of PAH from kidney cells (9). At this point we do not know which mechanisms account for the reduction of active PAH transport induced by amphotericin B. Since the drug does not induce lipid peroxidation in renal tissue (10) it seems likely that amphotericin B may have a direct influence on the PAH transport system and thus lead to an impairment of tubular transport.

REFERENCES

1. Sande MA, Mandell GL: Antimicrobial agents. In Gilman, Goodmann (eds); The pharmacological basis of therapeutics. Macmillan, New York, 1980, pp. 1222-1248.

2. Stamm AM, Diasio RB, Dismakes WE, Shadomy S, Cloud GA, Bowles CA, Karam GH, Espinel-Ingroff A: Toxicity of amphotericin B plus flucytosine in 194 patients with cryptococcal meningitis. Am J Med 83: 236-242, 1987.

3. Rhoades EG, Ginn HE, Mirchmore HG, Smith WO, Hammarsten JF: Effect of amphotericin B upon renal function in man. In: Gray, Tabenkin, Broadly (eds); Antimicrobiology agents annual 1960. New York, Plenum Press, 1961, pp 539-542.

4. Gerkens JF, Branch RA: The influence of sodium status and furosemide on canine acute amphotericin B nephrotoxicity. J. Pharmacol Exp. Ther 214: 306-311, 1980.

5. Thurau K, Boylan JW: Acute renal success: the unexpected logic of oliguria in acute renal failure. Am J Med 61: 308-315, 1976.

6. Heidemann HT, Gerkens JF, Jackson EK, Branch RA: Effect of aminophylline on renal vasoconstriction produced by amphotericin B in the rat. Naunyn- Schmiedeberg's Arch Pharmacol 324: 148-152, 1983.

7. Cross RJ, Taggart JV: Renal tubular transport: Accumulation of p-aminohippurate by rabbit kidney slices. Am J Physiol 161: 181-190, 1950.

8. Smith HW, Finkelstein F, Aliminosa L, Crawford B, Graber M: The renal clearances of substituted hippuric acid derivatives and other aromatic acids in dog and man. J Clin Invest 25: 388-404, 1945.

9. Fanestil DF: Amphotericin B inhibition of active PAH transport. J Lab Clin Med 71: 548-554, 1968.

10. Inselmann G, Kutzschbach A, Heidemann HTh: Amphotericin B (AmB)-induced alteration of PAH-transport in rat renal corticol slices. Eur J Clin Invest 19, A47, 1989.

3

EFFECT OF PARAQUAT-LIKE SUBSTANCES AND CEPHALOSPORINS ON ACCUMULATION OF p-AMINOHIPPURATE AND TETRAETHYLAMMONIUM IN RAT RENAL CORTICAL SLICES, AND ON LIPID PEROXIDATION IN RAT RENAL MICROSOMES AND CORTICAL SLICES

J. Duwe, C. Cojocel and K. Baumann

Department of Cell Physiology, Institute of Physiology, University of Hamburg, Grindelallee 117, D-2000 Hamburg 13, Germany

INTRODUCTION

Nephrotoxicity is one of the predominant side effects occurring in the extensive clinical use of cephalosporins. The nephrotoxicity of cephaloridine is characterized by acute proximal tubular necrosis in laboratory animals and in humans and is dependent upon its renal cortical accumulation and intracellular concentration (1-3). There is substantial evidence indicating that oxidative stress plays a major role in cephaloridine-induced nephrotoxicity (4-10). It is proposed that paraquat (11) and cephaloridine (7) undergo cyclic reduction-oxidation reactions with subsequent formation of superoxide anion and other activated oxygen species. These activated oxygen species are then very likely to react with cell membrane lipids to induce lipid peroxidation and toxicity. Regarding lipid peroxidation, the presence of pyridinium ring(s) in the molecular structure seems to play an important role (4,10). Results of previous studies suggest that the toxicity profile of cephalosporins could be altered by the increasing complexity of the chemical structure (10,12). In order to get more information about the relationship between the molecular structure and nephrotoxic potential, the peroxidative and the nephrotoxic potential was evaluated for chemicals containing one, two or no pyridinium, pyridine or piperidine ring(s).

METHODS

Male Wistar rats (Winkelmann, Kirchborchen, F.R.G.), weighing 240-280 g, were sacrificed, and kidneys were removed immediately to prepare renal cortical microsomes and renal cortical slices. In vitro, at an equimolar concentration of 24 mM in the incubation medium, the ability of the tested substances to generate superoxide anion (O_2-) in microsomes and to induce lipid peroxidation in microsomes and renal cortical slices was determined. Superoxide formation was measured using its ability to reduce acetylated cytochrome c (13). Lipid peroxidation was monitored by estimating the formation of malondialdehyde (MDA), using the thiobarbituric acid assay (14). Furthermore, the accumulation of tetraethylammonium (TEA) and p-aminohippurate (PAH) in renal cortical slices (15) was measured after preincubation of the slices with a test substance and used as a parameter of renal cortical cell function. Statistical analyses were carried out using Student's t-test. Other details of the methods used in this study have been described earlier (5-7,10).

Chemicals generating superoxide anions and/or inducing a significant increase in tissue content of MDA in renal cortical microsomes or slices, above the control value, were considered to have a peroxidative potential. Chemicals were considered to have a nephrotoxic potential when they induced a significant decrease in accumulation of TEA or PAH when compared to control value.

RESULTS

Paraquat induced the greatest microsomal superoxide anion formation. At an equimolar concentration of 24 mM in the incubation medium, cephaloridine, 1-(4-pyridyl)-pyridinium and cefsulodin were the next potent compounds to induce superoxide formation (Table 1). In addition, it is shown that for paraquat and cephaloridine the generation of superoxide increases in a dose-dependent fashion (Fig. 1).

Microsomal MDA production was increased by the tested beta-lactams, at an equimolar concentration of 24 mM, with the exception of aztreonam. Cephaloridine induced the greatest increase in MDA production followed by cefsulodin (Table 1). 4,4'-bipyridine, 4-piperidinopyridine and 4,4' bipiperidine caused no significant increase in microsomal MDA generation.

In the presence of paraquat, lower MDA contents were measured in the incubation medium as compared to controls.

At an equimolar concentration (24 mM) of the tested substances, MDA production in renal cortical slices was increased mainly by cephalosporins and paraquat. Cephaloridine caused the greatest increase in MDA production (Table 2).

Compared to control incubations, 4-piperidinopyridine and 4,4'-bipyridine induced, at an equimolar concentration of 24 mM, the greatest decrease in PAH accumulation by renal cortical slices. Aztreonam, paraquat, cephaloridine and ceftazidime were the next potent compounds to decrease PAH accumulation (Table 2).

At an equimolar concentration of 24 mM, the accumulation of TEA in renal cortical slices was decreased to the greatest extent by 4-piperidinopyridine and 4,4'-bipyridine, the next potent compounds were paraquat, 1-(4-pyridyl)-pyridinium and cephaloridine. Compared to cephaloridine, the other cephalosporins

Table 1. The peroxidative potential of paraquat (1,1'-dimethyl-4,4'- bipyridinium), cephaloridine and of other substances containing one, two or no pyridinium, pyridine or piperidine ring(s).

	O_2^- nmol/15min/ mg protein	MDA nmol/15 min/r protein
Control	a)	2.91 ±0.43
1,1'-Dimethyl-4,4'- bipyridinium	851.49 ±54.62	1.11 ±0.46[*]
4,4'-Bipyridine	14.69 ±1.27	2.27 ±0.16
1-(4-Pyridyl)-pyridinium	29.40 ±2.67	3.72 ±0.48[*]
4-Piperidinopyridine	4.30 ±1.11	2.45 ±0.26
4,4'-Bipiperidine	24.25 ±3.11	2.37 ±0.05
Cephaloridine	140.12 ±8.02	12.37 ±1.98[*]
Cefsulodin	28.85 ±4.23	9.11 ±1.69[*]
Ceftazidime	11.91 ±2.97	4.27 ±0.78[*]
Cefotaxime	11.13 ±4.55	7.32 ±0.93[*]
Mezlocillin	25.11 ±1.42	5.02 ±0.85[*]
Aztreonam	19.18 ±3.28	3.55 ±0.98

The peroxidative potential was determined by measuring both the generation of superoxide anions (O_2^-) and malondialdehyde (MDA) in renal cortical microsomes. Microsomes were incubated at 37°C for 15 min in a phosphate-buffered control medium or a medium containing the test substance at a concentration of 24 mM. The incubation media contained a NADPH regenerating system. Data represent x ± S.D. (n = 6). [*] (p< 0.05) as compared to controls. a) In control experiments, the incubation of renal cortical microsomes in the absence of a test compound did not cause formation of a detectable amount of O_2^-.

caused a lower decrease in TEA accumulation (Table 2).

DISCUSSION

Cephalosporins contain the 7-amino-cephalosporanic acid, the cephem nucleus, consistent of the β-lactam ring which is fused with the dihydrothiazine ring. The molecular structure of cephalosporins displays various side chains attached to the 3 and/or 7 position of the cephem nucleus. The molecular structure of paraquat, 1-(4-pyridyl)-pyridinium, cephaloridine, cefsulodin and ceftazidime have in

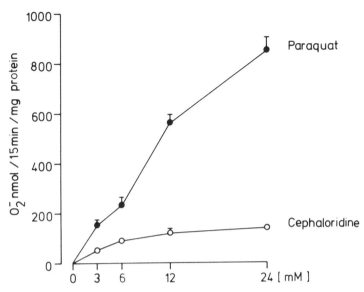

Fig. 1. Concentration-dependent increase of microsomal superoxide anion (O_2^-) generation caused by paraquat (1,1'-dimethyl-4,4' bipyridinium) and cephaloridine. Renal cortical microsomes were incubated at 37oC for 15 min in a phosphate-buffered medium containing the test substance at various concentrations and a NADPH regenerating system. In control experiments, the incubation of microsomes in the absence of a test compound did not cause formation of a detectable amount of superoxide. Data represent $\bar{x} \pm$ S.D. (n = 6).

common one or two pyridinium rings which carry a positive charge on the quaternary nitrogen. These compounds showed a nephrotoxic potential accompanied by the highest increase in superoxide generation and/or MDA tissue content. Formal charge of the pyridinium ring containing molecules seems to be important for the ability to undergo a redox cycle and to produce superoxide and subsequently lipid peroxidation. 4-piperidinopyridine and 4,4'-bipyridine, compounds which contain no pyridinium ring, revealed the highest nephrotoxic potential without induction of lipid peroxidation. The tested β-lactams which contain no pyridinium ring and 4,4'-bipiperidine showed a weak or no peroxidative and nephrotoxic potential. For β-lactams, the entire molecular structure seems to be important for the occurrence of lipid peroxidation and alterations in accumulation of organic ions by renal cortical slices.

ACKNOWLEDGEMENTS

A part of these studies was done in partial fulfillment of the requirements of the M.D. degree by J. Duwe. The authors thank Miss M. Kunkel and Mrs. G. Hacklaender for excellent technical assistance.

REFERENCES

1. Tune BM, Wu KY, Kempson RL: Inhibition of transport and prevention of toxicity of cephaloridine in the kidney. Dose-responsiveness of the rabbit and the guinea pig to probenecid. J Pharmacol Exp Ther 202: 466-471, 1977.

2. Tune BM, Fravert D: Mechanisms of cephalosporin nephrotoxicity: A comparison of cephaloridine and cephaloglycin. Kidney Int 18: 591-600, 1980.

Table 2. The peroxidative and the nephrotoxic potential of paraquat (1,1'- dimethyl-4,4'-bipyridinium), cephaloridine and of other substances containing one, two or no pyridinium, pyridine or piperidine ring(s).

	MDA nmol/h/g tissue	PAH S/M	TEA S/M
Control	30.64 ±3.39	24.17 ±2.37	21.13 ±1.96
1,1'-Dimethyl-4,4'-bipyridinium	46.53* ±3.72	7.87* ±1.12	5.82* ±0.71
4,4'-Bipyridine	38.31* ±3.50	3.53* ±0.49	1.73* ±0.34
1-(4-Pyridyl)-pyridinium	33.17 ±2.55	25.78 ±3.08	7.43* ±0.52
4-Piperidinopyridine	38.39* ±2.50	2.57* ±0.47	1.12* ±0.14
4,4'-Bipiperidine	29.01 ±2.26	15.07* ±1.00	15.10* ±2.36
Cephaloridine	81.88* ±5.34	11.63* ±1.51	9.43* ±1.64
Cefsulodin	50.15* ±4.69	25.48 ±1.37	15.34* ±0.92
Ceftazidime	39.56* ±3.21	11.51* ±3.21	14.06* ±1.10
Cefotaxime	51.22* ±2.89	26.34 ±1.01	16.24* ±2.17
Mezlocillin	33.23 ±3.31	23.52 ±2.83	14.67* ±2.77
Aztreonam	37.67* ±0.51	7.74* ±0.91	19.21 ±1.62

The peroxidative potential was determined by measuring the MDA content in renal cortical slices. The nephrotoxic potential was determined by measuring the decrease in accumulation of TEA and PAH in slices expressed as slice to medium ratio (S/M). Slices were incubated at 37°C for 60 min in a phosphate-buffered control medium or a medium containing the test substance at a concentration of 24 mM. At the end of that incubation, slices were either used to determine the slice content of MDA or were transferred for a subsequent incubation to a test substance-free medium to determine TEA or PAH accumulation. These slices were incubated for 90 min at 25°C in a TEA or PAH containing phosphate-buffered medium. Data represent x ± S.D. (n = 6) (p< 0.05) as compared to controls.

3. Wang PL, Prime DJ, Hsu CY, Tune BM: Effects of ureteral obstruction on the toxicity of cephalosporins in the rabbit kidney. J Infect Dis 145: 574-581, 1982.

4. Kuo CH, Maita K, Sleight SD, Hook JB: Lipid peroxidation: A possible mechanism of cepha-loridine-induced nephrotoxicity. Toxicol Appl Pharmacol 67: 78-88, 1983.

5. Cojocel C, Inselmann G, Laeschke KH, Baumann K: Species differences in cephalosporin-induced lipid peroxidation. Drugs Exptl Clin Res 10: 781-788, 1984.

6. Cojocel C, Laeschke KH, Inselmann G, Baumannn K: Inhibition of cephaloridine-induced lipid peroxidation. Toxicology 35: 295-305, 1985.

7. Cojocel C, Hannemann J, Baumann K: Cephaloridine-induced lipid peroxidation initiated by reactive oxygen species as a possible mechanism of cephaloridine nephrotoxicity. Biochim Biophys Acta 834: 402-410, 1985.

8. Goldstein RS, Pasino DA, Hewitt WR, Hook JB: Biochemical mechanisms of cephaloridine nephrotoxicity: Time and concentration dependence of peroxidative injury. Toxicol Appl Pharmacol 83: 261-270, 1986.

9. Goldstein RS, Smith PF, Tarloff JB, Contardi L, Rush GF, Hook JB: Biochemical mechanisms of cephaloridine nephrotoxicity. Life Sciences 42: 1809-1816, 1988.

10. Cojocel C, Göttsche U, Tölle KL, Baumann K: Nephrotoxic potential of first-, second-, and third-generation cephalosporins. Arch Toxicol 62: 458-464, 1988.

11. Bus JS, Aust SD, Gibson JE: Superoxide- and singlet oxigen-catalyzed lipid peroxidation as a possible mechanism for paraquat (methyl viologen) toxicity. Biochem Biophys Res Commun 58: 749-755, 1974.

12. Tune BM: The nephrotoxicity of cephalosporin antibiotics-structure- activity relationships. Comments Toxicol 1: 145-170, 1986.

13. Azzi A, Montecucco C, Richter C: The use of acetylated ferricytochrome c for the detection of superoxide radicals produced in biological membranes. Biochem Biophys Res Commun 65: 597-603, 1975.

14. Buege JA, Aust SD: Microsomal lipid per-oxidation. Methods Enzymol 52: 302-310, 1978.

15. Cross RJ, Taggart JV: Renal tubular transport: Accumulation of p-aminohippurate by rabbit kidney slices. Am J Physiol 161: 181-190, 1950.

4

DIFFERENTIAL URINARY EXCRETION OF PARAQUAT IN AVES FOLLOWING THE UNILATERAL MODE OF INTRAVENOUS ADMINISTRATION

R. O. Blackburn, D. N. Prashad and D. Chambers

School of Biological Sciences and Environmental Health, Thames Polytechnic, Woolwich, London SE18 6PF

INTRODUCTION

In mammals, renal excretion of the bipyridyl herbicide paraquat has been shown to involve the processes of glomerular filtration, tubular reabsorption and secretion (1-3), though the underlying mechanisms involved in renal 'handling' of paraquat remain largely unresolved. It has been shown that intravenous injections (20 mg/kg) of paraquat administered to hens with a mild diuresis resulted in a progressive reduction in both glomerular filtration rate (GFR) and urine flow with a concomitant increase in renal blood flow (RBF) to the kidneys (3). Probably paraquat-induced elevation of RBF in hens facilitates renal tubular secretion of the paraquat cation.

In order to evaluate the consequences of the increased blood flow to the kidneys use has been made of the functional renal portal system that exists in birds. In Aves, in addition to the renal arterial supply, each kidney receives a second, low pressure afferent blood input from the renal portal system via the external iliac and femoral veins. This latter system communicates directly with the peritubular areas of the kidneys, and has previously been used to evaluate tubular 'handling' of unilaterally injected exogenous substances, as the route isolates them from a significant glomerular component (4,5). In the current study, the differential excretion rates of paraquat from both kidneys are investigated, using para-amino hippuric acid (PAH) and inulin as markers for tubular secretion and GFR respectively.

METHODS

Eight adult Rhode Island Red cross Light Sussex hens of average weight 2.0kg were starved for 14 hr prior to the experiment. The left brachial vein of each hen was cannulated for continuous infusion of a mixture of 10% mannitol in isotonic saline solution (0.93%) at a constant rate of 0.25 ml/ min, to induce a mild diuresis.

After establishing an adequate urine flow, the ureters of each hen were cannulated, to permit collection of uncontaminated urine samples. The left external iliac vein was exposed, and a calibrated cannula inserted just proximal to the bifurcation of the caudal and cranial renal portal veins of the left (homolateral) kidney. This cannula was used for a bolus injection (1ml) of a mixture of 25mg paraquat dichloride, 2.5mg PAH and 25mg inulin in isotonic saline. Serial urine samples were collected from each ureter at 5 min intervals for 20 min following administration of the mixture. Inulin and PAH levels in the urine were determined by standard assay methods, and paraquat levels by a modification of the spectrophotometric methods of Calderbank and Yuen (6) and Berry and Grove (7).

RESULTS

Urinary excretion of paraquat and marker substances from the left kidney will be referred to as the homolateral excretion and that from the right kidney the contralateral excretion.

Following the bolus injection of the mixture containing paraquat, inulin and PAH, it was found that there was no significant difference p>0.1; n=32) between homolateral and contra-lateral excretion rates of inulin, despite the unilateral route of administration (Fig. 1). This finding suggests that the urinary excretion of inulin - a recognised marker for GFR - is not influenced by elevated peri-tubular levels, but appears in urine as a result of glomerular ultra-filtration alone. In addition, when the rates of urine flow from homolateral and contralateral kidneys were compared, no significant dif-ference (p>0.1; n=32) was detected (Fig. 1).

During the experimental period, a highly sig-nificant increase (p<0.001) in paraquat output from the homolateral kidney was observed within 5 min (0.65±0.1/mg/min) compared with that from the contralateral kidney (0.19±0.07mg/min) (Fig. 2). This increase, amounting to an overall excretion ratio of 3.4:1 over the experimental period of 20 min may be attributable to a rapid unilateral tubular secre-tion of paraquat.

In addition, urinary excretion of PAH from the homolateral kidney highly significantly ex-ceeded that from the contralateral kidney (p<0.001), reflecting an excretion ratio of 1.8:1 (Fig. 3). The rates of excretion of paraquat and of PAH from the homolateral kidney paralleled each other, and in the course of the experiment both excretion rates were found to be signifi-cantly correlated (r=0.67; n=32; p<0.001).

DISCUSSION

The urinary excretion of paraquat has pre-viously been shown to involve glomerular filtration together with simultaneous renal tubu-lar reabsorption and secretion (1,3). It has been demonstrated that following paraquat ad-ministration in the fowl, a decline in GFR was accompanied by an increase in RBF and a tubular secretion of paraquat into the urine (3). The present study has exploited the renal portal system to further investigate tubular secretion of paraquat, following its unilateral administra-tion simultaneously with markers for GFR (inulin) and tubular secretion (PAH). The results show that urinary inulin excretion from both

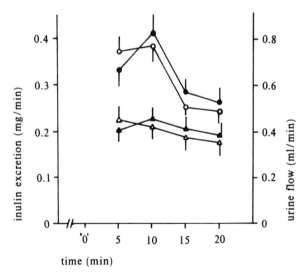

Fig.1 Rates of inulin excretion and urine output in 8 hens from homo- (empty circle-empty circle; empty triangle-empty triangle respectively) and contralateral (full circle-full circle; full triangle-full triangle respective-ly) kidneys (mean + se). 'O' corresponds to time of simultaneous administration of paraquat, inulin and PAH.

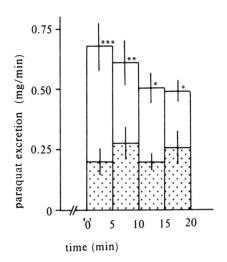

Figure 2. Urinary excretion of paraquat in 8 hens from homo- (clear) and contralateral (hatched) kidneys (mean ± se). 'O' corresponds to time of simultaneous administration of paraquat, inulin and PAH. *** p<0.001; ** p<0.002; * p<0.01 mark the levels of significance between homo- and contralateral paraquat excretion.

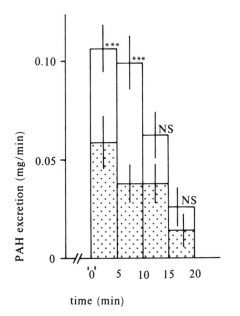

Figure 3. Urinary excretion of PAH in 8 hens from homo- (clear) and contralateral (hatched) kidneys (mean ± se). 'O' corresponds to time of simultaneous injection of paraquat, inulin and PAH. *** p<0.001 marks levels of significance between homo- and contralateral PAH excretion; NS indicates not significant.

kidneys was of similar magnitude, despite its unilateral mode of administration; indeed in mammals and birds, inulin output is influenced neither by renal tubular reabsorption nor by secretion, and appears in urine as a result of filtration alone (8,5).

In addition, urinary output of PAH by the homolateral kidney was found to be significantly raised (p<0.001) compared with that from the contralateral kidney, reflecting an excretion ratio of 1.8:1 over the experimental period. Furthermore, the homolateral excretion of PAH paralleled paraquat output (r = 0.67; n = 32; p<0.001) by the same kidney, indicating that the appearance of both substances in urine resulted from renal tubular secretion, perhaps augmented by the raised peritubular levels of these constituents. It is therefore likely that the increased renal blood flow, previously observed in the fowl (3) when the marker for renal plasma flow (PAH) and paraquat were administered systemically may have facilitated the enhanced tubular secretion of the herbicide, in spite of a reduction in glomerular filtration rate.

REFERENCES

1. Ecker JL, Gibson, JE, Hook, JB: In vitro analysis of the renal handling of paraquat. Toxicol Appl Pharmacol 34: 170-177, 1975.

2. Ferguson DM: Renal handling of paraquat. B J Pharmacol 42: 635, 1971.

3. Prashad DN, Chambers, D, Beadle, DJ: Changes in renal function associated with paraquat dichloride toxicity in the domestic fowl. Gen Pharmacol 12: 291-293, 1981.

4. Sperber I: Excretion. In: Marshall, AJ (ed) Biology and Comparative Physiology of Birds, New York, Academic Press, 1960, Chapter 12.

5. Sturkie PD: Reproduction in the female and egg production. In: Avian Physiology, Berlin, Springer-Verlag, 1976, pp 263-285.

6. Calderbank A, Yuen, SH: An ion exchange method for determining paraquat residues in food crops. Analyst, 90: 99-106, 1965.

7. Berry DJ, Grove, J: Determination of paraquat (1,1-dimethyl-4, 4-bipyridinium-cation) in urine. Clin Chim Acta 34: 5-11, 1971.

8. Pitts RF: Physiology of the kidney and body fluids, 3rd ed. Chicago Year Book Medical Publishers, 1974, pp 60-70.

5

EFFECT OF EXPERIMENTAL DIABETES ON THE NEPHROTOXIC RESPONSE TO CHEMICALS

C.-P.Siegers, A.Hattendorff, B.Raasch and G.Baretton (1)

Institutes of Toxicology and of Pathology (1), Medical University of Lübeck, D-2400 Lübeck, Germany

INTRODUCTION

Streptozotocin-induced diabetes has been shown to protect against gentamicin- and cisplatin-induced nephrotoxicity in rats (1-3). The aim of the present study was to investigate the influence of a diabetic statediabetic state on the nephrotoxic response to other drugs and chemicals, namely paracetamol, cyclosporin A and mercuric chloride.

MATERIALS AND METHODS

Male Wistar-rats (300-350 g) were kept for 3 days in metabolic cages with free access to food and tap water. Diabetes was induced by a single i.p. injection of 75 mg/kg streptozotocin 10 days before beginning of the experiments. Diabetic state was evidenced by significantly increased urinary and plasma glucose levels. The nephrotoxic agents paracetamol (1 g/kg p.o.)and mercuric chloride (1 mg/kg i.v.) were given once after the first blood sample (day 0), whereas cyclosporin A (30-120 mg/kg) was administered daily for 3 days. Nephrotoxicity was monitored by daily measurements of plasma creatinine and urea concentrations and urinary enzyme excretion of N-acetyl-β-glucosaminidase (NAG) using commercial reagent kits of Boehringer, Mannheim (Germany). At the end of the experiments the rats were killed by decapitation and the kidneys excised for light-microscopic morphometric and electron-microscopic evaluations.

RESULTS

Oral treatment with paracetamol caused a significantly higher urea retention and NAG-excretion in diabetic rats as compared to non-diabetics (data not shown). The kidney morphology, however, showed no differences between diabetic and non-diabetic animals.

Treatment with $HgCl_2$ caused significant increments of plasma urea and creatinine concentrations in non-diabetic rats which were markedly reduced in diabetic animals (Figure 1). $HgCl_2$-induced tubular necrosis was less extensive in diabetic as compared to normal rats (not shown).

Following oral treatment with cyclosporin A a dose-dependent retention of urea in plasma and an enhanced NAG-excretion was observed, which were more pronounced in diabetic rats (Figure 2). Kidney morphology as a consequence of cyclosporin A-treatment showed typical isometric tubular vacuolisation (Figure 3), by morphometric evaluation a significantly higher mean score of vacuolisation was calculated for diabetic rats (2.5$\pm$0.3) as compared to non-diabetic rats (1.3$\pm$0.3, p<0.05).

DISCUSSION

In this paper, further data are presented on the influence of diabetic state on the nephrotoxic response to chemicals. Published and own observations are compiled in Table 1.

For cisplatin and gentamicin an attenuated nephrotoxic response has been reported (1-4).

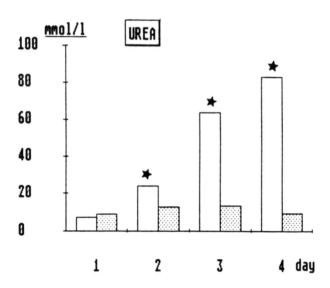

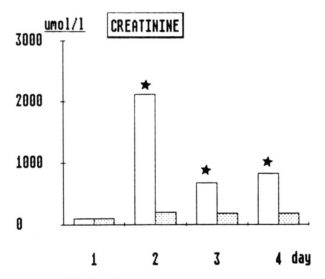

Figure 1. Effect of mercury (HgCl2: 1 mg/kg i.v. at day 1) on the plasma levels of urea and creatinine in normal (empty columns) and diabetic rats. Values represent means out of 6 animals each. * p<0.05 as compared to the corresponding value before treatment (day 1).

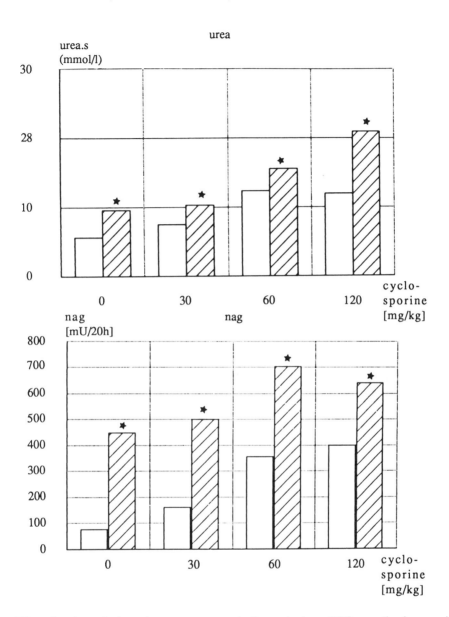

Figure 2. Effect of cyclosporin A on plasma urea concentration and urinary NAG-excretion in normal and diabetic rats (hatched columns). Values represent arithmetic means out of 5-6 rats each. * p<0.05 as compared to normal rats.

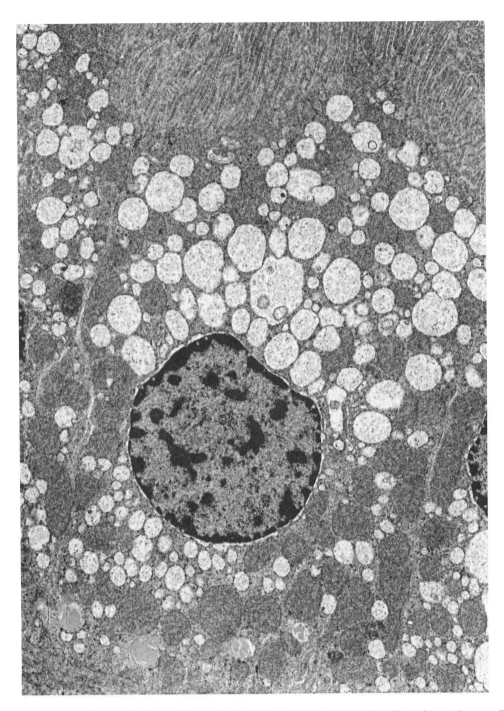

Figure 3. Electron-microscopic picture of a proximal tubular epithelial cell of a diabetic rat. Isometric vacuolisation of the cytoplasma is seen, the brush border is preserved (TEM, x 8500).

Table 1. Influence of diabetes on nephrotoxicity

nephrotoxic agent	Influence of diabetes	reference
Cisplatin	attenuation	(4)
Cyclosporin A	aggravation	
Gentamicin	attenuation	(1,2,3)
Mercuric chloride	attenuation	
Paracetamol	none	

Modulation of gentamicin nephrotoxicity is attributed to a diminished accumulation of the drug by the diabetic kidney (3); the same mechanism is proposed for the attenuation of cisplatin nephrotoxicity by diabetes (4). Our observations concerning mercuric chloride seem to fit into the same hypothesis, i.e. diminished tubular accumulation or increased renal clearance of HgCl2 during diabetes. For cyclosporin A, the opposite effect is postulated, which is now being investigated by measuring the renal concentration of cyclosporin A in diabetic and non-diabetic rats.

REFERENCES

1. Teixeira RB, Kelley J, Alpert H, Pardo V, Vaamode CA: Complete protection from gentamicin induced acute renal failure in the diabetes mellitus rat. Kidney Int 21:600-612, 1982.

2. Vaamonde CA, Bier RT, Gouvea W, Alpert H, Kelley J, Pardo V: Effect of duration of diabetes on the protection observed in the diabetic rat against gentamicin-induced acute renal failure. Miner Electrolyte Metab 10:209-216, 1984.

3. Elliot WC, Houghton DC, Gilbert DN, Baines-Hunter J, Bennett WM: Experimental gentamicin nephrotoxicity: Effect of streptozotocin induced diabetes. J Pharmacol Exp Ther 23:265-270, 1985.

4. Scott LA, Madan E, Valentovic MA: Attenuation of cisplatin nephrotoxicity by streptozotocin-induced diabetes. Fundam Appl Toxicol 12:530-539, 1989.

6

PARADOXICAL EFFECTS OF SUCCINYLACETONE ON RENAL HANDLING OF DELTA-AMINOLAEVULINIC ACID

K.S. Roth

Division of Genetics, Endocrinology and Metabolism, Department of Pediatrics, Medical College of Virginia, Richmond, VA 23298, USA

INTRODUCTION

Succinylacetone (SA) is a byproduct of tyrosine catabolism produced only by individuals affected by the inborn error of metabolism known as hereditary infantile tyrosinemia (1). Due to its unique presence in this disorder, urinary SA can be used as a biochemical marker for the disease. Since the enzyme defect is demonstrable in liver and kidney (2), it may be surmised that urinary excretion is a result of combined production by both organs. It has been well-documented that SA is a potent inhibitor of haem synthesis, exerting a strong competitive inhibitory effect on the enzyme delta-aminolaevulinic acid dehydratase (ALAD) in the liver (3). Due to this inhibitory effect, individuals who produce SA also excrete large quantities of delta-aminolaevulinic acid (ALA) in their urine (4). While the effect of SA on renal cortical ALAD activity has not been examined, it has been implicitly assumed that the increased urinary ALA excretion in these individuals is a result of the aggregate inhibitory effects on haem synthesis in both liver and kidney.

Our interest in the biochemical mechanisms underlying the human renal Fanconi syndrome (FS), with which hereditary infantile tyrosinemia is associated (5), led us into an extensive documentation of the effects of SA on renal cortical membrane transport of sugars and amino acids (6-8). Exposure of isolated renal tubules and brush border membrane vesicles, made from normal adult rat kidneys, to 4 mM SA results in substantial and easily reversible impairment of substrate uptake. SA treatment also results in increased membrane fluidity (8) and decreased oxygen consumption by the isolated renal tubules (7). These observations strongly suggest the possibility that in the genetically-affected kidney, endogenous production of SA plays a role in the genesis of a generalized renal tubular dysfunction (FS).

Since neither the effect of SA on renal ALAD activity nor the renal handling of ALA has been investigated, we speculated that any impairment in ALA uptake induced by SA could be augmented by concomitantly decreased renal ALAD activity, resulting in diminished heme, hence cytochrome, production by the renal tubular epithelial cell. Such effects would have significant consequences for energy production and might help to explain the impaired active transport observed in the presence of SA. Thus, we have studied the uptake of ALA in renal tubules and brush border vesicles, measuring the effect of SA thereon. We have also examined the effects of SA on renal cortical ALAD, thus addressing the speculation outlined above.

METHODS AND MATERIALS

Animals

Adult male Sprague-Dawley rats (150-175 g) were obtained from Charles River Breeding Labs (Wilmington, MA) and used in all experiments. Animals were housed separately and provided water and a standard chow diet <u>ad libitum</u> until sacrificed. Upon sacrifice, kidneys and liver were rapidly removed and placed in ice cold saline.

Tissue Preparations

Isolated renal tubules were prepared from minced cortical slices (9). Final suspensions contained approximately 10-12 mg/ml in Krebs-Ringer bicarbonate buffer, pH 7.4. Incubations were carried out in sidearm flasks at 37°C with continuous gassing with 95%O_2-5%CO_2. Experiments were begun by the addition of ^{14}C-labelled ALA (0.1 μCi/ml of suspension) plus unlabelled ALA to give the desired final concentration. Sufficient SA was added to the experimental flasks to yield a final concentration of 4 mM. Aliquots were processed as previously described (9). Total tissue water and extracellular fluid space determinations have been previously determined (9). Distribution ratios (cpm/microliter intracellular fluid:cpm/microliter extracellular fluid) were calculated (9). The data were analyzed by Student's "t-test" for significance and plotted as the distribution ratios vs time in minutes.

Brush border vesicles were prepared from cortical slices and purity assessed as previously described (8). Final preparations were suspended in sodium-free THM buffer, pH 7.4 (2 mM Tris/ HEPES + 100 mM mannitol) to a final protein concentration of 0.3 to 0.4 mg/ml as determined by the method of Lowry, et al (10). Uptake studies were carried out by addition of the membranes into tubes containing 3 micromolar ALA (0.1 μCi ^{14}C-labelled ALA/ml), with or without addition of 4 mM SA. Incubations were stopped by rapid filtration (8), the filters air-dried overnight and assayed for radioactivity. Data were expressed as uptake of ALA cpm/mg protein, analyzed by Student's "t-test" and plotted as mean values of uptake (cpm/mg) versus time of incubation in minutes.

Assay of ALAD activity was carried out in crude homogenates of liver and isolated renal tubules, prepared as described above. The homogenates were prepared in 100 mM sodium phosphate buffer, pH 5.8 (11). Homogenates were assayed for protein content (10), then divided into aliquots, incubated with and without

4mM SA and assayed for ALAD activity (11). Activities were expressed as micromoles of product formed/hr/gram tissue.

Delta-[4-^{14}C]-ALA (specific activity 55mCi/mmol) was purchased from New England Nuclear (Boston, MA). All chemicals were purchased from commercial sources and were of the highest degree of purity available.

RESULTS

Effect of SA on Substrate Uptake

Isolated tubules were observed to actively transport ALA (distribution ratio >1) after 1 min of incubation and to achieve an intracellular concentration more than 14-fold greater than that of the medium by 60 min. Addition of 4 mM SA to the medium resulted in significant impairment of ALA uptake after 5 min of incubation, with the tubules achieving a maximum distribution ratio of 3.9 thereafter.

Despite the dramatic decrease in steady-state level caused by the presence of SA, however, the early portion of the uptake curve appeared unaffected, suggesting that the difference might be attributable to more rapid efflux of accumulated substrate, rather than to reduced rate of influx. These data are shown in Figure 1.

ALA uptake by the vesicles occurred by a sodium-gradient dependent system, and showed a broad peak with the maximum solute uptake at 60 min of incubation. Addition of 4 mM SA reduced ALA entry into the vesicles to the level seen in the absence of a sodium gradient. By 120 min of incubation, control, SA-treated and sodium-equilibrated vesicles had reached a similar level of equilibrated uptake, indicating no significant differences in intravesicular volume. Initial rates of uptake over the first 3 min of study showed no significant difference between control and SA treated vesicles. These data are summarized in Figure 2.

Effect of SA on Renal Cortical ALAD

Under control conditions, renal ALAD activity was higher than that in liver. While addition of

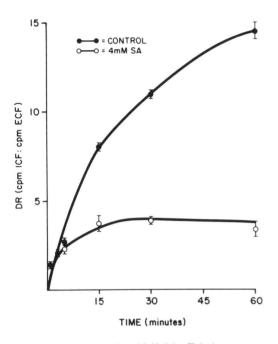

Figure 1-Uptake of 8mM ALA by Tubules

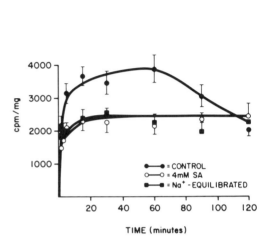

Figure 2-BBV Uptake of 3μM ALA

4 mM SA to liver homogenate resulted in approximately 67% inhibition, renal ALAD activity was enhanced 3-fold under the same conditions. Elevation of incubation temperature raised activity in both tissues, but addition of SA at 55°C produced the same divergent results in the two preparations (Table 1). Varying the concentration of SA from 0-10 mM resulted in a dose-related increase in renal ALAD activity (Table 2). Examination of the pH optima of liver and kidney ALAD showed different optima. The hepatic enzyme had a single pH optimum at pH 6.2-6.4, while renal cortical ALAD evidenced two separate optima, at pH 5.8 and 7.0-7.4. Addition of 4 mM SA enhanced renal ALAD activity throughout the entire pH range examined.

DISCUSSION

Hereditary infantile tyrosinemia is associated with increased urinary excretion of sugar, amino acids and phosphate (FS), as well as SA and ALA. Using a rat kidney model we have previously shown that the glucosuria and ami-noaciduria of the Fanconi syndrome can be explained by the effects of SA on the renal tubule (6-8). However, nothing is known of the association, at the renal tubular level, between endogenous synthesis of SA within the renal epithelium in which the enzymatic defect is expressed and membrane uptake of ALA. Moreover, while hepatic ALAD and the effects of SA thereon have been extensively studied, no examination of the effects of SA on renal cortical ALAD has been reported. Therefore, the present studies were undertaken to determine the nature of the interrelationship between SA, renal ALAD and membrane uptake of the substrate for this enzyme which represents the second step in haem biosynthesis.

Uptake of ALA by the renal tubule is clearly accomplished by means of active transport, the isolated tubules capable of achieving a distribution ratio of 14 by 60 min in our studies. SA caused a reduction in this capability, lowering the steady-state level reached by approximately 67% by a mechanism which appeared to depend upon increased efflux of accumulated substrate from the cell. Examination of the effects of SA on ALA uptake by brush border membrane vesicles confirmed a direct inhibition of the membrane transport system, reducing the ability of the vesicles to accumulate ALA to the same level as that of vesicles incubated under sodium-equilibrated conditions. However, control, SA-treated and Na-equilibrated vesicles all reached the same equilibrium value, suggesting that SA did not adversely affect the integrity of the membrane as represented by the intravesicular volume. These observations in toto suggest that SA reduces the amount of cytosolic ALA available to renal ALAD. Moreover, the data also suggest that the increased urinary excretion of ALA

TABLE 1 Temperature Dependence of Hepatic and Renal ALAD Activity

	Liver	Kidney
Control (37°C)	1.720($\pm$ 0.192)	2.503($\pm$ 0.207)
+ 4mM SA	0.414($\pm$ 0.091)	7.091($\pm$ 1.590)
Control (55°C)	3.210($\pm$ 0.221)	6.407($\pm$ 1.012)
+ 4mM SA	0.603($\pm$ 0.093)	13.610($\pm$ 0.979)
Control (37°C + 1%HgCl2)	0.748($\pm$ 0.102)	2.560($\pm$ 0.221)
+ 4mM SA	0.304($\pm$ 0.083)	6.841($\pm$ 0.984)

All results are the means ($\pm$ S.E.) of at least four triplicate determinations, expressed in units of enzyme activity (1U= 1μmol PBG formed/hr/g tissue at 37°C).

TABLE 2 Relationship of SA Concentration to Renal Cortical ALAD Activity

[SA](mM)	Activity (Units/gram)
0	2.502($\pm$ 0.207)
1	3.940($\pm$ 0.541)
2	5.843($\pm$ 0.155)
4	9.407($\pm$ 0.370)
8	11.150($\pm$ 0.735)
10	16.110($\pm$ 0.923)
12	16.860($\pm$ 0.952)

All results are the means ($\pm$ S.E.) of at least 4 triplicate determinations, carried out at 37°C with renal tubule homogenate in 8mM ALA.

seen in hereditary tyrosinemia is a combined result of increased hepatic release (due to hepatic ALAD inhibition) and decreased renal tubular reabsorption at the brush border surface.

Our observations regarding the effects of SA on renal cortical ALAD are particularly interesting. Enhancement of activity in kidney by the same substance which inhibits the hepatic enzyme suggests different molecular species in the two organs. Since the assay is carried out in homogenates, it is unlikely that the increased renal activity was attributable to induced protein synthesis. Further proof of distinct molecular species is offered by the differences in pH optima between the hepatic and renal enzymes. Although there are no data in the literature to suggest ALAD isozymes, this is the first report of any investigation into the comparative response of the two organs to SA. Further, more refined studies will be necessary to explore the differences between the molecular species.

Finally, we conclude that in the kidney affected by the genetic defect in hereditary tyrosinemia, an interesting physiologic paradox occurs. The metabolic byproduct of the enzyme defect, SA, inhibits transport of ALA, thus depriving the haem biosynthetic mechanism of substrate, while simultaneously enhancing the activity of ALAD in the renal epithelial cell. Hence, these two effects may offset each other, resulting in little or no overall deficit in haem synthesis. Studies of total haem production in control and SA-exposed renal tubules are currently underway, in order to assess this possibility. Alternatively, it is possible that there is a net decrease in haem synthesis which might be reflected in diminished cytochrome production by the cell, with a resultant decrease in oxygen consumption which we have previously reported (7).

ACKNOWLEDGEMENTS

This work was supported by Grant DK35319-05 from the National Institute of Health, Bethesda, MD.

REFERENCES

1. Foreman JW, Roth KS: Human renal Fanconi syndrome - then and now. Nephron 51:301-306, 1989

2. Berger R, van Faasen H, Taanman JW, de Vries H, Agsteribbe E: Type I tyrosinemia: lack of immunologically detectable fumaryl acetoacetase enzyme protein in tissues and cell extracts. Pediatr Res 22:394-398, 1987

3. Sassa S, Kappas, A: Hereditary tyrosinemia and the heme biosynthetic pathway: profound inhibition of delta-aminolevulinic acid dehydratase activity by succinylacetone. J Clin Invest. 71:625-634, 1983

4. Lindblad B, Linstedt S, Steen A: On the enzymic defects in hereditary tyrosinemia. Proc Natl Acad Sci (USA) 74:4641-4645, 1977

5. Roth KS, Foreman JW, Segal S: The Fanconi syndrome and mechanisms of tubular transport dysfunction. Kidney Int 20:705-716, 1981

6. Roth KS, Spencer PD, Higgins ES, Spencer RF: Effects of succinylacetone on methyl-alpha-D-glucoside uptake by the rat renal tubule. Biochim Biophys Acta 820:140-146, 1985

7. Spencer PD, Roth KS: Effects of succinylacetone on amino acid uptake in rat kidney. Biochem Med Metab Biol 27:101-109, 1987

8. Spencer PD, Medow MS, Moses LC, Roth KS: Effects of succinyl-acetone on the uptake of sugars and amino acids by brushborder vesicles. Kidney Int 34:671-677, 1988

9. Roth KS, Hwang SM, Segal S: The effect of maleic acid on the kinetics of alpha-methyl-D-glucoside uptake by isolated rat renal tubules. Biochim Biophys Acta 426:675-687, 1976

10. Lowry OH, Rosenbrough NJ, Fan AL, Randall RJ: Protein measurement with the Folin reagent. J Biol Chem 193:265-275, 1951

11. Sassa S: Delta-aminolevulinic acid dehydratase assay. Enzyme 28:133-145, 1982

7

RENAL FUNCTION IN THE SODIUM BICARBONATE INFUSED RAT: EFFECTS OF ALDOSTERONE AND OXYTOCIN

C.T. Musabayane (1), R.J. Balment (2) and M.J. Brimble (3)

Department of Physiology, University of Zimbabwe, P.O. Box 167, Mount Pleasant (1), Department of Physiological Sciences, University of Manchester, Manchester M13 9PT (2) and Department of Biological Sciences, Coventry Polytechnic, Coventry CV15 5FB (3)

INTRODUCTION

It has been suggested that high $NaHCO_3$ levels in the tubular lumen inhibit water and NaCl reabsorption by reducing the osmotic driving force across tight junctions (1). Micropuncture techniques in the rat have also established that the load of bicarbonate determines hydrogen ion secretion and HCO_3^- reabsorption in the distal tubule (2) and the rate of reabsorption in the papillary collecting ducts (3). High levels of HCO_3^- in the tubular lumen may lead to increases in urine flow, and the Na^+, K^+ and Cl^- excretion rates. However, these increases may be attributed to other factors, such as elevations in arterial blood pressure and glomerular filtration rate (GFR). Information on renal handling of HCO_3^- is available from scattered studies involving largely in vitro preparations. On this basis, we decided to investigate the renal effects of continuous $NaHCO_3$ infusion on water, Na^+, K^+ and Cl^- handling and on GFR and arterial blood pressure levels in vivo in an anaesthetised rat preparation. In view of the observations in preliminary experiments of the K^+ depletion resulting from HCO_3^- infusion, we have also examined the consequence of the induced hypokalaemia on plasma aldosterone levels. This preparation has been exploited in preliminary studies of the renal actions of aldosterone and oxytocin.

METHODS

Male Sprague-Dawley rats (300-450g) were used. The animals were maintained on a 12hr light/12hr dark regime and allowed free access to food (Mouse Comproids, National Foods, Harare) and water at all times. Rats were anaesthetised by intraperitoneal injection of Inactin, Byk Gulden (5-ethyl-5-(1 propyl)-2-thiobarbiturate) at 0.11g/kg body mass and tracheostomized.

Renal Excretion Studies

The right jugular vein was cannulated to allow intravenous infusion of $NaHCO_3$ (0.077M) at 150µl/min (Sage Syringe Pump model 351). The urinary bladder was also cannulated via an incision in the lower abdomen. An initial 4.5hr equilbration period was allowed to achieve stable urine flow, during which time urine was collected and the total volume, Na^+, K^+ and Cl^- excreted were determined. Following this, consecutive 20 min urine samples were collected into pre-weighed vials for 5hr. A terminal blood sample (2ml) was collected by cardiac puncture and Na^+ and K^+ were determined by flame photometry (Corning 435 flame photometer). Urinary Cl^- was determined by electrolytic chloridimetry (Corning Chloride Analyser 925). For the measurements of GFR and mean blood pressure, rats were prepared as for renal studies, except that a heparinized cannula (Portex, i.d. 0.86 mm, o.d. 1.27 mm) was also inserted into the femoral artery to record mean arterial blood pressure

(Gould Statham Physiological Pressure Transducer and Grass Model 7D Polygraph) and for withdrawal of blood samples. Animals were given a priming dose (0.3μCi of ^{3}H inulin in 0.3 ml of 0.077M NaHCO$_3$, Amersham International) and placed on continuous infusion at 150μl/min of NaHCO$_3$ (0.077M) containing inulin (0.14μCi/min). Urine collections were made every 30 min for 9hr and blood samples (200μl) were drawn at 2hr intervals into heparinized haematocrit tubes. Aliquots of urine (100 μl) and separated plasma (50μl) were counted for 10 min on a Minaxi a Tri-Carb 400 Series Liquid Scintillation Spectrometer using Lumax Scintillant (Lumac, BV, Holland) to allow calculation of inulin clearance as a measure of GFR.

For measurement of plasma pH and HCO$_3^-$ levels separate groups of rats were also prepared as for renal studies except that a cannula (Portex i.d. 0.86mm, o.d. 1.27mm) was also inserted into the left carotid artery for withdrawal of blood (200ml). Blood samples were withdrawn, each from a different group, to measure plasma pH and HCO$_3^-$ (ABL30 Acid Base Analyser) in the 1st, 3rd and 5th hour of the post equilibration period.

Plasma Hormone Assay

Further groups of animals were similarly prepared as for renal studies and decapitated after the end of the equilibration period and trunk blood was collected into pre-cooled containers. Blood for measuring aldosterone levels was similarly obtained from Inactin anaesthetised rats continuously infused with NaCl (0.077M). In all cases the plasma was separated, freeze-dried and stored at -20°C until dispatched by air to Manchester University for determination of aldosterone by radioimmunoassay (4).

Preliminary study of the renal action of aldosterone and oxytocin

The NaHCO$_3$ infused preparation for renal study described above was employed to examine the effect of addition of oxytocin (15μU/min, Sigma Grade V) and aldosterone (15ng/min, Sigma) to the infusate separately, or in combination. Aldosterone was administered throughout the whole period of infusion while oxytocin was added to the infusate for 2nd and 3rd hr of the post-equilibration period. Urinary excretion during these 2 hr is summarised in Table 3.

All values are presented as means ± SE and comparisons between infused groups are by unpaired t-test (*p<0.01).

RESULTS

Plasma HCO3-levels in the NaHCO$_3$ infused rats (Table 1) were, as anticipated, markedly elevated by comparison with the level of of 23μ1 mmol/l (n=6) in uninfused animals. The elevated plasma HCO$_3^-$ was associated with an alkalaemia compared with pH 7.31±0.01, (n=6) in the uninfused rat.

The mean femoral arterial blood pressure was well maintained throughout the 5hr period remaining in the range of 95 to 105 mmHg. GFR remained close to 2.5 ml/min throughout the 5hr period (Table 1).

In the 5hr post-equilibration period urine flow was maintained at approximately 140μl/min. The Na$^+$ excretion rate also did not differ significantly from the infusion rate, being maintained at approximately 10μmol/min (Figure 1). The Cl$^-$ excretion rate remained at

Table 1: Plasma HCO3-, Plasma pH, Mean arterial Blood Pressure, & GFR during the 5h post-equilibration period (n=6).

Time	HCO$_3$ mmol/l	pH	BP mmHg	GFR ml/min
1st hr	37±3	7.59±0.05	100±4	2.8±0.5
2nd hr	-	-	104±4	2.5±0.4
3rd hr	33±2	7.51±0.04	97±5	2.3±0.4
4th hr	-	-	95±5	2.6±0.5
5th hr	33±2	7.64±0.03	101±5	2.4±0.3

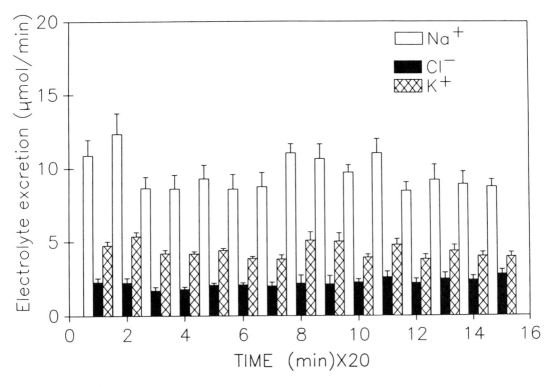

Figure 1. Na⁺, K⁺ and Cl⁻ excretion rates for 20 min collection periods throughout the 5hr post equilibration period in 0.077M NaHCO3 infused rats (n=10). Values are means, vertical bars indicate SE of means.

approximately 1.5µmol/min and that of K^+ was also constant at about 3.5µmol/min throughout.

Relative to NaCl infused animals, terminal plasma Na^+ and Cl^- concentrations were lower in the bicarbonate infused group (Table 2). In particular, the bicarbonate infused group was characterised by a marked hypokalemia. This was associated with considerably reduced plasma aldosterone levels. At the end of the equilibration period plasma and aldosterone in NaHCO3 infused rats was 0.85 ± 0.44 ng/ml (n=8) by comparison with 1.57 ± 0.26 ng/ml (n=7) in NaCl infused animals (p<0.01).

Neither the continuous adminstration of aldosterone nor the 2hr infusion of oxytocin altered urinary excretion rates during the 2nd and 3rd hr of the post equilibration period (Table 3).

However, when oxytocin administration was combined with aldosterone this resulted in a significant increase in sodium excretion (p<0.01). This natriuresis was not accompanied by significant increments in chloride excretion or by change in rates of urine production.

DISCUSSION

Bicarbonate infusion did not alter urine flow rates from those observed in animals receiving equivalent rates of NaCl infusion (5). The excretion of sodium similarly matched the rate of infusion as also occurs in preparations infused with NaCl (5). However, the low rate of chloride excretion observed in bicarbonate infused animals probably indicates that HCO_3^- is the major accompanying anion for the excreted sodium. The major difference in urinary excretion be-

Table 2: Terminal Plasma Electrolytes

	0.077M NaHCO$_3$ infused (n=8)	0.077M NaCl infused (n=13)
Na$^+$(mmol)	143±1 *	148 ±1
K$^+$(mmol)	3.0±0.2 *	4.6 ±0.2
Cl$^-$(mmol)	103±6 *	116±2

* p<0.01 by comparison with NaCl infused rats.

Table 3: Effect of aldosterone and oxytocin on urinary excretion during the 2nd and 3rd hour of the post-equlibration period

	Na$^+$ μmol	Cl$^-$ μmol	Urine Volume ml
Control (n=10)	1130±75	232±48	15.4±1.0
Aldosterone (n=8)	1242±154	313±53	15.4±1.4
Oxytocin (n=9)	1004±86	289±53	14.6±0.6
Aldosterone & Oxytocin (n=7)	1466±84 *	355±36	17.1±0.9

* p<0.01 by comparison with control (hormone-free) NaHCO$_3$ infused animals.

tween bicarbonate and previously observed saline infused animals, was the handling of potassium. In bicarbonate infused groups, potassium excretion rates remained at 4-5 mmol/min throughout the 9.5hr period of study. This contrasts with rates of only 1.8 mmol/min after 8hr of NaCl infusion in an equivalent preparation (5). The altered handling of K$^+$ was not associated with major change in GFR, which was similar to that measured in NaCl infused animals (5). This kaliuresis was reflected in the hypokalemia observed in the bicarbonate-infused groups. It was, perhaps then, not surprising to find that plasma aldosterone levels were reduced in the bicarbonate-infused groups relative to animals receiving saline. It is well established that plasma potassium concentration is a major determinant of aldosterone secretion (6), a rise in plasma potassium levels being a potent stimulus to secretion.

Thus the sodium bicarbonate-infused rat preparation provides a model in which arterial blood pressure, GFR and urine flow are maintained, but in which plasma aldosterone levels are lowered. This preparation is, therefore, of value for the study of renal actions of aldosterone, which are most clearly expressed where plasma aldosterone concentrations are reduced (7). This preparation would be preferred to the often used adrenalectomized animal (8) in which blood pressure and GFR are compromised.

Use of the bicarbonate-infused rat in preliminary studies does support a possible interaction between oxytocin and aldosterone in the regulation of renal sodium excretion as suggested by other workers (8). Using rates of oxytocin infusion, which would be expected to produce plasma oxytocin levels within the physiological range (5), there was no discernable effect on renal function. However, during aldosterone administration to supplement the lowered plasma aldosterone levels in the bicarbonate-infused animals, this same rate of oxytocin infused was natriuretic. Thus aldosterone may afford a permissive role in the natriuretic action of this neurohypophysial peptide. Clearly, the bicarbonate-infused rat preparation will be a valuable model with which to explore the mechanisms involved in this type of hormonal interaction.

REFERENCES

1. Ostensen J, Langberg H, Kiil F: How bicarbonate loading inhibits tubular reabsorption of NaCl in dog kidneys. Acta Physiol Scand 129: 35-46, 1987.

2. Malnic G, de Mello Aires G, Giebisch GJ: Micropuncture study of renal tubular hydrogen ion transport in the rat. Am J Physiol 222: 147-158, 1972.

3. Richardson RMA, Kanau RJ Jnr: Bicarbonate reabsorption in the papillary collecting duct: effect of acetazolamide. Am J Physiol 243: F74-F80, 1984.

4. Milne CM, Balment RJ, Henderson IW, Mosley W, Chester Jones I: Adrenocortical function in the Brattleboro rat Annal New York Acad Sci 394: 230-240, 1982.

5. Balment RJ, Brimble MJ, Forsling ML, Musabayane CT: The influence of neurohypophysial hormones on renal function in the acutely hypophysectomized rat. J Physiol 381: 429-452, 1986.

6. Blair-West JR, Coghlan JP, Denton DA, Goding JR, Munroe JA, Peterson RE, Wintour M: Humoral stimulation of adrenal cortical secretion. J Clin Invest 41: 1606-1627, 1982.

7. Burstyn PGR, Horrobin DF, Manku MS: Saluretic action of aldosterone in the presence of increased salt intake and restoration of normal action by prolactin or oxytocin. J Endocrinol 55: 369-376, 1977.

8. Morris DJ, Berek JS, Davis RP: The physiological response to aldosterone in adrenalectomized and intact rats and it sex dependence. Endocrinol 92: 989-993, 1973.

PART II
ACUTE RENAL FAILURE

8

EXPERIMENTAL ACUTE RENAL FAILURE INDUCED BY 3-AMINO-1-HYDROXYPROPYLIDENE- 1,1-BISPHOSPHONATE IN RODENTS

J.-C. Cal, A. Cockshott and P. T. Daley-Yates

Department of Pharmacy, University of Manchester, Manchester M13 9PL, United Kingdom

INTRODUCTION

3-Amino-1-hydroxypropylidene-1,1-bis-phos-phonate (APD), a potent inhibitor of osteoclast-mediated bone resorption, has over the past decade become the treatment of choice for Paget's disease and hypercalcaemia of malignancy (1-3). The relatively inert P-C-P bonds characterize all the bisphosphonates; the chemical formula of APD is:

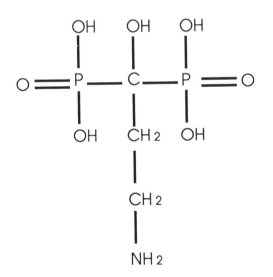

3-amino - 1- hydroxy propylidene-1, 1-bisphosphonate (APD)

Although bisphosphonates have been demonstrated to have numerous cellular effects, evidence still suggests that their action is due to their rapid binding to hydroxyapatite and the reduction of crystal solubility (4). When bisphosphonates are administered in vivo, a large proportion of that which is not excreted in the urine, is retained by bone. To date, no evidence of metabolism exists. However, it has been pointed out that the nephrotoxic potential of bisphosphonates could be a limiting factor in their clinical use (5-6). Since, to the best of our knowledge, no report has been published describing the nephrotoxicity of APD, the aim of this study has been to investigate the effect of APD on kidney function. To this end, we have explored the uptake of APD labelled with ^{14}C-APD by the kidney and other tissues and the elimination of the drug in the urine, in rats and mice. Several indicators of renal function were monitored including the plasma and urinary concentration of creatinine and urea, and enzymuria as an early and specific marker of tubular injury. The excretion of N-1-methylnicotinamide (NMN), an endogenous organic cation, was also monitored as a marker of tubular function (7). Morphological analysis of the kidneys by light microscopy was also performed in mice.

METHODS

Animals. Male Sprague-Dawley rats (180-200g) and Balb/c mice (23-25g) were allowed free access to food and water and housed in groups of 4 or 5 in temperature-controlled (22±1°C) rooms under a 12-hr light/dark cycle (0800/2000) during a standardization period of 10 days. The animals were weighed every day during the study.

Nephrotoxicity of APD in Mice. Groups of 10 mice received a single ip injection of either 0, 0.5, 2.5, 5, 10, 20 or 30 mg/kg APD labelled with ^{14}C-APD. Immediately after dosing, mice were placed in groups of 5 in metabolic cages for 24 hr for urine collection, then returned to standard cages for 24 hr. The final body weight was measured and blood was removed by cardiac puncture under halothane anaesthesia. Samples of bone (tibia), kidney and liver were collected and weighed.

Nephrotoxicity of APD in Rats. Groups of 6 rats were given a single ip dose of either 0, 1, 10, 20 or 40 mg/kg APD labelled with ^{14}C-APD. Rats were individually housed in metabolic cages 5 days before dosing, and the urine voided 24 hr before and 24 hr after dosing was collected. The final body weight was then measured and blood was removed as in mice. Samples of bone (tibia) and kidney were collected and weighed.

APD Assay. Samples of bone were first dissolved in 0.1 ml of 60% (v/v) $HClO_4$, then 1 ml Soluene-350 was added. The other samples were dissolved directly in 1 ml Soluene-350. Subsequently 1.5 ml 0.5 N HCl and 13.5 ml Insta-Gel liquid scintillator was added to each sample. Radioactivity was assessed using a Packard liquid scintillation counter.

Biochemical Analyses. Creatinine was determined in plasma and urine by the Jaffé's method and urea by enzymatic colorimetric method. Gamma- glutamyltranspeptidase (GGT), alkaline phosphatase (AlP) and N-ace-tyl-beta- D-glucosaminidase (NAG) were assayed using Boehringer Mannheim kits. NMN was determined fluorimetrically according to the method of Clark et al. (8) revised by Shim et al. (9).

Morphological Studies. The right kidney from mice injected with 0, 20 or 30 mg/kg APD was removed on the sixth day after dosing and placed in 5% sodium phosphate buffered (pH = 7.4) formaldehyde and embedded in paraffin. Sections (5μm) were stained with hematoxylin and eosin and examined by light microscopy.

Statistical Analysis. All data are reported as mean ± standard error. Analysis of variance followed by intergroup comparisons was used to estimate the effect of the dose on the different parameters studied. When these tests were not applicable, Kruskal-Wallis test or Mann and Whitney U-tests were used. Wilcoxon's tests or paired Student's t-tests were performed for comparing pre-dose and post-dose parameters.

RESULTS AND DISCUSSION

APD is linearly accumulated in bone and liver in both species with increasing doses, (Fig. 1) but the uptake of the drug by the kidney is significantly increased for the highest doses (p<0.0001). Moreover the renal elimination of APD fell gradually as a percentage of the administered dose (Table 1) indicating some changes in the renal handling of the drug.

When the animals were given high doses of APD, these events were accompanied by a striking increase of plasma creatinine from 39.78±1.7μmole/l in control mice to 61.38±4.9μmole/l in mice injected with 30 mg/kg APD (p<0.01) and from 40.7±5.4μmole/l in control rats to 97.7±17 μmole/l in rats injected with 40 mg/kg APD (p<0.01). The estimation of glomerular filtration rate from these data together with the data for the renal excretion of creatinine revealed a significant decrease. These results are in agreement with clinical data reported by Bounameaux et al. (5) on the increase of serum creatinine after a short term therapy with other bisphosphonates, especially etidronate and clodronate.

Additional information on the cause of this impairment of renal function is provided in this study by the analysis of the ratio of urine volume to water intake to compensate for the variability in drinking habits of the rats. In rats injected with 40 mg/kg APD, this ratio increased significantly from 35.9 ± 1.3% before injection to 53.5 ± 7.6% 24-hr after (p<0.05), indicating a loss of the concentrating ability. Moreover, the rise in urinary enzyme activity (Fig. 2) suggested that the proximal tubule was damaged

Mice

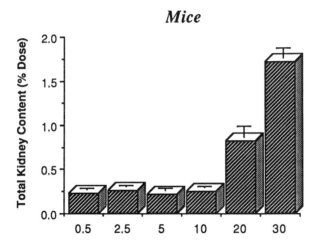

Rats

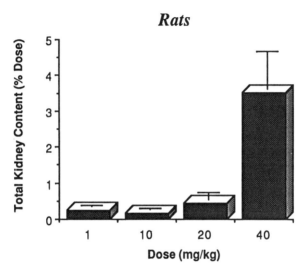

Figure 1. Total kidney content of APD as a percentage of the administered dose, 48-hr after a single ip injection of APD labelled in groups of 10 mice or 24-hr after in groups of 6 rats.

Table 1: Total amount of APD excreted in urine as a percentage of the dose during the first 24-hr after a single ip injection of APD in groups of 10 mice or 6 rats[a].

Doses	0.5	1	2.5	5	10	20	30	40
Mice	20.22 ±0.55	N.D.	17.08 ±2.5	14.37 ±1.9	13.1 ±2.4	9.05 ±1.7	4.44 ±0.8	N.D.
Rats	N.D.	20.52 ±1.26	N.D.	N.D.	17.23 ±0.92	14.88 ±2.97	N.D.	9.83 ±2.13

[a]: values are means ± S.E.; N.D.: no data

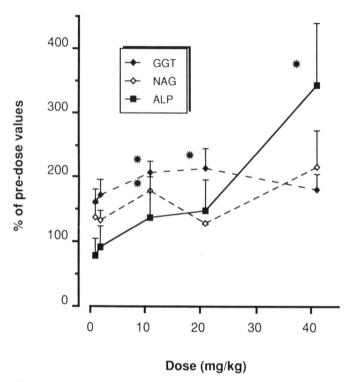

Figure 2. Urinary activity of gamma-glutamyltranspeptidase (GGT), alkaline phosphatase (AIP) and N-acetyl-beta-D-glucosaminidase (NAG) 24-hr after a single ip injection of APD in groups of 6 rats. The asterisks indicate a significant difference (p<0.05) between the pre- and post-dose values (Wilcoxon test).

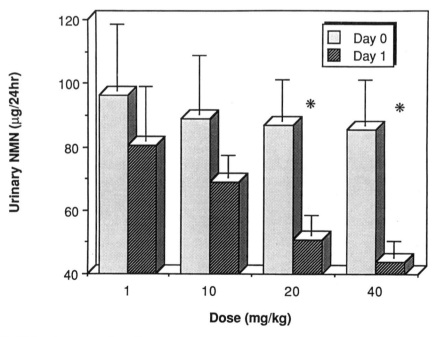

Figure 3. 24-hr urinary excretion of NMN before and after injection of APD. Each bar depicts the mean ± S.E. for 6 rats.

even at low doses of APD (10 mg/kg), taking into account the increase in GGT or NAG excretion for these doses.

Similarly, Fig. 3 shows a significant fall in the urinary excretion of NMN in groups of rats injected with 20 mg/kg ($p<0.02$) or 40 mg/kg APD ($p<0.05$). This is indicative of a functional loss of the nephron and especially a decrease in secretory capabilities of the proximal tubule (7).

Confirmation was provided by light microscopic evidence of focal cell necrosis with tubular obstruction in cortical areas of kidneys of mice injected with 20 or 30 mg/kg APD, 6 days after dosing. These data are consistent with other studies in which, for example, the intravenous bolus injection of large doses of Cl_2MDP was shown to induce structural renal abnormalities in dogs (10). In addition we have shown APD to be nephrotoxic at lower doses than other bisphosphonates.

The fall in the renal excretion of APD following high doses of this compound is easily explained in terms of the gross changes in renal function that occurred. In contrast, the fall in the renal excretion of APD at low doses is not accompanied by significant changes in the glomerular filtration rate. However, bisphosphonates have been shown to be eliminated partly by active renal secretion (11), data we have confirmed (unpublished). The increase in enzymuria and the fall in NMN excretion at low doses of APD show proximal tubular damage which may result in a reduction in the secretion of APD, and a consequent decrease in the renal elimination of this drug.

The mechanism of APD nephrotoxicity may relate to one of the main features of bisphosphonates, that is their ability to chelate metal ions such as calcium and iron. Other calcium chelating agents such as EDTA and DTPA are thought to be nephrotoxic due to their effects on mitochondrial function. Furthermore, redox cycling of chelated iron and the resulting free radical-mediated injury has already been postulated for clodronate. We are currently investigating these possible mechanisms. The significance of these results for patients receiving treatment especially with repeated doses of APD remains to be established.

ACKNOWLEDGEMENTS

The authors are indebted to Dr. Ray Bennett, head of the Department of Medical Physics, (for his expert work in the assay of ^{14}C-APD) and to Dr. R.S. Reeves, Department of Histopathology, Hope Hospital, Salford, U.K. (for his assistance in the preparation of kidney slices for microscopic examination). Mr. Michael Jackson, A.I.A.T., is also gratefully acknowledged for his excellent technical assistance. This work was funded by Ciba-Geigy Pharmaceuticals.

REFERENCES

1. Cantrill JA, Buckler HM, Anderson DC: Low dose intravenous 3-amino- 1-hydroxy-propylidene-1,1-bisphosphonate (APD) for the treatment of Paget's disease of bone. Ann Rheum Dis. 45: 1012-1018, 1986.

2. Thiébaud D, Jaeger P, Gobelet C, Jacquet AF, Burckhardt P: A single infusion of the bisphosphonate AHPrBP (APD) as treatment of Paget's Disease of bone. Am J Med 85: 207-212, 1988.

3. Morton AR, Cantrill JA, Pillai GV, McMahon A, Anderson DC, Howell A: Sclerosis of lytic bone metastases after disodium amino-hydroxypropylidene bisphosphonate (APD) in patients with breast carcinoma. Br Med J 297: 772-773, 1988.

4. Ieisch H: Experimental basis for the use of bisphosphonates in Paget's disease of bone. Clin Orth Rel Res 217: 72-78, 1987.

5. Bounameaux HM, Schifferli J, Montani JP, Jung A, Chatelanat F: Renal failure associated with intravenous diphosphonates. The Lancet 1: 471, 1983.

6. Alden CL, Englehart J, Eastman DF, Parker RD: Modulation of Cl_2MDP induced renal toxicity by sequestration of iron. In: Bach PH, Lock EA (eds.) Third International Symposium on

Nephrotoxicity Abstract Book. Guildford, 1987, pp. W5.

7. Cal JC, Maiza A, Daley-Yates PT: The clearance of endogenous N-1-methylnicotinamide: a new marker of nephrotoxicity ? In: Bach PH, et al (eds); Proceedings of the Fourth International Symposium on Nephrotoxicity. New York, Marcel Dekker, 1990.

8. Clark BR, Halpern RM, Smith RA: A fluorimetric method for quantitation in the picomole range of N-1-methylnicotinamide and nicotinamide in serum. Anal Biochem 68: 54-61, 1975.

9. Shim CK, Sawada Y, Iga T, Hanano M: Estimation of renal secretory function for organic cations by endogenous N-1-methylnicotinamide in rats with experimental renal failure. J Pharmacokin Biopharm 12: 23-42, 1984.

10. Hintze KI, D'Amato RA: Comparative toxicity of two diphosphonates. Toxicologist 2: 192, 1982.

11. Troëhler U, Bonjour JP, Fleisch H: Renal secretion of diphosphonates in rats. Kidney Int. 8: 6-13, 1975.

9

A COMPARISON OF THE GLYCEROL-INDUCED AND THE FIVE-SIXTHS NEPHRECTOMY MODELS OF RENAL FAILURE

T.R. McCappin (1), S.D. Heys (2), Y.A. Boateng (3), L. Smart (4), J.C. Petrie (3), H.E. Barber (1), P.H. Whiting (5)

Departments of Pharmacology (1), Surgery (2), Medicine and Therapeutics (3), Pathology (4) and Clinical Biochemistry (5), University of Aberdeen, Foresterhill, Aberdeen, AB9 2ZD, UK

INTRODUCTION

There are several animal models available for the study of renal failure. Two of the four most common models in the literature are surgically induced, either 5/6 nephrectomy or ligation of ureters and the other two are chemically induced (glycerol or uranyl nitrate). One model from each group, namely 5/6 nephrectomy and glycerol was chosen and fully characterised. It has been suggested that the glycerol model of acute renal failure (ARF) resembles the "crush syndrome" in man, since intramuscular injection of glycerol results in myohaemoglobinuria which leads to renal ischaemia (1). The 5/6 nephrectomy model has been useful in pre-clinical drug testing and can help in the prediction of changes in the kinetics of drugs caused by renal failure (2).

In this paper we describe the biochemical characterisation of these two models of renal dysfunction. Histological analysis of renal tissue from each animal model was also carried out to complete the characterisation.

MATERIALS AND METHODS

Male Sprague-Dawley rats, (initial weight 200-300g) were randomly assigned to glycerol (G) or nephrectomy (N) groups. Renal failure in the glycerol group was induced by a single i.m. injection of glycerol in normal saline (50% w/v) with a control group injected with saline only. All animals were used 48 hr after treatment. Animals in the nephrectomy group were anaes-thetised with ether followed by i.p. chloral hydrate after which a midline ventral incision was made to expose the intestines. The intestines were carefully moved to one side to expose the left kidney. This allowed ligation of two of the three branches of the renal artery supplying the organ. The right kidney was completely removed and the ureter ligated. Controls were sham-operated and all animals were used one week after surgery.

The animals were allowed a period of acclimatisation in the metabowls before the actual study days. Food consumption, water intake and urine flow rate were monitored. Blood samples were collected for analysis during each study period. Sodium, glucose, creatinine and urea content of serum and urine samples was estimated by standard laboratory techniques (3) using a Dimension Analyser (Du Pont Ltd). Urine N-acetyl-beta-D-glucosaminidase activity (NAG) was determined as described previously (4). Results (Tables 1 and 2) are expressed as units per mmol urinary creatinine, a measure independent of flow rate.

RESULTS

Renal structure and function was assessed in G and N animals after 48 hr and 7 days respectively and compared to values from appropriate controls. Table 1 is a summary of measured and calculated parameters obtained following the metabowl section of the study for G rats and Table 2 shows equivalent results from the N group.

TABLE 1. Metabowl data for the glycerol model of renal failure.

Measurement	G (n=6)	Control (n=6)	P-value
UFR (ml/hr/kg)	5.46 ± 3.30	1.74 ± 0.56	p<0.05
Cr.Cl . (ml/hr/kg)	41.50 ± 45.90	287.20 ±35.9	p<0.01
NAG (units/mmol)	789.02 ±315.41	72.61 ± 6.36	p<0.01
UREA (mmol/l)	64.70 ± 25.5	5.52 ± 1.3	p<0.01
FOOD (g)	2.67 ± 2.7	21.40 ± 2.6	p<0.01
WATER (ml)	41.67 ±16.9	38.80 ± 8.3	N.S.
SODIUM Cl. (ml/hr/kg)	3.60 ± 2.4	2.40 ± 0.6	N.S.
F.E. SODIUM	14.72 ± 9.1	0.82 ± 0.15	p<0.01

TABLE 2. Metabowl data for the 5/6 nephrectomy model of renal failure.

	N (n=6)	Control (n=6)	P-value
UFR (ml/hr/kg)	4.35± 0.85	1.46± 0.24	p<0.01
Cr.Cl. (ml/hr/kg)	146.61± 39.54	196.23±45.04	N.S.
NAG (units/mmol)	21.46± 7.15	28.79± 6.63	N.S.
UREA (mmol/l)	34.8 ± 26.3	7.9 ± 2.31	p<0.01
FOOD (g)	26.0 ± 15.7	29.3 ± 8.8	N.S.
WATER (ml)	57.5 ± 14.4	30.8 ±19.8	p<0.01
SODIUM Cl. (ml/hr/kg)	3.76± 3.01	2.3 ± 0.12	N.S
F.E. SODIUM	2.4 ± 1.6	1.22± 0.28	N.S.

Results are mean ± standard deviation.p-value from non-paired Student's t-test.
Legend: Cr.Cl. = creatinine clearance, UFR = urine flow rate, NAG = N- acetyl-B-D glucosaminidase, F.E. SODIUM = fractional excretion of sodium, N.S. = not significantly different.

The results presented in Table 1 illustrate the severe nature of glycerol induced acute renal failure. Glycerol injected rats only consumed one tenth of the food eaten by control animals. Urine production was significantly increased, but water intake did not change to a statistically significant degree. The animals were therefore dehydrated. In Table 2 the same parameters for N animals show there to be no change in food consumption while both water intake and urine production increased 2-fold compared to controls. Both models of renal failure resulted in elevated serum urea and creatinine levels, although it should be noted the changes in these parameters were most severe in the G animals. A comparison of creatinine clearance values clearly demonstrates the differences in severity of the two models. Glycerol injected animals demonstrated a 7-fold decrease in creatinine clearance compared to a slight insignificant decrease in N animals. Glycerol treated animals also demonstrated a 10-fold increase in urine NAG activity whilst following nephrectomy no increase in activity was observed.

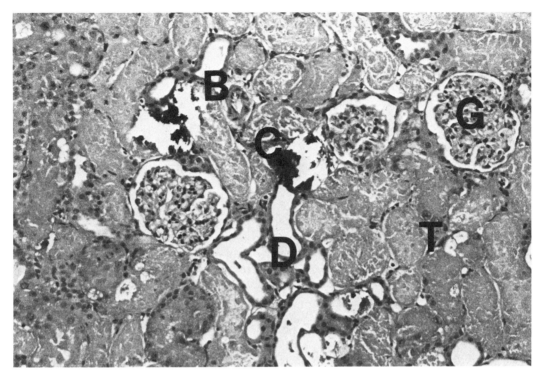

FIG. 1 Renal cortex showing necrotic tubules (T), tubular dilatation (D), focal calcification (C) and sparing of glomeruli (G) (H&E X300).

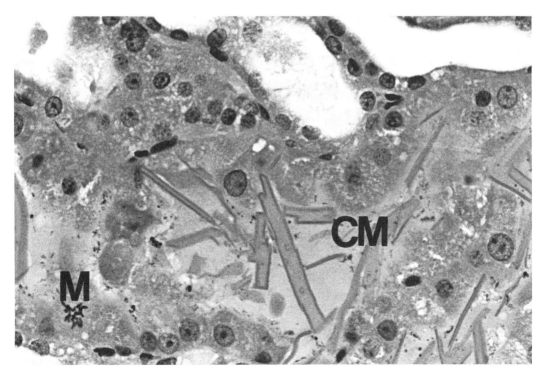

FIG 2. High power of damaged tubules showing regenerative mitotic activity (M). Crystalline material (CM) is present within the tubules (H&E X540).

Histological examination of kidneys from G animals (Figs. 1 & 2) revealed extensive tubular damage with many proximal tubules showing complete necrosis of the epithelium. In addition there was dilatation, focal calcification and early tubular regeneration. Large orangeophilic crystalloid deposits were conspicuous within damaged tubules. Distal tubules and collecting ducts contained large numbers of casts of a cellular and granular type. Glomeruli appeared spared and blood vessels were normal. Histology carried out on kidneys from N animals revealed normal tissue.

DISCUSSION

The highly significant differences in food consumption, creatinine clearance, urinary NAG and degree of uremia in G rats demonstrate the severe nature of this model at our chosen glycerol dose of 10 ml/kg. The extent and selective nature of the renal structural changes found suggest that, in addition to the known ischaemic and rhabdomyolytic effects of the glycerol model, there is also overlying nephrotoxic acute tubular necrosis.

The 5/6 nephrectomy model induces renal impairment 7 days post surgery as indicated by elevated serum urea and reduced creatinine clearance values (Table 2). At 14 or 21 days post surgery serum urea and creatinine levels in nephrectomy animals have been shown to be approaching normal values. Work in this laboratory (5) has shown there to be no differences in warfarin pharmacokinetics between nephrectomy and laparotomy rats 21 days post surgery. The return towards normal renal function after surgery results from compensatory hypertrophy of the remaining 1/6 kidney. Our data suggests one week post surgery as an acceptable time for experimental use of this model. After 7 days the animals have recovered from surgical stress and compensatory hypertrophy has not increased renal mass to any significant degree.

This study has shown the two chosen models of renal failure to be quite different. One requires a high degree of surgical skill (N) with associated equipment and facilities while the other (G) is very simple to induce. The resultant renal failure obtained with each model is also different. Nephrectomy results in a reduced mass of healthy tissue while glycerol produces ischaemic and nephrotoxic effects. Both models have been shown to alter pharmacokinetic parameters and hepatic uptake of several commonly prescribed drugs such as warfarin and sodium cromoglycate (6,7). In G rats hepatic uptake of sodium cromoglycate was significantly reduced while for warfarin the volume of distribution, volume of central compartment and the parameter Dose/Area under the curve (0-40 min) were all elevated. Most recent work carried out in this laboratory (8) has shown 5/6 nephrectomy to significantly alter the area under the curve (AUC), clearance, biological half-life and concentration at time zero of cyclosporin-A (CsA) in the rat whole animal pharmacokinetic model.

REFERENCES

1. Stein JH, Lifschitz MD, Barnes LD: Current concepts on the pathophysiology of acute renal failure. Am J Physiol 234: F171-181, 1978.

2. Moravek J, Schuck O, Hatala M, Priborsky J: Preclinical modeling of changes in drug kinetics caused by renal failure in rats. J Pharmacokinetics and Biopharm 15: 15-23, 1987.

3. Marsh WH, Fingerhut B, Miller H: Automated and manual methods for determination of blood urea. Clin Chem 11: 624-628, 1979.

4. Whiting PH, Ross IS, Borthwick LJ: N-acetyl-beta-D-glucosaminidase levels and diabetic microangiopathy. Clin Chem Acta 97: 191-195, 1979.

5. Boateng YA, McCappin TR, Barber HE, Heys SD, Whiting PH, Petrie JC: Pharmacokinetics of warfarin in nephrectomised rats. Europ J Clin Pharm 36 (Suppl): A127, 1989.

6. Barber HE, Buckley GA, McCappin TR, Petrie JC, Smith KJ: The effect of glycerol-induced acute renal failure on the hepatic uptake of sodium cromoglycate in the isolated perfused rat liver. Brit J Pharmacol 91:469P, 1987.

7. Barber HE, Boateng YA, McCappin TR, Petrie JC, Whiting PH: The effect of glycerol-induced acute renal failure on warfarin pharmacokinetics in the rat. Brit J Pharmacol 96: 291P, 1989.

8. McCappin TR, Boateng YA, Whiting PH, Barber HE, Petrie JC: The effect of glycerol-induced acute renal failure and 5/6 nephrectomy on the hepatic uptake and pharmacokinetics of cyclosporin-A. Unpublished Results.

10
ACUTE RENAL FAILURE FOLLOWING ACCIDENTAL CUTANEOUS ABSORPTION OF PHENOL

P.J.D. Foxall, M.R. Bending, K.P.R. Gartland and J.K.Nicholson

Department of Chemistry, Birkbeck College, University of London, Gordon House, 29 Gordon Square, London WC1H 0PP, UK

INTRODUCTION

Acute renal failure (ARF) due to cutaneous absorption of phenol is uncommon. We report here an unusual case of ARF following an industrial accident in which a male received burns following partial immersion in a solution of 20% phenol in dichloromethane. We were able to monitor the onset, progression and subsequent recovery from the nephrotoxic episode using a combination of conventional clinical chemistry assays and high resolution proton nuclear magnetic resonance (PMR) spectroscopic urinalysis, a technique which has proven very effective in the biochemical profiling of a variety of experimental toxicity states (1-4). The patient, a 41 year old married man, accidentally fell forward into a shallow vat of industrial solvent; he was partially immersed for only a few seconds and managed to avoid ingesting the fluid. He immediately showered, was subsequently found in a state of collapse and admitted to a local hospital. On examination he was found to have cold extremeties and 50% body surface burns involving the face, chest, genitals and both legs. Initial observations were stable, however, he developed nausea and vomiting after drinking fluids. Following admission he became anuric and plasma creatinine levels started to rise. He was transferred to the regional renal unit where he was diagnosed as suffering from phenol-induced burns, acute tubular necrosis and fluid overload. Intravenous furosemide was given and haemodialysis commenced on a daily basis for a period of seven days with decreasing intervals for a further 18 days until adequate urinary volumes were produced. The patient suffered discomfort from the skin burns and subsequently developed respiratory distress which required intensive care treatment. However following a period of polyuria, renal function improved 6 weeks after the accident. One year following the accident the patient was still showing marginal polyuria (1.5 - 3 l/day).

METHODS

Blood and Urine Samples. Venous blood (10ml into lithium heparinised tubes and 5 ml into EDTA tubes for haematological investigation) and urine samples were collected daily after admission. The plasma was separated by centrifugation and urea, electrolytes, calcium, creatinine, phosphate, total protein and albumin and glucose measured by multichannel autoanalysis. All urine produced by the patient was collected without the addition of a preservative, the volume recorded, an aliquot centrifuged for 5 min (3000 rpm, 4°C) and the supernatant used for analyses. A volume of 10 ml of each urine sample was frozen at -20°C for PMR analysis at a later date.

PMR spectroscopy. 2 ml of urine was lyophilised and redissolved in 0.75 ml ^2H_2O (to provide a spectrometer field/frequency lock) containing 1mg/ml 3-trimethylsilyl-[2,2,3,3-$^2H_4$]-1-propionate (TSP) as a chemical shift reference (d = 0 ppm) and added to 5mm tubes. Measurements were made at ambient probe temperature (298±1°K) using a 500 MHz (JEOL GSX500) PMR spectrometer operating at a

field strength of 11.8 Tesla. For spectra recorded at 500 MHz, 48 free induction decays
(FIDs) were collected into 32768 computer
points using 3us (40°) pulses, a sweep width of
6000 Hz and an acquisition time of 2.73 s. A
delay of 2 s was added to permit full T_1 relaxation. An exponential line broadening function of
0.6 Hz was applied prior to Fourier transformation. The residual water signal was suppressed
by a secondary irradiation field, the power being
gated off during acquisition.

RESULTS

Small volumes of urine were passed until day
21. There then followed a phase of polyuria in
which daily urine volumes of up to 11 litres were
produced (Figure 1a). Plasma creatinine rose
steadily to 1258 µmol/l (Figure 1b) on day 8
after the accident with a blood urea of 55 mmol/l
(Figure 1c) indicating poor renal function. The
fluctuating plasma creatinine and urea levels
are related closely to the haemodialysis treatment as indicated in Figure 1. Plasma
haemoglobin showed the patient to be anaemic
throughout the latter period of examination (Figure 1d).

For comparison a PMR spectrum of urine from
a healthy adult is shown in Figure 2. The dominant resonances arise from creatinine with
lesser contributions from hippurate, betaine
(N,N,N-trimethylglycine), citrate, dimethylamine (DMA) and 2-oxoglutarate (2-OG).
Spectra from urine collected soon after the
accident show intense signals corresponding to
very high levels of phenolic metabolites (not
shown) together with signals from infused dextran (Figure 3). Approximately 4 days after the
accident, elevated endogenous metabolites related to the toxic processes in the kidney were
observed. In particular, unusually strong signals from lactate, alanine, glutamine, valine,
glucose, succinate and acetate were observed
in addition to a decrease in creatinine excretion
(Figure 3). Phenol metabolites were still being
excreted at day 4 (data not shown). Throughout
the polyuric phase of the renal disease process
(days 26-28) the PMR metabolic profile of urine
had again changed dramatically with elevated
levels of acetate, DMG and DMA together with

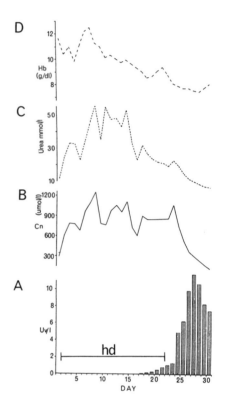

Figure 1. Time course of conventional clinical
chemistry data obtained from the subject over a period of 30 days following accidental exposure to phenol. A, urine volume (reference (ref.) range: 800-1800
ml/d); B, plasma creatinine (ref. range: 80-108
umol/l); C, plasma urea (ref. range: 2.5-6.4 mmol/l);
D, haemoglobin (ref. range:13.5-17.5 g/dl). hd,
haemodialysis.

an increase in creatinine relative to other metabolites (Figure 3). On release from hospital the
patient had a normal plasma creatinine of 115
µmol/l but the PMR urine profiles indicated
normal renal biochemistry and full function had
not yet been restored (Figure 3).

DISCUSSION

This report documents an unusual case of
ARF following a severe nephrotoxic episode
resulting from cutaneous absorption of phenol
and the subsequent clinical biochemical fol-
low-ups using conventional analytical methods
and PMR urinalysis - an advanced spectroscopic technique that has only recently been
used as a toxicological tool (1-4). Phenol is

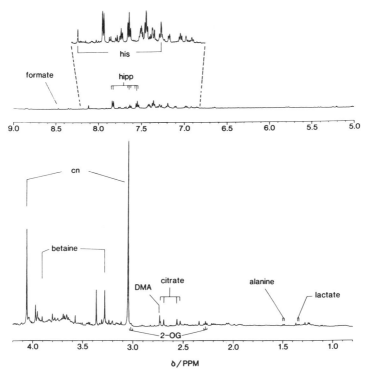

Figure 2. 500 MHz PMR spectrum of lyophilised urine obtained from a healthy male individual. cn, creatinine; DMA, dimethylamine; hipp, hippurate; his, histidine.

readily absorbed through the skin, the rate of absorption being proportional to the surface area involved and the duration of contact rather than phenol concentration (5). Local tissue damage is, however, dependant on concentration and with the intense necrosis that follows exposure to strong phenolic solutions, phenol absorption may be impaired (5). It has therefore been suggested that cutaneous exposure to dilute phenolic solutions may result in more serious systemic consequences (5). In the present case the patient was exposed to a 20% phenol concentration in dichloromethane, and showered shortly after exposure further diluting the surface phenol concentration and hence possibly enhancing absorption.

We have shown that highly abnormal metabolite profiles can be detected in the plasma and urine of patients who have experienced intentional overdoses of paracetamol through suicide attempts (6). In particular PMR has proven useful in the discovery of novel molecular markers for toxicity states and offers an efficient new means of obtaining toxicological information (1-4). In many ways PMR is uniquely suited to the study of toxicological events as rapid multi-metabolite analyses can be made which shed light on a range of biochemical pathways that are perturbed during a toxic process. The routine biochemical profiles obtained by conventional autoanalysis procedures assist in monitoring signs of water depletion, sodium and potassium balance, blood glucose control and provide a gross measure of renal functional capacity through creatinine and urea measurements. However, these measurements give very little information on the mechanism of action of a nephrotoxic agent, the site of the renal lesions or the biochemical function in different parts of the kidney. Conversely, PMR urinalysis

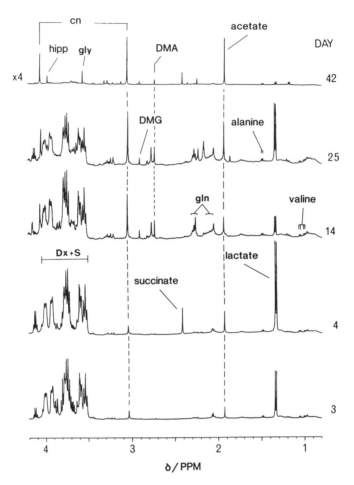

Figure 3. 500 MHz PMR spectra (region to low frequency of water) of urine obtained from the subject 3, 4, 14, 25 and 42 days following accidental exposure to phenol. cn, creatinine; DMA, dimethylamine; DMG, N,N-dimethylglycine; Dx, dextran; gln, glutamine; gly, glycine; hipp, hippurate; S, sugars (including glucose). The vertical scale of the top spectrum is expanded by a factor of 4.

can provide exactly this type of information in experimental animals exposed to different model nephrotoxins (1-4). Furthermore, PMR urinalysis can be at least as sensitive as an indicator of renal damage as conventional biochemical procedures such as urinary enzyme measurements (2). In the present investigation PMR urinalysis again proved useful in giving a more comprehensive biochemical description of the nephrotoxic process than can be given by conventional tests alone. In particular, recovery from the cortical lesions (with

associated lactic aciduria and amino aciduria) was rapid, leaving more persistent renal papillary lesions and a characteristically perturbed urine biochemistry. This study shows that PMR urinalysis offers an alternative and complementary means of following the time-course of biochemical perturbations after renal insult in clinical situations. Furthermore, PMR observations give greater insight into the toxicological processes involved and may be more sensitive than conventional clinical chemical approaches in the detection of residual renal damage.

ACKNOWLEDGEMENTS

We thank The Wellcome Foundation and The National Kidney Research Fund, for financial support and the MRC for the use of central NMR facilities.

REFERENCES

1. Nicholson JK, Timbrell JA and Sadler PJ: Proton NMR spectra of urine as indicators of renal damage. Mercury-induced nephrotoxicity in rats. Mol Pharmacol 27:644-651, 1984.

2. Gartland KPR, Bonner FW, Timbrell JA, et al.: The biochemical characterisation of p-aminophenol-induced nephrotoxic lesions in the F344 rat. Arch Toxicol 63:97-106, 1989.

3. Gartland KPR, Bonner FW, Nicholson JK: Investigations into the biochemical effects of region-specific nephrotoxins. Mol Pharmacol 35: 242-250, 1989.

4. Nicholson JK and Gartland KPR: A nuclear magnetic resonance approach to investigate the biochemical and molecular effects of nephrotoxins. In: Reid E, Cook, GMW, Luzio, JP (eds); Cells, Membranes and Disease Plenum Press, New York, 1987, pp. 397-408.

5. Pardoe R, Minami R, Sato R, Schlesinger S: Phenol burns. Burns 3 (1): 29-41, 1977.

6. Bales JR, Bell JD, Nicholson JK, et al.: Metabolic profiling of body fluids by proton NMR spectroscopy: Self poisoning episodes with acetaminophen Mag Res Med 6 (2) 301-309, 1988.

PART III
NATURAL TOXIC COMPOUNDS

11
EFFECTS OF THE FUNGAL TOXIN ORELLANINE ON RENAL EPITHELIUM

W. Pfaller, G. Gstraunthaler (1), H. Prast (2), L. Rupp (1), C. Ruedl (3), S. Michelitsch (3) and M. Moser (3)

(1) Institute of Physiology, (2) Institute of Pharmacokinetics and Toxicology and (3) Institute of Microbiology, University of Innsbruck, Austria

INTRODUCTION

Orellanine, a secondary metabolite of the mushroom Cortinarius orellanus, has been identified as the toxic principle which affected 102 inhabitants of Bygdosz in Poland (1). Individuals developed acute renal failure (ARF) and hepatic insufficiency and 20 persons died within 4-16 days after ingesting the mushrooms. The survivors developed chronic renal failure. Some years later, it became obvious that the closely related mushroom Cortinarius orellanoides (Kühn & Romagn) is also toxic, probably via the identic toxin (2-4).

Since the 1970s about 180 cases of intoxications with either Cortinarius orellanus or Cortinarius orellanoides have been reported from Switzerland, France, Germany, Czechoslovakia, Finland, Sweden, Norway and Scotland (5). Once the toxicity of these mushrooms had been recognized, several attempts to isolate and characterize the toxic principles were made (6-10) and 2,2'-bipyridine-3,3',4,4'-tetrol-1,1'dioxide was identified as the major toxin.

Confusion existed, however, regarding the organ specificity of orellanine, which has been reported to be hepato- (11-14), and nephrotoxic (15). A recent experimental study of Prast and Pfaller (5), however, clearly identified the kidney as the predominant target of orellanine.

In this presentation we summarize the effects of orellanine on renal epithelium in vivo and in vitro elaborated in our laboratory (5,10,16).

MATERIALS AND METHODS

In vivo studies

Male Sprague Dawley rats (250 ± 45 g) were fed with 2g dry weight of Cortinarius orellanus (25 mg orellanine /g dry mushroom) via gavage, following a starvation period of 12 hr. Controls received the same amount of the nontoxic Agaricus bisporus. Renal functional parameters, glomerular filtration rate, urine flow, Na-excretion, urine concentration capability, protein excretion and changes in renal morphology were followed in 12 hr intervals up to 72 hr after dosing. Morphologic studies were performed at the light- and electron microscopic level at 12, 24, 48 and 72 hr after administration of 2g/kg Cortinarius orellanus homogenate. For this purpose, kidneys were fixed by vascular perfusion of 1% glutaraldehyde, (17), postfixed with 1% OsO_4, dehydrated in graded series of acetone and embedded in Durcupan ACM[R] (Fluka AG. Switzerland).

In vitro studies

Orellanine extracted from Cortinarius orellanus and Cortinarius orellanoides as well as the synthetic version of orellanin (18) were administered in various concentrations over intervals of 24 and 48 hr to confluent layers of the established renal epithelial cell lines LLC-PK$_1$ (pig kidney cells) and OK (opossum kidney) or to the colonic carcinoma cell line CaCo-2 grown on impermeable supports. The parameters monitored were changes in monolayer morphology and changes in the activity of the apical membrane marker enzymes alkaline phosphatase (AP) and gamma-glutamyltranspeptidase (gamma-GT). AP and gamma-GT were assayed as described recently (19,20).

In addition, orellanine was added to LLC-PK$_1$ monolayer cultures grown on semipermeable supports (Millicell^{TM}-HA, Millipore Corp.) in order to test possible effects of the toxin on transcellular transport of the macromolecules ferritin, dextrane and horseradish peroxidase. Changes in transcytosis were determined by using electron microscopic morphometric methods (21,22).

RESULTS

In vivo studies:

Orellanine-induced changes in renal functional parameters are summarized in Table 1. The decrease in GFR was most pronounced between 36 and 72 hr after toxing. At 96 hr after dosing all animals were anuric. Urine output increased between 36 and 48 hr, indicating a polyuric phase of ARF before the onset of anuria between 72 and 96 hr after toxin administration. During the observation period the urine osmolality decreased to about 500 mOsmol/l. Fractional excretion of Na$^+$ and excretion of protein progressively increased 24 hr after toxin ingestion and reached maximum values 72 hr after dosing.

The first morphological changes can be recognized as early as 12 hr after 2 g orellanine/kg body weight. These changes are characterized by the appearance of vacuoles within proximal tubular epithelium of all segments (S1, S2, and S3). Furthermore, cytoplasmic protrusions into the lumen and irregularities of the brush border regions can be detected. Electron microscopy reveals deformation of microvilli and enhanced vacuolization of the luminal cell pole of proximal tubular cells. After 24 and 48 hr the whole renal cortex is affected (Fig. 1a,b) and in addition pre-necrotic and necrotic cells can be found. Brush border changes and apical cellular vacuolization are more pronounced and the

Table 1

hours after dosing	0	24	48	72
GFR [µl/min.g kidney]				
controls (n=3)	1057± 63	1012±103	959± 10	980± 38
2g Cortinarius orellanus (n=3)	1065± 22	885± 12	126± 66	33± 10
Urine flow [µl/min]				
controls (n=3)	6.1±0.2	6.8±0.2	7.8±0.8	7.6±0.6
2g Cortinarius orellanus (n=3)	6.3±0.3	5.9±0.2	14.6±4.6	8.2±2.9
Urine osmolality [mOsmol/l]				
controls (n=3)	1984±104	1872± 32	1805± 42	1750±176
2g Cortinarius orellanus (n=3)	1896±104	1355±167	876± 78	478± 58
Fractional excretion of Na± [%]				
controls (n=3)	0.13±0.01	0.11±0.06	0.10±0.01	0.78±0.02
2g Cortinarius orellanus (n=3)	0.13±0.01	0.23±0.05	2.26±0.60	16.31±3.65
Protein excretion [mg/24 h]				
controls (n=3)	1.91±0.1	1.94±0.1	1.38±0.1	0.44±0.1
2g Cortinarius orellanus (n=3)	1.76±0.1	6.80±0.6	19.15±2.4	27.57±0.5
Renal glutathione content [nmol/g kidney]				
controls (n=3)	2865± 50	--------	1390± 47	1875± 2
2g Cortinarius orellanus (n=3)	2865± 50	--------	859±112	447± 3

Values are means ± standard deviation (SD)

number of lysosomal transsection profiles is increased. Smooth endoplasmic reticulum is frequently found in form of big clusters, mitochondria are swollen and display disrupted innner membranes and flocculent electron dense precipitates. After 72 and 96 hr hardly any open proximal lumen can be detected and also distal tubular and cortical collecting duct cells show those changes described above for the proximal tubules, with the exception that lysosomal transsection profiles decrease in number. No changes could, however, be recognized in the glomerular ultrastructure.

In vitro studies

a) Renal epithelial cells (LLC-PK1 and OK cells)

LLC-PK1 monolayers incubated with varying concentrations of orellanine over a period of 24 or 48 hr show a dose-dependent inhibition of alkaline phosphatase (Fig. 2a,b), whereas under the same conditions no impairment of gamma-GT, another apical membrane marker enzyme expressed by LLC-PK1 cells, could be detected (Fig. 2c). At a concentration of 1 mM orellanine and an incubation time of 24 hours enzyme activity of AP is completely abolished in LLC-PK1 cells (Fig. 2a). The inhibitory effect is combined with severe morphologic alterations, characterized by a tremendous vacuolization of cells (Fig. 3b, d). A number of cells are injured and they detach from the culture substratum. OK cells expressing virtually no AP at their apical membrane show identical morphologic alterations (Fig. 3c).

LLC-PK1 cells grown on permeable supports also exhibit an enormous vacuolization, which is due to an increase in volume of the cisternae of the endoplasmic reticulum (Fig. 3d). The mean average cellular volume, $2300 \pm 300\,\mu m^3$ under control conditions increases to $2800 \pm 400\,\mu m^3$ after the action of 1 mM orellanine over 48 hr. This slight increase in volume is paralleled by an enlargement of the endoplasmic reticulum, which increases from $11 \pm 1,2$ to $450 \pm 12\,\mu m^3$. On the other hand, the total volume of endocytic or more specific transcytotic vacuoles labelled by either cationized ferritin or

horseradish peroxidase decrease by a factor of 1,4 as compared to the controls (Fig. 3d).

b) Colonic epithelial cells

Caco-2 cells containing the intestinal isoform of AP in their apical membrane also show a dose-dependent inhibition of the enzyme. However, they react less sensitively when compared to the renal cell lines (Fig. 2b).

The kinetics of inhibition of AP isoenzymes from LLC-PK1 and Caco-2 cells or the respective pure enzymes from either bovine kidney or bovine intestine and placenta, respectively, at substrate concentrations ranging from 0.125 to 2.0 mM and orellanine concentrations of 0.5 and 1.0 mM display distinct differences (Fig. 1b).

As shown (Fig. 2d,e) the intestinal isoenzyme is inhibited noncompetitively whereas the intestinal and placental isoforms of AP are inhibited competitively (16).

DISCUSSION

In the present investigation, Cortinarius orellanus homogenate was administered orally, which we think is the most realistic approach to experimentally study mushroom intoxication and ensures that orellanine is the only toxic principle (10). The LD_{50} of orellanin in rats appears to be 5 times that for humans and amounts to about 33 mg/kg body weight (10). The results show that the earliest alterations following orellanine refer to the luminal membrane and it later affects intracellular membrane systems of renal epithelial cells under both in vivo and in vitro conditions. The exact mechanism underlying the orellanine membrane interaction is not yet known. However, it might be assumed that it acts in a similar way to other cationic bipyridines, which once reduced to their radical form, start lipid peroxidation (15). This is supported by the finding that orellanin applied in vitro to kidney homogenate results in an enhanced formation of thiobarbituric acid reactive substances, predominantly malondialdehyde (Prast and Pfaller, unpublished observations).

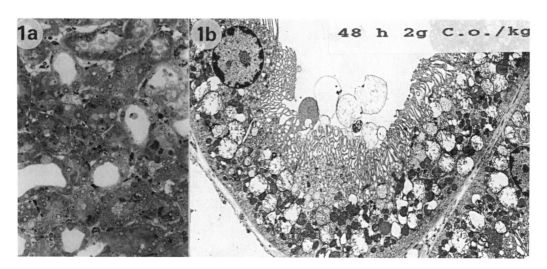

FIGURE 1. Early microscopic (a) and ultra structural (b)deformation of microvilli and enhanced vacuolization of the luminal cell pole of proximal tubular cells 48 hr after 2g orellanine.

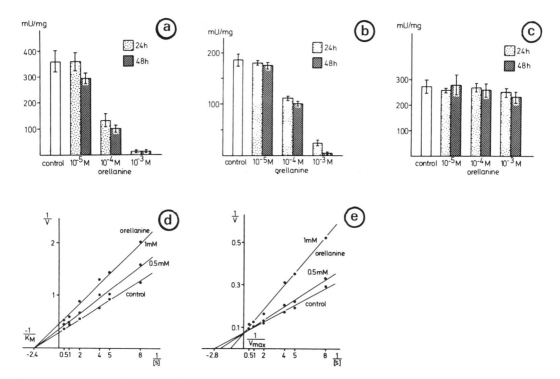

FIGURE 2. Effect of orellanine on alkaline phosphatase (a) and gamma- glutamyltranspeptidase (b) of LLC-PK$_1$ cells and alkaline phosphatase of Caco-2 cells. Noncompetitive inhibition of renal (c) and competititive inhibition of intestinal AP. Lineweaver-Burk gamma plots of alkaline phosphatase from LLC-PK$_1$ (d) and Caco-2 (e) cells.

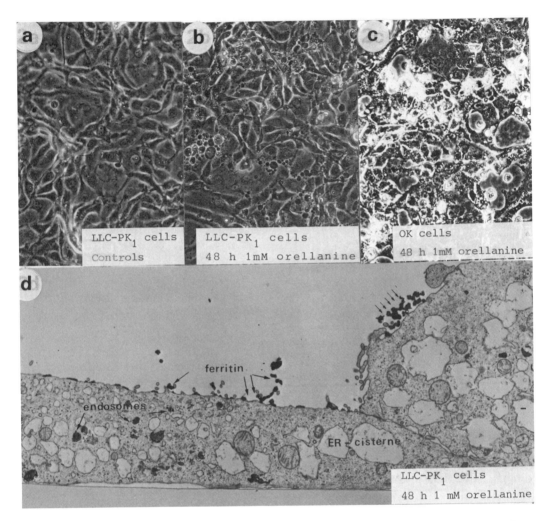

FIGURE 3. Comparison between LLC-PK$_1$ cells (a) control, (b) 1mM orellanine for 48 hr and (c) OK cells at the same concentration of orellanine as seen under phase microscopy, and the ultrastructural changes (d) in LLC-PK$_1$ cells exposed to 1mM orellanine for 48 hr

A membrane damage induced via radical chain reactions (23,24) will then lead to permeability changes of the membrane analogous to other nephrotoxins, resulting in cell injury and acute renal failure. The consequence will be an alteration of the intracellular ionic equilibrium causing disturbances in mitochondrial function and transepithelial transport. The morphologic changes within the kidney 48 hr after dosing, like mitochondrial swelling, the occurrence of mitochondrial flocculent densities, swelling of ER and disruption of mitochondrial inner membranes seem to support this hypothesis (Fig. 1). Another finding in support of peroxidative damage is the very low level of glutathione (Table 1), the kidney's major antioxidative compound

(25) which, when decreased, also may activate lipolysis (17).

Furthermore, the molecular architecture of orellanine, which is very similar to that of the herbicides paraquat and diquat, makes it likely that the compound is transported into the cell via the organic cation transporter and thereby exerts its detrimental action preferentially upon proximal tubular cell structures.

The effect of orellanine on AP is not necessarily linked to the development of cell injury, since the morphologic alterations triggered by the toxin are also found in OK cells (Fig. 2), which express no AP activity (26). The biologic relevance of AP inhibition by orellanine, and the molecular mechanism behind it, remains to be established. The fact that morphological alterations of cultured renal epithelial cells (with the exception of the increase in volume of endoplasmic reticulum) are less severe than those of cells in the kidney in vivo et situ, makes the data difficult to interpret, although high orellanine concentrations have been applied. One of the probable explanations may be the far lower transepithelial volume transport, the lower oxidative metabolism of epithelial monolayers regardless of whether or not they are grown on solid or permeable supports. The large increase in ER volume does not appear to be related to enhanced protein synthesis (27), since SDS-PAGE reveals no difference between controls and orellanine-treated tissue cultures. Whether or not ER swelling results from disturbed protein processing or osmotic effects must be clarified by studying the interaction of orellanine with transepithelial water and solute transport.

REFERENCES

1. Grzymala S: Massenvergiftungen durch den orangefuchsigen Hautkopf. Z Pilzkd 23:139-142, 1962.

2. Moser M: Gibt es neben dem orangefuchsigen Schleierling (Cortinarius orellanus) weitere giftige Schleierlinge? Z Pilzkde 39:29-34, 1969.

3. Hulmi S, Stipponen P, Forstroem J, Vilska J: Settikkisienen aheuttama vavka munaisvaurio. Duodecim (Finland) 90:1044-1050, 1974.

4. Gamper A: Untersuchungen ber die Giftstoffe der Pilze Cortinarius orellanus Fr. und Cortinarius speziocissimus Kühn & Romagn, doctoral thesis, University of Innsbruck, Austria, 1977.

5. Prast H, Pfaller W: Toxic properties of the mushroom Cortinarius orellanus (Fries). II. Impairment of renal function in rats. Arch Toxicol 62:89-96, 1988.

6. Antkowiak WZ, Gessner WP: The structures of orellanine and orelline. Tetrahedron Lett 21:1931-1934, 1979.

7. Testa E: I principi tossici del Cortinarius orellanus FR. Schweizer Z Pilkd 60:204-208, 1982.

8. Caddy BM, Kidd CBM, Robertson J, Tebbett IR, Tilstone WJ, Watling R: Cortinarius speciocissimus toxins - a preliminary report. Experientia 38:1439-1440, 1982.

9. Tebbett IR, Caddy B: Mushroom toxins of the genus Cortinarius. Experientia 40:441-446, 1984.

10. Prast H, Werner ER, Pfaller W, Moser M: Toxic properties of the mushroom Cortinarius orellanus. I. Chemical characterization of the main toxin of Cortinarius orellanus (Fries) and Cortinarius speciocissimus (Kühn & Romagn) and acute toxicity in mice. Arch Toxicol 62:81-88, 1988.

11. Grzymala S: L'isolement de l'orellanine poison du Cortinarius orellanus Fr. et l'etude de ses effects anatomapathologique. Bull Soc Myco Fr 78:394-404, 962.

12. Viallier J, Oddoux L, Palaird P, Lahneche J: Lesiones renales et hepatiques provoquees chez l'animal par ingestion de Cortinarius orellanus FR. et de quelques especes voisines. In: Les Hepatonephrites toxiques, Mason & Comp, Paris, 1968, pp. 79-84.

13. Marichal JF, Triby F, Wiederkehr JL, Carbiener R: Insuficiance renal chronique apres

intoxication par champignon de type Cortinarius orellanus Fries. Deux cas d'intoxication familiale. Nouv Presse Med (France) 6:2973-2975, 1977.

14. Flammer RG: Differentialdiagnose der Pilzvergiftungen. Gustav Fischer Verlag, Stuttgart, New York, 1980.

15. Schumacher T, Hoiland K: Mushroom poisioning caused by species of the genus Cortinarius Fries. Arch Toxicol 53:87-106, 1983.

16. Ruedl Ch, Gstraunthaler G, Moser M: Differential inhibitory action of the fungal toxin orellanine on alkaline phosphatase isoenzymes. Biochim Biophys Acta 991:280-283, 1989.

17. Pfaller W: Structure function correlation on rat kidney. Adv Anat Embryol Cell Biol 70:1-106, 1982.

18. Dehmlow EV, Schultz H: Synthesis of orellanine, the lethal poison of a toadstool. Tetrahedron lett 40:4903-4906, 1985.

19. Gstraunthaler G, Pfaller W, Kotanko P: Biochemical characterization of renal epithelial cell cultures (LLC-PK$_1$ and MDCK). Am J Physiol 248:F536-F544, 1985.

20. Gstraunthaler G, Handler JS: Isolation, growth, and characterzation of a gluconeogenic strain of renal cells. Am J Physiol 252:C232-C238, 1987.

21. Bonsdorff CH, Fuller SD, Simons K: Apical and basolateral endocytosis in Madin-Darby canine kidney (MDCK) cells grown on nitrocellulose filters. EMBO J 4:2781-2792, 1985.

22. Pfaller W, Gstraunthaler G, Loidl P: Morphology of the differentiation and maturation of LLC-PK$_1$ epithelia. J Cellular Physiol (submitted), 1989.

23. Halliwel B, Gutteridge JMC: Oxygen, free radicals and iron in relation to biology and medicine: some problems and concepts. Arch Biochem Biophys 246:501-514, 1986.

24. Pryor WA: Oxy-radicals and related species: their formation, lifetimes, and reactions. Ann Rev Physiol 48:657-667, 1986.

25. Chance B, Boveris A, Nakase Y, Sies H: Hydroperoxide Metabolism. An overview. In: Sies H, Wendel A (eds); Functions of glutathione in liver and kidney. Vol 3, Berlin, Heidelberg, New York, Springer Verlag, 1978, pp. 95-106.

26. Gstraunthaler GJA: Epithelial cells in culture. Renal Physiol Biochem 11:1-42, 1988.

PART IV
ANALGESICS AND PAPILLARY NECROSIS

12

NON-ASPIRIN NONSTEROIDAL ANTI-INFLAMMATORY DRUG USE AND CHRONIC RENAL DISEASE RISK

D. P. Sandler

Epidemiology Branch, National Institute of Environmental Health Sciences, Research Triangle Park, NC, USA

INTRODUCTION

An association between analgesic use and chronic renal disease was first noted in 1953 (1). Since that time there have been numerous reports linking phenacetin and other analgesic medications with chronic renal disease, but doubt remains about the nature of the relationship between analgesic use and renal disease risk and about the specific analgesics involved (2-4). More recently, there have been a number of reports linking use of NSAIDs to acute renal failure (5,6), and there is some suggestion that NSAIDs may increase the risk of chronic renal disease (7).

A few epidemiologic studies have evaluated chronic renal disease risk from analgesics, but these have had mixed results (3). One earlier case-control study from the USA was largely negative (8). Recent case-control studies from Germany (9) and Australia (10) have confirmed risks associated with both phenacetin and acetaminophen or with phenacetin alone, but neither presented data on NSAID use.

NSAIDs have been in use for many years, but only gained popularity in the late 1970s. Both the number of drugs and the indications for their use have increased substantially since 1971 when their effects on prostaglandin synthesis were reported (11). The present availability of these drugs in over-the-counter preparations calls for a better understanding of the benefits and risks of their use.

Regular heavy use of analgesics is reported to be common in the Southeastern USA, where analgesic abuse has been suggested as a cause of at least 10% of end stage renal disease (12). For the most part, this has been thought to be due to the widespread use of headache powders that once contained phenacetin, aspirin, and caffeine. These powders have now been replaced by mixtures containing acetaminophen, aspirin, and caffeine, without any apparent decrease in their popularity. Powders are available in vending machines, at checkout counters in many stores, and on coffee break carts at a number of local factories, and a social environment which encourages heavy use of analgesics has developed in some subgroups of the population. The increasing availability of NSAIDs, and the general impression that these offer more potent pain relief than other over-the-counter remedies may lead to inappropriate use of these drugs as well.

Because heavy analgesic use appears to be a regional problem, we evaluated the risk associated with regular use of analgesics, including NSAIDs, in a case-control study of risk factors for chronic renal disease in North Carolina.

METHODS

Cases were North Carolina residents hospitalized between September 1, 1980 and August 31, 1982 at one of four medical centers with a first diagnosis of chronic renal disease. Patients between 30 and 79 years, who had a renal problem mentioned somewhere on their discharge summary and had a sustained elevation in serum creatinine ≥ 1.5 mg/dl (130 μmol) that was not due to other causes were eligible for inclusion. Cases were excluded if they had certain hereditary or systemic conditions with known renal manifestations, but patients with hypertension and diabetes were not excluded.

The charts of over 4000 patients were reviewed to identify approximately 700 qualifying patients with newly diagnosed disease. Cases ranged in severity from minor renal insufficiency to end stage disease at diagnosis. Only 7% of patients had a biopsy, but using available clinical data, patients were classified by 3 nephrologists according to probable renal disease subtype. Approximately 28% of patients could not be classified beyond renal insufficiency or ESRD. 19% were classified as having hypertensive nephrosclerosis, 20% had diabetic nephropathy, 14% had glomerulonephritis, and 19% had interstitial nephritis.

Controls under age 65 were chosen by random telephone screening in North Carolina. We selected 360 potential controls who were local residents and were frequency matched to cases on age, race, sex and whether or not they lived near study hospitals. Because random telephone screening is not efficient for identifying older persons, 357 potential controls for cases older than 65 were chosen randomly from listings of Medicare recipients and were frequency matched in the same way.

About 15% of eligible cases and controls were lost, but we obtained telephone interviews for 90% of the cases and about 85% of the controls we located. About 1/2 (54.5%) of our case interviews and 10% of the control interviews were with proxy respondents. In all, we obtained data for 554 cases and 516 controls.

The interviewed cases and controls were similar on the study matching factors, but renal disease patients were less well educated and had lower incomes.

We obtained information about analgesic use in several ways. We first asked about specific symptoms and conditions such as arthritis or headaches for which analgesics may have been taken. We also asked about nonspecific reasons for analgesic use that are thought to be common among analgesic abusers, such as not feeling well other than because of a specific illness.

We then obtained detailed information about use of specific over-the-counter and prescription drugs. These drugs were classified as NSAIDs or other pain relievers. These other drugs were further classified as either single active ingredient agents - aspirin or acetaminophen (paracetamol) or as combination drugs - either combinations of phenacetin and aspirin, or other combinations.

For each drug, we considered subjects to have been daily users if they took an individual drug every day for at least 360 consecutive days. Weekly users were those who reported taking a pain reliever at least once a week for as long as a year.

Odds ratios (OR) and 95% confidence intervals (CI) were used to estimate the relative risk associated with weekly or daily analgesic use as compared to infrequent or never use of a particular analgesic. Adjusted odds ratios were calculated using Mantel Haenszel estimation and logistic regression. An odds ratio greater than one indicates an increased risk of renal disease associated with that drug.

Further details of study methods and results concerning use of phenacetin, aspirin, and acetaminophen have been published elsewhere (13).

RESULTS

Cases were significantly more likely than controls to be regular analgesic users, with odds ratios for weekly and daily use of any analgesic - excluding NSAIDs - of 1.5 (95% CI = 1.1-2.1) and 2.8 (1.9-4.2) after taking into account matching factors and other differences between cases and controls.

For individual analgesics, weekly and daily users of acetaminophen or phenacetin combinations appeared to be at increased risk of renal disease. After taking into account a number of potential differences between cases and controls, as well as the use of the other two analgesics, there appeared to be a 3-fold risk associated with daily use of acetaminophen (OR = 3.2, 95% CI = 1.1-9.8) and a 5-fold risk associated with daily phenacetin use (OR = 5.1, 95% CI = 1.8-14.9). After the same adjustments, there was little risk associated with daily aspirin use (OR = 1.3, 95% CI = 0.7-2.5).

These results were not changed by taking into account diabetes or hypertension or by taking into account indications for analgesic use such as headaches, backaches, or just not feeling well. Results were also not due to biased reporting by the relatives of subjects who were deceased or too ill to participate by themselves. Results were the same when we restricted our analysis to cases and controls who reported directly.

The data on phenacetin and acetaminophen seemed to suggest an overall risk that was not limited to one particular subgroup of patients. The data on NSAID use were somewhat different.

Overall, cases were twice as likely as controls to report daily use of NSAIDs, after taking into account both matching factors and potential confounding factors (Table 1). However, when we stratified by sex, it became apparent that risk was limited to men, among whom the risk was nearly 5-fold for daily users compared with never users (OR =4.6, 95% CI = 1.5-14.0). Stratifying even further, it was clear that only men over the age of 65 were at risk. The odds ratio of 16.6 associated with NSAID use in this group was statistically significant, although it was based on small numbers. This markedly increased risk for older men was not due to biased reporting by next-of-kin: the odds ratio was just about the same (OR = 18.9) when we adjusted for the source of the questionnaire data.

As with phenacetin and acetaminophen, results were not altered by adjusting for hypertension, diabetes, or symptoms for which NSAIDs might have been taken. Risks were also not altered by taking into account smoking, occupational exposures, or the use of phenacetin or acetaminophen.

While adjusting for other underlying conditions such as heart disease, ulcer, regular alcohol consumption, and diuretic use had little

Table 1. Chronic Renal Disease Risk Associated with Daily NSAID Use.

Sex and Age Group	Daily/Never Users		OR$^+$	(95% CI)
	Cases	Controls		
All Subjects	28/475	13/464	2.1	(1.1-4.1)
Men	17/265	4/267	4.6	(1.5-14.0)
<65 years	3/137	3/135	0.9	(0.2-4.6)
>65 years	14/128	1/132	16.6	(2.1-129)
Women	11/210	9/197	1.1	(0.4-2.7)
<65 years	5/106	5/100	0.9	(0.3-6.9)
>65 years	6/104	4/97	1.3	(0.4-4.9)

+ Adjusted for matching factors and income.

affect on the overall risk estimates, the NSAID-associated risk was greater among those with these conditions. This was especially true for younger men and for women, among whom there was no risk associated with NSAID use unless one of the other conditions was present.

Risk associated with NSAID use varied with probable disease subtype. The odds ratio was statistically significant only for interstitial nephritis (Table 2). When we limited the analysis to men, the confidence intervals were quite broad for all subgroups, but even so, the risk of interstitial nephritis was significantly increased (OR = 13.0, 95% CI = 3.4-50.8).

The numbers are even smaller for use of individual NSAIDs. Even so, chronic renal disease risk appeared to be elevated for daily users of ibuprofen (OR = 3.6, 95% CI = 1.2-11.0) and indomethacin (OR = 1.6, 95% CI = 0.6-4.2) - the more commonly used NSAIDs for this population. As in all comparisons, odds ratios were greater when the analysis was restricted to men. The odds ratio associated with ibuprofen was infinitely large (9 daily users among cases, but 0 among controls), and that for indomethacin was 3.7.

COMMENT

Our results confirm that daily use of analgesic mixtures containing phenacetin increases the risk of developing chronic renal disease, and suggest a similar risk for acetaminophen, which has replaced phenacetin in many popular over-the-counter analgesic mixtures. Since acetaminophen is the major metabolite of phenacetin, this is not an entirely unexpected finding. Because of this and the increasing use of acetaminophen, our observation of increased renal disease risk in acetaminophen users deserves more study.

Our data also suggest a risk of chronic renal disease associated with regular use of NSAIDs - at least for men or for other high risk groups. The NSAID findings are consistent with case-reports and with animal studies (5-7,14,15). The greater risk for interstitial nephritis is con-

Table 2. Daily NSAID Use and Risk of Specific Renal Diseases.

Diagnosis	OR[+]	(95% CI)
Hypertensive nephrosclerosis	1.8	(0.6-6.0)
Diabetic nephropathy	1.6	(0.5-4.8)
Glomerulonephritis	1.8	(0.5-6.6)
Interstitial nephritis	3.9	(1.6-9.7)
End-stage disease	1.5	(0.2-12.6)
Renal insufficiency	2.5	(0.9-6.9)

[+] Odds ratio, adjusted for matching factors and income.

sistent with several proposed mechanisms for renal injury from NSAIDs (16-18).

Our study is not alone in finding that certain subgroups - including older persons with age-related renal and vascular changes or those with certain conditions that indicate underlying renal impairment or poor renal circulation - are most at risk for renal damage due to NSAIDs use (18-20). We could find no easy explanation in our data for the difference between older men and older women, but it is possible that the men included in this study had a greater degree of unreported cardiovascular disease.

Although we included more than 500 renal disease patients in our study, we were hampered by small numbers for many specific comparisons. This was especially true for NSAIDs which were only available by prescription during the time-period of our study. Now that some of these drugs are available over-the-counter, and as experience with NSAID use accumulates, it will be possible and prudent to re-evaluate the potential for NSAID-induced chronic renal disease.

REFERENCES

1. Spuhler O, Zollinger HU. Die chronisch-interstitielle nephritis. Z Klin Med 151:1-50, 1953.

2. Prescott LF. Analgesic nephropathy: a reassessment of the role of phenacetin and other analgesics. Drugs 23:75-149, 1982.

3. Buckalew VM, Schey HM. Renal disease from habitual antipyretic analgesic consumption: an assessment of the epidemiologic evidence. Medicine 11:291-303, 1986.

4. Lanes SF, Delzell E, Dreyer NA, Rothman KJ. Analgesics and kidney disease. Int J Epidemiol 15:454-5, 1986.

5. Brandstetter RD, Mar DD: Reversible oliguric renal failure associated with ibuprofen treatment. Br Med J 2:1194-5, 1978.

6. Kimberly RP, Bowden RE, Keiser HR, Plotz PH: Reduction of renal function by newer nonsteroidal anti-inflammatory drugs. Am J Med 64:804-7, 1978.

7. Adams DH, Howie AJ, Michael J, McConkey B, Bacon PA, Abu D: Nonsteroidal anti-inflammatory drugs and renal failure. Lancet 1:57-59, 1986.

8. Murray TG, Stolley PD, Anthony JC, Schinnar R, Hepler-Smith E, Jeffreys JL. Epidemiologic study of regular analgesic use and end-stage renal disease. Arch Intern Med 143:1687-93, 1983.

9. Pommer W, Bronder E, Klimpel A, Molzahn M, Helmert U, Greiser E. Regular intake of analgesic mixtures and risk of end-stage renal failure. Lancet 1:381, 1989.

10. McCredie M, Stewart JH. Does paracetamol cause urothelial cancer or renal papillary necrosis? Nephron 49:296-300, 1988.

11. Vane JR: Inhibition of prostaglandin synthesis as a mechanism of action for aspirin-like drugs. Nature 231:232-5, 1971.

12. Gonwa TA, Hamilton RW, Buckalew VM: Chronic renal failure and end-stage renal disease in northwest North Carolina: the importance of analgesic associated nephropathy. Arch Intern Med 141:462-5, 1981.

13. Sandler DP, Smith JC, Weinberg CR, Buckalew VM, Dennis VW, Blythe WB, Burgess WP: Analgesic use and chronic renal disease. N Engl J Med 320:1238-43, 1989.

14. Wiseman EH, Reinert H: Anti-inflammatory drugs and renal papillary necrosis. Agents and Actions 5:322-5, 1975.

15. Nanra RS, Stuart-Taylor J, de Leon AH, White KH: Analgesic nephropathy: etiology, clinical syndrome, and clinico-pathologic correlations in Australia. Kidney Int 13:79-92, 1978.

16. Clive DM, Stoff JS: Renal syndromes associated with nonsteroidal antiinflammatory drugs. N Engl J Med 310:563-72, 1984.

17. Bender WL, Whelton A, Beschorner WE, Darwish MO, Hall-Craggs M, Solez K: Interstitial nephritis, proteinuria and renal failure caused by nonsteroidal anti-inflammatory drugs: Immunologic characterization of the inflammatory infiltrate. Amer J Med 76:1006-12, 1984.

18. Orme M L'E: Non-steroidal anti-inflammatory drugs and the kidney. Br Med J 292:1621-2, 1986.

19. Kincaid-Smith P: Renal toxicity of non-narcotic analgesics: At-risk patients and prescribing applications. Med Toxicol 1 (suppl 1): 14-22, 1986.

20. Blackshear JL, Davidman M, Stillman M: Identification of risk for renal insufficiency from nonsteroidal anti-inflammatory drugs. Arch Intern Med 143:1130-1134, 1983.

13

STRAIN DIFFERENCES IN MICE IN THEIR RESPONSE TO BROMOETHANAMINE

J.A. Scarlett, N.J. Gregg, S. Nichol and P.H. Bach

Nephrotoxicity Research Group, The Robens Institute, University of Surrey, Guildford, Surrey, GU2 5XH, UK

INTRODUCTION

One use of animals in nephrotoxicity studies is to develop reproducible models of the clinical situation in man. The use of genetically identical (inbred) animals in toxicology has been strongly advocated as a means of minimising the experimental variance attributed to the animals used (1). The exploitation of strains which are sensitive or resistant to particular drugs or chemicals may offer valuable information about the mechanism of toxicity which could be relevant to man (2).

C57Bl/6 mice have been reported to metabolise phenacetin via a similar pathway as in man, and are also prone to developing renal papillary necrosis (RPN) after dosing with phenacetin (3). An investigation into whether this mouse strain was sensitive to the papillo toxin, 2-bromoethanamine (BEA), was undertaken to determine if it would be a suitable animal model for studies into the pathogenetic mechanism of analgesic nephropathy. Obese mice (ob/ob) are a random bred mouse strain derived from C57Bl/6 mice which have the genetic potential to become obese, and they may also develop diabetes (4). Diabetics are prone to developing a number of nephropathies (including RPN). It was of interest to use the ob/ob strain to see whether they were more sensitive to BEA and whether there was any difference in sensitivity between the random outbred strain (ob/ob) and the inbred parent strain (C57Bl/6).

MATERIALS AND METHODS

Male Obese mice (University of Surrey strain) body weight: 30 ± 8 g; male Balb/c mice (Bantam and Kingman Ltd, Hull, E.Yorkshire, U.K.) body weight 20 ± 1.25 g and male C567Bl/6 mice (Bantam and Kingman Ltd.): body weight 22 ± 2 g were housed (10-12 animals per cage) in translucent shoe box type cages on sterile soft wood shavings in a controlled environment. Food and water was available ad libitum. One group was dosed with BEA 100 mg/kg i.p., (0.1 ml per 10 g body of a 10 mg/ml (w/v) solution in physiological saline and the controls received physiological saline only. Animals (n = 3) were housed in metal metabolism cages to allow the collection of urine after dosing for the 3, 6 and 12 hr groups, and 12 hr prior to sacrifice for the 24 and 48 hr groups. Water was available ad libitum, but no food was present. In individual animals any urine present in the bladder was aspirated using a 23g needle and placed in a microcentrifugation tube. Groups of animals (n=3) from treated and control groups were sacrificed by anaesthesia in diethyl ether, then cervical dislocation at 3, 6, 12, 24, 48 hr and 7, 14 and 21 days post BEA administration. Animals were weighed at sacrifice and kidney weight was recorded. Tissues were fixed in formal calcium at 4°C and embedded in glycol-methacrylate resin. Semithin (2 μm) sections were stained with H&E, Giemsa, PAS and enzyme histochemistry performed for acid (ACP) and alkaline phosphatase (ALP) and gamma-glutamyltranspeptidase (GGT) (5).

Urine samples: Individual urine samples were obtained at post mortem and immediately analysed for osmolality. Any urine remaining was placed in a microcentrifuge tube and stored at 4°C for urinary urea nitrogen determination at a later time. Pooled urine samples were stored at 4°C for the later determination of osmolality and urea nitrogen. Blood samples: These were centrifuged at 5,000 rpm for 3-4 minutes and serum stored at 4°C. Osmolality: the osmolality of both urine and serum samples (in mmol/kg) was analysed using a Wescor Inc. 5100C Vapour Pressure osmometer using standards from 290-1000 mmol/kg. Urea nitrogen: the urea nitrogen in urine (diluted 100-fold) and serum was determined using a blood urea nitrogen kit No. 535 (Sigma Diagnostics, Poole, Dorset, U.K.).

RESULTS

Functional results: The pooled urine results did not produce consistent results for osmolality, and the Balb/c strain did not produce sufficient urine to collect and analyse at any timepoint. It was for these reasons that the individual samples collected direct from the

bladder were used to produce mean values for each timepoint.

Mean control values for urine and serum osmolality, urea nitrogen and urine serum ratios are shown in Table 1.

Table 2 shows the mean control kidney weight/body weight ratio values for each strain.

Balb/c mice had a higher mean control kidney/body weight ratio value (0.0177 ± 0.0004), than either Obese (0.0158 ± 0.0008) or C57Bl/6 (0.0148 ± 0.0004) mice, n = 15 for all strains.

Histopathological results

Controls: There were no differences in morphology or histochemistry in any of the strains. In all the strains the proximal tubule segments in the outer cortex (predominantly P_1 and P_2) stained preferentially for ALP where as the P_3 segment stained most intensely for GGT. 3 hr: The initial changes in all strains were pyknotic interstitial cell nuclei (Figure 1) in the upper papilla region and areas of intensely staining interstitial cell matrix in the papilla with PAS and Giemsa. C57Bl/6 mice also had hydropic cyto-

Table 1. Mean Urine and Serum Control values for Urea Nitrogen and Osmolality

Strain	Urea Nitrogen			Osmolality		
	Urine (U) (mmol/kg)	Serum (S) (mg/dl)	U/S ratio	Urine (mmol/kg)	Serum (mg/dl)	U/S ratio
	Urine samples from metabolic cages			Urine samples direct from bladder		
Obese						
M	1496	18.28	81.84	1234	317.29	3.89
SD	675	6.39		397	87.0	
n	5	14		10	14	
Balb/c						
M				1304	295	4.42
SD	ND	ND	ND	387	82	
n				3	14	
C57Bl/6						
M	1069	16.92	63.18	991	292	3.39
SD	491	5.98		249	82	
n	9	15		8	15	

M = mean value, SD = standard deviation, n = number samples, ND = no data.

Table 2. Mean Control values of Kidney/Body Weight ratio

Strain	KW/BW ratio (g/kg)	SD	SE (x10-4)	95% cf (x10-4)	limits
Balb/c	0.0177	0.0004	1.03	±2.018	0.0179 - 0.0175
Obese	0.0158	0.0008	2.065	±4.047	0.0162 - 0.0154
C57Bl/6	0.0148	0.0004	1.03	±2.018	0.0150 - 0.0146

KW/BW ratio - kidney weight/body weight ratio, SD - standard deviation. SE - standard error, 95% cf - 95 % confidence limits. n = 15 for all groups.

plasmic changes in the S3 segment with some brush border disruption.

6 hr: All strains had adherent platelets and erythrocytes in the capillaries in the papilla (Figure 2). There was an increase in the number of pyknotic interstitial cell nuclei in Obese mice (upper papilla region) and C57BL/6 mice (papilla tip). Obese and C57Bl/6 mice had collecting duct cells which contained PAS positive staining granules within the cytoplasm. C57Bl/6 mice also had casts in the loop of Henle and intensely eosinophilic staining granules/droplets in the cytoplasm of the loop of Henle, collecting duct and proximal tubule. Some S3 segments had lost ALP brush border staining.

12 hr: Obese mice had enlarged vacuolated covering epithelium and pelvic epithelium cells in the fornices. All tubular lumen in the papilla were dilated with occasional ALP staining casts in the loop of Henle. Cortical changes were evident too, with PAS positive staining casts in the collecting duct. BALB/c mice had an increasing number of enlarged collecting duct cells with decreased interstitial cell matrix staining in the mid-papilla region. C57Bl/6 mice had enlarged collecting duct cells in papilla with more basophilic cytoplasmic granules (Figure 3), which were also PAS positive, cortical collecting duct cells were exfoliating into the lumen. PT brush border disruption and blebbing into the lumen was observed together with loss of ALP staining in both Obese and C57Bl/6 mice (S2 segment).

24 hr: Obese and C57Bl/6 mice showed the following changes; prominent interstitial cell

matrix staining in at the papilla tip, an influx of poly morphonuclear leucocytes in capillaries and interstitial cell matrix of papilla, covering epithelium cells in fornices were swollen and blebbing containing basophilic cytoplasmic granules (Figure 4) which were also PAS positive (C57Bl/6 Obese). Basophilic staining casts with exfoliated cells were seen in the loop of Henle and collecting duct in all regions of the kidney. BALB/c mice had a total loss of interstitial cell matrix staining in the upper papilla but the collecting duct and loop of Henle were still intact with no necrosis evident. A few basophilic casts present in the cortical collecting duct and occassional ALP staining casts in the papilla.

48 hr: C57Bl/6 mice had dilated tubular lumen in the papilla with many collecting duct cells containing PAS positive staining cytoplasmic granules, increased interstitial cell matrix staining at papilla tip, mild hyperplasia (2-3 cells thick) of the pelvic epithelium in the fornices with lobulated basophilic staining nuclei. Balb/c mice had pyknotic nuclei in the loops of Henle and collecting duct in upper papilla, enlarged basophilic interstitial cell nuclei adjacent to the vasa rectae, PAS positive staining casts in the cortical collecting duct. There was no noticeable progression in intensity of lesion at 48 hr in the Obese mice.

7 days: Obese mice had necrotic collecting ducts and loops of Henle with exfoliating cells, some proximal tubules which had basophilic staining nuclei and cytoplasm in a radiating pattern. Some glomeruli and Bowman's capsules had thickened basement membranes

and sclerosis particularly the juxtamedullary glomeruli. C57Bl/6 mice had intact collecting ducts and loops of Henle in the papilla, but the overall appearance of the lesion was worse with the changes described previously being more intense: many casts were seen throughout the kidney and more adherent platelets, accompanied by variable ALP and PAS staining of the proximal tubule brush border and displacement of collecting duct nuclei to luminal surface of cells.

14 days: C57Bl/6 mice had ALP staining casts in the papilla, in the cortex there were some proximal tubule segments which had flattened epithelial cells with basophilic staining cytoplasm. In Obese mice at 14 days there was no noticeable difference in the appearance of kidneys from BEA treated animals from the kidneys from control animals. Balb/c did not show any differences from control kidneys.

21 days: the C57Bl/6 mice had multiple casts within the papilla (Figure 5), but no gross total necrosis of the loop of Henle, collecting duct or covering epithelium usually found in the Wistar rat. There was focal interstitial nephritis with aggregates of monocytic leucocytes and basophilic staining atrophying tubules adjacent to juxtamedullary glomeruli (Figure 6), very prominent basement membrane staining (with PAS). Balb/c mice showed no gross necrosis in the papilla but prominent PAS staining casts were present in the vasae rectae vessels which also had thickened basement membranes, and some focal interstitial nephritis in the cortex but not to the same degree as C57Bl/6 mice. No slides from Obese animals were available for examination at the 21 day timepoint.

DISCUSSION

None of the mouse strains developed RPN to the same degree as in the W/A rat (6). However, based on the histopathological changes and failure to regain total concentrating capacity (up to 7 days after BEA treatment), the C57Bl/6 mice are more sensitive than Obese or Balb/c mice. Order of sensitivity: C57Bl/6 > Obese > Balb/c. Mice may have differing extrarenal or renal metabolism which could affect the re-

sponse of the mouse to BEA. The favoured hypothesis of BEA-induced RPN is via a prostaglandin hydroperoxidase mediated peroxidation within the interstitial cells (7,8). Differences in the medullary interstitial cells and the prostaglandin metabolism pathways between the mouse and rat may explain the differences observed. Functional changes may also explain why BEA fails to induce a frank RPN lesion in mice. C57Bl/6 mice had the lowest mean control urine osmolality value of all the strains. Their increased sensitivity to BEA would seem to provide evidence that the concentration of toxins in the papilla is not the primary mechanism for the initiation of RPN pathogenesis. This is in contrast to the findings of Sabatini et al, (1981), (9), who found that concentrating capacity was essential to produce BEA toxicity. One would of have expected the Balb/c mice to be more sensitive to BEA since this strain had the highest osmolality and produced very little urine. This provides additional evidence that differences in the metabolism of rats and mice is a likely explanation for the observed difference or other factors may be involved.

C57Bl/6 mice had the lowest kidney weight/body weight ratio value in control animals (Table 2). As dose is administered based on body weight, the C57Bl/6 received a larger renal dose relative to their body weight than did the Balb/c or Obese mice (see Table 3).

From Table 3 one can see that the order of renal dose received is C57Bl/6 > Obese >

Table 3. Renal dose* for each strain calculated for 100 mg/kg BW in a mouse of body weight 20 g

Strain	KW/BW ratio (g/kg)	KW (g)	Renal dose (mg/g)	Adjusted dose (mg/kg)
Balb/c	0.0177	0.354	282.48	100
Obese	0.0158	0.316	316.45	89
C57Bl/6	0.0148	0.296	337.83	83

Renal dose - dose of compound affecting kidney assuming 100% dose reaches kidney, **KW/BW** - kidney weight/body weight ratio. **Adjusted dose** - dose required administered as a mg/kg BW dose to give equal renal dose.

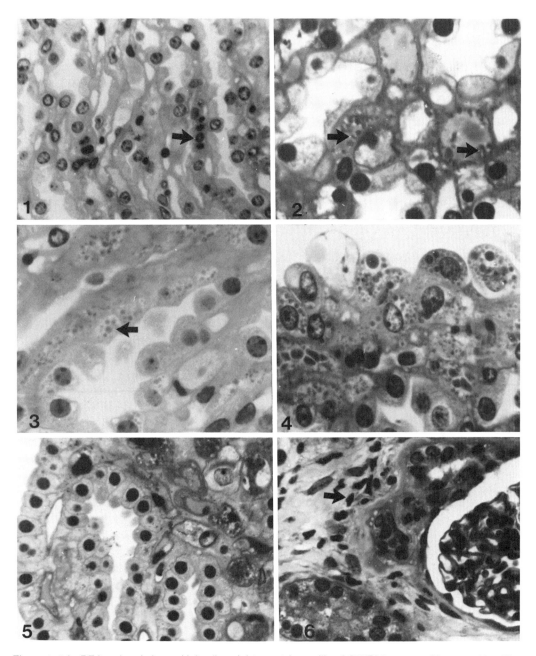

Figure 1. 3 hr BEA: pyknotic interstitial cell nuclei (arrow) in papilla of C57Bl/6 mouse, Giemsa x 430. Figure 2. 6 hr BEA: adherent platelets in capillaries in Obese mouse, Giemsa x 690. Figure 3. 12 hr BEA: enlarged collecting duct epithelial cells containing basophilic cytoplasmic granules (arrow). C57Bl/6 mouse, Giemsa x 690. Figure 4. 24 hr BEA: hyperplastic, blebbing covering epithelial cells with vacuoles and basophilic cytoplasmic granules. C57Bl/6 mouse, Giemsa x 690. Figure 5. 21 days BEA: casts and numerous platelets in capillaries and intact covering and collecting duct epithelia. C57Bl/6 mouse, Giemsa x 430. Figure 6. 21 days BEA: thickened basement membranes and atrophying tubules in focal interstitial nephritis. C57Bl/6 mouse, Giemsa x 430.

Balb/c, which is also the order of sensitivity to BEA. Thus, the effective renal dose may be a critical factor in strain sensitivity coupled with metabolic differences which account for the order of strain sensitivity observed.

In strain comparison experiments one may want to use historical control data for organ/body weight ratios to ensure that each strain receives the same effective organ dose (mg/g). This effective organ dose parameter assumes that 100% of administered dose reaches the target organ.

ACKNOWLEDGEMENTS

This work was supported in part by The Cancer Research Campaign, and a M.A.F.F. Research Fellowship for J.A.S..

REFERENCES

1. Festing, MFW: Inbred Strains in Biomedical Research. Macmillan Press, London, 1979.

2. Festing, MFW: The "Defined" Animal and the reduction of Animal Use. In: Sperlinger, D. (ed) Animals in Research: New perspectives in animal experimentation. John Wiley & Sons, Chichester, 1981.

3. Macklin, AW, Szot, RJ: Eighteen Month Oral Study of Aspirin, Phenacetin and Caffeine in C57Bl/6 mice. Drug Chem. Toxicol. 3: 135-163, 1980.

4. Flatt, PR, Bailey, CJ: Abnormal Plasma Glucose and Insulin Responses in Heterozygous Lean (ob/+) Mice. Diabetologia. 20: 573-577, 1981. 5. Bancroft, JB, Stevens, A: Theory and Practice of Histochemical Technique. 2nd Edition, Churchill Livingstone, 1982.

6. Gregg, NJ, Courtauld, EA, Bach, PH: High resolution microscopic changes in an acutely induced renal papillary necrosis: morphology and enzyme histo chemistry. In: Bach, P.H. and Lock, E.A. (eds) Nephrotoxicity: In vitro to In vivo, Animals to Man. Plenum Press, New York, 1989.

7. Bach, PH, Bridges, JW: The role of prostaglandin synthase mediated metabolic activation of analgesics and non-steroidal anti-inflammatory drugs in the development of renal papillary necrosis and upper urothelial carcinoma. Prost. Leuk. Med. 15: 251-274.

8. Bach, PH, Bridges, JW: Chemically induced renal papillary necrosis and upper urothelial carcinoma. CRC Crit. Rev. Toxicol. 15: 217-439.

9. Sabatini, S, Mehta, PK, Haye, S, Kurtzman, NA, Arruda, JAL: Drug-induced Papillary Necrosis: Electrolyte excretion and nephron heterogeneity. Am. J. Physiol. 241: F14-F22.

14
COCAINE NEPHROTOXICITY IN RATS

M.L. Kauker (1), P.J. Gisi (2), and E.T. Zawada (3)

Department of Physiology and Pharmacology (1,2) and Department of Internal Medicine (3), University of South Dakota School of Medicine, Vermillion, SD 57069, U.S.A.

INTRODUCTION

Consumption of large amounts of cocaine and its free base "crack" has contributed to the increased number of cocaine-related hospital admissions and deaths in recent years (1). The primary target organs for cocaine intoxication are the CNS and the cardiovascular system. The drug may produce stroke, myocardial infarction, pulmonary oedema, and death (1,2). Cocaine may also cause serious impairment of kidney function. In several recent reports (1,4-8) nontraumatic rhabdomyolysis has been associated with cocaine abuse. Rhabdomyolysis with myoglobinuria has long been recognized (3) as a cause of acute renal failure (ARF). In these clinical case studies, acute renal failure occurred in nearly 30% of the cases with a 45% mortality rate (1). These observations clearly identify the kidneys as important target organs of cocaine intoxication. Renal tubular necrosis in cocaine-induced rhabdomyolysis is usually considered to be secondary to myoglobinuria and hypotension (1,4,8). However, a direct toxic effect of cocaine on the kidney could not be excluded in these human case studies (1,8).

The renal vasculature and tubules receive a rich sympathetic innervation. Cocaine is known to inhibit the re-uptake of norepinephrine and cause a potentiation of the sympathetic nervous system. Enhanced renal sympathetic tone during cocaine intoxication may predispose the kidneys to myoglobin-induced renal failure by lowering renal blood flow (RBF) and glomerular filtration rate (GFR) and by inducing anoxic tubular necrosis (4). The direct toxic effects of cocaine on renal tubular and vascular functions have not been evaluated. Therefore, the present experiments were designed to examine the effects of an acute high dose of cocaine infused directly into the left renal artery on glomerular and tubular functions in rats under controlled experimental conditions. The results indicate that cocaine is capable of markedly lowering GFR and inhibiting tubular reabsorption of filtrate. This renal impairment may predispose the kidney to ARF which may be induced by cocaine through its effects on other organ systems such as the skeletal muscle (rhabdomyolysis) and the cardiovascular system (lowered BP, intravascular coagulation, myocardial failure, etc.)

METHODS

Experiments were performed in 13 adult male Sprague-Dawley rats with an average body weight of 336 ± 12 g. The animals had free access to food and water prior to the acute experiment. On the day of the experiment, the rats were anesthetized with an i.p. injection of a freshly prepared solution of Inactin, (100 mg/kg) and placed on a thermostatically controlled heated animal board to maintain body temperature between 36-37°C. The animals were then surgically prepared for renal clearance studies as described previously (9). Cannulae were placed in the trachea to maintain an open airway, into the right external jugular vein for fluid infusions, into the right common carotid artery for blood pressure recordings and periodic blood sampling, into the left renal artery (R.A.) for cocaine infusion, and into the left ureter for quantitative urine collections. Surgical areas were covered with Parafilm, to reduce evaporative fluid losses. The rats were maintained in saline diuresis by a continuous i.v. infusion of 0.89% NaCl at a rate of 4-6 ml/hr depending on the weight of the rat. ^{3}H-Inulin was also infused continuously at a rate of 100 μCi/hr after an appropriate priming dose to allow assessment of the glomerular filtration rate (GFR). After an equilibration period of 45-60 min, 2-3 control clearance periods of 30 min duration each were observed. During this time, an isotonic saline solution containing heparin was infused into the left R.A. Cocaine was then infused into the R.A. at an adjusted rate of 5-10 mg/kg (mean = 8.2 mg/kg). The dose of cocaine was adjusted to prevent generalized systemic hemodynamic effects. Experimental clearance periods began 20-40 min after the start of the cocaine infusion. In addition to the 13 rats that received cocaine infusion into the R.A., 3 rats were given only a continuous infusion of vehicle throughout the experiment. These animals served as time-controls. During each clearance period the following procedures were performed: collection of timed urine sample, collection of a small (200 μl) carotid blood sample, and recording of blood pressure, heart rate and body temperature as in our previous studies (10). All blood and urine samples were analyzed for ^{3}H-inulin activity using a liquid scintillation spectrometer and for sodium concentration using an ion analyzer. Urine volume was determined gravimetrically. Data were calculated using standard renal clearance formulas (9). Results are expressed as mean ± S.E. Statistical significance of the difference between two mean values was evaluated using the paired and unpaired Student's t-test and one way analysis of variance, as appropriate. A P-value of 0.05 was considered significant.

RESULTS

Mean blood pressure (BP) was not significantly altered by the infusion of cocaine into the R.A. Mean BP was 122 ± 4 mmHg during control periods and 118 ± 5 mmHg during cocaine infusion. Heart rate (HR) was also unchanged by cocaine. The lack of a cocaine effect on

systemic haemodynamic functions can be explained by the experimental design as the drug infusion into the R.A. was stopped at the first sign of changes in BP or HR. Such a design allowed the examination of the direct toxic effects of the drug on the kidney independent of its indirect renal effects mediated by systemic haemodynamic changes.

Glomerular filtration rate was markedly reduced in each rat but the magnitude of this effect varied markedly from one animal to another (Fig. 1). Mean GFR decreased from 951 ± 96 to 190 ± 80 μl.min^{-1}.kidney^{-1} (P) after cocaine administration indicating a marked renal hemodynamic response to the drug. The effects of the drug on urine flow and the percentage water excretion are shown in Fig. 2.

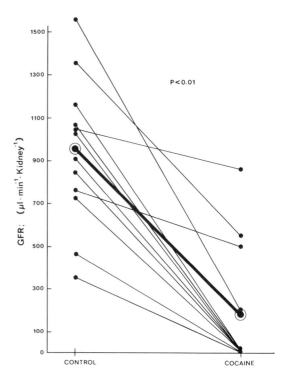

Figure 1. Effect of intrarenal cocaine administration on glomerular filtration rate (GFR) in rats as measured by inulin clearance. GFR declined in each animal. Dark line connects the mean values.

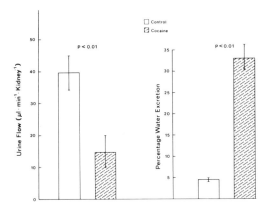

Figure 2. Mean urine flow and percentage of filtered water excreted in the urine during control
and cocaine infusion clearance periods.

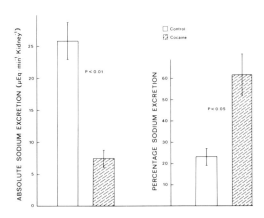

Figure 3. Effect of intrarenal cocaine infusion on
absolute and fractional sodium excretion. Data are
presented as mean + S.E.

Urine flow decreased significantly during cocaine infusion while the percentage of the
filtered water that appeared in the urine increased greatly suggesting that tubular
reabsorption was also inhibited by the drug.
The renal handling of sodium was also significantly altered by cocaine (Fig. 3). Absolute
sodium excretion was reduced while fractional
sodium excretion was increased in the
presence of the drug.

Tubular reabsorption of both sodium and
water were significantly inhibited by cocaine
whether the values are expressed as percentage of the amount filtered or as absolute
quantities (Table 1).

In the three vehicle-treated rats (data are not
presented), control values were similar to those
observed in the cocaine-treated rats during
control periods. None of the recorded parameters changed significantly during continued
vehicle infusion in these rats indicating that time
related changes did not influence the cocaine-
induced alterations in kidney function.

In summary, during control periods the rat
nephrons collectively filtered 951 µl/min. The
tubules reabsorbed 95.1% of this filtrate and
only 4.9% appeared in the urine (Fig. 4). During
cocaine administration, filtration decreased to

190 µl/min. Tubular reabsorption removed only
67.3% of the filtered water and a much greater
fraction of the filtrate (32.7%) appeared in the
urine (Fig. 4).

DISCUSSION

The observed marked reduction in GFR and
tubular reabsorption of filtrate after cocaine
treatment in the absence of systemic haemodynamic changes indicate that cocaine is capable
of exerting a direct renal effect. Reduced GFR
in these rats was most likely due to afferent
arteriolar constriction as a consequence of cocaine-induced enhancement of renal
sympathetic tone.

The marked reduction in renal blood flow may
have also contributed to the tubular damage
through anoxia. Alternatively, cocaine may
have a direct effect on the renal tubular epithelium or on the vascular smooth muscle cells.
The reduction in tubular reabsorption tended to
counteract the effect of lowered GFR on urinary
excretion of salt and water. Consequently,
oliguria was observed only in a few clearance
periods. Net urine flow and sodium excretion
were low after cocaine administration, but they
remained within normal physiological ranges.
These data suggest that cocaine may induce a

TABLE 1. COCAINE EFFECT ON THE REABSORPTION OF WATER AND SODIUM IN THE RAT NEPHRON

	Control	Cocaine	Change	P
Fractional Water Reabsorption (Percentage)	95.1±20.2	67.3±14.1	27.8±25.6	<0.01
Absolute Water Reabsorption ($\mu l \cdot min^{-1} \cdot kidney^{-1}$)	912.0±139	176.0±48	736.0±313	<0.01
Fractional Sodium Reabsorption (Percentage)	77.0±14.4	38.6±7.8	38.4±30.4	<0.05
Absolute Sodium Reabsorption ($\mu l \cdot min^{-1} \cdot kidney^{-1}$)	113.0±21.3	20.0±5	93.0±16	<0.01

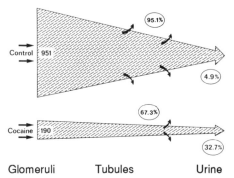

Figure 4. Comparison of glomerular filtration, tubular reabsorption and urinary excretion of fluid during control periods and after cocaine infusion.

In the present experiments, the mean dose of cocaine was high (8.2 mg/kg), perhaps higher than may be expected under clinical conditions. However, the kidneys receive a very high fraction of the cardiac output. Therefore, upon recirculation, the kidneys may be exposed to a very high percentage of the total drug entering the body. Even at lower exposure, the direct renal effects of the drug may be sufficient to predispose the kidneys to the nephrotoxic actions of cocaine that are consequent to rhabdomyolysis, volume depletion and hypotension. The combination of these factors have been associated with a high frequency of ARF and mortality in patients who used cocaine (1). Therefore, the kidneys should be considered as major target organs of acute cocaine intoxication.

The nature of the cocaine induced renal damage may be complex. Afferent arteriolar vasoconstriction is likely to play a primary role in the initiation of events. However, tubular obstruction (11), loss of epithelial cell integrity, local hormonal alterations, and cellular calcium overload may all contribute to the renal failure. Under the present experimental conditions, myoglobinuria, hypotension and volume depletion did not occur. Under clinical conditions, they appear to be primary contributors to the cocaine induced ARF (1,4,6,8).

hidden renal damage which may not be detected in a clinical setting unless ARF is produced. This may explain the lack of a frequent association between cocaine intoxication and renal dysfunction.

Cocaine would also be expected to increase renin release from the kidney due to elevated b-receptor activity. If it occurred, the consequent elevation in circulating angiotensin II levels may have contributed to the renal vasoconstriction and lowered GFR.

In conclusion, cocaine administered into the renal artery of rats in a dose of 8.2 mg/kg produced marked reductions in GFR and tubular reabsorption with a less remarkable inhibition of renal excretory functions. The results indicate a direct nephrotoxic action of the compound independent of its systemic hemodynamic and CNS effects. The drug acts on both renal vascular functions and tubular reabsorptive processes.

A rapid reduction in glomerular filtration rate and presumably renal blood flow appears to be the predominant initial renal alteration closely followed by an inhibition of tubular reabsorption of filtrate. The combination of reduced GFR and inhibited reabsorption leads to a relatively dampened reduction in urine flow and solute excretion. Cocaine is likely to cause a marked but largely hidden direct acute renal toxicity that may predispose the kidneys to the nephrotoxicities of the compound that result from its effects on other organ systems and may lead to acute renal failure.

ACKNOWLEDGEMENTS

These investigations were supported in part by USD General Research Fund and by V.A. Merit Review. The expert secretarial assistance of Michelle Delaney is appreciated.

REFERENCES

1. Roth D, Alarkon FJ, Fernandez JA, et al.: Acute rhabdomyolysis associated with cocaine intoxication. New Engl J Med 319: 673-677, 1988.

2. Billman GE and Hoskins RS: Cocaine-induced ventricular fibrillation: Protection afforded by the calcium antagonist verapamil. FASEB J 2: 2990-2995, 1988.

3. Grossman RA, Hamilton RW, Morse BM, et al.: Nontraumatic rhabdomyolysis and acute renal failure. New Engl J Med 291: 807-811, 1974.

4. Singhal P, Horowitz B, Quinones MC, et al.: Acute renal failure following cocaine abuse. Nephron 52: 76-78, 1989.

5. Krohn KD, Slowman-Kovacs S, Leapman SB: Cocaine and rhabdomyolysis. Ann Intern Med 108: 639-640, 1988.

6. Merigian KS, Roberts JR: Cocaine intoxication: Hyperpyrexia, rhabdomyolysis and acute renal failure. J Toxicol Clin Toxicol 25: 135-148, 1987.

7. Barrido DT, Joseph AJ, Rao, TKS, et al.: Renal disease associated with acute and chronic "crack" abuse. Kidney Int 33: 181 (Abstr.), 1988.

8. Herzlich BC, Arsura EL, Pagala M, et al.: Rhabdomyolysis related to cocaine abuse. Ann Intern Med 109: 335-336, 1988.

9. Kauker ML, Crofton JT, Share L, et al.: Role of vasopressin in regulation of renal kinin excretion in Long-Evans and Diabetes Insipidus rats. J Clin Invest 73: 824-831, 1984.

10. Kauker ML. Renal tubular effect of nisoldipine, a calcium channel blocker, in rats. J Cardiovas Pharmacol 9: 532-538, 1987.

11. Biber TUL, Mylle M, Baines AD, et al.: A study by micropuncture and microdissection of acute renal damage in rats. Am J Med 44: 664-705, 1968.

PART V
ANTIBIOTICS

15

EFFECT OF THE SCHEDULE OF ADMINISTRATION OF TWO AMINOGLYCOSIDES, NETILMICIN AND AMIKACIN, ON URINARY PHOSPHOLIPID EXCRETION IN HUMANS

S. Ibrahim (1), F. Clerckx-Braun (2), Ph. Jacqmin (2), J. Donnez (2), V. Brulein (2) and P.M. Tulkens (1)

Laboratory of Physiological Chemistry and International Institute of Cellular and Molecular Pathology (1), Laboratory of Pharmacokinetics (2), Department of Gynaecology (3); Catholic University of Louvain, Brussels, Belgium

INTRODUCTION

Aminoglycosides are very effective antibiotics, but also have the potential for producing nephro- and ototoxicity. On the average, 10 to 20% of patients treated with these drugs will experience a nephrotoxic reaction (1), but the incidence number varies from one study to another depending upon the criteria used to define this toxicity (2,3). Increase in serum creatinine is used clinically to detect aminoglycoside nephrotoxicity, but this change is a late event. Increase in the excretion of urinary markers such as low molecular weight proteins and lysosomal enzymes have been proposed to detect early renal damage including that induced by aminoglycosides (4), but these markers are nonspecific for aminoglycoside-induced alterations, and their increase can result from many other factors (5). The development of lysosomal phospholipidosis in proximal tubular cells is an early event in animals treated with low, therapeutic doses of aminoglycosides. This phospholipidosis is due to the inhibition of the activities of the lysosomal phospholipases and sphingomyelinase (6-8). Similar observations have been reported in humans treated with aminoglycosides (9,10). There is strong evidence that aminoglycoside-induced tubular necrosis is subsequent and correlated to lysosomal phospholipidosis (11,12). We have previously reported that animals treated with low doses of aminoglycosides

show a marked dose- and time-dependent rise in the urinary phospholipids excretion (13,14), which has also been reported at high doses (15). This increase is clearly related to the extent of the phospholipidosis observed in the renal cortex (16).

The purpose of the present study is to compare the effect of amikacin and netilmicin on the urinary excretion of phospholipids in treated patients. These aminoglycosides were selected, because they differ widely in the extent of the lysosomal phospholipidosis they cause both in rats and humans (9,17). Since a number of studies (reviewed in ref. 18) show that once-a-day (qd) administration of aminoglycoside reduces its toxic potential compared to standard regimens, such as twice-a-day (bid) and thrice-a-day (tid), we also examined the effect of schedule of administration on urinary phospholipids excretion.

MATERIALS AND METHODS

Four groups of 18 young (17-43 year) female patients suffering from pelvic inflammatory disease were included in our study. The 4 groups did not differ in mean age, weight and initial creatinine. Two groups of patients received netilmicin (6.6 mg/kg/day), and the two other groups recieved amikacin (14 mg/kg/day). For each drug, patients were randomly assigned either to the once-a-day (qd) schedule or the conventional mode of administration (tid, i.e. the daily dose split in 3 injections at 8 hr intervals, for netilmicin; bid, i.e. the daily dose split in 2 injections at 12 hr intervals for amikacin). Thus, the total dose of each drug was similar in groups treated qd or with intermittent dosing. All patients also received tinidazole (0.8 g/kg; qd) and ampicillin (4 g/day; bid) for 7 days. Phospholipids in urine samples taken from 24 hr collections at days 1, 4 and 7 were assayed, in addition to spot urine samples (available for only 60 patients) collected before therapy. Analyses were performed as described before (14), and results are expressed as µmol of phospholipid/g creatinine. Urine creatinine was measured by the method of Jaffe.

RESULTS

Table I shows the effect of amikacin and netilmicin given in one or multiple injection of the same daily dose on the urinary excretion of total phospholipids. Netilmicin tid induced a 2.8-fold increase after 7 days of treatment, but the increase was only 2.3-fold in patients treated qd, compared to day 0. These increases were significant in both groups (p<0.05) during the treatment (days 4 and 7). In contrast, only the group of patients treated with amikacin bid showed a significant increase of phospholipid excretion, whereas the slight increase ob-

served in patients receiving amikacin qd was not statistically significant.

Table II shows the results of the analysis of individual phospholipids for all patients at days 0, 4 and 7. For netilmicin, all individual phospholipids showed a significant increase as from day 4, with phosphatidylinositol being the most affected in relative, and phosphatidylcholine in absolute values. This pattern is similar to that observed in the renal cortex and urine of aminoglycoside-treated animals (13,14,19,20). Patients receiving netilmicin qd showed a somewhat lower excretion of all phospholipids, but the differences between groups was at the limit at the statistical significance. In contrast, only the excretion of phosphatidylinositol (at days 4 and 7) and of phosphatidylcholine and phosphatidylserine (at day 7) was increased in patients receiving amikacin bid, and that increase was lower than that observed in patients receiving netilmicin tid or even qd. Of all phospholipids measured, only phosphatidylinositol showed a significant increase compared to day 0 in the group of patients receiving amikacin on a qd schedule.

DISCUSSION

Aminoglycosides induce a marked increase of the urinary excretion of phospholipids in

Table I: Urinary excretion of total phospholipids in patients treated with amikacin and netilmicin

Duration of treatment (day)	Treatment group[b]			
	A-qd (n=18)	A-bid (n=18)	N-qd (n=18)	N-tid (n=18)
0[c]	3.0±1.8[d]	3.4±1.5	3.8±2.0	4.1±3.8
1	3.2±1.8	2.8±1.4	3.5±2.0	2.9±1.0
4	3.8±1.9	4.2±1.7*	5.6±5.0*	7.2±4.4*
7	3.9±1.8	5.9±3.6*	8.9±4.1*	11.5±6.1*

* significantly different from day 1 values (p<0.05);a Phospholipid excreted in umol per g creatinine and per day;b A, amikacin; N, netilmicin; qd, once-a-day; bid, twice-a-day; tid, thrice-a-day;c no. of patients at day 0 are A-qd (13); A-bid (12); N-qd (17); N-tid(18);d no significant difference between day 1 and day 0

Table II: Urinary excretion of individual phospholipids in amikacin- and netilmicin-treated patients after 7 days of treatment

drug[a]	Sched[b].	day	Phospholipids excreted (umol/g creatinine)				
			PI	PS	PC	PE	SM
Baseline[d]		0	0.20±0.19	0.46±0.29	0.62±0.40	0.75±0.46	0.97±0.74
A	qd	4	0.22±0.16[*]	0.57±0.31	0.55±0.29	0.58±0.24	0.68±0.24
		7	0.28±0.23[*]	0.57±0.30	0.54±0.43	0.66±0.38	0.63±0.38
A	bid	4	0.27±0.12[*]	0.61±0.30	0.71±0.43	0.58±0.29	0.87±0.36
		7	0.50±0.35[*]	0.97±0.40[*]	1.18±1.26[*]	0.98±0.46	0.94±0.43
N	qd	4	0.71±0.75[*]	0.77±0.53[*]	1.08±1.12[*]	1.00±1.03[*]	1.37±1.15[*]
		7	1.22±0.70[*]	1.13±0.49[*]	1.70±1.07[*]	1.54±0.63[*]	2.20±1.08[*]
N	tid	4	0.92±0.65[*]	1.06±0.76[*]	1.78±1.86[*]	1.50±0.98[*]	1.69±1.10[*]
		7	1.79±1.06[*]	1.43±0.87[*]	2.55±2.10[*]	2.01±1.38[*]	2.38±1.16[*]

[*] $p < 0.05$ compared to day 0 in same group of patients.a A, amikacin; N, netilmicin.b qd, once-a-day; bid, twice-a-day; tid, thrice-a-day.c PI, phosphatidylinositol; PS, phosphatidylserine; PC, phosphatidylcholine; PE, phosphatidylethanolamine; SM, sphingomyelin.d values for all patients for which pre-therapy samples were available (n=60)

treated rats (13), probably due to exocytosis and/or regurgitation of excess of phospholipids stored in lysosomes, or, in part, to focal tubular necrosis (14). Our present results show this observation can be extended to humans treated with netilmicin or amikacin, and that it depends on the drug given, and the duration and the schedule of the treatment. In particular, amikacin induces a significantly lower increase compared to that netilmicin. Yet, in both cases, phosphatidylinositol is the most affected phospholipid in relative values. In fact, phosphatidylinositol also manifested the greatest fractional increase among the different phospholipid classes in the renal cortex (19) and the urine (13) of treated rats. Our study also clearly demonstrates a constant trend towards less excretion of phospholipids in patients treated qd compared to bid (for amikacin) or tid (for netilmicin). The effect was similar for total and the individual phospholipids assayed.

The nephrotoxicity risk associated with aminoglycoside administration is difficult to estimate in patients since they are always exposed to factors that may affect the intrinsic toxicity of the drug (12). This may make clinical ranking of different aminoglycosides contradictory, especially with a late parameter of toxicity such as a rise in serum creatinine. Lysosomal phospholipidosis is an early index of aminoglycoside nephrotoxicity and has been observed in both animals and humans (7,9,10). As pointed out in a separate paper (16), phospholipiduria is related to the severity of this phospholipidosis in rats. Moreover, the difference between netilmicin- and amikacin-induced urinary excretion of phospholipids in this study is consistent with the difference reported for those two aminoglycosides with respect to lysosomal phospholipidosis in human cortex (9). Assuming that phospholipidosis and phospholipiduria are related, it can be concluded that the qd schedule, by causing less phospholipidosis, will also be less toxic. This difference could be the result of a decreased renal accumulation of aminoglycosides in the cortex of patients treated qd due to the saturable character of the uptake of these drugs by proximal tubular cells (18). Measurement of urinary excretion of phospholipids may therefore be a sensitive and reliable index to monitoring aminoglycoside-induced early renal alterations.

ACKNOWLEDGEMENTS

S.I. is recipient of a fellowship from the Ministry of Higher Education and Scientific Research of the Republic of Iraq and P.M.T. is Maître de Recherches of the Belgian Fonds National de la Recherche Scientifique. This work was supported in part by the Belgian Fonds de Recherche Scientifique Medical (grant no. 3.4553.88).

REFERENCES

1. Kahlmeter G, Dahlager JI: Aminoglycoside toxicity: a review of clinical studies published between 1975 and 1982. J Antimicrob Chemoth 13 suppl A:9-22, 1984.

2. Lane AZ, Wright GE, Blair DC: Ototoxicity and nephrotoxicity of amikacin. An overview of phase II and phase III. Experience in the United States. Am J Med 62:911-918, 1977.

3. Gatell JM, SanMiguel JG, Zamora L, Araujo V, Castells C, Moreno A, Jimenez de Anta MT, Marin JL, Elena M, Ballesta: Tobramycin and amikacin in nephrotoxicity. Values of serum creatinine verus urinary concentration of beta-2-microglobulin. Nephron 41:337-343, 1985.

4. Piscator M: Markers of tubular dysfunction. Toxicol Lett 46:197-204, 1989.

5. Bernard A, Viau C, Ouled A, Tulkens P, Lauwerys R: Effects of gentamicin on the renal uptake of endogenous and exogenous proteins in conscious rats. Toxicol Appl Pharmacol 84:431-438, 1986.

6. Kosek JC, Mazz RI, Cousins MJ: Nephrotoxicity of gentamicin. Lab Invest 30:48-57, 1974.

7. Laurent G, Carlier MB, Rollman B, Van Hoof F, Tulkens P: Mechanism of aminoglycoside-induced lysosomal phospholipidosis: in vitro and in vivo studies with gentamicin and amikacin. Biochem Pharmacol 31:3861-3870, 1982.

8. Mingeot-Leclercq MP, Laurent G, Tulkens PM: Biochemical mechanism of aminoglycoside-induced inhibition of phosphatidylcholine hydrolysis by lysosomal phospholipases. Biochem Pharmacol 37:591-599, 1988.

9. De Broe ME, Paulus GJ, Verpooten GA, Giuliano RA, Roels F, Tulkens PM: Early toxicity of aminoglycosides in human kidney: a prospective, comparative study of amikacin, gentamicin, netilmicin and tobramycin. In: Spitzy KH, Karrer K (eds); Proceedings of the 13th International Congress of Chemotherapy, Vienna, 1983, Vol 86, pp. 11-24.

10. De Broe ME, Paulus GJ, Verpooten GA, Roels F, Buyssens N, Weeden R, Van Hoof F, Tulkens P: Early effects of gentamicin, tobramycin and amikacin on the human kidney. Kidney Int 25:643-652, 1984.

11. Tulkens PM: Experimental studies on nephrotoxicity of aminoglycosides at low doses: mechanisms and perspectives. Am J Med 80 (6B): 105-114, 1986.

12. Tulkens PM: Nephrotoxicity of aminoglycosides. Toxicol Lett 46:107-123, 1989.

13. Ibrahim S, Tulkens PM: Increased urinary excretion and change of patterns of phospholipids in gentamicin-treated rats. In: 26th Intersc Conf Antimicrob Agents Chemother, New Orleans, Abstract no 27, 1986.

14. Ibrahim S, Kallay Z, Clerckx-Braun F, Donnez J, Tulkens PM: Urinary phospholipids pattern after treatment with aminoglycoside antibiotics and cis-platinum. In: Bach PH, Lock EA (eds); Nephrotoxicity: Extrapolation from in vitro to in vivo, and animals to man. London, Plenum Press, 1989, pp. 177-182.

15. Josepovitz C, Levine R, Farruggella T, Kaloyanides GJ: Comparative effects of aminoglycosides on renal cortical and urinary

phospholipids in rat. Proc Soc Exp Med 182: 1-5, 1986.

16. Ibrahim S, Kishore BK, Lambricht P, Laurent G, Tulkens PM: Effect of aminoglycosides and of coadministration of poly-L-aspartic acid on urinary phospholipids excretion: A comparative study. Proceedings of 4th Int Symposium on Nephrotoxicity, Guildford, 1989.

17. Tulkens P, Laurent G, Carlier MB, Toubeau G, Heuson-Stiennon J, Maldague P: Comparative study of the alterations induced in rat kidney by gentamicin, dibekacin, netilmicin, tobramycin and amikacin at low doses. In: Spitzy KH, Karrer K (eds); Proceedings of the 13th International Congress of Chemotherapy, Vienna, 1983, Vol 86, pp. 30-35.

18. Tulkens PM, Clerckx-Braun F, Donnez J, Ibrahim S, Kallay Z, Delmee M, Jacqmin Ph, Lesne M, Gersdorff M, Kaufman L, Derde MP: Safety and efficacy of aminoglycosides once-a-day: experimental data and randomized, controlled evalution in patients suffering from pelvic inflammatory disease. J Drug Devel 1 (suppl 3): 71-82, 1988.

19. Ibrahim S, Carlier MB, Laurent G, Tulkens PM: Quantitative analysis of phospholipids composition of rat kidney cortex after treatment with gentamicin, debekacin, netilmicin and tobramycin at low doses (10 mg/kg/day). In: 25th Intersc Conf Antimicrob Agents Chemother, Minneapolis, Abstract no 708, 1985.

20. Josepovitz C, Farruggella T, Levine R, Lane B, Kaloyanides GJ: Effect of netilmicin on the phospholipid composition of subcellular fractions of rat renal cortex. J Pharmacol Exp Ther 235:810-819, 1985.

16

ASSESSMENT OF THREE THERAPEUTIC INTERVENTIONS FOR MODIFYING GENTAMICIN NEPHROTOXICITY IN THE RAT

G. J. Kaloyanides, L. Ramsammy and C. Josepovitz

Division of Nephrology and Hypertension, Department of Medicine, State University of New York at Stony Brook, Stony Brook, New York 11794 and Department of Veterans Affairs Medical Center, Northport, New York 11768

INTRODUCTION

During the past few years three distinctively different therapeutic interventions have been reported to be efficacious in either preventing or ameliorating experimental aminoglycoside-induced nephrotoxicity in the rat. These interventions consist of the administration of hydroxyl radical scavengers (1), pyridoxal-5-phosphate (2) or polyaspartic acid (3) given simultaneously with the aminoglycoside. In this paper we describe the results of experiments in which we examined the relative efficacy of these three interventions in modifying the expression of gentamicin nephrotoxicity in the rat, a model we have studied extensively over the years (4-8).

METHODS

Experiments were performed on male Sprague-Dawley rats housed in metabolic cages and provided with access to food and water ad libitum.

I. Hydroxyl radical scavengers: Eight groups of rats were injected for 8 days with 0.9% saline at 2.5 ml/kg/day sc; gentamicin at 100 mg base/kg/day sc; dimethylthiourea (DMTU) at 500 mg/kg ip as the initial dose followed by 125 mg/kg ip bid; gentamicin plus DMTU; dimethyl-sulfoxide (DMSO) at 4 g/kg ip bid; gentamicin plus DMSO; sodium benzoate (NaBNZ) at 150 mg/kg ip bid; or gentamicin plus NaBNZ.

II. Pyridoxal-5-phosphate (P-5-PO$_4$): Rats were injected for 6 days with saline, gentamicin,

P-5-PO$_4$ at 250 mg/kg per day ip or gentamicin plus P-5-PO$_4$.

III. Polyaspartic acid (PAA): Rats were injected for 6 days with either saline, gentamicin, PAA (mol. wt. 15,000) at 500 mg/kg per day or gentamicin plus PAA.

Twenty-four hours after the last injection the rats were sacrificed and the renal cortex was assayed for malondialdehyde (MDA), catalase, total phospholipid and gentamicin. In selected rats, kidneys were processed for light and electron microscopy. Urine was collected daily on ice and assayed for alanine aminopeptidase (AAP) and N-acetyl-beta-D-glucosaminidase (NAG). Urine creatinine in the last collection was also measured. Serum creatinine was measured at the time of sacrifice. The methods for processing tissue and performing the biochemical analyses have been reported previously (4-8).

RESULTS

Hydroxyl radical scavengers: These experiments are summarized in Table 1. Gentamicin nephrotoxicity was manifested by increased urinary excretion of AAP and NAG, increased MDA, an end product of lipid peroxidation, in the renal cortex, depression of renal cortical catalase activity, elevation of serum creatinine and depression of creatinine clearance. These biochemical and functional changes were accompanied by the typical pattern of histopathology consisting of loss of brush bor-

Table 1. Effect of co-administration of hydroxyl radical scavengers on the expression of gentamicin (G) toxicity in the rat.[1]

	Saline	G	DMTU	DMTU + G	DMSO	DMSO + G	NaBNZ	NaBNZ + G
Delta Urinary AAP unit/8 days	0.10 ±0.24	3.50** ±0.27	-1.54** ±0.59	2.30** ++ ±0.45	1.85** ±0.40	3.61** + ±0.70	2.24** ±0.21	3.18** ±0.71
Delta Urinary NAG units/8 days	1.8 ±5.6	142.8** ±9.6	-2.6 ±4.8	89.0**++ ±17.6	26.3** ±9.6	209.6** ++ ±37.2	33.1** ±1.6	190.6** ++ ±9.8
MDA n mol/mg protein	0.67 ±0.02	1.14** ±0.08	0.69 ±0.04	0.70 ±0.04	0.59 ±0.04	0.73 ±0.02	0.58 ±0.02	0.60 ±0.02
Catalase k/min	0.129 ±0.007	0.060** ±0.004	0.125 ±0.009	0.019** ±0.006	0.106 ±0.009	0.011** ±0.007	0.088** ±0.009	0.032** ±0.009
Gentamicin ug/mg protein	-	7.9 ±0.4	-	5.6** ±0.6	-	4.5** ±0.3	-	7.2 ±0.7
Serum Creatinine mg/dl	0.23 ±0.04	0.65** ±0.07	0.22 ±0.01	1.31** ±0.15	0.23 ±0.02	1.50** ±0.20	0.24 ±0.01	0.64** ±0.14
Creatinine Clearance ml/min/100 g bw	0.54 ±0.03	0.25** ±0.04	0.55 ±0.04	0.11** ±0.04	0.63 ±0.04	0.09** ±0.03	0.60 ±0.03	0.30** ±0.04

[1]. Data represent mean ± SE, N=6-12. G, gentamicin; DMTU, dimethylthiourea; DMSO, dimethylsulfoxide; NaBNZ, sodiu benzoate AAP alanin aminopeptidase NAG n-acetyl-β-d-glucosaminidase; MDA, malondialdehyde.*,**: significantly different from saline, p<0.05 and p<0.01, respectively. +,++: significantly different from preceding value; p<0.05 and p<0.01,

der membrane, increased number and size of inclusion bodies and proximal tubular cell necrosis. Rats injected with gentamicin plus one of the scavengers of hydroxyl radicals showed no increase in MDA compared to saline rats, a finding which signifies that these agents were effective in scavenging free radicals and preventing lipid peroxidation. However, these agents were ineffective in preventing the other biochemical or functional derangements induced by gentamicin. In fact, DMTU and DMSO accentuated the gentamicin-induced changes in urinary enzyme excretion, catalase, serum creatinine and creatinine clearance. This accentuation was also manifested by more severe proximal tubular cell injury and necrosis in rats injected with gentamicin plus DMTU or DMSO. Moreover, these changes occurred despite the fact that the amount of gentamicin accumulated in the renal cortex of rats injected with DMTU or DMSO was significantly less than that of rats injected only with gentamicin. The lower drug level in renal cortex may reflect the greater

degree of proximal tubular cell necrosis in rats injected with gentamicin plus DMTU or DMSO and the resulting greater loss of drug-ladened cells into the urine.

P-5-PO4: The results of these experiments are summarized in Table 2. The administration of P-5-PO4 with gentamicin had no significant beneficial effects in terms of preventing increased urinary enzyme excretion, increased renal cortical phospholipids or MDA or depression of catalase activity. However, these rats experienced significantly less elevations of serum creatinine and BUN, less depression of creatinine clearance and less proximal tubular cell necrosis than rats injected with gentamicin alone. This protective influence of P-5-PO4 could not be explained by an effect on the renal cortical accumulation of drug which was not different from that of rats injected with gentamicin alone. The renal cortical concentration of P-5-PO4 was depressed in rats injected with gentamicin alone whereas it was not different

Table 2. Effect of co-administration of pyridoxol-5-phosphate (P-5-PO4) on the expression of gentamicin (G) nephrotoxicity in the rat.[1]

	Saline	P-5-PO4	G	G+P-5-PO4
Delta Urinary AAP (U/6 days)	-0.26 ±0.24	-0.05 ±0.4	1.50 ±0.24 **	1.60 ±0.37 **
Delta Urinary NAG (U/6 days)	-0.42 ±1.9	15.60 ±2.0 *	43.10 ±7.2 **	60.20 ±5.9 **
Phospholipid (nmol/mg protein)	211.00 ±1.0	196.00 ±13	290.00 ±23 **	273.00 ±22 *
MDA (nmol/mg protein)	0.590±.03	0.59 ±.05	0.97 ±.05 **	0.87 ±.09 **
Catalase (k/min)	0.205±.022	0.167±.018	0.067±.015 **	0.070±.013 **
Gentamicin (ug/mg protein)	-	-	7.7±0.5	7.50 ±0.7
Serum Creatinine (mg/dl)	0.246±.006	0.277±.013	1.095±.257 **	0.481±.058 * +
Creatinine Clearance (ml/min/100 g b.w.)	0.513±.014	0.463±.038	0.146±.034 **	0.332±.065 *+
BUN (mg/dl)	14.90 ±1.1	16.50 ±0.7	50.3±10.1 **	23.60 ±3.1 * +
P-5-PO4 (ng/mg protein)	41.60 ±3.1	50.80 ±2.1 *	27.5±1.7 **	39.00 ±2.6

[1]. Data represent mean ± SE, N=8. AAP, alanine aminopeptidase; NAG, n- acetyl-β-d-glucosamidase; MDA, malondialdehyde; BUN, blood urea nitrogen. *,**: significantly different from saline, $p<0.05$ and $p<0.01$, respectively. + : significantly different from G, $P<0.05$.

from controls in rats injected with gentamicin plus P-5-PO4.

PAA: These experiments are summarized in Table 3. Rats injected with PAA alone showed no changes in any of the parameters measured. Rats injected with gentamicin plus PAA demonstrated significantly less elevation of NAG excretion, less elevation of renal cortical phospholipids and MDA, less depression of catalase compared to rats injected with gentamicin alone and no significant changes in serum creatinine or creatinine clearance when compared to the data of saline-injected control rats. Histopathological changes were also significantly less pronounced in rats injected with gentamicin plus PAA compared to the changes observed in rats injected with gentamicin alone.

DISCUSSION

Walker and Shah reported that gentamicin augmented the generation of hydrogen peroxide by renal mitochondria in vitro (9). Subsequently these investigators reported that treatment of rats with a variety of hydroxyl radical scavengers conferred significant protection against gentamicin-induced acute renal failure in the rat (1). Stimulated by the latter report, we sought to confirm the protective effects of hydroxyl radical scavengers. Our experimental protocols were identical to those described by Walker and Shah (1). However, in contrast to their observations, we found that the co-administration of hydroxyl radical scavengers with gentamicin not only afforded no protection against gentamicin nephrotoxicity, but the severity of the renal injury was magnified in two of the three scavengers tested. The reason for this marked difference between the two studies

Table 3. Effect of polyaspartic acid (PAA) on the expression of gentamicin (G) nephrotoxicity in the rat.[1]

	Control	PAA	G	G+PAA
Delta Urinary AAP units/6 days	(6) 0.21 ±.12	(6) 0.48 ±.36	(6) 1.40 ±.30[**]	(6) 1.47 ±.12[**]
Delta Urinary NAG units/6 days	(6) -2.90 ±2.6	(6) -3.20 ±1.8	(6) 48.80 ±3.9[**]	(6) 15.60 ±6.8[*a]
MDA nmol/mg protein	(12) 0.70 ±.03	(6) 0.69 ±.03	(12) 1.14 ±.04[**]	(12) 0.75 ±0.04[a]
Catalase k/min	(12) 0.144±.010	(6) 0.148±.009	(12) 0.090±.004[**]	(12) 0.114±.006[**a]
Total Phospholipid nmol/mg protein	(6) 333.00 ±13	(6) 338.00 ±17	(6) 431.00 ±36[**]	(6) 360.00 ±13[*a]
Gentamicin ug/mg protein	-	-	(12) 12.60 ±1.0	(12) 14.50 ±1.5
Serum Creatinine mg/dl	(12) 0.23 ±.01	(6) 0.23 ±.01	(12) 0.32 ±.02[**]	(12) 0.26 ±.01[a]
Creatinine Clearance ml/min	(6) 0.569±.020	(6) 0.481±.036	(6) 0.364±.043[**]	(6) 0.480±.035[a]

[1]. Data represent mean ± SE. Numbers in parentheses equal N. AAP, alanine aminopeptidase; NAG, n-acetyl- b -d-glucosaminidase; MDA, malondialdehyde.   , significantly different from control, P<0.01 [*a], significantly different from G, P<0.05.

remains obscure. Nevertheless our results are in agreement with two previous studies reported from our laboratory in which it was shown that two free radical scavengers, diphenyl phenylenediamine (7) and vitamin E (8) were highly effective in preventing gentamicin-induced lipid peroxidation in the renal cortex of the rat as assessed by MDA levels, but that neither agent protected against the development of acute renal failure and proximal tubular cell necrosis. Thus, the results of the experiments involving hydroxyl radical scavengers reinforce the conclusion of our earlier studies (7,8), i.e. that free radical mediated lipid peroxidation is a consequence and not the cause of gentamicin-induced acute renal failure.

Kacew (2) recently reported that the co-administration of P-5-PO$_4$ (250 mg/kg/day) with gentamicin (60 mg/kg/day) for 14 days to rats prevented enzymuria, depression of renal cortical enzymes and the development of the typical phospholipidosis. The same dose of P-5-PO$_4$ was ineffective in rats injected with gentamicin at 100 mg/kg per day for 4 days. In neither protocol did Kacew measure glomerular filtration rate or examine the kidney for histopathological evidence of injury. In our study we used the high dose of gentamicin (100 mg/kg per day) for 6 days and found that although P-5-PO$_4$ did not prevent the typical changes in enzymuria, the elevations of renal cortical phospholipid and MDA or the depression of catalase, it did result in significantly less depression of creatinine clearance and less proximal tubular cell necrosis. The protective effect of P-5-PO$_4$ most likely is exerted at a step distal to the uptake and accumulation of gentamicin since the renal concentration of drug was not reduced by P-5-PO$_4$. Our findings are sufficiently encouraging to warrant further investigation to determine if a higher dose of P-5-PO$_4$ might confer complete protection against gentamicin-induced nephrotoxicity.

Williams et al. (3) reported that PAA conferred complete protection of rats against the development of aminoglycoside nephrotoxicity as assessed by histopathological scoring. Biochemical and functional correlates of nephrotoxicity were not examined in their study. We have shown that the injection of PAA significantly reduced gentamicin- induced alterations of NAG excretion, renal cortical phospholipid, MDA and catalase and completely prevented the depression of creatinine clearance and greatly attenuated the severity of proximal tubular cell necrosis. In our experience no other intervention has provided such an impressive degree of protection against gentamicin nephrotoxicity. Recently Gilbert et al. (10) have also confirmed the protective effect of PAA as assessed by functional, biochemical and morphological criteria. In agreement with the original observation of Williams et al. (3) we also found that PAA protection was not mediated by depression of the renal cortical accumulation of gentamicin. This observation indicates that PAA must inhibit gentamicin from disrupting one or more critical intracellular processes causally linked to the initiation and propagation of the injury cascade. In two companion papers (11,12) we present evidence that the protection afforded by PAA is related to its capacity to serve as an anionic substrate for the cationic aminoglycosides and thereby prevent these antibiotics from interacting electrostatically with membrane anionic phospholipids, especially the phosphoinositides. It is noteworthy that P-5-PO$_4$ is also an anionic compound that has been shown to form a complex with aminoglycoside antibiotics (13). Taken together, these data suggest that the testing of other anionic compounds for their capacity to form complexes with aminoglycosides would likely be a fruitful strategy for identifying new therapies to protect against the development of nephrotoxicity.

ACKNOWLEDGMENTS

This research was supported by a grant from the NIH, AM-27061 and from the Medical Research Service, Department of Veterans Affairs. The authors express their appreciation to Pamela Geller for expert secretarial assistance in preparing this manuscript for publication.

REFERENCES

1. Walker PD, Shah SV: Evidence suggesting a role for hydroxyl radical in gentamicin-induced acute renal failure in rats. J Clin Invest 81:334-341, 1980.

2. Kacew S: Inhibition of gentamicin-induced nephrotoxicity by pyridoxal-5'-phosphate in the rat. J Pharmacol Exp Ther 248:360-366, 1989.

3. Williams PD, Hottendorf GH, Bennett DB: Inhibition of renal membrane binding and nephrotoxicity of aminoglycosides. J Pharmacol Exp Ther 237:919-925, 1986.

4. Soberon L, Bowman RL, Pastoriza-Munoz E, Kaloyanides GJ: Comparative nephrotoxicities of gentamicin, netilmicin and tobramycin in the rat. J Pharmacol Exp Ther 210:334-343, 1979.

5. Feldman S, Wang MY, Kaloyanides GJ: Aminoglycosides induce a phospholipidosis in the renal cortex of the rat: an early manifestation of nephrotoxicity. J Pharmacol Exp Ther 220:514-520, 1982.

6. Ramsammy L, Ling KY, Josepovitz D, Levine R, Kaloyanides, GJ: Effect of gentamicin on lipid peroxidation in the rat renal cortex. Biochem Pharmacol 34:3895-3988, 1985.

7. Ramsammy LS, Josepovitz C, Ling KY, Lane BP, Kaloyanides GJ: Effects of diphenylphenylenediamine on gentmaicin-induced lipid peroxidation and toxicity in rat renal cortex. J Pharmacol Exp Ther 238:83-88, 1986.

8. Ramsammy LS, Josepovitz C, Ling KY, Lane BP, Kaloyanides GJ: Failure of inhibition of lipid peroxidation by vitamin E to protect against gentamicin nephrotoxicity in the rat. Biochem Pharmacol 36:2125-2132, 1987.

9. Walker PD, Shah SV: Gentamicin enhanced production of hydrogen peroxide by renal cortical mitochondria. Am J Physiol 253:C495-C499, 1987.

10. Gilbert DN, Wood CA, Kohlhepps SJ, Kohner PW, Houghton DC, Finkbeiner HC, Lindsley J, Bennett WM: Polyaspartic acid pre-

vents experimental aminoglycoside nephrotoxicity. J Inf Dis 159:945-953, 1989.

11. Kaloyanides GJ, Ramsammy L, Josepovitz C: Polyaspartic acid inhibits gentamicin-induced perturbation of phospholipid metabolism in cultured renal cells. In: Bach PH, Delacruz L, Gregg NJ, Wilks MF (eds); Proceedings of the Fourth International Symposium on Nephrotoxicity. New York, Marcel Dekker, 1990, this volume.

12. Kaloyanides GJ, Ramsammy L: Alterations of biophysical properties of liposomes predict aminoglycoside toxicity: inhibitory effect of polyaspartic acid. In: Bach PH, Delacruz L, Gregg NJ, Wilks MF (eds); Proceedings of the Fourth International Symposium of Nephrotoxicity. New York, Marcel Dekker, 1990, this volume.

13. Kenniston RC, Calbellon Jr S, Yarbrough KS: Pyrodixal-5-phosphate as an antidote for cyanide, spermine, gentamicin and dopamine toxicity: an in vivo rat study. Toxicol Appl Pharmacol 88:433-441, 1987.

17

EFFECT OF AMINOGLYCOSIDES AND OF COADMINISTRATION OF POLY-L-ASPARTIC ACID ON URINARY PHOSPHOLIPIDS EXCRETION: A COMPARATIVE STUDY

S. Ibrahim, B.K. Kishore, P. Lambricht, G. Laurent and P.M. Tulkens

Laboratory of Physiological Chemistry, Catholic University of Louvain, and International Institute of Cellular and Molecular Pathology, Brussels, Belgium

INTRODUCTION

Aminoglycoside nephrotoxicity in animals and humans is associated with the selective accumulation of these drugs in the lysosomes of proximal tubular cells and the development of a lysosomal phospholipidosis resulting from drug-induced inhibition of the catabolism of phospholipids (1-5). Significant differences among aminoglycosides can be observed in this respect. Comparative studies suggest that the toxicity of a given aminoglycoside is related to the extent of the lysosomal phospholipidosis (see 6,7 for review). Moreover, substances such as piperacillin and poly-L-aspartic acid, which protect against aminoglycoside-induced nephrotoxicity (8,9), also protect aganist aminoglycoside-induced lysosomal phospholipidosis (10). In previous studies, we have reported that gentamicin administration at low, clinically relevant doses in rats, induces a marked increase of the urinary excretion of all major phospholipids in a pattern similar to the increase in phospholipid content of the renal cortex (11-13). Similar effects have been reported at high doses (14). In the present study, we examine the effect of five aminoglycosides (netilmicin, gentamicin, tobramycin, amikacin and isepamicin) and the influence of the coadministration of poly-L-aspartic acid on urinary phospholipids excretion in rats.

MATERIALS AND METHODS

Female Sprague-Dawley rats were used throughout. In the first series of experiments, rats were treated for 10 days with gentamicin (4, 10, 20 and 50 mg/kg/day), netilmicin (10 mg/kg/day), tobramycin (10 mg/kg/day), amikacin (40 mg/kg/day) or isepamicin (40 mg/kg/day), for 10 days. The daily dose of drug was administered in two equally divided injections. In the second series of experiments, rats were treated for 4 days with gentamicin (20 mg/kg/day; administered intraperitoneally) given either alone or concomitantly with poly-L-aspartic acid (250 mg/kg/day; 10-20KDa; Sigma Chem. Co., St-Louis, MO, USA; administered by subcutaneous injection). The drug and poly-L-aspartic acid were administered once a day. Rats injected with 0.9% NaCl on the same schedules were included as controls in each series of experiments. Each experimental group contained at least 5 rats. Twenty four hr urine samples were collected by housing the animals individually in metabolic cages. Urine samples of each animal were centrifuged, and phospholipids were extracted, separated by thin-layer chromatography and measured as previously described (13). Animals were sacrificed by decapitation either 12 hr (first series) or 24 hr (second series) after the last drug injection, and exactly 1 hr after injection of 200 µCi/rat of [methyl-^{3}H] thymidine. Blood was collected and analyzed for creatinine by the Jaffe's reaction.

Table I. Effect of gentamicin given alone or with poly-L-aspartic acid on urinary total phospholipids excretion

Treatment[a]	Schedule[b]	daily dose mg/kg	Phospholipids excreted per day[c]	
			4 days	10 days
GM	bid	4	132± 10[*]	339± 45[*]
GM	bid	10	253±116[*]	544± 66[*]
GM	bid	20	477±177[*]	1041±336[*]
GM	bid	50	624± 47[*]	459±343[*]
GM	qd	20	223± 41[*]	-----
GM+ pASP	qd	20	94± 25	-----

[*] significantly different from control values (p< 0.05);[a] GM, gentamicin; pASP, poly-L-aspartic acid (250 mg/kg.day)[b] bid, twice-a-day; qd, once-a-day[c] Total phospholipids excreted per 24 hr in percent of the values of control rats (n=5)

RESULTS

Several doses and time schedules were used to characterize the relative effect of gentamicin. As shown in Table I, the effect of gentamicin on urinary phospholipids excretion was already detectable even at a dose as low as 4 mg/kg/day, and was dose-dependent after 4 days of treatment, reaching values approximately 6-fold those of controls after administration of 50 mg/kg/day. As the treatment was prolonged from day 4 to day 10, the increase became more pronounced for the doses of 4 to 20 mg/kg.day, reaching values approximately 10-fold those of controls for the latter dose. At a higher dose (50 mg/kg.day), however, phospholipiduria decreased from day 4 to day 10, and these animals concomitantly showed a significant rise in their terminal serum creatinine which rose from 0.60±04 (controls) to 2.25±1.3 mg % (treated rats).

Table I also shows that the increase in phospholipiduria induced by gentamicin was completely suppressed when the aminoglycoside was given together with poly-L-aspartic acid (250 mg/kg/day). It can also be observed that the increase of urinary phospholipids excretion after 4 days of treatment with gentamicin at 20 mg/kg/day in this experimental series was lower than that observed in animals treated at the same dose and for the same duration in the first experimental series. This difference could result from the schedule of administration (once-a-day vs twice-a-day) choosen for each series (7).

Table II shows the urinary excretion of total and individual phospholipids in rats treated for 10 days with low and equitherapeutic doses of gentamicin, netilmicin, tobramycin, amikacin, and isepamicin. The highest increases were induced by netilmicin (6 to 10-fold, except for sphingomyelin), whereas isepamicin induced only modest increases. For all aminoglycosides tested, phosphatidylinositol showed the highest, and sphingomyelin the lowest increase in relative values. In absolute values, however, phosphatidylcholine was the most abundant phospholipid excreted.

DISCUSSION

The present study demonstrates that different aminoglycosides induce an increase of the urinary excretion of total phospholipids. This observation extends our previous study (12), which showed an association between gentamicin treatment and increase in phospholipiduria. The importance of the effect, however, varies markedly among the drug studied, with a rank order of netilmicin >

Table II. Effect of aminoglycosides on urinary excretion of phospholipids after 10 days of treatment

Drug[a]	daily dose mg/kg	Phospholipids excreted (% of control)[*]					
		TPL[b]	PI	PS	PC	PE	SM
GM	10	544± 66	1009± 99	609± 70	711± 28	565±27	240±20
NT	10	620± 33	1050± 73	797± 25	740± 40	579±21	289±22
TO	10	306±167	606±127	358± 64	500± 88	253±69	167±17
AK	40	303±131	538±371	280±191	500±332	261±84	178±40
IP	40	264± 76	238±139	154± 56	234±133	208±74	139±39

[*] all values are different from controls (p< 0.05); absolute value for control rats were (in nmol/24hr) for TPL, 70.6±17.4; PI, 2.3±.6; PS, 4.6± 0.7; PC, 10.61±1.2; PE, 11.8±1.1; SM, 14.8±1.6[a] given in two injections at 12 h interval (bid).[b] TPL, total phospholipids; PI, phosphatidylinositol; PS, phosphatidylserine; PC, phosphatidylcholine; PE, phosphatidylethanolamine; SM, sphingomyelin.[c] GM, gentamicin; NT, netilmicin; TO, tobramycin; AK, amikacin; IP, isepamicin

gentamicin > tobramycin > amikacin > isepamicin. Analysis of individual phospholipids leads to similar conclusions while demonstrating also that, as for gentamicin, phosphatidylinositol shows the highest increase in relative values for all drugs tested. These observations are consistent with the hypothesis that the increased phospholipiduria is related to the lysosomal phospholipidosis induced by these drugs. We previously reported that the different aminoglycosides induce lysosomal phospholidosis in a similar rank order as that found here (2,15,16). Moreover, the cortex of aminoglycoside-treated animals has been shown to be enriched in acidic phospholipids (11,17). The present data, therefore, strongly support our previous conclusions about the origin of phospholipids found in excess in urine (13), which could be released from proximal tubular cells by exocytosis. Yet, we do not exclude the possibility that phospholipiduria could also partly result from focal tubular necrosis. The fact, however, that netilmicin causes conspicuous phospholipidosis and phospholipiduria but is reported to cause less necrosis than gentamicin, indicates that necrosis may not be the main cause of phospholipiduria. Interestingly enough, phospholipiduria induced by gentamicin is dose- and

time-dependent up to a certain threshold. Phospholipiduria (and phospholipid accumulation in renal cortex; data not shown) decreased when the treatment was prolonged from day 4 to day 10 with a daily dose of 50 mg/kg/day. This observation could be related to the fact that treatment with such a high dose of gentamicin is likely to produce acute necrosis, as evidenced from the rise of serum creatinine (1), exhausting the kidney stores of phospholipids, followed by extensive renal tissue repair (see ref. 18 for review).

Another important observation made in the present study was that the effect of gentamicin on urinary phospholipids excretion was completely suppressed by the coadministration of poly-L-aspartic acid. Poly-L-aspartic acid has been reported to protect against gentamicin-induced nephrotoxicity (9,19) and gentamicin-induced phospholipidosis (10,20). The mechanism involved in this protective effect could be related to binding of gentamicin to poly-L-aspartic acid in lysosomes, thereby interfering with the sequence of events leading from drug uptake to lysosomal phospholipidosis (20,21).

In conclusion, urinary excretion of phospholipids appears a sensitive index of aminoglycoside-induced early renal alterations and its measurement could replace that of less specific markers such as urinary enzymes or low molecular weight proteins (beta-2-micro-globulin, lysozyme). However, it must be emphasized that this determination appears useful only if performed before serum creatinine rises.

ACKNOWLEDGEMENTS

SI is the recipient of a fellowship from the Ministry of Higher Education and Scientific Research of the Republic of Iraq, and BKK. of an ICP-followship. PMT is Maître de Recherches of the Belgian Fonds National de la Recherche Scientifique. This work was supported in part by the Belgian Fonds de la Recherche Scientifique Medicale (grant no. 3.4553.88).

REFERENCES

1. Kosek JC, Mazz RI, Cousins MJ: Nephrotoxicity of gentamicin. Lab Invest 30: 48-57, 1974.

2. Laurent G, Carlier MB, Rollman B, Van Hoof F, Tulkens P: Mechanism of aminoglycoside-induced lysosomal phospholipidosis: in vitro and in vivo studies with gentamicin and amikacin. Biochem Pharmacol 31: 3861-3870, 1982.

3. Carlier MB, Laurent G, Claes PJ, Vanderhaeghe HJ, Tulkens PM: Inhibition of lysosomal phospholipases by aminoglycosides antibiotics: comparative studies in vitro. Antimicrob Agents Chemother 23: 440-449, 1983.

4. De Broe ME, Paulus GJ, Verpooten GA, Roels F, Buyssens N, Weeden R, Van Hoof F, Tulkens P: Early effects of gentamicin, tobramycin and amikacin on the human kidney. Kidney Int 25: 643-652, 1984.

5. Giurgea-Marion L, Toubeau G, Laurent G, Heuson-Stiennon J, Tulkens PM: Impairment of lysosome-pinocytic vesicle fusion in rat kidney proximal tubules after treatment with gentamicin at low doses. Toxicol Appl Pharmacol 86: 271-285, 1986.

6. Tulkens PM: Experimental studies on nephrotoxicity of aminoglycosides at low doses: mechanisms and perspectives. Am J Med 80 (6B): 105-114, 1986.

7. Tulkens PM: Nephrotoxicity of aminoglycosides. Toxicol Lett 46: 107-123, 1989.

8. Carlier MB, Kallay Z, Rollmann B, Tulkens PM: Reduction of aminoglycoside-induced renal alterations in rats by co-administration of piperacillin at clinically-relevant doses. In: Progress in Antimicrobial and Anticancer Chemotherapy (Proceedings of 15th International Congress Chemotherapy, Istanbul, Turkey), Ecomed, pp 873-875, 1987.

9. Gilbert DN, Wood CA, Kohlhepp SJ, Kohnen PW, Houghton H, Finkbeiner HC, Lindsley J, Bennet WM: Polyaspartic acid prevents experimental aminoglycoside nephrotoxicity. J Infect Dis 159:945-953, 1989.

10. Beauchamp D, Laurent G, Maldague P, Tulkens PM: Reduction of gentamicin nephrotoxicity by the concomitant administration of poly-L-aspartic acid and poly-L-asparagine in rats. Arch Toxicol (Suppl) 9:306-309, 1986.

11. Ibrahim S, Carlier MB, Laurent G, Tulkens PM: Quantitative analysis of phospholipids composition of rat kidney cortex after treatment with gentamicin, debekacin, netilmicin and tobramycin at low doses (10 mg/kg/day). In: 25th Intersc Conf Antimicrob Agents Chemother, Minneapolis, Abstract no 708, 1985.

12. Ibrahim S, Tulkens PM: Increased urinary excretion and change of patterns of phospholipids in gentamicin-treated rats. In: 26th Intersc Conf Antimicrob Agents Chemother, New Orleans, Abstract no 27, 1986.

13. Ibrahim S, Kallay Z, Clerckx-Braun F, Donnez J, Tulkens PM: Urinary phospholipids pattern after treatment with aminoglycoside antibiotics and cis-platinum. In: Bach PH, Lock EA (eds); Nephrotoxicity: Extrapolation from in vitro to in vivo, and animals to man. London, Plenum press, 1989, pp. 177-182.

14. Josepovitz C, Levine R, Farruggella T, Kaloyanides GJ: Comparative effects of aminoglycosides on renal cortical and urinary phospholipids in rat. Proc Soc Exp Med 182: 1-5, 1986.

15. Tulkens P, Laurent G, Carlier MB, Toubeau G, Heuson-Stiennon J, Maldague P: Comparative study of the alterations induced in

rat kidney by gentamicin, dibekacin, netilmicin, tobramycin and amikacin at low doses. In: (Spitzy K, Karrer K (eds); Proc 13th Internat Congress Chemotherapy, Vienna, Vol. 86. pp. 30-35, 1983.

16. Matsumoto K, Lambricht P, Kishore BK, Ibrahim S, Rollmann B, Laurent G, Tulkens PM: In vitro and in vivo evalution of the early renal alterations induced by HAPA-gentamicin B (isepamicin). In: 28th Intersc Conf Antimicrob Agents Chemother, Los Angeles, Abstract no. 1503, 1988.

17. Josepovitz C, Farruggella T, Levine R, Lane B, Kaloyanides GJ: Effect of netilmicin on the phospholipid composition of subcellular fractions of rat renal cortex. J Pharmacol Exp Ther 235: 810-819, 1985.

18. Laurent G, Maldague P, Toubeau G, Heuson-Stiennon JA, Tulkens PM: Kidney tissue repair after nephrotoxic injury: biochemical and morphological characterization. CRC Crit Rev

Toxicol 19:147-183, 1988.

19. Williams PD, Hottendorf GH, Bennet DB: Inhibition of renal membrane binding and nephrotoxicity of aminoglycosides. J Pharmacol Exp Ther 237:919-925, 1986.

20. Kishore BK, Mingeot-Leclercq MP, Kallay Z, Beauchamp D, Tulkens PM: Mechanism of the protection afforded by poly-L-aspartic acid against gentamicin-induced nephrotoxicity: poly-L-aspartic acid binds gentamicin in lysosomes. In: 28th Intersc Conf Antimicrob Agents Chemother, Los Angeles, Abstract no 293, 1988.

21. Kishore BK, Lambricht P, Ibrahim S, Laurent G, Tulkens PM: Inhibition of aminoglycoside-induced nephrotoxicity in rats by polyanionic peptides. I. In vitro and in vivo biochemical studies. In: 6th International Symposium of Nephrology at Montecatini. Kidney, Proteins and Drugs, Montecatini Terme, Italy, p. 58, 1989.

18

POLYASPARTIC ACID INHIBITS GENTAMICIN-INDUCED PERTURBATION OF PHOSPHOLIPID METABOLISM IN CULTURED RENAL CELLS

G. J. Kaloyanides, L. Ramsammy and C. Josepovitz

Division of Nephrology and Hypertension, Department of Medicine, State University of New York at Stony Brook, Stony Brook, New York 11794, and Department of Veterans Affairs Medical Center, Northport, New York 11768

INTRODUCTION

The pathogenesis of aminoglycoside antibiotic-induced acute renal failure involves a two-step process consisting of the transport and accumulation of the drug by renal proximal tubular cells followed by an adverse interaction of these polycationic compounds with one or more critical intracellular processes (1). Recently, polyaspartic acid (PAA) a polymer of the anionic amino acid aspartate, has been shown to protect rats against the development of aminoglycoside nephrotoxicity without reducing the amount of drug accumulated by renal proximal tubular cells (2). From this observation it follows that PAA must interfere with a pathogenic step distal to the uptake of drug. Among the numerous metabolic derangements in renal proximal tubular cells caused by these drugs, the most prominent is altered phospholipid metabolism (3). We have previously reported that these drugs induce a phosphatidylinositol (PI) enriched phospholipidosis in renal cortical cells in vivo (4) and in culture (5) and that the phospholipidosis reflects primarily the accumulation of phospholipid within lysosomes in the form of myeloid bodies (6) consequent to impaired phospholipid degradation (5) which, as others have shown, is due to inhibition of lysosomal phospholipase activity (7,8). More recently we have presented evidence that gentamicin disrupts agonist activation of the PI cascade in renal proximal tubular cells by a mechanism most likely involving electrostatic binding between the polycationic drug with the polyanionic phosphatidylinositol-4-5'- bisphosphate (9). Disruption of phospholipid metabolism has been advanced as the fundamental pathogenic mechanism underlying aminoglycoside nephrotoxicity (10). Thus, we decided to investigate whether PAA has the capacity to inhibit gentamicin-induced perturbations of phospholipid metabolism in cultured renal proximal tubular cells.

METHODS

Experiments were performed in OK_1 cells, an established line derived from the proximal tubule of opossum kidney (11), grown in Eagle's minimal essential medium containing Earle's balanced salt solution and supplemented with 10% fetal calf serum under 5% CO_2 and room air at $37^{\circ}C$. Primary cultures of rabbit proximal tubular cells were prepared as previously reported from this laboratory (5). Cells were incubated in medium containing PAA (3×10^{-4}M), gentamicin (10^{-3}M) or both for 6 days at which time gentamicin accumulation and total phospholipid were determined (5). Other cells were incubated with [^{3}H]myoinositol to label the phosphoinositide pool following which we examined the effects of PAA, gentamicin and gentamicin plus PAA on the degradation of phosphoinositides assayed as the rate of disappearance of label from the phospholipid pool (5). In other experiments we examined whether PAA prevented gentamicin from inhibiting bradykinin (BK) stimulation of protein kinase C. Monolayers were incubated in control medium or in medium containing PAA, gentamicin or gentamicin plus PAA for 48 hr. Then half the cells were stimulated with BK (10^{-6}M) for 3 min following which the cells were processed and analyzed for the redistribution of protein kinase C from the cytosolic to the membrane fraction (9). The above experiments were performed on OK$_1$ cells. In primary cultures of rabbit proximal tubular cells we examined whether PAA prevented gentamicin from inhibiting BK generation of IP$_3$. The experimental methods were identical to those previously reported (9).

RESULTS

The results are summarized in Table 1. After 6 days of incubation there was no difference between the accumulation of gentamicin by OK$_1$ cells grown in medium with PAA and that of cells grown in medium without PAA. OK$_1$ cells exposed to gentamicin developed a marked increase in total phospholipid in association with the appearance of lysosomal myeloid bodies. In OK$_1$ cells exposed to gentamicin plus PAA total phospholipid was not different from control. Moreover these cells contained only rare lysosomal myeloid bodies; however, large cytoplasmic vacuoles with a coarsely granular matrix were evident. In cells exposed to PAA the $t_{1/2}$ for the degradation of phosphoinositides was 2.6 days, which is not different from that of control cells. In cells exposed to gentamicin the $t_{1/2}$ was prolonged to 6.9 days. In the presence of gentamicin plus PAA the $t_{1/2}$ was reduced to 3.3 days. BK stimulated a two-fold increase of IP$_3$ whereas in cells exposed to gentamicin for two days IP$_3$ did not rise above baseline following stimulation by BK. In cells exposed to gentamicin plus PAA, BK stimulated a significant increase of IP$_3$ equal in magnitude to that observed in cells exposed to PAA alone. In control cells BK stimulated a decline of protein kinase C activity in the cytosolic fraction in association with a reciprocal rise of protein kinase C activity in the membrane fraction. No redistribution of protein

kinase C activity was detected in cells exposed to gentamicin alone; however, in the presence of gentamicin plus PAA there was a significant BK-stimulated redistribution of protein kinase C from the cytosolic to the membrane fraction equal in magnitude to that observed in cells exposed to PAA alone.

DISCUSSION

The purpose of these experiments was to determine whether PAA has the capacity to inhibit gentamicin-induced perturbations of phospholipid metabolism. We chose to examine this question in cultured proximal tubular cells, because we have utilized this model previously to characterize the alterations of phospholipid metabolism caused by gentamicin (5,9). As a first step it was necessary to document that PAA did not inhibit the accumulation of gentamicin by cultured renal proximal tubule cells. This finding in cell culture is in agreement with in vivo studies showing that PAA does not depress the renal accumulation of aminoglycoside antibiotics in the rat (2,12). From this observation we have inferred that the protective effects of PAA must be exerted at a step distal to the uptake and accumulation of antibiotic. A corollary of this conclusion is that PAA is also accumulated by renal proximal tubular cells in vivo and in vitro. Although we have not directly tested this assumption, Kallay and Tulkens (13) have presented evidence that PAA, like gentamicin, is accumulated by renal proximal tubular cells. We suspect that the large cytoplasmic vacuoles with coarsely granular matrix observed in our cultured cells exposed to PAA reflects the uptake and accumulation of this amino acid peptide.

The results of our experiments confirm the findings of our previously reported cell culture studies (5,9) in which it was shown that renal proximal tubular cells grown in medium containing gentamicin manifest a time-dependent increase of phospholipid in association with the appearance of lysosomal myeloid bodies, impaired degradation of phospholipid as assessed by the delayed disappearance of labeled phospho-inositides and disruption of

Table 1. Effect of polyaspartic acid (PAA) on gentamicin (G)-induced perturbations of phospholipid metabolism in cultured renal cells.1

	Control	PAA	G	G+PAA
Gentamicin Uptake ug/mg protein	-	-	(5) 26.0±1.0	(5) 29.7±1.4
Total Phospholipid nmol/mg protein	(5) 242±4	(5) 261±6	(5) 414±8**	(5) 251±6
PI Degradation t 1/2 (days)	(5) 2.4	(5) 2.6	(5) 6.9	(5) 3.3
IP3 (baseline) dpm	(5) 1344±133	(5) 1290±72	(5) 1723±139	(5) 1389±115
IP3 (bradykinin) dpm	(5) 2638±191[b]	(5) 2146±96[b]	(5) 1720±175	(5) 2191±177[b]
PKCcyt(baseline) pmol Pi/mg protein	(5) 1199±40	(5) 864±40	(5) 1204±44	(5) 900±16
PKCcyt(bradykinin) pmol Pi/mg protein	(5) 894±40[b]	(5) 735±29[a]	(5) 1203±61	(5) 784±45[a]
PKCmemb(baseline) pmol Pi/mg protein	(5) 507±24	(5) 868±35	(5) 483±27	(5) 642±33
PKCmemb.(bradykinin) pmol Pi/mg protein	(5) 819±20[b]	(5) 956±47[b]	(5) 551±24	(5) 850±36[b]

1. Data represent mean ±SE. Numbers in parenthesis = N. PI, phosphatidylinositol; IP₃, inositol phosphates; PKC, protein kinase C. **, significantly different from control, $P<0.01$. "a", "b", significantly different from baseline, $P<0.05$ and P <0.01 respectively.

the PI cascade as assessed by the failure of BK to stimulate increased generation of IP3 and redistribution of protein kinase C. These alterations in phospholipid metabolism were either completely or almost completely prevented in cells grown in medium containing gentamicin plus PAA at a molar concentration ratio similar to that we administered to rats in vivo (14). Since PAA by itself had no detectable influence on phospholipid metabolism, we conclude that PAA inhibited gentamicin from perturbing phospholipid metabolism in cultured renal proximal tubular cells.

Previous investigators have established that aminoglycoside antibiotics, being organic polycations, bind electrostatically to anionic phospholipids of biological and model membranes (15-20) and alter their biophysical properties (21-24). For example we have previously reported that gentamicin depresses the glycerol permeability of phosphatidylcholine: phosphotidylinositol (PC:PI) liposomes (23), and stimulates liposomal aggregation (24). Both effects are a consequence of an electrostatic interaction between the cationic gentamicin and the anionic PI. In a companion paper (25) we report that PAA inhibits these actions of gentamicin by a mechanism most likely involving an electrostatic interaction between the anionic PAA and the cationic gentamicin. Since anionic phospholipids have been shown to be the preferred membrane binding sites of aminoglycoside antibiotics (16,19,20,22,26), the results of our experiments support the hypothesis that the toxicity of aminoglycosides is causally linked to the electrostatic interaction between these organic polycations and membrane anionic phospholipids and the resulting disturbances of phospholipid metabolism and membrane function related thereto.

ACKNOWLEDGMENT

This research was supported by NIH grant AM-27061 and a grant from the Medical Research Service, Department of Veterans Affairs. The authors express their appreciation to Pamela Geller for expert secretarial assistance in preparing this manuscript for publication.

REFERENCES

1. Kaloyanides GJ, Pastoriza-Munoz E: Aminoglycoside Nephrotoxicity. Kidney Int 18:571-582, 1980.

2. Williams PD, Hottendorf GH, Bennett DB: Inhibition of renal membrane binding and nephrotoxicity of aminoglyocisdes. J Pharmacol Exp Ther 237:919-925, 1986.

3. Kaloyanides GJ: Aminoglyocside-induced functional and biochemical defects in the renal cortex. Fund Appl Toxicol 4:930-943, 1984.

4. Feldman S, Wang M-Y, Kaloyanides GJ: Aminoglyocsides induce a phospholipidosis in the renal cortex of the rat: an early manifestation of nephrotoxicity. J Pharmacol Exp Ther 220:514-520, 1982.

5. Ramsammy LS, Josepovitz C, Lane B, Kaloyanides GJ: Effect of gentamicin on phospholipid metabolism in cultured rabbit proximal tubular cells. Am J Physiol 256: C204-C213, 1989.

6. Josepovitz C, Farruggella T, Levine R, Lane B, Kaloyanides GJ: Effect of netilmicin on the phospholipid composition of subcellular fractions of rat renal cortex. J Pharmacol Exp Ther 235:810-819, 1985.

7. Laurent G, Carlier M-B, Rollman B, Van Hoof F, Tulkens P: Mechanism of aminoglycoside-induced lysosomal phospholipidosis: in vitro and in vivo studies with gentamicin and amikacin. Biochem Pharmacol 31:3861-3870, 1982.

8. Hostettler KY, Hall LB: Inhibition of kidney lysosomal phospholipases A and C by aminoglycoside antibiotics: possible mechanisms of aminoglycoside toxicity. Proc Natl Acad Sci USA 79:1663-1667, 1982.

9. Ramsammy LS, Josepovitz C, Kaloyanides GJ: Gentamicin inhibits agonist stimulation of the phosphatidylinositol cascade in primary cultures of rabbit proximal tubular cells and in rat renal cortex. J Pharmacol Exp Ther 247:989-996, 1988.

10. Tulkens PM: Nephrotoxicity of aminoglycoside antibiotics. Tox Lett 46:107-123, 1989.

11. Teitelbaum AP, Strewler GJ: Parathyroid hormone receptors coupled to cyclic adenosine monophosphate formation in an established renal cell line. Endocrinol 114:980-985, 1984.

12. Gilbert DN, Wood CA, Kohlhepps SJ, Kohnen PW, Houghton DC, Finkbeiner HC, Lindsley J, Bennett WM: Polyaspartic acid prevents experimental aminoglycoside nephrotoxicity. J Inf Dis 159:945-953, 1989.

13. Kallay Z, Tulkens PM: Uptake and subcellular distribution of poly-L-aspartic acid. A protectant against aminoglycoside-induced nephrotoxicity in rat kidney cortex. In: Bach PH, Lock EA (eds); Nephrotoxicity: In Vitro to In Vivo, Animals to Man. New York, Plenum Press, 1989, pp 189-192.

14. Kaloyanides GJ, Ramsammy L, Josepovitz C: Assessment of three therapeutic interventions for modifying gentamicin nephrotoxicity in the rat. In: Bach PH, Delacruz L, Gregg NJ, Wilks MF (eds); Proceedings of the

Fourth International Symposium on Nephrotoxicity. New York, Marcel Dekker, 1990, this volume.

15. Kirschenbaum BB: Interactions between renal brush border membranes and polyamines. J Pharmacol Exp Ther 229:409-416, 1984.

16. Schacht J, Weiner ND, Lodhi S: Interaction of aminocyclitol antibiotics with polyphosphoinositides in mammalian tissues and artificial membranes. In: Wells WW, Eisenberg F (eds); Cyclitols and Phosphoinositides. New York, Academic Press, 1978, pp 153-165.

17. Brasseur R, Laurent G, Ruysschaert JM, Tulkens P: Interactions of aminoglycoside antibiotics with negatively charged lipid layers. Biochem Pharmacol 33:629-637, 1984.

18. Chung L, Kaloyanides GJ, McDaniel R, McLaughlin A, McLaughlin S: Interaction of gentamicin and spermine with bilayer membranes containing negatively charged phospholipids. Biochemistry 24:442-452, 1985.

19. Sastrasinh M, Knauss TC, Weinberg JM, Humes DM: Identification of the aminoglycoside binding site in rat renal brush border membranes. J Pharmacol Exp Ther 222:350-358, 1982.

20. Gabev E, Kasianowica J, Abbott T, McLaughlin S: Binding of neomycin to phosphatidylinositol 4,5-bisphosphate (PIP_2). Biochem Biophys Acta 979:105-112, 1989.

21. Au S, Weiner ND, Schacht J: Aminoglycoside antibiotics preferentially increase permeability in phosphoinositide-containing membranes: a study with carboxyfluorescein in liposomes. Biochem Biophys Acta 902:80-86, 1987.

22. Wang BM, Weiner ND, Takada A, Schacht J: Characterization of aminoglycoside-lipid interactions and developoment of a refined model for ototoxicity testing. Biochem Pharmacol 33:3257-3262, 1984.

23. Ramsammy LS, Kaloyanides GJ: Effect of gentamicin on the transition temperature and permeability to glycerol of phosphatidylinositol containing liposomes. Biochem Pharmacol 36:1179-1181, 1987.

24. Ramsammy LS, Kaloyanides GJ: The effect of gentamicin on the biophysical properties of phosphatidic acid liposomes is influenced by the 0-C=0 group of the lipid. Biochem 27:8249-8254, 1988.

25. Kaloyanides GJ, Ramsammy L: Alterations of biophysical properties of liposomes predict aminoglycoside toxicity: inhibitory effect of polyaspartic acid. In: Bach PH, Delacruz L, Gregg NJ, Wilks MF (eds); Proceedings of the Fourth International Symposium on Nephrotoxicity. New York, Marcel Dekker, 1990, this volume.

26. Williams SE, Schact J: Binding of neomycin and calcium to phospholipids and other anionic compounds. J Antibiotics 39:457-462, 1986.

19

ALTERATIONS OF BIOPHYSICAL PROPERTIES OF LIPOSOMES PREDICT AMINOGLYCOSIDE TOXICITY: INHIBITORY EFFECT OF POLYASPARTIC ACID

G. J. Kaloyanides and L. Ramsammy

Division of Nephrology and Hypertension, Department of Medicine, State University of New York at Stony Brook, Stony Brook, New York 11794, and Department of Veterans Affairs Medical Center, Northport, New York 11768

INTRODUCTION

The toxicity of aminoglycoside antibiotics resides in the potential of these drugs to be transported and accumulated by renal proximal tubular cells (1) where they bind to and alter the function of plasma and subcellular membranes (2-11). Several lines of evidence indicate that these organic polycations preferentially bind to anionic phospholipids (12), especially phosphoinositides (13-15). This finding has stimulated investigations using model membranes into the mechanism by which aminoglycoside antibiotics bind to anionic phospholipids (15-20) and the effects of such binding on the biophysical properties of the membrane (15,17,18,20-26). Recently we presented evidence that the binding of gentamicin to anionic phospholipid involves not only an electrostatic interaction between the positively charged amino groups of the antibiotics and the negatively charged phosphate head group of the phospholipid, but also hydrogen bonding between the cationic amino groups and carbonyl groups of the glycerol backbone of the lipid (18). Furthermore, we presented evidence that hydrogen bonding was an important determinant of the effect of gentamicin on glycerol permeability and aggregation of liposomal membranes (18). In this paper we report that the relative potentials of aminoglycoside antibiotics to depress glycerol permeability and promote aggregation of phosphatidylinositol (PI)-containing liposomes

correlate with a high degree of precision with the established clinical nephrotoxicity potentials of these drugs. In addition we report that polyaspartic acid (PAA) inhibits gentamicin from altering these biophysical properties of PI-containing liposomes and that this action probably explains the protective effect of this polypeptide.

METHODS

Phosphatidylcholine (PC) and PI at a molar ratio of 1:1 were dispersed in 0.15 M KCl, 10 mM Tris HCl, pH 7.0 by means of a Vortex to form multilamellar liposomes. Liposomes (15 mmoles lipid/ml) were incubated with and without polycation at 50°C for 1 hr and stored under N_2 at room temperature for 20 hr. The polycations studied were spermine (10^{-4}M), netilmicin (10^{-4}M), tobramycin (10^{-4}M), gentamicin (10^{-4}M) and neomycin (5×10^{-5}M). Glycerol permeability was measured by adding 20 ml of liposomes to 1.0 ml of 0.3 M glycerol and monitoring at 450 nm the change in absorbance due to liposome swelling. The relative permeability ($p^{\sim}$) was calculated using the formula:

$$p^{\sim} = dA/A_o^2 \, t_1$$ where dA equals the change in absorbance over time (t) and A_o equals the initial absorbance (18). Measurements were performed between 20° and 33°C. The energy of activation (E_a) for glycerol permeation was calculated from the Arrhenius plot of the data.

117

Unilamellar liposomes of phosphatidyethanolamine (PE):PI and PC:PI were prepared in 5 mM HEPES, 0.2 mM Tris and 0.2 mM Na$_2$EDTA, pH 7.0 (18) and surface electrostatic potential was calculated from the partitioning of methylene blue (MB) (18). Liposomes were incubated with varying concentrations of polycations at 37°C for 1 hr prior to incubation with MB (2x10^{-5}M) for 30 min at room temperature following which an absorbance spectrum between 725 and 560 nm was obtained with a Beckman scanning spectrophotometer. Aggregation was measured by the turbidity method as previously reported (18).

RESULTS

Each aminoglycoside depressed the glycerol permeability of PC:PI liposomes whereas the organic polycation spermine was without effect (Figure 1). The rank order for aminoglycoside-induced depression of glycerol permeability was neomycin > gentamicin > tobramycin > netilmicin. Clear differences between these drugs were evident at the lower temperatures of 20° and 24°C. At 27°C differences between tobramycin and netilmicin were abolished. At 33°C all antibiotics were equivalent and only slight depression of glycerol permeability were detected.

The permeability data were subjected to an Arrhenius plot from which we calculated the energy of activation (E$_a$) for glycerol permeation (Figure 2). Neomycin, gentamicin and tobramycin significantly increased E$_a$ for glycerol permeation of PC:PI liposomes above the control value. Netilmicin and spermine had no effect on E$_a$. Since neomycin at 5x10^{-5}M had the same effect as gentamicin at 10^{-4}M, the rank order of the polycations with respect to their effects on E$_a$ for glycerol permeation was neomycin > gentamicin > tobramycin > netilmicin = spermine = control.

We measured the aggregation threshold, defined as the lowest concentration of cation at which a measurable change in OD is detected, for the various cations. The aggregation threshold concentrations were (μM): calcium, 1000; spermine, 80; netilmicin, 80; tobramycin, 20; gentamicin, 15; neomycin, 3. The relative effects of these cations at 8x10^{-4}M on liposome aggregation were examined (Figure 3). With the exception of spermine the same relative potencies were observed as for the threshold concentrations.

Whereas there were clearly identifiable differences among these organic polycations with respect to their effects on glycerol permeability and aggregation of liposomes, no significant

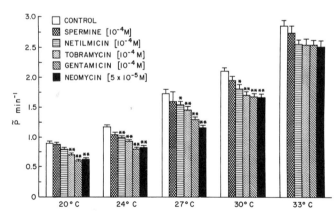

Figure 1. Effect of organic polycations on the relative permeability coefficient (p~) for glycerol permeation in PC:PI liposomes. Data represent mean ± SE, N8. *,**, significantly different from control, p<0.05 and p<0.01, respectively.

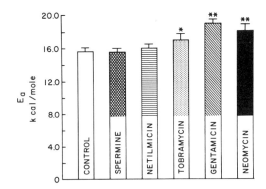

Figure 2. Effect of organic polycations on the energy of activation (Ea) for glycerol permeation in PC:PI liposomes. Data represent mean ± SE, N=8. Kcal, kilocalories. *,**, significantly different from control, p<0.05 and p<0.01, respectively.

differences among gentamicin, tobramycin, netilmicin and spermine were detected with respect to the concentration dependent effects of these agents on the membrane surface potential of PE:PI liposomes (Figure 4). Of all the agents examined, neomycin showed the greatest potential to neutralize membrane surface charge (Figure 4).

Incubation of liposomes with PAA (3×10^{-4}M) resulted in inhibition of gentamicin (10^{-3}M) induced depression of glycerol permeability (Figure 5). PAA was also effective in inhibiting gentamicin-induced aggregation of liposomes (Figure 6) but only if added prior to gentamicin. If aggregation was initiated by the prior addition of gentamicin to liposomes, the subsequent addition of PAA was unable to stop or reverse aggregation (data not shown). The molar concentration ratio of gentamicin/PAA was a critical determinant of the observed response. As shown in the right panel of Figure 6, when liposomes were exposed to a lower concentration of PAA (2×10^{-5}M), the subsequent addition of gentamicin (1.65×10^{-5}M) provoked an immediate and maximal rise in absorbance, a pattern strikingly different from that observed when gentamicin was added to liposomes in the absence of PAA (see left panel of Figure 6). This finding suggested that gentamicin was forming an aggregating complex with PAA. This suspi-

cion was confirmed by subsequent experiments in which gentamicin was mixed with PAA in the absence of liposomes. When the gentamicin/PAA molar concentration ratio exceeded 8.25, a maximal rise in absorbance was seen in association with the development of a cloudy solution. Further evidence of a direct electrostatic interaction between gentamicin and PAA was provided by the experiment illustrated in Figure 7. Addition of 8×10^{-4}M PAA to 2×10^{-5}M methylene blue (MB) sharply depressed the maximal absorbance of MB (compare curves a and b). The amplitude of the MB absorbance is directly related to the free MB concentration in solution (18). The fall in MB absorbance in response to the addition of PAA signifies a decline in the free concentration of MB secondary to the formation of an electrostatic complex between the cationic dye and the anionic PAA as PAA does not absorb at this wave length. Addition of gentamicin restored the absorbance of MB in a concentration-dependent manner (curves c-f) and reflects the ability of this organic polycationic drug to form an electrostatic complex with PAA.

DISCUSSION

The results of our experiments demonstrate that aminoglycoside antibiotics depress glycerol permeability and cause aggregation of PI-containing liposomes. Since previous studies have established that these drugs do not bind to PC or PE (15,20), it follows that these changes are related to an electrostatic interaction between the polycationic aminoglycosides and the anionic phospholipid PI. The results demonstrate, however, that the rank order with respect to the relative potentials of these drugs to depress glycerol permeability (neomycin> gentamicin > tobramycin > netilmicin = spermine) does not coincide with their net cationic charge (Table 1). This rank order also does not coincide with the relative potentials of these drugs to neutralize membrane surface charge. As shown in Figure 4, with the exception of neomycin the remaining organic polycations were equally effective in neutralizing surface charge whereas they had differing effects on glycerol permeability. A similar pat-

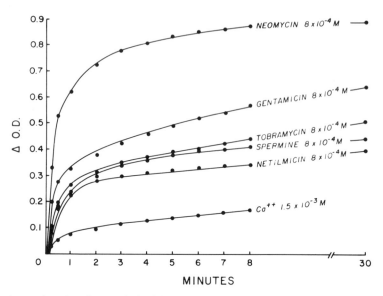

Figure 3. Effect of organic polycations and of calcium on the aggregation of PE:PI liposomes. The data points represent the mean of four determinations at each time point. The SE estimates were omitted for clarity. The lines were drawn by visual inspection.

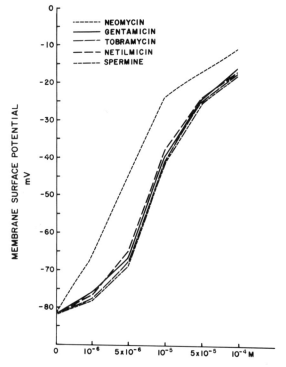

Figure 4. Influence of increasing concentrations of organic polycations on the membrane surface potential of PE:PI liposomes. Lines represent mean data derived from four replications; the SE estimates were omitted for clarity.

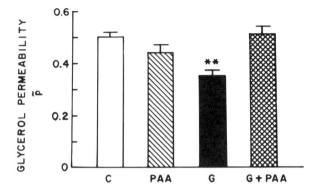

Figure 5. Effect of polyaspartic acid (PAA), gentamicin (G) and gentamicin plus polyaspartic acid on glycerol permeability of PC:PI liposomes. Data represent the mean $\pm$ SE, N=5. ** signifies significantly different from control (c). $\tilde{p}$ equals the relative permeability coefficient.

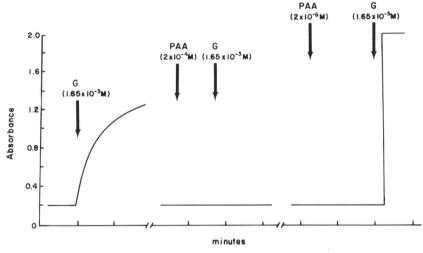

Figure 6. Prior addition of polyaspartic acid (PAA) inhibits gentamicin (G)-induced aggregation of PC:PI liposomes. This representative tracing demonstrates that addition of $1.65 \times 10\text{-}3M$ G (left panel) caused aggregation of PC:PI liposomes whereas no aggregation was seen when PAA was added to liposomes prior to the addition of G (middle panel). The right panel demonstrates that when the concentration of PAA was reduced to $2 \times 10\text{-}5M$ while holding G constant, it provoked a maximal rise in absorbance, a pattern distinctly different from that seen in the left panel.

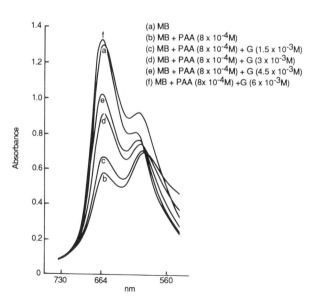

(a) MB
(b) MB + PAA ($8 \times 10^{-4}M$)
(c) MB + PAA ($8 \times 10^{-4}M$) + G ($1.5 \times 10^{-3}M$)
(d) MB + PAA ($8 \times 10^{-4}M$) + G ($3 \times 10^{-3}M$)
(e) MB + PAA ($8 \times 10^{-4}M$) + G ($4.5 \times 10^{-3}M$)
(f) MB + PAA ($8 \times 10^{-4}M$) + G ($6 \times 10^{-3}M$)

Figure 7. Reversal of polyaspartic acid (PAA)-induced depression of methylene blue (MB) absorbence by gentamicin (G). This representative tracing demonstrates that PAA sharply depressed the absorbance of MB (compare curves a and b) which signifies a reduction of the free concentration MB consequent to the electrostatic binding of the cationic MB to the anionic PAA. Addition of G raised the absorbance of MB in a concentration dependent manner (curves c to f) which signifies that G competed with MB for binding to PAA.

Table 1. Ranking of aminoglycosides and spermine according to charge.

	maximum charge	net charge at pH 7.4
Neomycin	+6.0	+4.37
Netilmicin	+5.0	+3.48
Gentamicin	+5.0	+3.46
Tobramycin	+5.0	+3.10
Spermine	+4.0	+3.62

tern was observed with respect to the rank order of these drugs in initiating liposomal agregation: neomycin > gentamicin> tobramycin> netilmicin> spermine. Except for the minor reversal of spermine and netilmicin, the same rank order was observed with respect to the magnitude of aggregation induced by these agents at 8×10^{-4}M.

It is evident that close apposition of liposomal membranes is an obligatory step in aggregation. Membranes containing PI have a negative surface potential that generates a strong repulsive force, therefore membrane surface charge must be neutralized for liposomal aggregation to occur. While neutralization of membrane surface charge may be a necessary condition for aggregation, the data depicted in Figure 4 indicates that neutralization of charge is not sufficient to explain the differences in the relative aggregation potentials of these drugs illustrated in Figure 3. Thus, some other interaction between these drugs and PI must be operating. We postulate that the ability of these drugs to engage in hydrogen bonding with the carbonyl group of the glycerol backbone is a major determinant of their effects on glycerol permeability and aggregation of liposomes (18). Hydrogen bonding requires precise spatial orientation of donor groups and acceptor groups. Thus, the lack of a tight correlation between net charge and the effects of these organic polycations on the biophysical properties of model membranes may be related to the orientation of specific protonated amino groups. In this regard it is noteworthy that netilmicin has a net charge equivalent to that of gentamicin (Table 1) but its effects on glycerol

permeability and aggregation of liposomes are substantially less than those of gentamicin. Netilmicin is a semi-synthetic analogue of gentamicin C_{1a}; it differs from the parent compound by the acetylation of a primary amino group located on the central aminocyclitol ring (27) which could limit netilmicin's capacity to engage in hydrogen bonding.

Although the rank order describing the potentials of these aminoglycosides to depress glycerol permeability and cause aggregation of liposomes does not correlate with their net cationic charge, it does correlate precisely with the established toxicity potentials of these agents in man (28) and in experimental animals (29). These findings suggest that the toxicity of these drugs is intimately linked with their propensity to interact electrostatically and by hydrogen bonding with anionic phospholipids of biomembranes. Inhibition of phospholipid degradation with the accumulation of phospholipid in the form of myeloid bodies (30,31), disruption of the PI cascade (32), inhibition of mitochondrial respiration (6-8), and disturbance of lysosomal integrity (8-10) are several of the more obvious consequences of aminoglycoside-membrane interactions. Although the temporal order of involvement and the relative importance of these specific drug-membrane interactions in the pathogenesis of aminoglycoside-induced proximal tubular cell injury and necrosis remain to be established, it appears highly likely that the fundamental mechanism underlying the toxicity of these drugs is their potential to interact electrostatically and by hydrogen bonding with anionic phospholipids of cell membrane.

This concept of the pathogenesis of aminoglycoside toxicity is strengthened by the experiments with PAA. We and others have shown that this polyanionic peptide confers protection against aminoglycoside nephrotoxicity in the rat (5,33,34). In a companion paper we reported that PAA inhibited gentamicin from perturbing phospholipid metabolism in cultured renal cells (35). Now we have demonstrated that PAA inhibited gentamicin from depressing liposomal glycerol permeability and from aggregating liposomes. The mechanism of inhibition appears to involve the formation of an electrostatic complex between the polyanionic peptide and the polycationic gentamicin. Evidence for this conclusion includes the test tube demonstration that when the gentamicin/PAA molar concentration ratio exceeded 8.25, a cloudy precipitate formed. Even more convincing is the MB experiment which indicates that gentamicin interacts electrostatically with PAA at all concentrations. We suspect that the optimal concentration for completely preventing aminoglycoside nephrotoxicity is that which is sufficient to neutralize the net charge of the polycation. In other words PAA functions as an anionic substrate competing with anionic phospholipid as a binding site for aminoglycoside antibiotics.

ACKNOWLEDGEMENT

This research was supported by a grant from the NIH, AM-27061 and from the Medical Research Service, Department of Veterans Affairs. The authors express their appreciation to Pamela Geller for expert secretarial assistance in preparing this manuscript for publication.

REFERENCES

1. Kaloyanides GJ: Renal pharmacology of aminoglycoside antibiotics. In: Berlyne CM, Giovannetti S (eds); Contr Nephrology, vol 42. Basel, Karger, 1984, pp. 148-167.

2. Kaloyanides, GJ: Aminoglycoside-induced functional and biochemical defects in the renal cortex. Fund Appl Toxicol 4:930-943, 1984.

3. Williams PD, Holoham PD, Ross CR: Gentamicin nephrotoxicity. I. Acute biochemical correlates in rats. Toxicol Appl Pharmacol 61:234-242, 1981.

4. Williams PD, Holohan PD, Ross CR: Gentamicin nephrotoxicity. II. Plasma membrane changes. Toxicol Appl Pharmacol 61:243-251, 1981.

5. Williams PD, Hottendorf GH, Bennett DB. Inhibition of renal membrane binding and nephrotoxicity of aminoglycosides. J Pharmacol Exp Ther 237:919-925, 1986.

6. Mela-Riker LM, Widener LL, Houghton CD, Bennett WM: Renal mitochondrial integrity during continuous gentamicin treatment. Biochem Pharmacol 35:979-984, 1986.

7. Weinberg JM, Humes HD: Mechanisms of gentamicin-induced dysfunction of renal cortical mitochondria. I. Effects on mitochondrial respiration. Arch Biochem Biophys 205:222-231, 1980.

8. Fillastre JP, Kuhn JM, Bendirdjian JP, Foucher B, Lesuer J.P., Rollin P, Vaillant R: Prediction of antibiotic nephrotoxicity. In: Hamburger J, Crosnier J (eds); Advances in Nephrology, vol 6. Year Book Med Pub, 1976, pp 148-167.

9. Powell JH, Reidenberg MM: Further studies on the response of kidney lysosomes to aminoglycosides and other cations. Biochem Pharmacol 32:3213-3220, 1983.

10. Tulkens PM: Nephrotoxicity of aminoglycoside antibiotics. Tox Let 46:107-123, 1989.

11. Buss WC, Piatt MK: Gentamicin administered in vivo reduces protein synthesis in microsomes subsequently isolated from rat kidneys but not from rat brains. J Antimicrob Chemother 15:715-721, 1985.

12. Williams SE, Schacht J: Binding of neomycin and calcium to phospholipids and other anionic compounds. J Antibiotics 39:457-462, 1986.

13. Sastrasinh M, Knauss TC, Weinberg JM, Humes DM: Identification of the aminoglycoside binding site in rat renal brush border membranes. J Pharmacol Exp Ther 222:350-358, 1982.

14. Schacht J: Isolation of an aminoglycoside receptor from guinea pig inner ear tissues and kidney. Arch Oto-Rhino-Laryngol 224:129-134, 1979.

15. Gabev Z, Kasianowicz J, Abbott T, McLaughlin S: Binding of neomycin to phos-

phatidylinositol 4,5-bisphosphate (PIP2). Biochim Biophys Acta 979:105-112, 1989.

16. Brasseur R, Laurent G, Ruys-Schaert JM, Tulkens P: Interactions of aminoglycoside antibiotics with negatively charged lipid layers. Biochem Pharmacol 33:629-637, 1984.

17. Chung L, Kaloyanides, GJ, McDaniel R, McLaughlin A, McLaughlin S: Interaction of gentamicin and spermine with bilayer membranes containing negatively charged phospholipids. Biochemistry 24:442-452, 1985.

18. Ramsammy LS, Kaloyanides GJ: The effect of gentamicin on the biophysical properties of phosphatidic acid liposomes is influenced by the 0-C=0 group of the lipid. Biochemistry 27:8249-8254, 1988.

19. Mingeot-Leclercq MP, Schanck A, Ronvaux-Dupals MF, Deleers M, Brasseur R, Ruys-Schaert JM, Laurent G, Tulkens P: Ultrastructural, physico-chemical and conformational study of the interactions of gentamicin and bis (beta-diethylaminoethylether) hexestrol with negatively charged phospholipid layers. Biochem Pharmacol 38:729-741, 1989.

20. Auslander DE, Felmeister A, Sciarrone BJ: Drug-biomolecule interactions: interaction of gentamicin with lipid monomolecular films. J Pharmaceut Sci 64:516-519, 1975.

21. Ramsammy LS, Kaloyanides GJ: Effect of gentamicin on the transition temperature and permeability to glycerol of phosphatidylinositol containing liposomes. Biochem Pharmacol 36:1179-1181, 1987.

22. Lullmann H, Vollmer B: An interaction of aminoglyocisde antibiotics with Ca binding to lipid monolayers and to biomembranes. Biochem Pharmacol 31:3769-3773, 1982.

23. Wang BM, Weiner ND, Takada A, Schacht J: Characterization of aminoglycoside-lipid interactions and development of a refined model for ototoxicity testing. Biochem Pharmacol 33:3257-3262, 1984. 24. Wang BM, Weiner ND, Ganesan MG, Schacht J: Interaction of calcium and neomycin with anionic phos-

pholipid-lecithin liposomes: a differential scanning calorimetry study. Biochem Pharmacol 33:3787-3791, 1984.

25. Au S, Schacht J, Weiner N: Membrane effects of aminoglycoside antibiotics measured in liposomes containing the fluorescent probe, 1-anilino-8-naphthalene sulfonate. Biochem Biophys Acta 862:205-210, 1986.

26. Au S, Weiner ND, Schacht J: Aminoglyocisde antibiotics preferentially increase permeability in phosphoinositide-containing membranes: a study with carboxylfluorescein in liposomes. Biochim Biophys Acta 902:80-86, 1987.

27. Wright JJ: Synthesis of 1-N-ethyl-sisomicin: a broad spectrum semi-synthetic aminoglycoside antibiotic. J Chem Soc Chem Commun 6:206-208, 1975.

28. Smith CR, Lietman PS: Comparative clinical trials of aminoglycosides. In: Whelton A, Neu H (eds); The Aminoglycosides: Microbiology, Clinical Use and Toxicology. New York, Marcel Dekker, 1982, pp 497-509.

29. Kaloyanides, GJ, Pastoriza-Munoz E: Aminoglycoside nephrotoxicity. Kidney Int 18:571-582, 1980.

30. Laurent G, Carlier MB, Rollman B, Van Hoof F, Tulkens P: Mechanism of aminoglycoside-induced lysosomal phospholipidosis: in vitro and in vivo studies with gentamicin and amikacin. Biochem Pharmacol 31:3861-3870, 1982.

31. Ramsammy LS, Josepovitz C, Lane BP, Kaloyanides GJ: Effect of gentamicin on phospholipid metabolism in cultured rabbit proximal tubular cells. Am J Physiol 256: C204-C213, 1989.

32. Ramsammy LS, Josepovitz C, Kaloyanides GJ: Gentamicin inhibits agonist stimulation of the phosphatidylinositol cascade in primary cultures of rabbit proximal tubular cells and in rat renal cortex. J Pharmacol Exp Ther 247:989-996, 1988.

33. Gilbert DN, Wood CA, Kohlhepps SJ, Kohnen PW, Houghton DC, Finkbeiner HC, Lindsley J, Bennett WM: Polyaspartic acid prevents experimental aminoglycoside nephrotoxicity. J Inf Dis 159:945-953, 1989.

34. Ramsammy LS, Josepovitz C, Lane BP, Kaloyanides GJ: Polyaspartic acid protects against gentamicin nephrotoxicity in the rat. J Pharmacol Exp Ther 250:149-153, 1989.

35. Kaloyanides GJ, Ramsammy L, Josepovitz C: Polyaspartic acid inhibits gentamicin-induced perturbations of phospholipid metabolism in cultured renal cells. In: Bach PH, Delacruz L, Gregg NJ, Wilks MF (eds); Proceedings of the Fourth International Symposium on Nephrotoxicity. New York, Marcel Dekker, 1990, this volume.

20

AMELIORATION OF GENTAMICIN NEPHROTOXICITY BY MAGNESIUM-L-ASPARTATE-HYDROCHLORIDE

H. McGlynn, B. Kavanagh and M.P. Ryan

Department of Pharmacology, University College Dublin, Dublin 4, Ireland

INTRODUCTION

Gentamicin, one of the aminoglycoside anti-biotics, has an established role in the treatment of gram-negative sepsis. The nephrotoxicity of gentamicin has encouraged several workers to develop less toxic antibiotics such as tobramycin, the monobactams and the third generation cephalosporins.

An alternative approach is to examine ways in which the toxicity of gentamicin can be reduced. Several workers have developed experimental models of gentamicin nephrotoxicity, and using these models have examined compounds which may be co-administered with gentamicin in order to ameliorate nephrotoxicity. Studies using polyamino acids, particularly polyaspartic acid, have shown protective effects on gentamicin nephrotoxicity in rats (1).

Magnesium depletion has been described through excessive renal loss following gentamicin therapy, both in humans and in experimental rats (2,3). Furthermore gentamicin nephrotoxicity was significantly worse in experimental rats rendered hypomagnesaemic prior to treatment (4).

We investigated if a preparation of magnesium-l-aspartate- hydrochloride given with gentamicin would have protective effects on renal toxicity, as assessed by biochemical and histopathological criteria .

METHODS

Male Sprague Dawley rats (n=64), weighing approximately 200-250g were used in this study. All animals had free access to water throughout the course of the experiment and were maintained on a standard rat chow diet. The animals were housed in individual metabolic cages for urine collection and were exposed to a 12hr light/ dark cycle. The animals were divided into 4 groups of 16 animals per group.

Group 1 were given saline, group 2 were given magnesium -l-aspartate- hydrochloride 4.98 mmoles/kg, group 3 were given gentamicin sulphate 60 mg/kg, and group 4 were given gentamicin and magnesium-l-aspartate -hydrochloride.

All injections were given by the intraperitoneal route twice a day for 5 days.

A 'run in' period of 2 days was allowed for all groups, the urine was collected daily and stored at $4^{\circ}C$ for subsequent enzymatic analysis. All rats were sacrificed by cervical dislocation on the 6th day 12 hr after the last drug administration.

Urinary analysis. N-acetyl-beta-D-glucosaminidase (beta-NAG) estimation was assayed as described by (5), Leucine aminopeptidase (LAP) activity was quantified by measuring the release of p-nitroaniline from the substrate leucine-p-nitroaniline. Both enzymes were expressed as units per mg urinary creatinine, which was measured by the Jaffe reaction.

Plasma analysis. Plasma creatinine and blood urea nitrogen levels were determined using standard kits (Sigma Ltd.). Plasma magnesium was monitored using atomic absorption spectrophotometry and plasma chloride using the corning 925 chloride analyser.

Histopathological analysis. Light microscopic examination and assessment of renal morphology were performed by a pathologist in a blind study. Proximal tubular and glomerular epithelial changes were graded according to the following scale.

I = normal, II = degranulation of proximal tubules and capsular adhesions, and III = diffuse tubular necrosis and focal necrosis of glomerular tufts.

Statistics. All data was compared using the students (unpaired) t-test and a value of p <0.05 was deemed significant.

RESULTS

Urinary parameters. Urinary excretion of N-acetyl-beta-D-glucosaminidase, a marker for lysosomal damage, and leucine aminopeptidase, a marker for brush border membrane damage, were measured on days 0, 2 and 4 of the study. The results for day 2 are shown in Table 1.

Table 1. Excretion of urinary enzymes N-acetyl-beta-D-glucosaminidase and leucine aminopeptidase on day 2 following treatment.

Group	N-acetyl-beta-D-glucosaminidase (units/mmol creatinine)	Leucine aminopeptidase (units/mmol creatinine)
Control (1)	0.048 ± 0.03	0.015 ± 0.008
magnesium-aspartate -hydrochloride (2)	0.024 ± 0.07	0.012 ± 0.005
gentamicin (3)	0.024 ± 0.085	0.121 ± 0.017
gentamicin + magnesium-aspartate-hydrochloride (4)	0.11 ± 0.022	0.040 ± 0.004
p value	1 v 2 N.S.	N.S.
	1 v 3 $p<0.05$	$p<0.005$
	3 v 4 $p<0.05$	$p<0.005$

Gentamicin significantly increased the urinary excretion of both these marker enzymes. It was demonstrated that the concurrent administration of magnesium-l-aspartate-hydrochloride significantly ameliorated the enzymuria induced by gentamicin.

Plasma parameters. A number of plasma measurements providing indices of renal functional damage were carried out. Results for these measurements are provided in Table 2.

Gentamicin treatment produced a significant elevation in plasma creatinine. Co-administration of magnesium-l-aspartate-hydrochloride resulted in significantly lower levels of serum creatinine. Similar trends were seen in values for blood urea nitrogen. Gentamicin caused significant hypomagnesaemia ($p<0.05$), which was prevented by the co-administration of magnesium-l-aspartate-hydrochloride. Similar results were also shown for plasma chloride with a reduction in values following gentamicin treatment and correction by co-administration of magnesium-l-aspartate-hydrochloride. Some changes were also seen in the packed cell volume.

Gentamicin treatment resulted in a packed cell volume ($66.5\pm1.5\%$) which was significantly greater than the control ($50.8\pm2.5\%$, $p<0.005$). Magnesium-l-aspartate-hydrochloride co-administration resulted in maintenance of the packed cell volume (49.2 ± 0.2 %) at control levels.

Histopathological changes. Gentamicin administration was seen to induce histopathological changes in the kidneys of the treated animals, evidenced by diffuse tubular necrosis and focal necrosis of glomerular tufts which were prominent in the kidneys of gentamicin treated animals indicated by Grade II (n=6)and Grade III (n=8). Treatment with magnesium-l-aspartate-hydrochloride alone (n=10)and magnesium-l-aspartate-hydrochloride with gentamicin(n=10) showed a reduced histopathological profile similar to that observed in the controls (n=7) indicated by Grade I (normal) in all cases.

Table 2. Plasma creatinine, blood urea nitrogen and magnesium on day 5 following treatment.

Group	Plasma creatinine (mg %)	Blood Urea Nitrogen (mg %)	Magnesium (mmol/L)
Control (1)	0.37 ± 0.04	6.7 ± 1.12	1.2 ± 0.15
magnesium-aspartate -hydrochloride (2)	0.36 ± 0.09	6.8 ± 0.5	1.25 ± 0.06
gentamicin (3)	0.81 ± 0.04	12.7 ± 3.9	0.86 ± 0.08
gentamicin + magnesium-aspartate -hydrochloride (4)	0.65 ± 0.003	6.31 ± 3.1	1.08 ± 0.08
p value	1 v 2 N.S.	N.S.	N.S.
	1 v 3 $p<0.0005$	$p<0.01$	$p<0.05$
	3 v 4 $p<0.005$	N.S.	$p<0.05$

CONCLUSION

Gentamicin, when given alone, caused significant nephrotoxicity as indicated in the urinary, plasma and histopathological criteria examined. Magnesium-l-aspartate-hydrochloride when given alone was shown to have no adverse effects in all the indices of nephrotoxicity assessed. Concurrent administration of gentamicin and magnesium-l-aspartate-chloride was shown to produce a significant amelioration of gentamicin nephrotoxicity as compared to gentamicin alone. The mechanism of amelioration is as yet not fully understood but may relate to a reduction in accumulation of the gentamicin moiety into the renal proximal cell or the intracellular accumulation into the lysosome.

ACKNOWLEDGEMENTS

This work was supported by Eolas, the Irish Science and Technology Agency.

REFERENCES

1. Williams PD and Hottendorf GH. Inhibition of renal membrane binding and nephrotoxicity of gentamicin by polyaspartic acid in the rat. Res Commun Chem Path and Pharmacol 47:317-320, 1985.

2. Bar RS, Wilson HE and Mazzaferri EL. Hypomagnesaemic hypocalcemia secondary to renal magnesium wasting. A possible consequence of high-dose gentamicin therapy. Ann Int Med 82:646-649, 1979.

3. Nanji AA and Denegri JF. Hypomagnesaemia associated with gentamicin therapy. Drug Intell Pharm 18:596-598, 1984.

4. Rankin LI, Krous H, Fryer AW, Whong R. Enhancement of gentamicin nephrotoxicity by magnesium depletion in the rat. Gen Electrol Metab 10:199-203, 1984.

5. Jones BR, Bhalla RR, Mladek J, Kaleya RN, Gralla RJ, Schwartz MK, Young CW and Reidenberg MM. Comparison of methods of evaluating the nephrotoxicity of cisplatin. Clin Pharmacol Ther 27:557-562, 1980.

21

MORPHOLOGICAL EVIDENCE OF NEPHROTOXICITY OF POLY-D-GLUTAMIC ACID IN RATS

P. Maldague (1), B.K. Kishore (2), P. Lambricht (2), S. Ibrahim (2), G. Laurent (2) and P.M. Tulkens (2)

Unit of Pathology and Experimental Cytology (1) and Laboratory of Physiological Chemistry (2), Catholic University of Louvain and International Institute of Cellular and Molecular Pathology (2), Bruxelles, Belgium

INTRODUCTION

The kidney is one of the main sites of uptake and metabolism of circulating low molecular weight proteins and peptides (1), and therefore plays a major role in their turnover. These constituents are usually taken up by the proximal tubular cells by endocytosis after being filtered through the glomeruli. Tubular absorption of proteins is a selective process that is determined by the nature of the protein molecule such as size, compactness, net charge, type of positively charged groups etc. The endocytosed proteins are generally hydrolysed by lysosomal enzymes after the fusion of the endosomes with primary lysosomes. There is, however, a wide variation in the rate at which different types of absorbed proteins are hydrolysed by the lysosomal enzymes and it can vary from hours to days (1).

It is widely believed that polycationic peptides such as polylysine are nephrotoxic because they damage the tubular cells (1,2), after binding to the brush border and/or during their intracellular uptake. However, to our knowledge no report exists on the renal safety of polyanionic peptides. In fact, in recent years, poly-L-aspartic acid, a polyanionic peptide, emerged as a protectant against aminoglycoside antibiotics-induced nephrotoxicity (3-5). During the course of a research to use other polyanionic peptides, such as poly-L-glutamic and poly-D-glutamic acids as nephroprotectants, we discovered that the latter produces

hitherto undescribed lesions in the renal cortex of rats.

MATERIALS AND METHODS

Animals: Female Sprague Dawley rats (Iffa Credo, L'Arbresle, France), weighing between 180-200 g were used throughout.

Peptides and Other Products: Poly-D-glutamic acid (20 kDa, lots 84F-5031 and 104F-50451) and poly-L-glutamic acid (15,850 Da, lot 118F-5010 and 14,300 Da, lot 127F-5008) were purchased from the Sigma Chemical Co., St. Louis, MO, USA. Gentamicin sulfate (Geomycine[R]) as supplied for clinical use was a gift from the Schering Corp., NJ, USA. ^{3}H-thymidine was purchased from the Amersham International plc, Amersham, UK.

Treatment of Animals: In the first series of experiments, animals were given the polyanionic peptides at a dose of 250 mg/kg body weight per day subcutaneously for 3 days, during which they were challenged by a single toxic dose of gentamicin (100 mg/kg body weight intraperitoneally) on the second day. In the second series of experiments, the animals received gentamicin (20 mg/kg body weight per day intraperitoneally) together with polyanionic peptides (250 mg/kg body weight subcutaneously) for 4 consecutive days. Control animals received saline (0.9% NaCl) injections. Two groups of animals were also administered with poly-L-glutamic or poly-D-glutamic acids

(250 mg/kg body weight per day subcutaneously) without gentamicin for 1 to 4 days. Animals were sacrificed by decapitation 24 hr after the last injection. For histo-autoradiographic studies, the animals were dosed with 200 or 300 µCi of ^{3}H-thymidine per animal intraperitoneally 1 hr before sacrifice.

Morphological Studies: Kidney cortical specimens were processed for optical and electron microscopy by embedding in paraffin and plastic (epoxy resin) as described by Toubeau et al (6). Sections for optic microscopy were stained with the Periodic acid-Schiff reagent combined with hematoxylin-eosin or with the Giemsa stain. Histoautoradiography was performed on paraffin sections as described previously (7).

RESULTS AND DISCUSSION

In control rats treated with saline only, lysosomes were normal both in appearance and size (Figures 1A & 2A). In gentamicin-treated rats (4 days of treatment) many so-called 'myeloid bodies', heavily stained by toluidine blue were observed within the lysosomes of the proximal tubular cells (Figures 1B & 2B). When co-administered with poly-L-aspartic acid, a protectant against aminoglycoside-induced nephrotoxicity, the myeloid bodies were less numerous and looked smaller in size, demonstrating a reduction in the gentamicin-induced phospholipidosis (data not shown). The renal cortex of rats injected with poly-D-glutamic acid and gentamicin, and stained by the Periodic acid-Schiff method, revealed an interstitial cell proliferation (not depicted in figures). In sections treated by the Giemsa stain, conspicuous lysosomal alterations were observed in the proximal tubular cells (Figure 1C). These lysosomes were enlarged, displayed an elongated shape and were all situtated at the basal pole of the cells. In electron microscopy, these very large lysosomes appeared to be filled with an electron dense, non-lamellar, but granular and osmophilic material, which apparently became pulverised during cutting (Figures 2C & 2D). Concurrently, using biochemical criteria, (total lipid phosphorus; activity of acid sphingomyelinase), we found that poly-D-glutamic acid

effectively blocked the development of the gentamicin-induced lysosomal phospholipidosis. Poly-D-glutamic acid, when given alone without gentamicin, also was capable of inducing lysosomal alterations of similar nature with respect to size and shape (Figure 1E). However, these lysosomes never contained the electron dense and osmophilic material (Figure 2E) that was observed in animals with co-administered gentamicin. We therefore believe that this material is a complex of gentamicin and poly-D-glutamic acid formed within the lysosomes. We could not observe such lysosomal alterations in animals treated with poly-L-glutamic acid with or without gentamicin (Figures 1D & 1F).

On histoautoradiography, less than 2 nuclei per thousand (1.72 ± 0.62, mean ± SD) were labelled in animals receiving saline (Figure 3A). After treatment with gentamicin (20 mg/kg body weight per day for 4 days), this labelling index was more than doubled with most of the increase being localised in the proximal tubules (Figure 3B). Co-administration of poly-L-aspartic acid (a protectant), but not poly-L-glutamic acid (a non-protectant), brought down this labelling index to control values (not depicted in the figure). On the other hand, administration of poly-D-glutamic acid, with or without gentamicin, caused a dramatic 12 to 16-fold increase in the labelling index of the cortex, with more than 80% of the label being localised in the interstitium (Figures 3 C to E).

In vitro, we found that poly-L-glutamic acid was rapidly hydrolysed by lysosomal extracts whereas poly-D-glutamic acid was not (data not shown). Thus, we suggest that poly-D-glutamic acid induces an acute lysosomal storage disease in the renal cortex. This acute storage disease is apparently not due to the direct inhibition of lysosomal proteinases by poly-D-glutamic acid, since in vitro poly-D-glutamic acid (up to 100 µg/ml) did not inhibit the activity of these enzymes (data not shown). Most probably, the storage disease is due to the accumulation of large amounts of non-digestible poly-D-glutamic acid. Yet, the relation

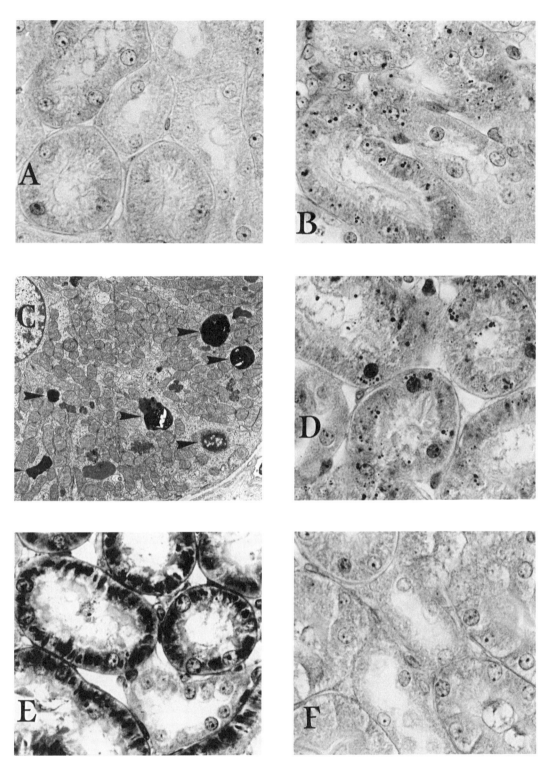

Figure 1. Optic microphotographs of Giemsa-stained kidney cortex sections from rats injected with saline (A), gentamicin (B), gentamicin plus poly-D-glutamic acid (C), gentamicin plus poly-L-glutamic acid (D), poly-D-glutamic acid (E) and poly-L-glutamic acid (F).

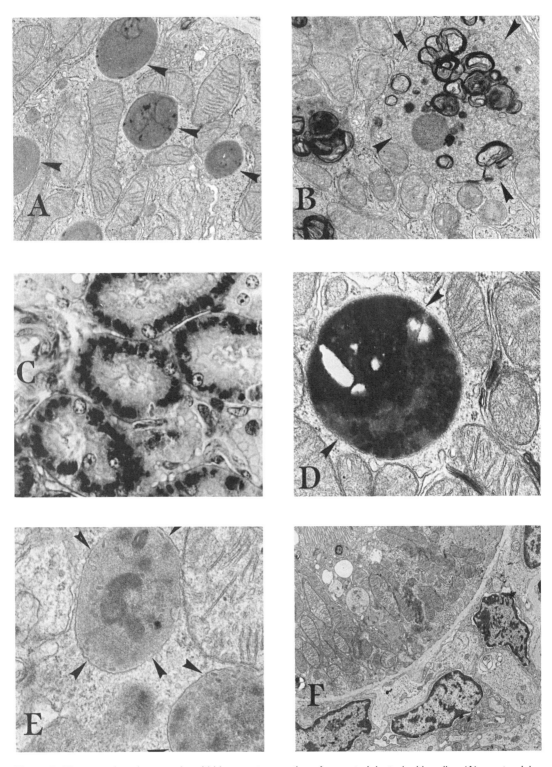

Figure 2. Electron microphotographs of kidney cortex sections from rats injected with saline (A), gentamicin, showing typical 'myeloid bodies' (B), gentamicin plus poly-D-glutamic acid, showing electron dense material in enlarged lysosomes under low magnification (C) and high magnification (D), poly-D-glutamic acid alone, showing enlarged and less denser lysosomes (E) and interstitial cell proliferation (F). The location and boundaries of lysosomes are indicated by arrow heads.

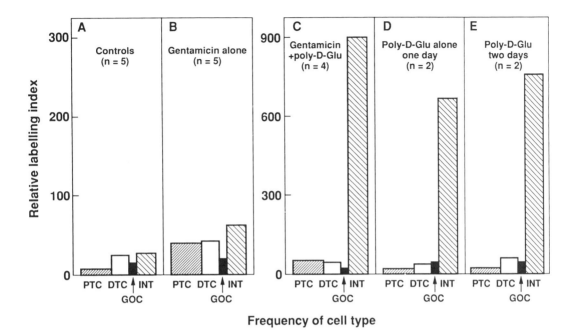

Figure 3. Quantitative evaluation of histoautoradiographic labelling of kidney cortex cells in rats injected with saline (A), gentamicin for 4 days (B), gentamicin + poly-D-glutamic acid for 4 days (C), poly-D-glutamic acid for 1 day (D) and for 2 days (E). The figure gives a quantitative estimate of the distribution of nuclear labelling among the main cell types of the cortex (PTC, proximal tubular cells; DTC, distal tubular cells; GOC, glomerular cells; INT, interstitial cells). The abscissa represents the frequency of each cell type as a proportion of total cortical nuclei. The ordinate shows the relative labelling index of each cell type. Thus the area within each block is equal to the absolute number of labelled nuclei for each cell type, and the sum area of the blocks for each group of rats depicts the global labelling index for that group. Note that the scale on the ordinate is enlarged 3-times for A and B. For further details of this method of representation, see reference (7).

between tubular thesaurismosis and interstitial cell proliferation remains unclear.

In conclusion, poly-D-glutamic acid can produce a previously undescribed acute lysosomal storage disease in the kidney cortex of rats, associated with an extensive proliferation of interstitial cells, but no direct or indirect evidence of marked tubular necrosis.

ACKNOWLEDGEMENT

B.K.K. is recipient of an ICP-Fellowship and S.I. of a Fellowship from the Ministry of Higher Education and Scientific Research of the Republic of Iraq. P.M.T. was Maître de Recherches of the Belgian Fonds National de la Recherche Scientifique.

REFERENCES

1. Maack T, Park CH and Camarge MJF. Renal filtration, transport and metabolism of proteins. In: Seldin DW, Giebisch G (eds); The Kidney: Physiology and Pathophysiology. Raven Press, New York, 1985, pp. 1773-1803.

2. Renal Pathogenicity of Cationic Compounds. In: Lambert PP, Bergmann P, Beauwens R (eds); The Pathogenicity of Cationic Proteins. New York, Raven Press, 1983, pp. 272-337.

3. Williams PD, Hottendorf GH and Bennett DB: Inhibition of renal membrane binding and nephrotoxicity of aminoglycosides. J Pharmacol Exptl Ther 237: 919-925, 1986.

4. Beauchamp D, Laurent G, Maldague P and Tulkens P: Reduction of gentamicin nephrotoxicity by the concomitant administration of poly-L-aspartic acid and poly-L-aspargine in rats. Arch Toxicol 9 (Suppl): 306-309, 1986.

5. Gilbert DN, Wood CA, Kohlepp SJ, Kohnen PW, Houghton DC, Finkbeiner HC, Lindsley J and Bennett WM: Polyaspartic acid prevents experimental aminoglycoside nephrotoxicity. J Infect Dis 159: 945-953, 1989.

6. Toubeau G, Laurent G, Carlier MB, Abid S, Maldague P, Heuson-Stiennon JA, Tulkens PM: Tissue repair in rat kidney cortex after short treatment with aminoglycosides at low doses. Lab Invest 54: 385-393, 1986.

7. Laurent G, Maldague P, Carlier MB, Tulkens P: Increased renal DNA synthesis in vivo after administration of gentamicin to rats. Antimicrobial Agents Chemother 24: 586-593, 1983.

22
EFFICACY AND RENAL EFFECTS OF CEFONICID IN PATIENTS WITH URINARY TRACT INFECTION

C. Donadio (1), G. Tramonti (1), G. Garcea (1), M. Costagli (1), A. Lucchetti (1), R. Giordani (1), G. Paizis (2), R. Pierotti (3), G. Falcone (3), C. Bianchi (1)

Nefrologia Medica, Istituto di Clinica Medica 2, University of Pisa, I-56100 Pisa, Italy (1), Smith Kline & French Spa, Milano (2), Istituto di Microbiologia, University of Pisa, Pisa, Italy (3)

INTRODUCTION

Cefonicid (CEF) is a second generation parenteral cephalosporin active against most Gram-negative aerobic bacteria and Gram-positive cocci (1-3). CEF is highly bound to plasma proteins (approximately 98%) and has a prolonged half life (1). Due to these pharmacokinetic characteristics, the drug can be administered once daily. It is eliminated unmodified almost exclusively by the kidney (4-6). More than 80% of the injected dose is excreted with the urine in the 24 hr following the iv injection. Its renal clearance accounts for approximately 90% of total plasma clearance (4-6). Tubular secretion is probably the main mechanism of renal excretion (4).

Despite the important role of the kidney in the excretion of CEF, no exhaustive data are available concerning effects on renal function and nephrotoxicity of CEF in man. This study evaluates efficacy, renal effects and nephrotoxicity of CEF in patients with difficult urinary tract infection (UTI) and different renal function.

MATERIAL AND METHODS

Eleven adult patients participated in this study. Their main clinical data are reported in Table I.

All patients had significant bacteriuria (>100,000 cfu/ml urine, by the dilution pourplate method) in 3 clean-catch midstream urine samples. The isolated bacteria were suscep-

tible to CEF (disk sensitivity test). No antimicrobial drug had been given within 1 month before the beginning of the study. Cefonicid (Monocid-SK&F SpA, Milano, Italy) was administered intramuscularly once daily at dosage adjusted to renal function: 1 g a day in 8 patients with plasma creatinine ≤ 2 mg/dl; 0.25 g a day (0.5 g on the first day of treatment) in 3 patients with renal failure and plasma creatinine between 3 and 5 mg/dl. The length of treatment was 7 days in all patients. No other medication was given in 6 patients, while another 2 patients were treated with clonidine and nicardipine, 1 with clonidine, 1 with insulin and long-acting nitrates, 1 with thyroxine.

Table I. Clinical data

Sex	10 F;1 M
Age (years)	23-71, mean 47
Plasma creatinine (mg/dl)	0.7-4.6, mean 1.8
Creatinine clearance (ml/min)	19-161, mean 75
Recurrent UTI	7
Upper UTI	9
Lower UTI	2
Isolated bacteria	
Escherichia coli	7
Proteus mirabilis	2
Pseudomonas aeruginosa	1
Citrobacter freundii	1

Urinalysis, urine culture, plasma concentration of creatinine, urea and uric acid, renal clearances of creatinine, urea and uric acid, urinary enzyme activities of alanine-aminopeptidase (AAP), gamma-glutamyltransferase (GGT), alkaline phosphatase (ALP), N-acetyl-beta-D-glucosaminidase (NAG), and lysozyme (LZM) were determined twice in the week preceding the treatment, again on the 4th day and at the end of treatment and 10 days after completion of therapy (7-11). Bacteriuria was checked daily in the study period by means of the Ortho Bacteriuria Detection Test (12). Glomerular filtration rate (GFR) and effective renal plasma flow (ERPF) were measured in the pre-treatment period and at the end of therapy by means of the non-invasive bladder cumulative method, using diethylene-triamine-pentaacetic acid (DTPA) labelled with Tc99m and hippuran-I^{131} respectively (13, 14).

Statistical analysis was performed by paired Student t-test. A p value of <0.05 was considered statistically significant.

RESULTS

Efficacy.

The therapeutic effect of CEF was quite rapid and satisfactory. In fact, after 2 days of treat-

ment bacteriuria test was negative in 10/11 patients.

The results of urine cultures are reported in Fig 1.

No failure was observed. On the fourth day and at the end of treatment urine cultures were sterile in all patients, even the one with isolated Pseudomonas aeruginosa. Ten days after the completion of therapy a relapse was observed in 4 patients: all these patients had difficult and/or recurrent UTI.

Renal effects.

The results of renal function tests performed before, during and after treatment with CEF are shown in Table II.

No sign of renal damage was demonstrated by common urine parameters. CEF did not modify plasma concentrations of creatinine, urea and uric acid, as well as their renal clearances. GFR did also not change. Only a very modest decrease of ERPF, statistically not significant, was observed. Filtration fraction was unmodified. Urine enzymes were measured to detect any toxic effect of CEF on proximal tubular cells. Only the brush border enzyme AAP increased slightly at the end of therapy. The increase was not statistically significant. AAP returned to base-line values in the post-treat-

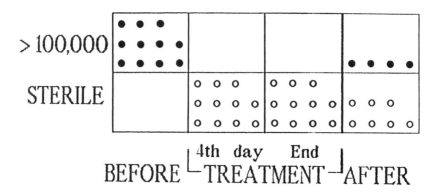

Fig 1. Therapeutic effect of cefonicid: urine cultures (cfu/ml) before, during and 10 days after completion of treatment.

Table II. Renal effects of cefonicid (mean $\pm$ SD; *$p<0.05$)

	n	Before	4th day	End	10 days after
URINE					
Output (L/12 hr)	10	1.23 ± 0.46	1.07 ± 0.59	1.36 ± 0.47	1.48 ± 0.62
Specific gravity	10	1.008± 0.006	1.008± 0.006	1.008± 0.007	1.008± 0.006
Proteins (mg/dl)	10	23.7 ±39.1	21.5 ±26.0	16.0 ± 24.5	20.0 ± 23.9
PLASMA					
Creatinine (mg/dl)	11	1.80 ± 1.40	1.64 ± 1.24	1.67 ± 1.33	1.71 ± 1.31
Urea (mg/dl)	11	51.5 ±39.0	49.5 ±32.3	48.2 ±30.8	45.7 ±25.1
Uric acid (mg/dl)	11	5.3 ± 1.6	5.1 ± 1.7	5.1 ± 1.8	5.1 ± 1.8
CLEARANCES					
Creatinine (ml/min)	10	74.6 ±51.0	70.9 ±42.7	82.9 ±63.1	72.2 ±45.8
Urea (ml/min)	10	30.6 ±19.0	28.3 ±15.9	30.5 ±17.5	34.6 ±22.3
Uric acid (ml/min)	9	6.3 ± 3.1	5.5 ±2.9	6.6 ± 5.1	6.8 ± 5.0
RENAL HEMODYNAMICS					
GFR (ml/min)	9	45.3 ± 28.3		41.0 ± 24.1	
ERPF (ml/min)	9	251.0 ±180.0		205.6 ±109.8	
FF (percent)	9	19.5 ± 3.4		20.0 ± 3.7	
URINE ENZYMES					
AAP (U/g creat)	8	2.6 ± 1.6	2.3 ± 2.4	5.0 ± 5.8	2.2 ±1.6
GGT (U/g creat)	10	34.9 ±10.5	32.7 ±15.2	28.1 ±16.3	38.5 ±23.6
ALP (U/g creat)	11	23.0 ±11.0	14.4 ± 6.7*	16.2 ±11.8	21.8 ±14.3
NAG (umol/h/g creat)	11	35.2 ±19.5	36.4 ±21.6	37.0 ±22.3	45.7 ±32.0

ment period. The other two brush border enzymes GGT and ALP, as well as the lysosomal enzyme NAG, and low molecular weight protein lysozyme remained stable during treatment with CEF.

DISCUSSION

The kidney has a prominent role in the excretion of CEF, which is eliminated unmodified with the urine via tubular secretion (4-6). Because of this pharmacokinetic characteristic, CEF is effective in the treatment of both lower and upper UTI (15-17). The results of this study, performed in patients with different impairment of renal function, indicate that CEF is effective also in the treatment of difficult and recurrent UTI. On the other hand, due to its extensive excretion through the kidney, CEF could be nephrotoxic. Therefore, a careful evaluation of its renal effects, prior to a wide clinical use, is necessary. The results of this study indicate that CEF, in spite of its extensive renal handling, has no effect on the most common clinical tests of renal function (plasma concentrations and clearances of creatinine, urea and uric acid). Also GFR and ERPF are not affected by CEF. Finally, CEF has no potential of tubular toxicity, as demonstrated by the stability of urinary enzyme activities during the treatment.

In conclusion, cefonicid is effective in the treatment of UTI, even in patients with renal failure. It does not influence renal function nor cause nephrotoxic effects.

ACKNOWLEDGEMENTS

This research has been supported in part by a research fund from Ministero Pubblica Istruzione, Italy. Mr. Joseph Franceschina is gratefully acknowledged for his valuable help in the preparation of this paper.

REFERENCES

1. Actor P, Uri JV, Zajac I, Guarini JR, Phillips L, Pitkin DH, Berges DA, Dunn GL, Hoover JRE, Weisbach JA: SK&F 75073, new parenteral broad-spectrum cephalosporin with high and prolonged serum levels. Antimicrob Agents Chemother 13: 784-790, 1978.

2. Hamilton-Miller JMT, Patel R, Brumfitt W: Cefonicid, a long acting cephalosporin: in vitro activity compared with three cephalosporins and gentamicin. Drugs Exp Clin Res 12: 861-869, 1986.

3. Saltiel E, Brogden RN: Cefonicid. A review of its antibacterial activity, pharmacological properties and therapeutic use. Drugs 32: 222-259, 1986.

4. Pitkin D, Dubb J, Actor P, Alexander F, Ehrlich S, Familiar R, Stote R: Kinetics and renal handling of cefonicid. Clin Pharmacol Ther 30: 587-593, 1981.

5. Barriere SL, Hatheway GJ, Gambertoglio JG, Lin ET, Conte JE Jr: Pharmacokinetics of cefonicid, a new broad-spectrum cephalosporin. Antimicrob Agents Chemother 21: 935-938, 1982.

6. Blair AD, Maxwell BM, Forland SC, Jacob L, Cutler RE: Cefonicid kinetics in subjects with normal and impaired renal function. Clin Pharmacol Ther 35: 798-803, 1984.

7. Peters JE, Schneider I, Haschen RJ: Bestimmung der I-Alanyl-Peptidhydrolase (Alanyl-Aminopeptidase, Aminosäure-Arylamidase) im menschlichen Harn. Clin Chim Acta 36: 289-301, 1972.

8. Szasz G: Gamma-Glutamyltranspeptidase-Aktivität im Urin. Z Klin Chem Klin Biochem 8: 1-8, 1970.

9. Amador E, Wacker WEC: Enzymatic methods used for diagnosis. Methods Biochem Anal 13: 265-356, 1965.

10. Merle LJ, Reindenberg MM, Camacho MT, Jones BR, Drayer DE: Renal injury in patients with rheumatoid arthritis treated with gold. Clin Pharmacol Ther 28: 216-222, 1980.

11. Prockop DJ, Davidson WD: A study of urinary and serum lysozyme in patients with renal disease. N Engl J Med 270: 269-274, 1964.

12. Wallis C, Melnick JL, Longoria CJ: Colorimetric method for rapid determination of bacteriuria. J Clin Microbiol 14: 342-346, 1981.

13. Bianchi C: Noninvasive methods for the measurement of renal function. In: Duarte CG (ed); Renal function tests. Clinical laboratory procedures and diagnosis. Boston, Little Brown, 1980, pp. 65-84.

14. Bianchi C, Donadio C, Tramonti G: Noninvasive methods for the measurement of total renal function. Nephron 28: 53-57, 1981.

15. Pontzer RE, Krieger RE, Boscia JA, McNamee W, Levison ME, Kaye D. Single-dose cefonicid therapy for urinary tract infections. Antimicrob Agents Chemother 23: 814-816, 1983.

16. Morgan SI, Pontzer RE, Cortez LM, Guice SL, Brannan W, Krieger RE, McNamee W, Boscia JA, Levison ME, Kaye D: Single-dose regimen of cefonicid for the treatment of uncomplicated infections of the lower urinary tract. Rev Infect Dis 6 (Suppl 4): S844-S846, 1984.

17. Cox CE, Jacob LS: Treatment of urinary tract infections in hospitalized patients: a double-blind comparison of cefonicid and cefamandole. Rev Infect Dis 6 (Suppl 4): S839-S843, 1984.

23

INTERACTIONS AMONG NEPHROTOXICANTS: CEPHALORIDINE AND N-(3,5-DICHLOROPHENYL)SUCCINIMIDE

G.O. Rankin (1), V.J. Teets (1), D.W. Nicoll (1) and P.I. Brown (2)

Departments of Pharmacology (1) and Anatomy (2), Marshall University School of Medicine, Huntington, West Virginia 25755-9310, U.S.A.

INTRODUCTION

Several recent studies have examined the effects of exposure to combinations of drugs and/or other chemicals on renal function in man or animals. In many cases, combination exposure to two drugs, solvents or environmental contaminants resulted in a potentiation of the nephrotoxic effects induced by one or both of the compounds (1-5). In other studies, combination exposure to two agents resulted in an attenuated nephrotoxic response following administration of a nephrotoxic dose of one or both of the compounds (6-8). Since combination drug therapy is quite common and exposure to two or more chemicals in the workplace or through the environmental route occurs daily for many individuals, continued efforts to understand the interactive potential of drugs and other chemicals remains an important area of research.

N-(3,5-Dichlorophenyl)succinimide (NDPS) was developed during the 1970s as an agricultural fungicide. However, use of NDPS as a fungicide has been limited in part because of potential health hazards associated with exposure to the compound. Acute exposure to NDPS has been shown to induce acute tubular necrosis (9), while chronic exposure to NDPS resulted in the development of interstitial nephritis (10). Although NDPS is not a carcinogen, NDPS does promote the nephrocarcinogenesis induced by other compounds (11,12). The mechanism by which NDPS induces nephrotoxicity is unknown, but studies in our laboratory have demonstrated that one or more NDPS metabolites are responsible for mediating the renal effects observed following NDPS administration (13,14).

Cephaloridine (CPH) is a first generation cephalosporin antibiotic which has been replaced clinically by less toxic drugs. Nephrotoxicity is a major toxicity of high dose CPH use in man, with renal effects in man and animals characterized as acute proximal tubular necrosis. Although several mechanisms have been proposed to explain this drug-induced toxicity, induction of lipid peroxidation appears to be the most likely mechanism of CPH-induced nephropathy (15). CPH and other cephalosporin antibiotics can also alter the nephrotoxic potential of other drugs. For example, combination administration of CPH or cephalothin with another proximal tubular toxicant, gentamicin, resulted in a synergistic nephrotoxic response (16). Therefore, it is also possible that CPH could interact with other nephrotoxicants to potentiate or attenuate the nephrotoxic responses observed with the individual compounds.

The purpose of this study was to examine the interactive potential of the two nephrotoxicants, NDPS and CPH. Experiments were conducted with combinations of marginally or subnephrotoxic doses of NDPS (0.2 mmol/kg) and CPH (500 mg/kg) and with combinations of subtoxic doses of the two compounds with nephrotoxic doses of the alternate chemical (NDPS, 0.4 or 1.0 mmol/kg; CPH, 1000 mg/kg). The results of these studies demonstrate the interactive potential of two model nephrotoxicants.

METHODS

Male Fischer 344 rats (220-250 g) were housed individually in stainless steel metabolism cages. Following 2 control days, rats (4 rats/group) were given an intraperitoneal (i.p.) injection of CPH (500 mg/kg), NDPS (0.2 mmol/kg), CPH vehicle (0.9% saline, 2.0 ml/kg) or NDPS vehicle (sesame oil, 2.5 ml/kg) 1 hr before the i.p. administration of NDPS (0.2, 0.4, or 1.0 mmol/kg), CPH (1000 mg/kg) or the appropriate NDPS or CPH vehicle. Renal function was monitored at 24 and 48 hr as previously described (14). Tail blood samples were obtained prior to individual housing and

again just prior to killing (48 hr) for the determination of the blood urea nitrogen (BUN) concentration. Kidney weights and accumulation of [^{14}C]-p-aminohippurate (PAH) and [^{14}C]-tetraethylammonium (TEA) by renal cortical slices were determined at 48 hr.

RESULTS

Pretreatment with CPH (500 mg/kg) did not substantially potentiate NDPS (0.2 mmol/kg)-induced effects. No increases in BUN concentration or kidney weight were observed when CPH (500 mg/kg) and NDPS (0.2 mmol/kg) were administered alone or in combination (Table 1). Also, organic ion accumulation by renal cortical slices was not altered except for a decrease in basal PAH

Table 1. Effect of CPH and NDPS Combinations on BUN Concentration and Kidney Weight[a]

Compound	Dose	BUN Concentration		Kidney Weight
		0 hr	48 hr	(g/100g body weight)
CPH	500 mg/kg	29 ± 3^c	24 ± 1	0.43 ± 0.01
NDPS	0.2 mmol/kg	18 ± 1	20 ± 1^c	0.41 ± 0.01
CPH +	500 mg/kg +	23 ± 1	23 ± 1	0.45 ± 0.01
NDPS	0.2 mmol/kg			
CPH	500 mg/kg	27 ± 1^c	22 ± 2^b	0.43 ± 0.01
NDPS	0.4 mmol/kg	15 ± 1^c	133 ± 35^c	0.68 ± 0.03^c
CPH +	500 mg/kg +	23 ± 1	26 ± 1^b	0.42 ± 0.01
NDPS	0.4 mmol/kg			
CPH	500 mg/kg	25 ± 1	18 ± 1^b	0.38 ± 0.01^c
NDPS	1.0 mmol/kg	19 ± 1^c	$187 \pm 20^{b,c}$	0.59 ± 0.04^c
CPH +	500 mg/kg +	26 ± 1	24 ± 1	0.45 ± 0.01
NDPS	1.0 mmol/kg			
NDPS	0.2 mmol/kg	19 ± 1	18 ± 1^c	0.43 ± 0.02^c
CPH	1000mg/kg	18 ± 1	$82 \pm 8^{b,c}$	0.56 ± 0.01
NDPS +	0.2 mmol/kg +	19 ± 1	143 ± 25^b	0.59 ± 0.05
CPH	1000 mg/kg			

[a] Values are means $\pm$ S.E. for N=4 rats per group.
[b] Significantly different (P<0.05) from the appropriate 0 hr value.
[c] Significantly different (P<0.05) from the appropriate CPH+NDPS or NDPS+CPH group value.

TABLE 2. Effect of CPH and NDPS Combinations on Organic Ion Accumulation by Renal Cortical Slices[a]

Compound	Dose	PAH	S/M Ratio PAH + Lactate	TEA
CPH	500 mg/kg	4.87 ± 0.23	11.06 ± 0.59	19.53 ± 0.77
NDPS	0.2 mmol/kg	3.59 ± 0.07^b	11.99 ± 0.93	18.96 ± 1.10
CPH + NDPS	500 mg/kg + 0.2 mmol/kg	4.94 ± 0.24	10.10 ± 0.68	16.63 ± 0.15
CPH	500 mg/kg	4.78 ± 0.22	10.38 ± 0.41	18.40 ± 0.98
NDPS	0.4 mmol/kg	2.19 ± 0.30^b	6.15 ± 0.81^b	11.55 ± 1.64^b
CPH + NDPS	500 mg/kg + 0.2 mmol/kg	4.42 ± 0.13	10.25 ± 0.12	20.51 ± 0.58
CPH	500 mg/kg	3.63 ± 0.02	5.51 ± 0.40^b	16.01 ± 0.63
NDPS	1.0 mmol/kg	1.50 ± 0.14^b	2.69 ± 0.16^b	13.20 ± 1.53
CPH + NDPS	500 mg/kg + 1.0 mmol/kg	3.94 ± 0.39	8.63 ± 0.37	16.53 ± 0.69
NDPS	0.2 mmol/kg	3.36 ± 0.30^b	8.70 ± 1.15^b	18.30 ± 0.80^b
CPH	1000 mg/kg	1.47 ± 0.14	1.57 ± 0.09	6.65 ± 0.10
NDPS + CPH	0.2 mmol/kg + 1000 mmol/kg	1.24 ± 0.11	1.41 ± 0.26	7.76 ± 0.58

[a]Values are means $\pm$ S.E. for N=4 rats per group.
[b]Significantly different (P<0.05) from the appropriate CPH+NDPS or NDPS+CPH group value.

uptake in the NDPS (0.2 mmol/kg) group when compared to the CPH and NDPS group (Table 2). Renal morphological changes were minor in all three groups and restricted to some vacuolization in proximal tubular cells.

Pretreatment with CPH (500 mg/kg) markedly attenuated NDPS (0.4 or 1.0 mmol/kg)-induced nephrotoxicity. The large NDPS-induced increases in BUN concentration were prevented by CPH pretreatment at both NDPS dose levels (Table 1). NDPS-induced increases in kidney weight (Table 1) and decreases in organic ion accumulation were also markedly attenuated by CPH pretreatment. Renal morphological changes induced by NDPS (0.4 mmol/kg) were reduced by CPH pretreatment, although excessive vacuolization was still evident in some proximal tubular cells. Rats treated with CPH

and NDPS (1.0 mmol/kg) exhibited extensive tubular damage with occlusion of some lumina. These changes were similar to the renal morphological changes observed following NDPS (1.0 mmol/kg) alone, but the extensive accumulation of erythrocytes noted with NDPS alone was not seen in renal tissue from rats administered CPH (500 mg/kg) and NDPS (1.0 mmol/kg).

Pretreatment with NDPS (0.2 mmol/kg) potentiated the CPH (1000 mg/kg)-induced elevation in BUN concentration (Table 1), but not the CPH-induced changes in kidney weight (Table 1) or organic ion accumulation. Proximal tubular damage induced by CPH also was potentiated by NDPS (0.2 mmol/kg) pretreatment. Although both proximal and distal tubular cells had increased vacuolization and some lumina were occluded with CPH alone, when animals were pretreated with NDPS followed by CPH administration, numerous proximal and distal tubular cells were severely damaged with debris from necrotic cells occluding lumina throughout the cortex.

DISCUSSION

Combination exposure to two or more nephrotoxicants can result in potentiation or attenuation of the nephrotoxic potential of one or more of the nephrotoxicants (1-8). If potentiation occurs, then administration of borderline nephrotoxic doses of the chemicals can result in an enhanced nephrotoxic response. For example, exposure to styrene and toluene in combination can induce nephrotoxicity at concentrations of the individual compounds which do not induce nephropathy (3). However, the results obtained in the present study indicate that a nonnephrotoxic or borderline nephrotoxic dose of CPH (500 mg/kg) does potentiate the renal effects induced by a borderline nephrotoxic dose of NDPS (0.2 mmol/kg). CPH (500 mg/kg) pretreatment does markedly attenuate the nephrotoxic effects induced by nephrotoxic doses of NDPS (0.4 or 1.0 mmol/kg). Therefore, the interactions between CPH and NDPS observed when CPH is administered first results in a decrease in the nephrotoxic potential of NDPS.

When rats were pretreated with a non-nephrotoxic dose of NDPS (0.2 mmol/kg), CPH (1000 mg/kg)-induced renal effects were slightly enhanced. The most dramatic effect was observed on the CPH-induced increase in BUN concentration (Table 1) where the combination of NDPS and CPH induced a 174% increase in BUN concentration compared to CPH alone. Therefore, the interaction between CPH and NDPS observed when NDPS is administered first results in an increase in the nephrotoxic potential of CPH.

The mechanism for these interactions are unknown at the present time. CPH, an organic acid, could be attenuating NDPS-induced nephropathy by decreasing the renal accumulation of acidic, nephrotoxic NDPS metabolites. This hypothesis is supported by the observation that probenecid, an inhibitor of renal organic anion transport systems, also attenuated NDPS-induced nephrotoxicity (17). Alternatively, CPH could be inhibiting biotransformation of NDPS to nephrotoxic metabolites. This hypothesis is supported by the report that CPH (500 mg/kg) can inhibit microsomal enzyme activity (18), and NDPS requires activation via microsomal enzyme-mediated oxidation to induce significant nephrotoxicity (13,14). NDPS could be worsening CPH-induced renal effects by interfering with the ability of the kidney to respond to damage. This possible explanation is supported by preliminary studies which have suggested that NDPS metabolites might be able to inhibit the formation of vasodilatory prostaglandins (unpublished observations). However, further studies are necessary to determine the mechanisms responsible for the interactions between CPH and NDPS.

ACKNOWLEDGEMENTS

The authors would like to thank Joyce Stern for her excellent technical assistance and Darla Kuryla for her help in the preparation of this manuscript. This work was supported by NIH grant DK 31210.

REFERENCES

1. Haberman PJ, Baggett JMcC, Berndt WO: The effect of chromate on citrinin-induced renal dysfunction in the rat. Toxicol Lett 38: 83-90, 1987.

2. Goren MP, Wright RK, Pratt CB, Horowitz ME, Dodge RK, Viar MJ, Kovnar EH: Potentiation of ifosfamide neurotoxicity, hematotoxicity, and tubular nephrotoxicity by prior cis-diamminedichloroplatinum (II) therapy. Cancer Res 47: 1457-1460, 1987.

3. Chakrabarti S, Tuchweber B: Studies of nephrotoxicity due to mixed exposure to styrene and toluene. Toxicol Lett. 39: 27-34, 1987.

4. Bernard AM, de Russis R, Ouled Amor A, Lauwerys RR: Potentiation of cadmium nephrotoxicity by acetaminophen. Arch Toxicol 62: 291-294, 1988.

5. Avent CK, Krinsky D, Kirklin JK, Bourge RC, Figg WD: Synergistic nephrotoxicity due to ciprofloxacin and cyclosporin. Amer J Med 85: 452-453, 1988.

6. Sparrow S, Magos L, Snowden R: The effect of sodium chromate pretreatment on mercuric chloride-induced nephrotoxicity. Arch Toxicol 61: 440-443, 1988.

7. Hayashi T, Watanabe Y, Kumano K, Kitayama R, Yasuda T, Saikawa I, Katahira J, Kumanda T, Shimizu K: Protective effect of pipericillin against the nephrotoxicity of cephaloridine and gentamicin in animals. Antimicrob Agents Chemother 32: 912-918, 1988.

8. Hayashi T, Watanabe Y, Kumano K, Kitayama R, Muratani T, Yasuda T, Saikawa I, Katahira J, Kumada T, Shimizu K: Protective effect of pipericillin against the nephrotoxicity of cisplatin in rats. Antimicrob Agents Chemother 33: 513-518, 1989.

9. Rankin GO: Nephrotoxicity following acute administration of N-(3,5-dichlorophenyl)succinimide in Sprague-Dawley rats. Toxicology 23: 21-31, 1982.

10. Sugihara S, Shinohara Y, Miyata Y, Inoue K, Ito N: Pathologic analysis of chemical nephritis in rats induced by N-(3,5-dichlorophenyl)succinimide. Lab Invest 33: 219-230, 1975.

11. Ito N, Sugihara S, Makiura S, Arai M, Hirao K, Denda S, Nishio O: Effect of N-(3,5-dichlorophenyl)succinimide on the histological pattern and incidence of kidney tumors in rats induced by dimethylnitrosamine. Gann 65: 131-138, 1974.

12. Shinohara Y, Arai M, Hira K, Sugihara S, Nakanishi K, Tsunoda H, Ito N: Combination effect of citrinin and other chemicals on rat kidney tumorigenesis. Gann 67: 147-155, 1976.

13. Rankin GO, Snib AC, Yang DJ, Richmond CD, Teets VJ, Wang RT, Brown PI: Effect of microsomal enzyme activity modulation on N-(3,5-dichlorophenyl)succinimide-induced nephrotoxicity. Toxicology 45: 269-289, 1987.

14. Rankin GO, Snib AC, Yang DJ, Richmond CD, Teets VJ, Brown PI: Nephrotoxicity of N-(3,5-dichlorophenyl)succinimide metabolites in vivo and in vitro. Toxicol Appl Pharmacol 96: 405-416, 1988.

15. Goldstein RS, Smith PF, Tarloff JB, Contardi L, Rush GF, Hook JB: Biochemical mechanisms of cephaloridine nephrotoxicity. Life Sci 42: 1809-1816, 1988.

16. Gamarellou H, Petrikkos G, Doudoulaki P, Diakos GK: Prospective comparative evaluation of gentamicin alone and gentamicin plus various cephalosporins with respect to nephrotoxicity in human. In: Siegenthaler W, Luthy R (eds); Current Chemotherapy. Washington, American Society for Microbiology, 1978, pp 968-970.

17. Rankin GO, Yang DJ, Teets VJ, Lo HH, Brown PI: The effect of probenecid on acute N-(3,5-dichlorophenyl)succinimide-induced nephrotoxicity in the Fischer 344 rat. Toxicology 44: 181-192, 1987.

18. Cojocel C, Kramer W, Mayer D: Depletion of cytochrome P-450 and alteration in activation of drug metabolizing enzymes induced by cephaloridine in the rat kidney cortex. Biochem Pharmacol 37: 3781-3785, 1988.

24

DIRECT RENAL TOXICITY OF CEPHALORIDINE IN NORMOGLYCAEMIC AND DIABETIC RATS

M.A. Valentovic, J.G. Ball, D. Bailly, M. Morenas, B. Jeffrey and J.W. Kinder

Department of Pharmacology, Marshall University School of Medicine, 1542 Spring Valley Drive, Huntington, WV 25755-9310, USA

INTRODUCTION

The cephalosporin antibiotic, cephaloridine, is acutely toxic in humans (1) as well as experimental animals (2). Administration of cephaloridine to Fischer 344 (F344) rats results in increased kidney weight, BUN levels and serum glutamic-pyruvic transaminase (SGPT) values. Proximal tubular function is impaired by cephaloridine administration since anion and cation transport systems are diminished within 48 hr after cephaloridine injection (3). Histological examination has confirmed that the primary target of cephaloridine toxicity (4) is the S_2 segment of the proximal convoluted tubule.

The specific events involved in cephaloridine mediated cell damage are not entirely understood. However, lipid peroxidation (5,6) has been implicated as a mechanism of nephrotoxicity. Kuo and associates (5) suggested that lipid peroxidation may be involved in cephaloridine nephrotoxicity since renal damage was potentiated in animals fed a selenium and vitamin E deficient diet.

Cephaloridine is also known to be directly toxic to the renal cortex. The addition of cephaloridine to renal cortical slices (7) or microsomes (6) induced lipid peroxide formation in a concentration and time dependent manner. Goldstein and associates have also shown that renal cortical slice uptake of organic ions was diminished as a function of the cephaloridine concentration (7).

Previous work in the investigator's lab has shown that the nephrotoxicity of cephaloridine is attenuated in streptozotocin (STZ)-induced diabetic rats. The administration of 750-1500 mg/kg cephaloridine to normoglycaemic rats produced increased kidney weight, decreased renal cortical slice uptake of p-aminohippurate (PAH) and tetraethylammonium (TEA) as well as proximal tubular necrosis. BUN levels and renal cortical slice uptake of organic ions, however, were not altered in the diabetic rats treated with 1500 mg/kg cephaloridine. The diabetic state is associated with numerous physiological changes which could contribute to reducing cephaloridine nephrotoxicity. Consequently, the purpose of the following studies was to compare the direct toxicity of cephaloridine between normoglycaemic and diabetic rats.

MATERIALS AND METHODS

Animals and induction of diabetes: Male F344 rats (230-380 gm) were housed at a constant ambient temperature (21-23°C) and light period (0600-1800 hr). Animals were permitted a 5 day minimum acclimatization prior to initiation of any experimental procedures. Rats were injected with 35 mg/kg STZ freshly prepared in citrate buffer (pH 4.6) to induce diabetes. Vehicle treated rats were injected with citrate buffer pH 4.6. Diabetes was confirmed by glucosuria and serum glucose (Sigma, #510) levels in excess of 225 mg/dl.

Lipid peroxidation: The kidneys were decapsulated, excised and placed in ice cold Krebs Ringer buffer (pH 7.4). The kidneys were cut longitudinally and renal cortex slices were prepared freehand. Renal slices (70-100 mg) were equilibrated in Krebs Ringer buffer for 15 min at 37°C under an oxygen atmosphere. Samples were then incubated for 30, 90 or 120 min with cephaloridine at a final concentration of 0, 2.5 or 5 mM in a total volume of 3 ml Krebs Ringer buffer. At the end of the incubation period, the tissues were blotted, weighed and homogenized in 2 ml Krebs Ringer. Lipid peroxides were determined as the reactive products of thiobarbituric acid and designated malonaldehyde (MDA) products using a molar extinction coefficient of 1.56×10^5 (8).

Organic ion transport: In a separate series of experiments, the direct toxicity of cephaloridine on renal cortical slice accumulation of TEA was compared between normoglycaemic and diabetic rats. Renal cortical slices were prepared from kidneys obtained 14 days post STZ or vehicle administration. The tissues were allowed to equilibrate for 15 min at 25°C in an oxygen atmosphere. The samples were then incubated for 30 min with 0, 2.5, 5 or 7 mM cephaloridine. Upon completion of the incubation period, renal cortical slice accumulation of PAH or TEA was determined (9). Renal cortical slice accumulation of PAH was expressed as the slice to media (S/M) ratio where S denotes the radioactivity in the tissue (dpm/g tissue) while M represents the radioactivity in the media (dpm/ml).

Statistical analysis: Values were reported as the Mean± S.E. All experiments contained N = 4-8 per group. Differences between various concentrations of cephaloridine within groups were quantitated using an Analysis of Variance (ANOVA) followed by a Dunnett's test with a 95% confidence interval. Comparisons between normoglycaemic and diabetic rats were made using an ANOVA followed by a Newman Keuls test.

RESULTS

The diabetic state protected against the direct renal toxicity of cephaloridine. The doses of cephaloridine employed in these studies were toxic in the normoglycaemic rats since free radical generation was increased in cortical

tissue following a 90 min incubation with cephaloridine. A 90-120 min pre-incubation with 2.5 or 5 mM cephaloridine stimulated lipid peroxide formation in the normoglycaemic rats (Table 1). However, lipid peroxidation was not significantly increased after a 120 min incubation with 5 mM cephaloridine in renal cortical tissue obtained from diabetic rats.

Direct toxicity was produced in the normoglycaemic group by pre-incubating renal cortical slices with 0-7 mM cephaloridine. Cephaloridine induced a concentration dependent decrease in basal and lactate stimulated renal cortical slice accumulation of PAH (Table 2) in the normoglycaemic tissue. Basal PAH uptake by renal cortical slices obtained from normoglycaemic animals were statistically different (p) in the presence of 7 mM cephaloridine. Lactate stimulated PAH uptake in the normoglycaemic tissue was diminished in a concentration dependent manner as indicated in Table 2. Lactate stimulated PAH accumulation in the normoglycaemic group was significantly decreased (p) in the presence of 5 and 7 mM cephaloridine. In contrast, basal and lactate stimulated PAH uptake were not altered in renal cortical slices obtained from diabetic animals. Cephaloridine diminished renal cortical slice accumulation of TEA (Table 2) in a concentration dependent manner in normoglycaemic and diabetic tissue. A higher concentration of cephaloridine was required to inhibit renal cortical uptake of TEA in the diabetic group. TEA accumulation was decreased in the presence of 2.5, 5 or 7 mM cephaloridine in the normoglycaemic group while the diabetic group was decreased in the presence of 5 and 7 mM cephaloridine. These results indicate that the direct toxicity of cephaloridine is attenuated in the diabetic rat.

DISCUSSION

It is well established that the diabetic state produces many physiological and biochemical alterations. Diabetes is also associated with enhanced urine output, increased kidney weight and an elevated glomerular filtration rate (10). The renal damage occurring subsequent

Table 1. Cephaloridine Mediated In Vitro Lipid Peroxidation In Normoglycaemic and Diabetic Renal Cortical Slices

Group	Serum Glucose (mg/dl)	Cephaloridine (mM)		
		0	2.5	5
		30 min		
Normoglycaemic	136± 18	74.3± 9.6[a]	70.5± 8.7	92.3±18.3
Diabetic	383± 20[b]	53.9± 5.1	54.5± 4.0	51.6± 4.7
		90 min		
Normoglycaemic	133± 7	37.8± 5.1	49.2± 6.4[*]	58.5± 4.2[*]
Diabetic	420± 24[b]	47.4± 7.8	64.0±17.2	68.3±13.7
		120 min		
Normoglycaemic	133± 7	39.2± 5.1	53.8± 4.4[*]	63.0± 3.3[*]
Diabetic	304± 31[b]	69.8± 3.8[b]	88.4± 7.3b	89.1± 5.4[b]

[a]Values reported as Mean± S.E.; all groups contained an $N \geq$ 4-6 animals/group. Renal cortical slices were pre-incubated for 30-120 min with cephaloridine prior to determination of lipid peroxidation. Denotes different from respective vehicle p<0.05. [b]Denotes different (p<0.05) from respective normoglycaemic group.

Table 2. Direct Effect of Cephaloridine on Organic Ion Transport In Tissue Derived from Normoglycaemic and Diabetic Rats

Group	Cephaloridine (mM)			
	0	2.5	5	7
	PAH			
Normoglycaemic	2.64± 0.28[a]	2.51± 0.21	2.32± 0.33	1.88± 0.11[*]
Diabetic	2.96± 0.31	3.63± 0.11[b]	3.18± 0.16	2.01± 0.34
	PAH + LAC			
Normoglycaemic	8.55± 0.74	8.37± 0.81	6.88± 0.66[*]	6.65± 0.10[*]
Diabetic	9.70± 0.78	10.84± 0.75	9.48± 1.18	8.10± 0.44[b]
	TEA			
Normoglycaemic	19.90± 3.10	14.80± 1.76[*]	14.80± 1.99[*]	13.00± 1.59[*]
Diabetic	24.86± 2.14	20.56± 1.69	17.90± 1.14[*]	17.02± 0.44[*]

[a]Values are expressed as the Mean± S.E. with an $N \geq$ 4 per group. Tissues were pre-incubated for 30 min with 0-7 mM cephaloridine and then incubated for 90 min with TEA or PAH. PAH was measured in the presence of 0 or 10 mM lactate. [*]Values are different (p<0.05) from respective vehicle. [b]Denotes different (p<0.05) from normoglycaemic group.

to in vivo administration of cephaloridine is attenuated in the diabetic state. The ability of the experimental diabetic state to reduce cephaloridine nephrotoxicity may be due to gross alterations in renal function. Consequently, this study examined only the direct toxicity of cephaloridine in order to eliminate the physiological changes that occur in the diabetic kidney.

The results of our studies indicate that the in vitro toxicity of cephaloridine is attenuated in the diabetic rat. Lipid peroxidation was produced in a dose- and time-dependent manner in the renal cortex of normoglycaemic rats (Table 1). However, cephaloridine induced lipid peroxidation was not significantly increased in diabetic tissue even after exposure to very toxic doses of the antibiotic. Since the proposed mechanism for cephaloridine toxicity involves lipid peroxide formation, the reduced level of lipid peroxidation in the diabetic rats would indicate diminished cellular toxicity.

Renal cortical slice accumulation of organic ions was also measured since this procedure is a very sensitive parameter for detection of proximal tubular damage (11). Cephaloridine induced a concentration dependent decrease in renal cortical slice accumulation of PAH and TEA in the normoglycaemic group (Table 2). These results are in agreement with previous studies by other investigators (7) which observed a decrease in organic ion uptake as a function of in vitro exposure to cephaloridine. Cephaloridine, however, was less toxic in the diabetic group (Table 2) since basal and lactate stimulated PAH uptake were not altered in the presence of 0-7 mM cephaloridine. The diabetic state did not totally attenuate toxicity since TEA uptake was diminished in the presence of 5 and 7 mM cephaloridine.

The results of this study show that the in vitro toxicity of cephaloridine is reduced in tissues derived from diabetic animals. These data suggest that diabetes induces a cellular alteration which influences the direct toxicity of cephaloridine. Additionally, these data indicate the ability of diabetes to reduce nephrotoxicity can-

not be entirely attributed to increases in urine output or glomerular filtration rate.

The experimental diabetic state has been reported to reduce gentamicin induced renal damage (12). Although gentamicin and cephaloridine are structurally unrelated chemicals, similarities do exist for the site of renal damage. Studies conducted by other investigators showed gentamicin accumulation was less marked in the experimental diabetic state. Another possibility for reduced toxicity is an alteration in the phospholipid composition of membranes in diabetic kidneys. Gentamicin selectively binds to phosphatidylinositol located on the brush border (13). The diabetic state may accumulate less gentamicin since diabetes is associated with a decrease in renal phosphatidylinositol levels (14).

The diabetic state may attenuate cephaloridine induced renal damage by modifying the subcellular changes produced by cephaloridine. Since lipid peroxidation is involved in the cellular damage of cephaloridine (5-7), diabetes may reduce the severity of renal damage by inhibiting the cellular lipid peroxide formation. Further studies are needed to determine if the mechanisms responsible for reducing in vitro renal damage in diabetes is due to alterations in accumulation of the toxin or if its is due to a decreased susceptibility to lipid peroxide formation.

ACKNOWLEDGEMENT

This work was supported in part by NIH RR05870.

REFERENCES

1. Foord RD: Cephaloridine, cephalothin and the kidney. J Antimicrob Chemother 1:119-133, 1975.

2. Atkinson RM, Currie JP, Davis B, Pratt DA, Sharpe HM, Tomich EG: Acute toxicity of cephaloridine, an antibiotic derived from cephalosporin. Toxicol Appl Pharmacol 8:398-406, 1966.

3. Kuo CH, Hook JB: Depletion of renal glutathione content and nephrotoxicity of cephaloridine in rabbits, rats and mice. Toxicol Appl Pharmacol 292-302, 1982.

4. Silverblatt F, Turck M, Bulger R: Nephrotoxicity due to cephaloridine: a light and electron microscopic study in rabbits. J Infectious Dis 122: 33-44, 1970.

5. Kuo CH, Maita K, Sleight SD, Hook JB: Lipid peroxidation: a possible mechanism of cephaloridine induced nephrotoxicity. Toxicol Appl Pharmacol 67:78-88, 1983.

6. Cojocel C, Hannemann J and Baumann K: Cephaloridine-induced lipid peroxidation initiated by reactive oxygen species as a possible mechanism of cephaloridine nephrotoxicity. Biochim Biophys Acta 834:402-410, 1985.

7. Goldstein RS, Pasino DA, Hewitt WR, Hook JB: Biochemical mechanisms of cephaloridine nephrotoxicity: time and concentration dependence of peroxidative injury. Toxicol Appl Pharmacol 83:261-270, 1986.

8. Ottolenghi A: Interaction of ascorbic acid and mitochondrial lipids. Arch Biochem Biophys 79:355-363, 1959.

9. Rankin GO: Nephrotoxicity following acute administration of N-(3,5- dichlorophenyl)succinimide in rats. Toxicology 23:21-31, 1982.

10. Jensen PK, Christiansen JS, Steven K, Parving HH. Renal function in streptozotocin-diabetic rats. Diabetologia 21:409-414, 1981.

11. Kluwe WM: Renal function tests as indicators of kidney injury in subacute toxicity studies. Toxicol Appl Pharmacol 57: 414-424, 1981.

12. Teixeira RB, Kelley J, Alpert H, Pardo V, Vaamonde CA: Complete protection from gentamicin induced acute renal failure in the diabetes mellitus rat. Kidney Int 21:600-612, 1982.

13. Sastrasinh M, Knauss TC, Weinberg JM, Humes HD: Identification of the aminoglycoside binding site in rat renal brush border membranes. J Pharmacol Exp Ther 222:350-358, 1982.

14. Kaloyanides GJ, Wang M, Govea W, Alpert H, Vaamonde CA: Altered phosphatidylinositol metabolism in diabetic rats confers resistance to gentamicin induced acute renal failure. Kidney Int 21:219A, 1982.

PART VI
CYCLOSPORINE A

25

ALTERATIONS IN RENAL TUBULAR FUNCTION FOLLOWING CALCIUM CHANNEL BLOCKADE IN LONG-TERM RENAL ALLOGRAFT RECIPIENTS

D.J. Propper (1), P.H. Whiting (2), D.A. Power (1), G.R.D. Catto (1)

Departments of Medicine and Therapeutics (1), and Clinical Biochemistry (2), University of Aberdeen, Polwarth Building, Foresterhill, Aberdeen, AB9 2ZD, UK

INTRODUCTION

Cyclosporin A has revolutionised organ transplantation. However, its nephrotoxicity, particularly that affecting renal allograft recipients, remains a serious problem. One of the main components of cyclosporin A nephrotoxicity is afferent renal arteriolar vasoconstriction, but what mediates this component is unknown (1). Recently a number of reports have suggested that renal allograft recipients receiving cyclosporin A and calcium channel antagonists have better graft function than those receiving cyclosporin A alone (2-4). Others, however, have failed to confirm these observations (5).

The effect of nifedipine on renal function has not been investigated in cyclosporin A-treated patients with stable graft function. We therefore assessed the effect of nifedipine on glomerular and tubular function in patients with stable allograft function at least one year after transplantation.

METHODS

Two groups of renal allograft recipients with stable renal function were studied (Table 1). Group 1 comprised 10 patients receiving low dose prednisolone and cyclosporin A. Group 2 comprised 9 patients receiving low dose prednisolone and azathioprine (0.75-1.5mg/kg/day). Measurement of lithium clearance was assessed by the method of Thomsen (6), and was performed before, and at the end of an eight day course of nifedipine 10 mg three times per day. Clearance rates for creatinine (C.Cr), sodium (C.Na) and lithium (C.Li) and urinary flow rates (UFR) were derived by the usual methods and expressed as ml/min/100 kg body weight. For each subject the following derived measurements of tubular function were calculated:- (1) Fractional lithium excretion (Fe.Li). (2) Fractional sodium excretion (Fe.Na). (3) The absolute proximal tubular reabsorption of iso-osmotic fluids (C.Cr-C.Li). (4) The absolute reabsorption of sodium from the distal nephron was expressed as (C.Li-C.Na). (5) The absolute reabsorption of water from the distal nephron (C.Li - UFR). (6) The fractional reabsorption of sodium from the distal tubule relative to the delivery of sodium from the proximal tubule (1-C.Na/C.Li). (7) The fractional reabsorption of water from the distal tubule relative to the

Table 1. Details of the patient groups studied

Treatment	GROUP 1 Cyclosporin A	GROUP 2 Azathioprine
Sex	8M 2F	5M 4F
Mean age (years)	55.1 $\pm$ 19.9	45.5 $\pm$ 14.3
Mean time since transplant (months)	20.5 $\pm$ 8.5	77.2 $\pm$ 27.3
Mean prednisolone dose (mg/24 hrs)	10 $\pm$ 0	8.6 $\pm$ 1.3

delivery of water from the proximal tubule (1-UFR/C.Li).

Intergroup comparison of clearance rates, fractional excretions, urinary flow rates and the derived measurements of tubular function was by Mann-Whitney U-tests. Within both groups clearance rates, fractional excretions and the derived measurements of tubular function were compared at the beginning and end of the study period by paired Student's t-tests.

RESULTS

At the beginning of the study creatinine clearance rates did not differ significantly between the two groups. Lithium clearance rates were, however, significantly lower (p< 0.01) in the cyclosporin A treated patients (Group 1) than in those receiving azathioprine, as were fractional lithium excretions (p<0.01). Sodium clearance rates and the fractional sodium ex-

cretions did not differ significantly between the two groups.

Of the derived values of tubular function, the absolute reabsorption of sodium from the distal nephron (C.Li-C.Na) (p<0.01), the absolute reabsorption of water from the distal nephron segment (C.Li - UFR) (p< 0.01), and the fractional reabsorption of sodium from the distal tubule relative to the delivery of sodium from the proximal tubule (1- C.Na/C.Li) (p<0.01) were significantly lower in the cyclosporin A treated group than in the azathioprine treated group. Other values did not differ significantly.

After treatment with nifedipine (Table 2) there was a significant fall in sodium clearance, (p<0.01) and fractional excretion of sodium (p<0.05) in the cyclosporin A treated patients, which was accompanied by increases in the fractional distal reabsorption of sodium relative to the delivery of sodium from the proximal tubule (1-C.Na/C.Li) (p< 0.01), and the fractional distal reabsorption of water

Table 2. Effect on renal function after 7 days nifedipine treatment

	GROUP 1		GROUP 2	
	Pre-nifedipine treatment	During nifedipine	Pre-nifedipine treatment	During nifedipine
UFR ml/min	2.18 ± 1.37	1.48 ± 0.95	2.72 ± 1.28	2.76 ± 1.11
C.Cr ml/min	73.6 ± 33.2	67.10 ± 28.9	107.70 ± 37.9	92.30 ± 44.2
C.Na ml/min	1.43 ± 0.95	$0.78 \pm 0.69^{+}$	1.77 ± 0.89	1.56 ± 0.75
C.Li ml/min	11.59 ± 5.87	11.08 ± 5.19	26.40 ± 9.1	26.60 ± 12.5
FeNa %	2.21 ± 1.90	$1.45 \pm 1.23^{*}$	1.80 ± 0.99	2.15 ± 1.43
FeLi%	16.02 ± 6.05	16.86 ± 6.38	26.12 ± 4.55	$29.65 \pm 4.31^{*}$
C.Cr-C.Li mL/min	62.01 ± 28.87	55.75 ± 24.98	79.70 ± 33.6	$65.80 \pm 32.5^{+}$
C.Li-C.Na ml/min	9.95 ± 5.08	10.41 ± 5.29	24.50 ± 8.6	24.80 ± 12.2
C.Li-UFR ml/min	9.45 ± 5.4	9.91 ± 5.4	23.80 ± 8.6	24.30 ± 12.4
1-C.Na/C.Li %	0.87 ± 0.07	$0.92 \pm 0.01^{+}$	0.93 ± 0.03	0.93 ± 0.05
1-UFr/C.Li%	0.79 ± 0.12	$0.86 \pm 0.08^{**}$	0.90 ± 0.04	0.89 ± 0.08

Mean values shown * p< 0.05, ** p< 0.02, + p< 0.01. All values expressed per 100 kg body weight.

relative to the delivery of water from the proximal tubule (1-UFR/C.Li)(p < 0.02). Treatment of patients in the azathioprine group with nifedipine (Table 2) produced a significant rise in the fractional excretion of lithium (p<0.05), and a significant fall in the absolute proximal tubular reabsorption of iso-osmotic fluids (C.Cr-C.Li) (p<0.01).

DISCUSSION

The results of this study confirm previous investigations from our group, and others, which have shown that proximal tubular reabsorption of sodium and water is increased in patients or rats treated with cyclosporin A, and that distal tubular reabsorption of sodium is impaired (7-9). In rats these changes are accompanied by a decrease in GFR, and because they occur acutely it has been suggested that they are secondary to alterations in renal blood flow (10). In our study nifedipine therapy had no effect on GFR or the increased proximal reabsorption of lithium (and therefore sodium), which was apparent prior to commencing treatment in the cyclosporin A treated group. Tests of distal tubular function, however, showed that nifedipine therapy induced a significant rise in both sodium and water reabsorption from the distal tubule in the cyclosporin A treated patients but not in those patients given azathioprine.

The lack of improvement in GFR in the cyclosporin A treated patients cannot, however, be taken to imply that nifedipine did not improve renal blood flow. Nifedipine may cause efferent as well as afferent arteriolar vasodilation, thus increasing renal blood flow without affecting GFR (11-13). Furthermore, at the start of the study distal tubular reabsorption of sodium (as shown by 1-C.Na/C.Li) was significantly lower in the cyclosporin A treated patients than in those given azathioprine. During nifedipine treatment, distal reabsorption of sodium increased only in the cyclosporin A treated patients. In acute experiments on rats it was shown that nifedipine could prevent such cyclosporin A induced distal tubular abnormalities; because of the rapidity of the

distal tubular changes it was postulated that they were secondary to improvements in renal blood flow (9). The same study, however, showed that the acute fall in GFR induced by cyclosporin A cannot be reversed by calcium channel blockade. Thus the rise in distal sodium reabsorption in our patients may have been the only manifestation of enhanced renal blood flow.

At present it is not known whether the morphological and functional tubular changes of chronic cyclosporin A nephrotoxicity are secondary to haemodynamic alterations or due to a direct tubulotoxic affect (14). Therefore an alternative explanation may be that the changes in distal tubular function were due to a reduction in cyclosporin A tubulotoxicity, as calcium channel blockade reduces uptake of cyclosporin A into renal tubular cells (15). Furthermore it has been suggested that by a direct effect on the renal tubules, cyclosporin A activates tubuloglomerular feedback to cause a fall in GFR (8,16,17). If this were the case, the rise in distal tubular sodium reabsorption observed during nifedipine therapy could have modified such cyclosporin A mediated activation.

In conclusion, this study shows that nifedipine can ameliorate functional changes in distal tubular handling of sodium due to cyclosporin A therapy. The lack of improvement in GFR after nifedipine treatment was, perhaps, not surprising, as all the patients studied had been transplanted for at least one year, by which time cyclosporin A associated arteriolopathy would have been well established (18). The implications of these changes remain to be ascertained in longer term studies.

REFERENCES

1. Racusen LC, Solez K: Cyclosporine nephrotoxicity. Int Rev Exp Path 30: 107-157, 1988.

2. Feehally J, Walls J, Mistry N, Hosburgh T, Taylor J, Veitch PS, Bell PR: Does nifedipine ameliorate cyclosporin A nephrotoxicity. Br Med J 295: 310-311, 1987.

3. Wagner K, Albrecht S, Neumayer HH: Prevention of post-transplant acute tubular necrosis by the calcium antagonist diltiazem: A prospective randomized study. Am J Nephrol 7: 287-294, 1987.

4. Neumayer HH, Wagner K: Prevention of delayed graft function in cadaver kidney transplants by diltiazem: outcome of two prospective, randomised clinical trials. J Cardiovasc Pharmacol 10 (Suppl 10): S170-S177, 1987.

5. Hwan JTC, Foxall PJD, Townend JN, Bending MR, Eisinger AJ: Does nifedipine ameliorate cyclosporin A nephrotoxicity? Brit Med J 295: 851, 1987.

6. Thomsen H: Lithium clearance: a new method for determining proximal and distal tubular reabsorption of sodium and water. Nephron 37: 217-223, 1984.

7. Wheatley HC, Datzmann M, Williams JW, Miles DE, Hatch FE: Long-term effects of cyclosporine on renal function in liver transplant recipients. Transplantation 43: 641-647, 1988.

8. Whiting PH, Simpson JG: Lithium clearance measurements as an indication of cyclosporin A nephrotoxicity in the rat. Clin Sci 74: 173-178, 1988.

9. Dieperink H, Leyssac PP, Starklint H, Jorgensen HA, Kemp E: Antagonist capacities of nifedipine, captopril, phenoxybenzamine, prostacyclin and indomethacin on cyclosporin A induced impairment of rat renal function. Eur J Clin Invest 16: 540-548, 1986.

10. Dieperink H, Leyssac PP, Kemp E, Steinbrucke L, Starklint H: Glomerulotubular function in cyclosporine treated rats. Clin Nephrol 25 Suppl 1: 70-74, 1986.

11. Sterzel RB: Renal actions of calcium antagonists. J Cardiovasc Pharmac 10 (suppl 10): 17-21, 1987.

12. Loutzenhiser R, Epstein M: Effects of calcium antagonists on renal haemodynamics. Am J Physiol 249: F619-F629, 1985.

13. Krussell LR, Christensen CH, Pedersen OL: Acute natriuretic effect of nifedipine in hypertensive patients and normotensive controls - a proximal tubular effect. Eur J Clin Pharmacol 32: 121-126, 1987.

14. Thiel G: Experimental cyclosporine A nephrotoxicity: A summary of The International Workshop (Basle, April 24-26 1985). Clin Nephrol 25: 205-210, 1986.

15. Naginemi CN, Misra BC, Lee DBN, Yanagawa N: Cyclosporine A - calcium channels interaction: A possible mechanism of nephrotoxicity. Transplant Proc 19: 1358-1364, 1987.

16. Gerkens JF, Bhagwandeen SB, Dosen PJ, Smith AJ: The effect of salt intake on cyclosporine-induced impairment of renal function in rats. Transplantation 38: 412-417, 1984.

17. Gnutzmann KH, Hering H, Gutsche H-V: Effect of cyclosporine on the diluting capacity of the rat kidney. Clin Nephrol 25 (Suppl 1): S5l-56, 1986.

18. Myers BD, Nehdon L, Bashkos C, Macoviak JA, Frist WH, Derby GC, Perlroth MG, Sibley RK: Chronic injury of human microvessels with low-dose cyclosporine therapy. Transplantation 46: 694-703, 1988.

26
INTERACTION OF CALCIUM ANTAGONISTS AND CYCLOSPORINE A

H.-H.Neumayer (1)[*], J. Brockmöller (2), U. Kunzendorf (1), I. Roots (2), K. Wagner (1)

Departments of Internal Medicine and Nephrology (1) and Clinical Pharmacology (2), Klinikum Steglitz, Free University of Berlin, Germany

INTRODUCTION

Our group has previously demonstrated that perfusion of the donor kidney or the combined treatment of donor kidney and recipient with the calcium antagonist (CA) diltiazem (Dil) reduces the incidence of delayed graft function or rejection episodes in cadaveric kidney transplants, despite significantly elevated cyclosporine A (CyA) whole blood trough levels (1,2). By contrast, some authors found worsening of some CyA side-effects under the Dil treatment associated with elevated CyA-levels (3,4). However, the CyA concentration had been analysed by unspecific radioimmunoassay (RIA) (5) not permitting to differentiate between the parent substance and its metabolites. It was therefore the aim of the present studies to investigate retrospectively the influence of initiation or discontinuation of two different CA (Dil) and nifedipine (Nif) on CyA-therapy. In a second prospectively performed clinical trial, the effect of Dil on kidney graft function and CyA pharmacokinetics has been investigated in patients with stable graft function to elucidate a possible mechanism of this drug interaction.

METHODS

In a retrospective investigation of nonhospitalized patients, at least three months after kidney transplantation, CyA-whole blood trough levels, CyA-doses and CyA-clearances

were recorded before the start of therapy with either Dil (n=23) or Nif (n=24) and after achieving CyA blood levels comparable to those before the initiation of CA. The same parameters were determined after withdrawal of Dil or Nif, and after stable CyA blood levels had been achieved without further dose adjustment. Patients (n=20) receiving no CA were used as a reference group. After informed consent and according to the guidelines of the declaration of Helsinki, 22 non-hospitalized patients without previous CA therapy and with stable graft function (at least 6 months after cadaveric kidney transplantation, plasma creatinine levels below 150 Mol/l and no changes exceeding 10% and no rejection episodes during the last three months) were included in this prospective study. Initially, a pharmacokinetic profile of the orally applied maintenance dose of CyA was obtained together with measurements of glomerular filtration rate (GFR) and renal blood flow (RBF), using single shot techniques with inulin and PAH (6). Thereafter, Dil-therapy was initiated at a dose of 2 x 60 mg/d orally. After 1 and 4 weeks pharmocokinetic investigations and measurements of renal function were repeated. Subsequently, over a period of 3 weeks, CyA-dose was tapered down to achieve CyA whole blood trough levels comparable to those before start of Dil-therapy. CyA whole blood trough levels were determined by RIA using polyvalent and monovalent unspecific antibodies according to the method of Donatsch (5). In addition, CyA blood levels and concentrations of the metabolites M1, M17, M18, and M21 were measured by HPLC ac-

[*]New address: Transplantationszentrum der Universität Erlangen-Nürnberg, 4 Medizinisch Klinik Kontumazgarte 14-18 850 Nürnberg Germany

cording to the method of Christians et al (7). In addition, the inhibition of CyA metabolism by Dil was investigated "in vitro", using human liver microsomes coincubated with different concentrations of Dil. Data are given as means $\pm$ SD or SEM. Statistical significance was accepted at the 5% level. (Student's t-test, Wilcoxon test).

RESULTS

Initiation of Calcium Antagonists: Therapy with CA was initiated 349$\pm$63 days (Dil, n=23) and 164$\pm$27 days (Nif, n=24) after renal transplantation. In all patients, the occurrence of mild or moderate arterial hypertension was the indication for the application of CA. CyA-parameters were recorded before and

after 214$\pm$40 (Dil) or 169$\pm$42 (Nif) days of continuous intake of the drugs. In the control group, the same parameters were recorded 311$\pm$41 days after renal transplantation and after an additional period of 185$\pm$4 days. No significant changes (Table 1) in plasma creatinine levels or plasma concentrations of liver enzymes (GOT, GPT, AP) occurred in any of the groups. During the observation periods, CyA was reduced by 16$\pm$2 % in controls (p<0.001), by 21$\pm$4% in patients receiving Nif (p<0.01) and by 435% in the Dil-treated individuals (p<0.0001). CyA whole blood levels (RIA) remained stable in the Dil-group (+5$\pm$3%), whereas there was a fall of 15$\pm$6% in the Nif-group and of 7%$\pm$4% in controls. These findings were reflected by

Table 1. Influence of Calcium Antagonists (CA) on Cyclosporin-A Therapy (CsA)

		Diltiazem	Nifedipin	Control
Initiation of CA				
Patients	(n)	23	24	20
CsA parameters before initiation of CA				
dose	(mg/kg/d)	4.47$\pm$0.3	5.62$\pm$0.4	4.57$\pm$0.3
blood level	(ng/mL)	404.00$\pm$50	472.00$\pm$41	375.00$\pm$32
clearance	(mL/min/kg)	8.60$\pm$0.6	9.10$\pm$0.8	9.80$\pm$1.2
CsA parameters under therapy with CA				
dose	(mg/kg/d)	2.55$\pm$0.2*	4.4$\pm$0.2[+]	3.85$\pm$0.3[++]
blood level	(ng/mL)	425.00$\pm$29	403.00$\pm$25	350.00$\pm$27
clearance	(mL/min/kg)	4.30$\pm$0.3[#]	8.10$\pm$0.5	8.10$\pm$0.7[++]
Discontinuation of CA				
Patients	(n)	20	13	20
CsA parameters before discontinuation of CA				
dose	(mg/kg/d)	3.47$\pm$0.4	5.21$\pm$0.5	4.57$\pm$0.3
blood level	(ng/mL)	493.00$\pm$50	399.00$\pm$43	375.00$\pm$32
clearance	(mL/min/kg)	5.20$\pm$0.5	11.10$\pm$2.2	9.80$\pm$1.2
CsA parameters after discontinuation of CA				
dose	(mg/kg/d)	3.96$\pm$0.4	4.27$\pm$0.4[#]	3.85$\pm$0.3
blood level	(ng/mL)	319.00$\pm$26[#]	405.00$\pm$35	350.00$\pm$27
clearance	(mL/min/kg)	9.20$\pm$0.8[#]	8.10$\pm$1.2*	8.10$\pm$0.7*

Note: Results are mean, SEM. P values reflect comparison to initial values. [#]P<.05, [+]P<.01, [++]P<.001, *P<.0001.

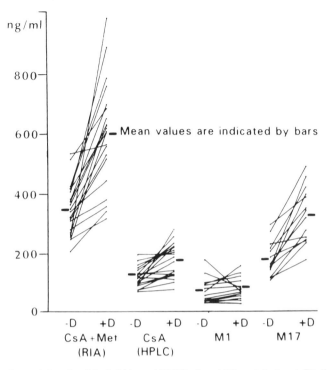

Figure 1. Whole blood trough levels of CsA, M1, and M17 before (-D) and during (+D) diltiazem application.

changes in CyA-clearances: -50±9% in the Dil-treated patients (p<0.05), -11±3% in the Nif-group (ns) and -17±4% in controls (p<0.001).

Discontinuation of Calcium Antagonists: (Table I) Dil (n=20) was given for 206±39 days and Nif (n=13) for 272±50 days. The indications for discontinuation of Dil and Nif were retrospectively not established in most cases. Parameters of CyA-therapy were recorded 103±16 (Dil) or 146±28 (Nif) days after termination of calcium blocker therapy. CyA-dose was raised by 14±3% in patients after discontinuation of Dil, but significantly reduced by 17±4% in patients after withdrawal of Nif (p<0.05). An analogous dose reduction of 16±2% was observed in the control group (p<0.001). In contrast to a significant reduction of CyA whole blood trough levels in the Dil-treated patients by 37±6% (p<0.001)   only minor changes occurred after abandonment of Nif (+2±5%, ns)

and in controls (-7±4%, ns). This was also confirmed by the calculated alterations of CyA-clearances in all three groups: Dil: +77±11% (p<0.05), Nif: -37±4% (p<0.0001), controls: -17±4% (p<0.001). During the observation period, 6 rejection episodes occurred in the Dil group compared to only 3 in the Nif group. Corrected for an equivalent period of 100 days, 0.29 rejection episodes per patient occurred in the Dil group compared to 0.15 episodes in the Nif group (p<0.05).

Influence of Dil on CyA Pharmacokinetics and Kidney Function: After one week of Dil application (2 x 60 mg/d), CyA blood trough levels (Figure 1) were raised from 350±18 ng/ml to 595±35 ng/ml (p<0.0 05). HPLC showed an increase in native CyA from 117±8 to 170±12 ng/ml (p<0.005) after Dil comedication. Mean trough levels of metabolite M17 increased from 194±13 to 336±25 ng/ml (p<0.005), whereas the concentrations of metabolite M1 (70±9 vs

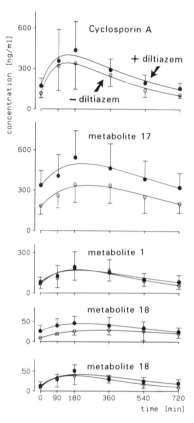

Figure 2. Concentration profiles of CyA and metabolites in 22 patients after kidney transplantation with (black circle) and without diltiazem.

than at the starting point (435±32 vs 350±16 ng/ml, p<0.05.). It was calculated that a dose reduction by 40% (2.02±0.2 mg/kg/min) would bring about the same CyA blood levels. At the end of the investigation, neither GFR nor RBF nor plasma creatinine (128±4 mol/l) levels differed from initial values.

In vitro Metabolism Experiments.

In order to experimentally verify the inhibition of CyA metabolism by Dil, microsomes metabolizing CyA were co-incubated with different concentrations of Dil. Human liver microsomes prepared from 4 different tisssue samples were used as well as rat liver microsomes from phenobarbital-pretreated rats. Similar values for formation of M1 and M17 were found in liver microsomes from phenobarbital-treated rats and in human liver microsomes (Figures 3,4). Comparison of the inhibitory effects of the three CA Dil, Nif and verapamil showed the highest degree of inhibition for verapamil (Ki=10 mol/l). An analogous high degree of inhibition of CyA metabolism was measured for Dil (Ki=15 mol/l). Both compounds showed the non-competitive type of inhibition. In contrast, Nif showed much less inhibition (ki 100 mol/l), and inclusion of Nif in these CyA-metabolizing assays led to competitive inhibition according to Lineweaver-Burk and Dixon-Plot analysis. Formation of M1 and M17 was inhibited in the same manner.

80±8 ng/ml), M18 and M21 were found unchanged.

There was a clear trend towards an increase in the maximal concentration (C_{max}) (Figure 2) from 1,638±200 to 2,035±304 ng/ml with Dil, while no change was detectable in the invasion (K_{inv}) or elimination rate (K_{elim}). One week after Dil application and in parallel with the increase in CyA blood levels, RBF was slightly but significantly reduced from 324±17 to 295±16 ml/min (91±4%, p<0.05). There was also a tendency of a moderate decrease in GFR (57±5 vs 64±6 ml/min, ns). After 4 weeks of Dil therapy, the initial CsA dose was reduced by 29±3% from 3.62±0.2 to 2.61±0.2 mg/kg/d (p<0.0001), but CyA blood levels remained significantly higher

DISCUSSION

In contrast to our findings with Nif, the results of the retrospective investigation revealed a striking effect of Dil, a CA of the benzodiazepine- type, on CyA pharmacokinetics. After initiation of Dil, a dramatic drop of CyA-clearance by 50±9% occurred, which led to a reduction of the CyA dose by 43±5%. This dose reduction was twice as high as in controls and might at least reduce the costs of aftercare in organ transplantation. It must, however, be mentioned that due to the reversibility of this interaction, an untoward situation may occur after discontinuation of Dil. Since CyA clearance increased by 77±11% and CyA dose was only augmented by 14±3% in our patients, a clinically relevant decrease in CyA blood levels

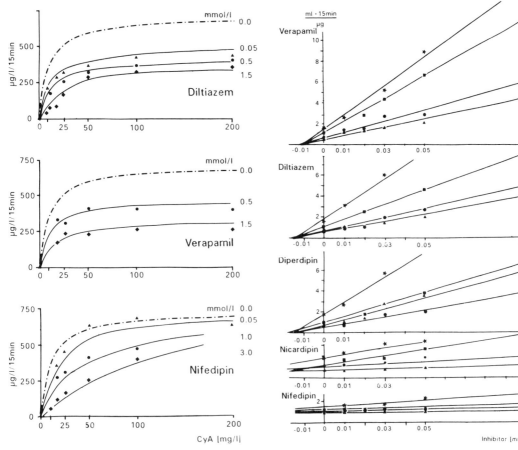

Figure 3. Formation rate of metabolite 1 in human liver microsomes during incubation with different concentrations of various calicium antagonist.

Figure 4. Dixon-plots, demonstrating the inhibition of various calcium antagonist on CyA-metabolism (phenobarbital-treated rat liver micromes).

occurred. Consecutively, the incidence of rejection episodes was twice as high as in the group after withdrawal of Nif. It is therefore mandatory to intensify CyA blood level control, in transplant recipients receiving CA like nicardipine (8), verapamil (9) or Dil, especially when those drugs are discontinued. The observed increase of CyA blood levels with mono- and polyclonal RIA-kits and HPLC after application of Dil might in part be due to alterations in the metabolite composition, since the concentration of M17 determined by HPLC was markedly increased, whereas M1, M18, M21 remained mainly unchanged. The main mechanism of

this drug interaction seems to be an inhibition of hepatic CyA metabolism by Dil. This is confirmed by our in vitro studies with human liver microsomes, which showed a dose-dependent non-competitive inhibition of CyA metabolism by Dil.

In summary, the present data, as well as previous results of CyA level determination in our study on the prevention of delayed graft function by Dil using HPLC (10,11) clearly demonstrate that the elevated CyA blood levels are caused, at least in part, by the accumulation of CyA metabolites. This might be of great clinical relevance, since the inhibitory potency of M 17 on interleukin-2 formation is comparable with that of native CyA (12), while its nephrotoxic activity seems to be less pronounced (13). This would also explain the results of our previous clinical trial, where we demonstrated a reduced incidence of rejection episodes under concomitant therapy with Dil and CyA, although CyA blood levels were in the same range due to a drastic dose reduction of CyA (1). One possible explanation for these results would be that Dil application had led to an accumulation of metabolites with less pronounced nephrotoxicity but equivalent immunosuppressive activity (14).

REFERENCES

1. Neumayer HH, Wagner K: Prevention of delayed graft function in cadaver kidney transplants by diltiazem: Outcome of two prospective, randomized cinical trials. J Cardiovasc Pharmacol 10: S170-S177, 1987.

2. Neumayer HH, Schreiber M, Wagner K: Prevention of delayed graft function by diltiazem and iloprost. Transplant Proc 21: 1221-1224, 1989.

3. Pochet JM, Pirson Y: Cyclosporine-diltiazem interaction. Lancet 1: 979, 1986.

4. Grino JM, Sabate I, Castelao AM, Alsina J: Influence of diltiazem on cyclosporine clearance. Lancet 1: 1387, 1986.

5. Donatsch P, Abisch E, Homberger M, Trabar R, Trapp M: A radio-immunoassay to measure cyclosporine A in plasma and serum samples. J Immunoassay 2: 19-32, 1981.

6. Hall JE, Guyton AC, Farr BM: A single-injection method for measuring glomerular filtration rate. Am J Physiol 232: 72-76, 1977.

7. Christians U, Zimmer KO, Wonigeit K, Sewing KF: Measurements of cyclosporine A and of four metabolites in whole blood by high-performance liquid chromatography. J Chromatogr 413: 121-129, 1987.

8. Bourqbigot B, Giuserix J, Airiau J, Bressollette L, Morin JF Cledes J: Nicardipine increases cyclosporine blood levels. Lancet 2: 1447, 1987.

9. Lindholm A, Henricsson S: Verapamil inhibits cyclosporin metabolism. Lancet 2: 1262-1263, 1987.

10. Kunzendorf U, Walz G, Neumayer HH, Wagner K, Keller F, Offermann G: Einfluss von Diltiazem auf die Ciclosporin-Blutspiegel. Klin Wochenschr 65:1101-1103, 1987.

11. Walz G, Kunzendorf U, Keller F, Neumayer HH, Offermann G: Cyclosprine blood levels in diltiazem-treated kidney graft recipients. Clin Transplantation 2: 21-25, 1988.

12. Freed BM, Rosano TG, Lempert N: In vitro immunosuppressive properties of cyclosporine metabolites. Transplantation 43: 123-127, 1987.

13. Ryffel B, Hiestand P, Foxwell B, Donatsch P, Boelsterli HJ, Maurer G, Mihatsch MJ: Nephrotoxic and immunosuppressive potentials of cyclosporine metabolites in rats. Transplant Proc 18: 41-45, 1986.

14. Kunzendorf U, Brockmöller J, Jochimsen F, Roots I, Offermann G. Immunosuppressive properties of cyclosporin metabolites. Lancet ii: 734-735, 1989.

27

THE USE OF LITHIUM CLEARANCE MEASUREMENTS TO ASSESS RENAL TUBULAR DYSFUNCTION OF CYCLOSPORIN TREATED UVEITIS PATIENTS

P. H. Whiting (1), H. M. A. Towler (2), A. M. Cliffe (2) and J. V. Forrester (2)

Departments of Clinical Biochemistry (1) and Ophthalmology (2), University of Aberdeen, Medical Buildings, Foresterhill, Aberdeen AB9 2ZD, UK

INTRODUCTION

The use of CsA in the treatment of autoimmune disease (1) in general, and intraocular inflammatory disease in particular, is becoming more widespread following the initial studies of Nussenblatt et al (2). However, the potential therapeutic benefits to these patients, who usually present with normal renal function, may be limited by CsA-induced nephrotoxicity. It is, therefore, important to regularly monitor renal function, both glomerular and tubular, in patients treated with CsA for autoimmune disease to provide early indications of renal dysfunction. The biochemical parameters most commonly used include serum urea and creatinine concentrations, and estimations of creatinine clearance rate. However, reliable and sensitive indicators of early CsA-nephrotoxicity have not yet been established.

Previous work from both this and other laboratories (3-5) has demonstrated that lithium clearance, as a measure of overall renal proximal fluid and sodium delivery (6-7), may provide a method for estimating and monitoring the degree of CsA-induced renal tubular dysfunction in renal allograft recipients. This study describes the use of lithium clearance measurements in 12 patients treated with CsA for chronic intraocular inflammatory disease as an estimate of drug-induced nephrotoxicity.

PATIENTS AND METHODS

Patients: Twelve patients (7 males and 5 females, mean age 43.8 years, range 8.5 - 66.9 years) with chronic posterior uveitis of various aetiologies, whose control of ocular disease activity with systemic steroids alone had been unsatisfactory, were treated with low dose oral CsA for 6-48 months (mean maintenance dose 4.0 ± 1.1mg/kg body weight; mean ± SD). Seven of the 12 patients also continued to receive oral prednisolone (15mg/day or less). Clinical evaluation included visual acuity (Snellen), slit-lamp biomicroscopy, fluorescein angiography and indirect ophthalmoscopy.

Lithium clearance. At 10pm on day 1 patients received 750mg Li_2CO_3 (Camcolit, Norgine Ltd). On day 2, venous blood (10ml) was collected at 9am and 4pm and all urine passed between these times was collected (7 hours). In addition, at 9am a pre-dose whole blood sample was obtained for measurement of trough CsA concentration. This procedure was performed at 3-4 monthly intervals over the treatment period of up to 48 months (64 determinations). Lithium and creatinine clearance rates and fractional clearance values were also obtained over the treatment period from 40 healthy volunteers (23 males and 17 females, mean age 35, aged 16-68 years).

Analyses. Serum and urine concentrations of sodium, lithium and creatinine were measured as previously described (3) and whole blood trough CsA levels using radioimmunoassay kits

(Sandoz Ltd.). The polyclonal antibody used in the kits was unable to distinguish between CsA and certain of its metabolites.

Calculations. The clearance rates of lithium (CLi) and creatinine (CCR) and the fractional clearance rate of lithium (FELi, %) were calculated as previously described (6). CLi and FELi reflect the delivery of isoosmotic fluid from the end of the proximal tubule to the loop of Henle and the proximal fractional reabsorption, respectively.

Statistics. Results, presented as mean $\pm$ SD from CsA-treated patients and those from normal volunteers, were compared using the Mann-Whitney U test and probability values of < 0.05 were considered significant. Linear regression analysis was also performed and, where indicated, regression lines were compared using Snedecor's F-test (8).

RESULTS

Clinical Response to CsA Therapy

Visual acuity was improved in 10 of the 12 patients studied, both at 6 and 12 months and this improvement corresponded well with a measureable decrease in intraocular inflammation. This visual improvement has been maintained in these patients over the study period.

Renal function

Although CCR was measured in all 12 patients prior to initiation of CsA treatment (128.4$\pm$42.3 ml/min/100 kg body weight), CLi measurements were only obtained in 6 patients before initiation of treatment. Over the treatment period, CCR remained relatively constant or improved by between 8 and 48% in 3 cases, but fell by 9-70% in the remaining 9 patients. Values for both CLi and FELi fell significantly over the treatment period in all 12 patients. For the 6 patients with pretreatment values, CLi and FELi both fell 2 to 3-fold after 6-8 months of CsA treatment although CCR values were not significantly altered (Table 1). In patients treated with CsA for between 12 and 15 months, values of CCR, CLi and FELi (available for 7 patients) were consistently reduced compared to values obtained from healthy volunteers. The presence of renal impairment was managed initially by CsA dose reduction and finally by withdrawal of treatment if required. Improvements in CCR, CLi and FELi were usually observed following such CsA dose modifications.

Within the patient and normal volunteer groups, and considering all available measure-

Table 1. The effect of CsA treatment on renal function.

Group	CCR ml/min/100kg	CLi ml/min/100kg	FELi %
1. Pretreatment (6)	136.9$\pm$53.9	34.1$\pm$8.1	26.2$\pm$4.7
2. CsA for 6-8 months (6)	115.3$\pm$50.3	12.3$\pm$8.2**	10.4$\pm$3.7**
3. Healthy controls (40)	178.7$\pm$9.4	43.2$\pm$12.7	25.9$\pm$3.9
4. CsA for 12-15 months (7)	110.9$\pm$45.8#	19.4$\pm$10.3**	18.9$\pm$3.9#

Results expressed as mean$\pm$SD and the number of determinations is given in parentheses. Groups 1 v 2, **, p<0.001 and 3 v 4, #, p<0.05; *, p<0.01.

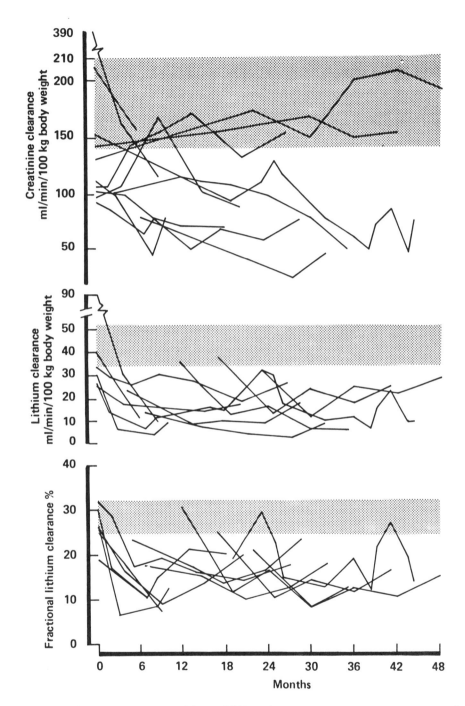

Figure 1. The effect of CsA treatment on creatinine and lithium clearance rates and the fractional excretion of lithium. Shaded area represents the reference range (95%) derived from 40 normal volunteers.

ments, there were similar linear relationships between CLi and CCR (r=0.4566, p<0.01 and r=0.8215, p<0.001 respectively), and CLi and FELi (r=0.7655 and r=0.5720 respectively, both p<0.001).

Trough CsA concentrations were usually maintained within the therapeutic window published by Sandoz Ltd. at 425 ± 223 µg/l, although on two occasions 8 weeks apart, values of 1055 and 938 for one patient were observed. However, there was no apparent temporal relationship between CsA levels, GFR or the observed changes in CLi or FELi.

DISCUSSION

The results of the present study clearly demonstrate that renal tubular dysfunction, with respect to the handling of water and electrolytes, as reflected by reduced lithium clearance rates and fractional excretion of lithium values, was present in all the patients treated with CsA. Furthermore, tubular dysfunction was also observed in patients who maintained creatinine clearance rates within the reference range of the laboratory. These reductions in both glomerular and tubular function were observed in patients treated with a low dose CsA/steroid regimen when previous studies had indicated that the incidence of nephrotoxicity was of significance only when higher doses of the drug were used (10). Although similar observations using stable renal transplant patients have also been noted (3,5), uveitis patients provide a unique opportunity to study CsA-nephrotoxicity in non-transplant patients.

Deray et al (11) have also suggested that the renal dysfunction associated with CsA after 9 months of treatment and characterised by increased serum creatinine concentrations was reversible on drug withdrawal. Some evidence of reversibility following either drug withdrawal or dose reduction was also observed in the present study following up to 40 months of treatment. Interestingly, reduction in administered dose, but not circulating CsA levels, was associated with improved renal function. This may be consistent with the development of a

chronic rather than acute (circulating CsA concentration-dependent) nephrotoxicity.

Studies from this and other laboratories using experimental animals and patients (12,13) suggest that the increased reabsorption of lithium by the proximal renal tubule observed in these patients reflects a decreased ultrafiltration pressure, produced as a result of an afferent arteriolar or glomerular haemodynamic effect, followed by an inadequate adaptive reduction in absolute proximal tubular reabsorption. Although the mechanism underlying this haemodynamic effect remains unclear, altered renal prostaglandin metabolism (13-16) and/or stimulation of the renin-angiotensin-aldosterone system (17), or CsA induced damage to the proximal tubule with consequent alteration to tubulo-glomerular feedback mechanisms (3,18) have all been implicated.

Although the use of CsA as an effective treatment for autoimmune diseases offers potential advantages to the patient, the benefits to one particular organ or organ system may not be achieved without detriment to the kidney. It must also be remembered that the traditional treatment regimes using azathioprine and/or steroids are also not without serious side effects. Although structurally CsA-induced renal dysfunction falls into several categories it is the non-dose dependent progressive chronic damage (19) which may ultimately limit its use as an effective therapeutic agent. The nephrotoxic properties of CsA cannot then be ignored when treating diseases affecting other organ systems and it is in this context that the regular monitoring of both glomerular and tubular function, using lithium clearance measurements, provides obvious benefits to the patient by potentially allowing dose adjustment to compensate for the renal functional deficit.

REFERENCES

1. Schmitz-Schumann M: Interim Report of Clinical Studies Presented at the International Symposium on Ciclosporin in Autoimmune Diseases. In: Borel J (ed); Ciclosporin: Progress in Allergy. Basel, Karger, 1986, vol 38, pp 436-446.

2. Nussenblatt RB, Palestine AG, Chan CC, Leak WC, Rook AH, Scher I, Gery I: Cyclosporine Therapy in Uveitis. Transplant Proc 15 (suppl 1): 2914-2922, 1983.

3. Whiting PH, Propper DJ, Simpson JG, McKay J, Jones MC, Catto GRDC. The use of lithium clearance measurements to assess renal tubular function in experimental and clinical cyclosporin nephrotoxicity. Transplant Proc 20 (suppl. 3): 845-849, 1988.

4. Dieperink H, Starklint H, Kemp E, Leyssac P. Comparative Pathophysiology and Histopathology of Cyclosporine Nephrotoxicity. Transplant Proc 20 (suppl. 3): 785-791, 1988.

5. Vincent HH, Wenting GJ, Schalenkamp MA, Jeekel J, Weimar W. Impaired fractional excretion of lithium: a very early marker of cyclosporine nephrotoxicity. Transplant Proc 19: 4147-4148, 1987.

6. Thomsen K. Lithium clearance: a new method for determining proximal and distal tubular reabsorption of sodium and water. Nephron 37:217- 223, 1984.

7. Thomsen K, Oleson OV. Renal lithium clearance as a measure of the delivery of water and sodium from the proximal tubule in humans. Am J Med Sci 288:158-161, 1984.

8. Snedecor GW. In: Statistical Methods (6th Ed). Iowa: Iowa State University Press, pp 432-466, 1967.

9. Levey AS, Perrone RD, Madias NE. Serum Creatinine and Renal Function. Ann Rev Med 39: 465-480, 1988.

10. Klintmalm G, Sawe J, Ringden O, von Bahr C, Magnusson A. Cyclosporin plasma levels in renal transplant patients. Association with renal toxicity and allograft rejection. Transplantation 39:132-137, 1985.

11. Deray G, Le Hoang P, Cacoub P, Aupetit B, Mertani A, Martinez F, Rottemburg J. Renal function and Blood Pressure in Patients Treated with Cyclosporin A for Uveitis. Eur J Clin Pharm 34: 601-604, 1988.

12. Dieperink H, Starklint H, Leyssac PP. Nephrotoxicity of cyclosporin - an animal model: study of the nephrotoxic effect of cyclosporine on overall renal and tubular function in conscious rats. Transplant Proc 15 (suppl 1): 2736-2741, 1983.

13. Dieperink H, Leyssac PP, Kemp E, Steinbruckl D, Starklint H. Glomerulotubular function in cyclosporin A treated rats. Clin Nephrol 25 (suppl 1):S70-S74, 1986.

14. Stahl RAK, Kudelka S. Chronic cyclosporine A treatment reduces prostaglandin E_2 formation in isolated glomeruli and papilla of rat. Clin Nephrol 25 (suppl 1):S78-S82, 1986.

15. Perico N, Benigni A, Zoja C, Delaini F, Remuzzi G. Functional significance of exaggerated renal thromboxane A_2 synthesis induced by cyclosporin A. Am J Physiol 251:F581-F587, 1986.

16. Kawaguchi A, Goldman MH, Shapiro R, Foegh M, Ramwell PW, Lower RR. Increase in urinary thromboxane B_2 in rats caused by cyclosporine. Transplantation 40:214-216, 1985.

17. Duggin GC, Baxter C, Hall B, Horvath JS, Tiller DJ. Influence of cyclosporine A on intrarenal control of GFR. Clin Nephrol 25 (suppl 1):S43-S45, 1986.

18. Gerken JF, Bhagwandeen SB, Dosen PJ, Smith AJ. The effect of salt intake on cyclosporine-induced impairment of renal function in rats. Transplantation 38:412-417, 1984.

19. Mihatsch MJ, Thiel G, Ryffel B. Morphology of Ciclosporin Nephropathy. In: Borel J (ed); Ciclosporin. Progress in Allergy, vol 38. Basel: Karger, 1986. pp 447-465.

28

CYCLOSPORIN REDUCES RENAL BLOOD FLOW THROUGH VASOCONSTRICTION OF ARCUATE ARTERIES IN THE HYDRONEPHROTIC RAT MODEL

L. B. Zimmerhackl*, M. Fretschner and M. Steinhausen,with technical assistance of R. Dussel and H. Filsinger

Department of Pediatrics*, University Freiburg, D-7800 Freiburg, and 1. Physiologisches Institut, University Heidelberg, D-6900 Heidelberg, Germany

INTRODUCTION

In transplant recipients as well as in patients receiving Cyclosporin A (CyA) for treatment of autoimmune disease, the drug may cause nephrotoxicity as indicated by an acute reduction in glomerular filtration rate and increase in serum creatinine values (1-3). Human renal biopsy specimens may exhibit nephrotoxic signs such as unspecific glomerular sclerosis, tubulo-interstitial fibrosis and occasionally as preglomerular vasculopathy (1,6). Recently Mihatsch and coworkers proposed arteriolar dysfunction as a mediator of disturbed glomerular filtration rate (4). This observation is in agreement with the experience of the Stanford heart transplant group (1).

From micropuncture studies in rats, Barros et al. (6) described increased afferent and efferent resistance in combination with a reduction in the ultrafiltration coefficient K_F (10). Thomson et al. (7) hypothesized that CyA causes preglomerular vaso-constriction without decrease in K_F. Murray et al. suggested that increased alpha-receptor mediated vasoconstriction is of importance (8). The exact vasoconstrictory site, vas afferens or other preglomerular arterioles, could not be specified, however.

The hydronephrotic kidney model permits direct visualization of the complete renal vascular system for microcirculatory observation (13). In the present study we used this model to determine the site of change in vascular resistance after acute administration of CyA.

MATERIAL AND METHODS

Wistar Furth rats (n=27) were prepared for microscopic observation as described (9,10). The left hydronephrotic kidney was prepared and displayed in a bathing chamber (9). Twenty recordings were taken: recordings #1-3 were taken in an initial control period where the animals received saline infusion; #4-8 were taken in the vehicle (solvent 1) period; recordings #9-17 were done in the experimental period during and after CyA or solvent 2, respectively; #18-19 after local application of nitrendipine $(2.8 \times 10^{-6}$ Mol) and #20 after local acetylcholine addition $(2.8 \times 10^{-6}$ Mol). In groups I and II, in addition to diameter measurements, blood velocity in microvessels was detected using the double slit technique as described earlier (10,11). Single vessel blood flow was calculated from diameter and velocity with correction for the Fahraeus effect (11).

Experimental groups: Group I (n=7): CyA dissolved in cremophore (50mg/ml) was administered in a dosage of 30mg/kg.

Vascular diameters and single vessel erythrocyte velocity were determined and apparent blood flow was then calculated according to standard formula (11).

Group II (n=5): Time Control 1, the solvent "cremophore", dissolved in rat plasma as described in group I, was administered instead of CyA in the experimental period.

Group III (n=8): CyA was dissolved in ethanol + 5% Tween-80 and administered intravenously in a dosage of 30 mg/kg in 30 min followed by a second administration of 20mg/kg 60 min after the end of the first infusion. Only diameters were determined. The protocol was otherwise identical to the groups I and II.

Group IV (n=3): Time Control 2; the solvent ethanol + 5% Tween-80 was administered instead of CyA. The protocol was otherwise identical to group III.

Group V (n=4): CyA, dissolved in cremophore, was added in increasing concentrations (10^{-7} to 10^{-5}) to the bathing chamber of the displayed kidney and after a stabilization period of 15 min intrarenal microvessel diameters were determined.

Statistics: Statistical analysis was done using analysis of variance with the Bonferoni-Holmes correction. Variation with time and difference in absolute values were compared and eleven contrasts were calculated and F-values corrected acccording to Bonferoni-Holmes.

RESULTS

General parameters: The body weight of animals ranged from 250-310g and the duration of hydronephrosis ranged between 110 and 170 days, respectively.

Renal vessel diameters: Diameters of group I and II are given in Figure 1 and 2. Infusion of CyA was associated with a preferential decrease in luminal diameter in arcuate arteries, reversible by the calcium channel-blocker nitrendipine (2.8×10^{-6}M). Maximal vasodilatation achieved with acetyl choline (2.8×10^{-6} M) was similar in both groups.

The diameters in efferent arterioles near the welling point decreased slightly, but significantly after CyA infusion in group III. CyA infusion was again associated with a significant vaso-

constriction of preglomerular vasa arcuata. Increasing the dosage of CyA did not cause further vasoconstriction (group III, Figure 3). On the contrary, the degree of vasoconstriction decreased in some animals during the course of the experiment.

Local administration of CyA (Group V), which was achieved by adding CyA in increasing concentrations to the perfusion chamber, did not demonstrate vasoconstriction (Table 1).

Glomerular blood flow: Blood flow decreased significantly after CyA by 70% (Figure 3). The glomerular blood flow decreased immediately after initiation of the CyA infusion as shown in figure. Neither drug, nitrendipine nor acetylcholine, could reverse the blood flow to the initial control levels or to levels comparable to the control group.

DISCUSSION

Effects of Cyclosporin on renal microvessels: CyA decreases renal blood flow immediately after acute intravenous administration. CyA infusion is associated with a marked vasoconstriction of arcuate arteries and a slight diminution in diameters of efferent arterioles in the hydronephrotic kidney model. Vasoconstriction of arcuate arteries without vasoconstriction of interlobular arteries and afferent arterioles is in contrast to the "classical" vasoconstrictors investigated in our laboratory such as angiotensin, norepinephrine, epinephrine or dopamine. The latter hormones cause vasoconstriction in different, more distant locations of renal vessels (12). Thus, in contrast to the observations of Perico et al. (13) increased renin-angiotensin-system activity does not seem to be the mediator in the CyA-induced vasoconstriction, at least not in the present model.

The vasoconstriction is inhibited by the calcium channel blocker nitrendipine. As shown earlier, nitrendipine dilates preglomerular vessels in the hydronephrotic kidney model (12). This indicates that a Ca^{++}-entry activating step is involved in the transcellular signal transmission causing arterial vasoconstriction. The

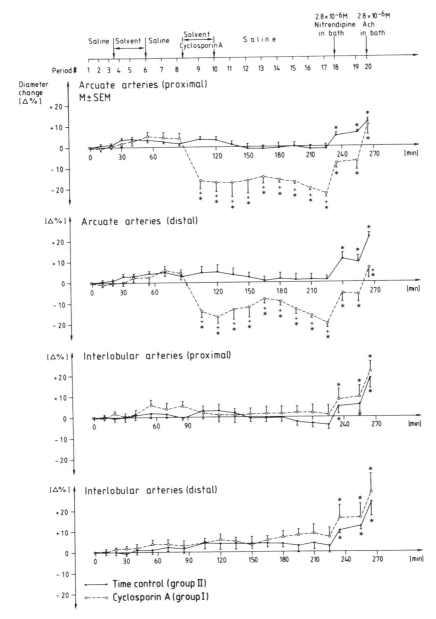

Figure 1. Relative change in vascular diameter of respective vessels in the hydronephrotic kidney model. Relative change in % to initial value. Group I receiving CyA 30mg/kg i.v. dashed line. Time-control, group II, solid line. The vertical arrows in the top line indicate the time of the infusion for the respective drug, the horizontal arrows indicate application of the drug to the kidney chamber (local application). Relative values of the control period (recording #1-3), after CyA or solvent, respectively (#17-18). Significance to control value of the same group is indicated by "*", significant difference in between groups by "+".

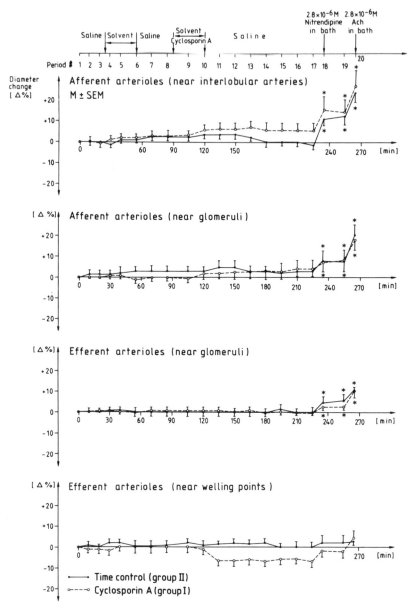

Figure 2. Relative change in diameter of respective vessels in the hydronephrotic kidney model. Relative change in % to initial value. See legend to Figure 4 for further explanation.

vasoconstriction is completely reversible with acetylcholine, which implies that CyA does not functionally damage the myocytes within the time period of this experiment.

The slight decrease in efferent arteriolar artery diameter near the welling point may be secondary to CyA. Any decrease in glomerular blood flow would cause a passive decrease in efferent arteriolar diameters (12).

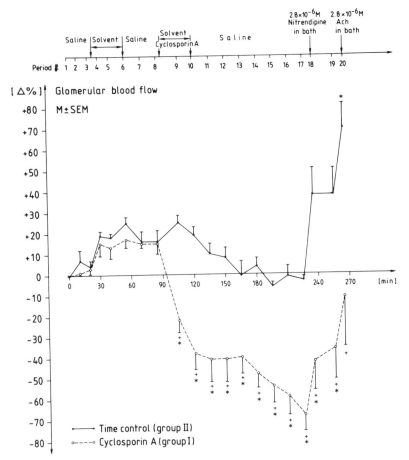

Figure 3. Glomerular blood flow. Relative values are given for the control period (#1-3), the solvent period (#7-8) and CyA or solvent 2 (#17-18), respectively.

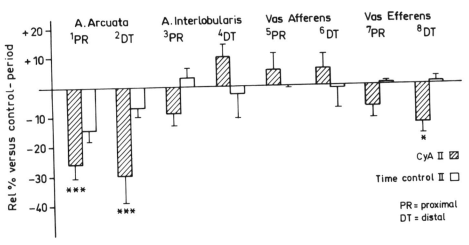

Figure 4. Effect of CyA 50mg/kg i.v. on renal vessel diameters (Groups III & IV). Relative changes compared to control period of each animal are given.

TABLE 1: Results of Group V: Effect of CyA added to the kidney chamber (local application). Diameters and glomerular blood flow are given as absolute value in control period. The following data are given as relative changes to the initial value.

	CONTROL (μm)	SOLVENT (%)	CYA (35') (%)	CYA (120') (%)
arcuate artery (proximal)	63.4±4.5	3.9±2.3	-29.3±4.5 *** +++	-26.2±4.6 **
arcuate artery (distal)	42.5±3.3	3.3±3.6	-33.0±5.23 *** +++	-29.8±8.7 *
interlobular artery (proximal)	23.2±1.4	2.4±3.1	-4.4±6.5	-9.1±4.4
interlobular artery (distal)	12.7±0.8	1.5±3.2	4.2±3.3	10.3±4.2
afferent artery (near interlobular artery)	9.5±1.10	0.3±2.8	0.4±4.0	5.7±6.1
afferent artery (near glomeruli)	9.4±0.7	-3.6±1.7	0.3±3.9	6.4±3.7
efferent artery (near glomeruli)	13.3±1.0	-3.4±3.3	-4.1±4.6	-7.4±4.7
efferent artery (near welling point)	18.3±1.3	-3.6±1.5	-13.2±3.1 * +	-13.6±3.4 *

Values are means ± SD, with significant differences shown * P < 0.05, **P < 0.01, and *** P < 0.001 for control period , and + P < 0.05, ++P < 0.01, and +++ P < 0.001 compared to control group.

CyA did not exhibit any vasoactive effect when administered from the tissue compartment (group V, Table 1).

Solvent effects: It has been suggested that the dissolution of CyA is critical. Cremophore solvent itself may alter renal blood perfusion (14). We used two different solvents to dissolve CyA: cremophore and ethanol/Tween. Using either solvent CyA caused similar responses (groups I+III). Therefore, the present results strongly indicate that CyA itself, and not the solvent, caused the vasoconstriction of arcuate arteries in this particular animal model.

ACKNOWLEDGEMENTS

Dr. N. Parekh gave valuable advice during the course of the experiments. Cyclosporine, cremophore and ethanol/Tween solutions were a gift from SANDOZ, Basel, Suisse. Dr. B. Ryffel (Sandoz) gave valuable advice concerning the dissolution of cyclosporine and the experimental protocol. This study was supported by the German Research Foundation (Forschergruppe Niere, Heidelberg) and Zi 314/1-1.

REFERENCES

1. Myers BD, Sibley R, Newton L, Tomlanovich SJ, Boshkos C, Stinson E, Luetscher JA, Whitney DJ, Krasny D, Coplon NS, Perlroth MG: The long-term course of cyclosporine associated chronic nephropathy. Kidney Int 33: 590-600, 1988.

2. Miescher PA, Favre H, Chatelanat F, Mihatsch MJ: Combined Steroid- Cyclosporin Treatment of Chronic Autoimmune Diseases. Klin Wochenschr 65: 727-736, 1987.

3. Zimmerhackl LB, Klein W, Helmchen U, Brandis M: Cyclosporin-trial in children with nephrotic syndrome: evaluation of nephrotoxicity. Eur J Pediatr 147: 218, 1988.

4. Miehatsch MJ, Thiel G, Spichtin HP, Oberholzer M, Brunner P, Harder F, Olivieri V, Bremer R, Ryffel B, Stocklin E, Torhorst J, Gudat F, Zollinger H, Loertscher R: Morphological findings in kidney transplants after treatment with cyclosporine. Transplant Proc 15 (Suppl 1): 2821-2825, 1983.

5. Steinhausen M, Parekh N, Zimmerhackl B: Pathophysiology of acute renal failure. In: (Seybold D, Gessler U (eds); Acute renal failure. Basel, Karger, 1982, pp. 9-22.

6. Barros EJG, Boim MA, Ajzen H, Ramkos OL, Schor N: Glomerular hemodynamics and hormonal participation on cyclosporine nephrotoxicity. Kidney Int 32: 19-25, 1987.

7. Thomson S, Tucker BJ, Blantz RC: Functional effects of chronic cyclosporine on glomerular hemodynamics. Kidney Int 33: 368, 1988.

8. Murray BM, Paller MS, Ferris TF: Effect of cyclosporine administration on renal hemodynamics in conscious rats. Kidney Int 28: 767-774, 1985.

9. Steinhausen M, Snoei H, Parekh N, Baker R, Johnson PC: Hydronephrosis: A new method to visualize vas afferens, efferens, and glomerular network. Kidney Int 23: 794-806, 1983.

10. Steinhausen M, Zimmerhackl B, Thederan H, Dussel R, Parekh N, Esslinger HU, Von Hagens G, Komitowski D, Dallenbach FD: Intraglomerular microcirculation: measurements of single glomerular loop flow in rats. Kidney Int 20: 230-239, 1981.

11. Zimmerhackl B, Tinsman J, Jamison RL, Robertson CR: Use of digital cross-correlation for on-line determination of single-vessel blood flow in the mammalian kidney. Microvasc Res 30: 63-74, 1985.

12. Steinhausen M: Physiologie und Pathophysiologie der Nierendurchblutung. Z Kardiol 76: Suppl 4, 71-79, 1987.

13. Perico N, Benigni A, Bosco E, Orisio S, Ghilardi F, Piccinelli A, Remuzzi G: Acute cyclosprine A nephrotoxicity in rats: which role for renin-angiotensin system and glomerular prostaglandins? Clin Nephrol 25: S83-S88, 1986.

14. Thiel G, Hermle M, Brunner FP: Acutely impaired renal function during intravenous administration of cyclosporine A: a cremophore side-effect. Clin Nephrol 25: S40-42, 1987.

29

EVIDENCE SUGGESTING A ROLE FOR PAF IN CYCLOSPORIN NEPHROTOXICITY IN RATS – EFFECT OF BN 52063 AND VERAPAMIL

J. Egido, A. Mendiluce, E. González, F. Mampaso, M. Gómez-Chiarri, A. Rivero, A. Ortiz, C. Gómez, L. Hernando

Laboratory of Nephrology, Fundación Jiménez Díaz, Universidad Autónoma, Madrid, Spain

INTRODUCTION

Cyclosporin A (CyA) is a potent immunosuppressant and its effectiveness in suppressing allograft rejection is well established. However, its use is associated with various side effects, the most important of which is nephrotoxicity. The pathophysiological mechanisms of renal damage induced by CyA are unclear. It has been suggested that damage by CyA may be initiated by haemodynamic alterations due to intrarenal vasoconstriction (1). A number of mediators have been implicated in the regulation of this phenomenon, among which, various fatty acids and more specifically the metabolites of arachidonic acid appear to play a role (2-4). Indeed, increased production of renal thromboxane under CyA treatment has been recently demonstrated (4).

Platelet activating factor (1-0-alkyl-2-acetyl-sn-glycero-3-phosphocholine; PAF) is a biologically active phospholipid that is synthetized by several cell types including neutrophils, monocytes-macrophages and renal cells (5). PAF infusion into the renal artery induces a dose-dependent reduction of the renal plasma flow, glomerular filtration rate, urinary volume and sodium excretion (6-7). For those reasons, PAF is thought to be one of the mediators of CyA-induced kidney damage.

In the present paper we have compared in a rodent model, with several features of chronic CyA toxicity, the effects of a specific PAF receptor antagonist BN-52063, and verapamil, a calcium entry blocker, which seems to reduce some of the in vivo effects of CyA (8,9).

MATERIAL AND METHODS

Materials The PAF receptor antagonist BN-52063, was prepared by Institut Henri-Beaufour, and a gift from Dr. P. Braquet. Cyclosporin (CyA) and Verapamil were kindly provided by Sandoz, Ltd., Basel, Switzerland and Knoll-Iberica, Madrid, Spain.

Experimental design Sprague-Dawley rats weighing 200-225 g were kept in metabolic cages with a standard diet and water ad libitum. Two days later rats were allocated randomly to 3 groups. In group I, rats received single, daily injections of CyA (25 mg/kg) i.p. mixed in olive oil for 4 weeks. In group II, rats received the same dose of CyA plus the PAF antagonist BN-52063, 50 mg/kg/day by oral route. In group III, rats received the same dose of CyA plus verapamil, 10 mg/kg/day by oral route.

The measurements of serum creatinine and BUN were done on 7, 15 and 28 days by means of a standard Coulter technique. Serum levels of CyA were determined by radioimmunoassay by employing polyclonal antibodies (Cyclo-Trac, Inestar, Co., Minnesota, USA).

Histologic and immunohistochemistry study of the kidney Kidneys perfused with normal saline were processed for histologic and immunohistochemistry studies as previously published (10).

To identify lymphohaemopoietic cell surface markers in frozen kidney tissue sections, we used a panel of monoclonal antibodies (Serotec, Oxford, England) and the avidin-biotinperoxidase (ABC) technique. The characteristic cell binding pattern of these monoclonal antibodies has been extensively described (11).

Incubation of isolated glomeruli and PAF assay. Renal glomeruli were isolated based on the ability of glomeruli to pass through a 105 μm sieve and to be retained in a 75 μm sieve. The production of PAF by glomerular cells was based upon the ability of incorporating ^{3}H-acetate substrate for lyso-PAF acetyl-CoA acetyltransferase into phospholipids including PAF (12). Samples were subjected to thin-layer chromatography on analytical silica gel plates of 2 mm thickness, Merck, Darmstadt, Germany, as previously described. The area of the plates migrating with a standard of synthetic PAF were scrapped off and counted for radioactivity. Bioassay for PAF was performed, in samples of which no ^{3}H acetate was added,

by measuring the release of ^{3}H-serotonine from rabbit platelets as previously described (12).

Statistical analysis The results are expressed as the mean ± SD. Significance was established using the Student's t-test.

RESULTS

Animals injected with CyA for 4 weeks presented elevated levels of serum creatinine (1.3 ± 0.4 mg/dl) in relation to the basal levels (0.70 ± 0.15). By contrast, animals treated with BN-52063 (group II) or Verapamil (group III) had lower levels of creatinine than those not treated, with values in the normal range (0.8 ± 0.2; 0.85 ± 0.18, respectively).

Tubular vacuolization was a prominent feature in CyA treated rats (group I). Small areas of interstitial atrophy with a moderate and focal interstitial mononuclear cell infiltration was also seen in these animals (Fig. 1).

Furthermore, some pre-glomerular arterioles presented exudative lesions with lumen reduction.

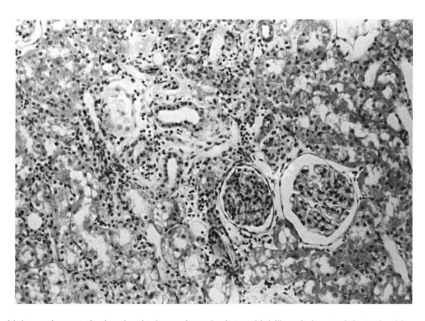

Figure 1. Light   micrograph showing lesions of patchy interstitial fibrosis in rats injected with cyclosporin for 4 weeks.

Rats from treated groups (II and III) depicted a striking amelioration in the renal histological lesions, with absence of minor changes of tubular vacuolization, diminution in the interstitial cell infiltrates and no lesions of fibrosis.

The identification of renal interstitial cells was performed by using a panel of monoclonal antibodies (Table I).

The protection afforded by BN-52063 and by Verapamil was not due to changes in the pharmacokinetics of the CyA, since mean serum levels of the drug were similar to those observed in non-treated rats (data not shown).

Glomeruli from normal rats incubated with CyA incorporated ^{3}H-acetate into a polar lipid that co-migrated with authentic PAF on thin layer chromatography. Maximal incorporation was seen with 10^{-8}M CyA, that corresponds to a 90% increase in relation to basal values. Samples processed without labeled acetate contained a lipid which stimulated the release of serotonine from rabbit platelets in a dose-dependent manner similar to that of synthetic PAF. This release was inhibited when platelets were pre-incubated with specific PAF receptor antagonists.

The pre-incubation of glomeruli from normal rats with Verapamil inhibited ^{3}H-acetate incorporation into PAF induced by CyA in a dose dependent manner. Maximal inhibition was

TABLE I Phenotypic characterization of interstitial cell infiltrates in CyA-nephrotoxicity

Group	Cell surface markers		
	0X1	0X6	W 3/13
Normal rats	23 ± 4//	15 ± 3	16 ± 3
Group I	85 ± 10*	49 ± 7*	37 ± 8**
Group II	47 ± 12	26 ± 6	24 ± 4
Group III	54 ± 9	32 ± 6	27 ± 5

//mean $\pm$ SD of cells/10 fields; *p<0.01. 0X1 reacts wtih leucocyte common antigen; 0X6 reacts with Ia bearing cells; W3/13 reacts with T cells and neutrophils. The number of animals in each group ranges from 5 to 7.

noted with 10^{-5}M of Verapamil (25% of that observed with 10^{-8}M CyA).

DISCUSSION

We have established a suitable rodent model to study chronic CyA nephrotoxicity. Together with the histologic features described, most often in rats administered CyA, as proximal tubular vacuolization, we have also observed an interstitial lesion dominated by the presence of an infiltrate of mononuclear cells that have been identified as Ia$^+$ cells and T cells by means of specific monoclonal antibodies. The existence of focal areas of interstitial fibrosis, though moderate, and the occasional presence of arteriolar hyperplasia, further support the resemblance of the histological lesions in this rat model with chronic CyA nephrotoxicity in humans. Our results are in agreement with those recently published using the same schedule (13).

In this paper we have also shown that the PAF antagonist, BN-52063, and the calcium channel blocker, Verapamil, reduce, to a large extent, CyA nephrotoxicity in rats. This beneficial effect was seen on renal function abnormalities and on histological lesions.

The results obtained with BN-52063 in our chronic model of nephrotoxicity confirm previous studies by Pirotzky et al. (14) in a model of CyA- nephrotoxicity in spontaneous hypertensive rats, and by our group in Sprague-Dawley rats injected with CyA for 15 days (15) using the same PAF antagonist. These data strongly implicate PAF in the pathogenesis of CyA-induced renal damage. This mediator exerts important changes on the renal haemodynamics. Thus, systemic PAF infusion is associated with profound diminution of renal blood flow, glomerular filtration rate (GFR) and urinary sodium excretion (6,7). In vitro, PAF contracts mesangial cells and stimulates PGE$_2$ synthesis (16). PAF also decreased the glomerular surface and thus the ultrafiltration coefficient (8,16), suggesting that the local generation of PAF by glomerular cells could explain some of the functional alterations observed in renal physiopathological situations. In fact, this mediator can be produced by endothelial, mesangial and interstitial renal cells upon appropriate stimuli (16). Since endothelium is considered a target cell in the early stages of CyA nephrotoxicity, it is possible that PAF released by endothelial or glomerular cells upon stimulation by CyA might provoke the renal hemodynamic alterations commented above. Recent in vitro studies have shown that CyA could reduce GFR by decreasing the glomerular ultrafiltration coefficient (8), perhaps as a consequence of the contraction of mesangial cells (16,17). The production of significant amounts of PAF by glomeruli of normal rats upon in vitro stimulation with CyA, observed in this paper, and recently published by other authors (17), further support the potential role of PAF in CyA nephrotoxicity.

The reduction in the severity of CyA renal damage afforded by the administration of Verapamil in this chronic model agrees with that observed by Iaina et al (18) in an acute renal failure in rats induced by CyA plus ischemia. In this regard, the same calcium-channel blocker prevented ischemic acute renal failure provoked by various injuries (19,20). Furthermore, Verapamil attenuated CyA effects on renal vascular resistance and renal plasma flow in rats studied by micropuncture (8), and by an in vivo fluorescence microscopy technique (9).

The mechanism of protection by the calcium channel blocker, Verapamil, could be related to an alteration of the vasoconstrictive ischaemic effect, due directly to CyA or indirectly through the release of a mediator substance like PAF. A direct CyA cellular effect inducing sublethal or lethal cell injury facilitating the entrance of calcium into the cells cannot be discarded (21). The results presented in this paper on the inhibition by verapamil of the CyA-induced glomerular synthesis of PAF suggest a novel mechanism, by which calcium channel blockers can ameliorate toxic renal failure. The similar beneficial effects observed in our model of CyA nephrotoxicity, by BN-52021 and Verapamil, on clinical and histological features, included the striking diminution in the interstitial cell infiltrates, suggest that PAF could be the final

common pathway of this injury. These data suggest that PAF antagonists and calcium channel blockers, probably in combination, could be useful in the prevention and treatment of CyA-induced nephrotoxicity.

ACKNOWLEDGEMENTS

This work was supported in part by grants from FISss and Fundación Iñigo Alvarez de Toledo (FIAT). A. Mendiluce, M. Gómez-Chiarri, C. Gómez and A. Rivero are fellows from FIAT, MEC, Fundación Conchita Rábago and FISss.

REFERENCES

1. Murray BM, Paller MS, Ferris TF. Effect of cyclosporin administration on renal hemodynamics in conscious rats. Kidney Int 28: 767-774, 1985.

2. Experimental cyclosporin A nephrotoxicity. An international workshop. Clin. Nephrol. 25:S 2-205, 1986.

3. Bennett WM, Elzinga L, Kelley V. Pathophysiology of cyclosporine nephrotoxicity: Role of eicosanoids. Transplant. Proc. 20:628-633, 1988.

4. Benigni A, Perico N, Remuzzi G. Abnormalities of arachidonate metabolism in experimental cyclosporin nephrotoxicity. Am. J. Nephrol. 9:72-77, 1989.

5. Pinckard RN, Ludwig JC, McManus LM. Platelet activating factors. In: I.I. Gallin, I.M. Goldstein, R. Snyderman (eds). Inflammation: Basic principles and clinical correlates. Raven Press Ltd, New York, 1988, pp 139-167.

6. Pirotzky E, Page CP, Morley C, Bidault J, Benveniste J. Vascular permeability induced by PAF acether in the isolated perfused rat kidney. Agents and Actions 16:17-18, 1985.

7. Scherf H, Nief AS, Schwertschlag V, Hughes M, Gerber JE. Hemodynamic effects of platelet activating factor in the dog kidney in vivo. Hypertension 8:737-741, 1986.

8. Barros EJG, Boim MA, Ajzen H, Ramos OL, Schor N. Glomerular hemodynamics and hormonal participation on cyclosporine nephrotoxicity. Kidney Int. 32:19-25, 1987.

9. Rooth P, Dawidson I, Diller K, Tljedal IB. Protection against cyclosporin-induced impairment of renal microcirculation by Verapamil in mice. Transplantation 45:433-437, 1988.

10. Mampaso F, Wilson CB. Characterization of inflammatory cells in autoimmune tubulointerstitial nephritis in rats. Kidney Int. 23:448-454, 1983.

11. Eddy AA, Crary GS, Michael AF. Identification of lymphohemopoietic cells in the kidney of normal rats. Am. J. Pathol. 129: 335-342, 1986.

12. Sánchez-Crespo M, Iñarrea P, Alvarez V, Alonso F, Egido J, Hernando L. Presence in normal human urine of a hypotensive and platelet activating phospholipid. Am. J. Physiol. 244:F706-711, 1983.

13. Gillum DM, Truong L, Tasby J, Migliore P, Suki WN. Chronic cyclosporin nephrotoxicity. A rodent model. Transplantation 46: 285-292, 1988.

14. Pirotzky E, Colliez PH, Guilmar C, Schaeverbeke J, Braquet P. Cyclosporin-induced nephrotoxicity: preventive effect of PAF acether antagonist BN-52063. Transplant. Proc. 20:665-669, 1988.

15. Egido J, Mampaso F, Rodríguez MJ, Martínez JC, Mendiluce A, Hernando P, Hernando L. Papel de los antagonistas del factor activador de las plaquetas (PAF) en la nefrotoxicidad inducida por la ciclosporina en ratas. Nefrología 8:S,30-37, 1988.

16. Schlondorff D, Neuwirth R. Platelet activating factor and the kidney. Am. J. Physiol. 25I:F1-F11, 1986.

17. Rodríguez Puyol D, Lamas S, Olivera A, López Farré A, Ortega G, Hernando L, López Novoa JM. Actions of cyclosporin A on cultured rat mesangial cells. Kidney Int. 35:632-637, 1989.

18. Iaina A, Herzog D, Cohen D, Gavendo S, Kapuler S, Serban I, Schiby G, Eliahou HE. Calcium entry blockade with verapamil in cyclosporin A plus ischemia induced acute renal failure in rats. Clin. Nephrol. 25:S168-S170, 1986.

19. Malis CD, Cheung JY, Alexander L, Bonventre J. Effects of verapamil in models of ischemic renal failure in the rat. Am. J. Physiol. 245:F735-F742, 1983.

20. Humes HD, Hunt DA, Clark MJ, White MP, Weinberg JM. Several mechanisms of protection in nephrotoxic and ischemic acute renal failure. In: R.R. Robinson (ed). Nephrology. Springer-Verlag New York, 1984. pp 776-783.

21. Farber JL. The role of calcium in cell death. Life Science 29:1289-1296, 1981.

30

CYCLOSPORINE-INDUCED NEPHROTOXICITY IN THE RAT IS PREVENTED BY THE GINKGOLIDE MIXTURE BN 52063

Ph. Colliez, C. Guilmard, E. Pirotzky and P. Braquet

Institut Henri Beaufour Research Labs, ZA de Courtaboeuf - 1, ave des Tropiques, 91952 LES ULIS CEDEX - France

INTRODUCTION

The therapeutic use of Cyclosporine (CsA) is limited because of its nephrotoxicity, the mechanism of which is not fully understood. Recent evidence suggests that nephrotoxicity may be initiated by haemodynamic alterations due to intrarenal vasoconstriction (1). A number of mediators have been implicated in the regulation of this phenomenon, among which, various fatty acids and more specifically the metabolites of arachidonic acid appear to play a role. Indeed increased production of renal thromboxane under CsA treatment has recently been demonstrated (2).

Platelet-activating factor (PAF) is a phospholipid mediator endowed with inflammatory and anaphylactic properties (3, 4). The production of PAF from various kidney cell types has indicated a role for this mediator in renal physiopathological processes (5, 6). In the present study spontaneously hypertensive rats (SHR) were treated with CsA and the creatinine clearance (CCr), blood urea nitrogen (BUN) and body weight were measured. Renal tissues were sampled and analyzed by light microscopy. Urinary thromboxane was also measured. Furthermore, in view of the possible role of PAF, the possible protection against CsA-induced nephrotoxicity afforded by the PAF-antagonist, BN 52063, was examined.

MATERIALS AND METHODS

Male spontaneously hypertensive rats (SHR) were treated for 21 days with CsA (Sandoz Pharmaceuticals, Basel, Switzerland). A group of animals received the vehicle of CsA and BN 52063 (IHB, Le Plessis-Robinson, France). A group of animals received CsA treatment (25 mg/kg/day, per os). A third group of rats is similarly treated with CsA but also received BN 52063 (50 mg/kg/day, per os).

Rats were placed in individual metabolic cages for 24 hr at day 12 and 21. Urine was collected free of food and faeces and blood samples were obtained at the midpoint of each period by retroorbital puncture. Serum and urine creatinine and BUN concentrations were determined with commercial kits (Abbot Laboratories, Rungis, France).

Fragments of renal cortex were fixed in Dubosq-Brazil fluid (80 % alcohol, 150 ml ; 40 % formol, 60 ml ; acetic acid, 0.5 ml ; picric acid 1 g) and embedded in paraffin. Sections of 4 μm were prepared and stained with chromotrope aniline blue and PAS. Tubular atrophy and interstitial fibrosis were graded on a scale ranging from 1 (+) to 3 (+++). 1 represents minimal focal alterations, 3 represents widely distributed lesions.

Immunoperoxidase labeling of infiltrated cells was performed on frozen sections using monoclonal antibodies (Serotec) recognizing a specific antigen in each cell subset. Briefly, OX6, W3/13, W3/25, OX8, ED1 monoclonal antibodies react respectively with Ia bearing cells, T cells and neutrophils, T helper cells, cytotoxic suppressor T cells and macrophages. The quantitative assessment of cellular infiltrate was performed by determining the total number of positively labeled cells for each antibody in 10 randomly selected areas for each rat using a light microscope (LEITZ Aristoplan X63).

Urinary thromboxane levels were assessed by an RIA test (NEN KIT Dupont).

RESULTS

Administration of CsA caused a significant decrease of body weight at day 21 associated with significant increase in BUN (Table 1). Throughout the time course, rats treated with CsA and receiving BN 52063 exhibited values of CCr, BUN and body weight similar to those of the control animals.

On day 21, the rats were killed and the kidneys processed for histological studies. The morphological changes caused by CsA were mainly located in the outer renal cortex. These changes were time dependent and consisted in tubular atrophy and dilatation, cell infiltration and slight fibrosis (Table 1).

The administration of BN 52063 markedly reduced the tubular and interstital damages.

Characterization of cell infiltrates: In rats receiving CsA, the cytoimmunological labeling of inflammatory cells present in the renal interstitium revealed focal infiltrations of a small number of cells. The cells were more frequently located in the areas of tubular atrophy, and were mainly Ia-bearing cells, macrophages and T lymphocytes as described in Figure 1.

All these cell types were present in control rats but they significantly increased in the treated rats. In this study, we failed to detect B lymphocytes as well as polymorphonuclear leukocytes. Co-treatment with BN 52063 significantly reduced the number of Ia-bearing cells and macrophages, but T cell infiltrates remained elevated (Figure 1).

Thromboxane excretion: The urinary excretion of TxB_2 was significantly increased in group 3 (CsA, 25 mg/kg/day) (Table 2). BN 52063

reduced the urinary excretion of TxB_2 induced by CsA.

DISCUSSION

The results suggest that BN 52063 prevents the nephrotoxic effects of CsA treatment. This prevention was evidenced by histological and physiological improvement. In fact, only minimal alterations in tubular cells were observed in the group of animals treated with CsA (25 mg/kg/day) and BN 52063 (50 mg/kg/day). The slight discrepancies between our results and those reported by Mihatsch et al. (8) can be attributed to differences in experimental protocol. Although the physiopathological mechanism of renal alterations after CsA treatment remains unclear, haemodynamic alterations may initiate tissue lesions. Indeed, a single injection of CsA in rats decreases renal plasma flow consistent with a vasoconstrictor mechanism in nephrotoxicity (7, 8). In our experiments, CsA administration reduced C_{Cr} after 21 days of treatment, but the variation is not significant. At 12 days, values of C_{Cr} were normal in all groups of animals. The lack of significant alteration in C_{Cr} probably reflects the fact that C_{Cr} is not the best indicator of nephrotoxicity. Serum BUN was significantly higher after 12 days. At this latter time, changes in body weight were also observed. Previous reports indicate that in experimental studies, it is very difficult to induce chronic renal failure after CsA treatment. Only prolonged administration of a high dose of the drug results in impairment of kidney function, while there is no effect with lower doses (1). In fact, the absence of severe renal failure throughout the experiment reported here may be due to the short duration of treatment.

Moreover, the increased number of inflammatory cells in the renal cortex (9, 10) was confirmed in this study. There appeared to be a correlation between the presence of infiltrating inflammatory cells and the increased urinary excretion of TxB_2 in rats receiving CsA.

TxB_2 could be synthetized by glomerular cells as well as by macrophages. There is evidence suggesting an implication of TxB_2 in CsA ne-

Table 1: TREATMENT EFFECT OF CYCLOSPORINE AND BN 52063

GROUP	GFR (ML/MIN)	SERUM BUN (MG/L)	MORPHOLOGICAL ALTERATIONS	
			TUBULAR ATROPHY	INTERSTITIAL FIBROSIS
VEHICLE ALONE				
day 12	1.06± 0.062	0.25 ± 0.016	ABSENT	ABSENT
day 21	1.15 ± 0.132	0.23 ± 0.017		
CYCLOSPORINE (25 mg/kg)				
day 12	0.86 ± 0.048	0.32 ± 0.029*	++	+
day 21	0.90 ± 0.101	0.33 ± 0.035*		
CYCLOSPORINE (25 mg/kg) + BN 52063				
day 12	1.07± 0.139	0.25 ± 0.017	ABSENT	ABSENT
day 21	1.17± 0.168	0.26 ± 0.017		

The results are means $\pm$ 1 SD. * p 0.05 ; ** p 0.01 ; *** p 0.001. Significance was calculated against the control group values. Values at day 0 were 1.03 $\pm$ 0.06 for GFR, 0.22 $\pm$ 0.01 for serum BUN and 207.5 $\pm$ 3.9 for body weight. Groups comprised 10 animals.

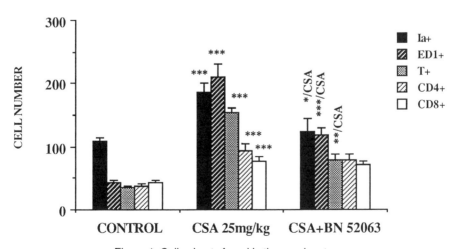

Figure 1: Cell subsets found in the renal cortex

Table 2: URINARY EXCRETION OF TXB$_2$

DAY 21	TXB$_2$ (ng/mg/creat)
CONTROL	2.22 ± 0.107
BN 52063 alone 50 mg/kg/day	2.48 ± 0.317 NS
CYCLOSPORINE 25 mg/kg/day	5.65 ± 0.492 *
CYCLOSPORINE + BN 52063	3.57 ± 0.486 NS

phrotoxicity. The results of Konieczkowski et al. (11) showed an increased synthesis of TxB$_2$ in normal SHR, which may partially account for the increased vascular resistance, and thus, could explain susceptibility of SHR rats to CsA (11).

A role for PAF has been suggested in the pathogenesis of a variety of experimental and human diseases (12). Recent data indicate that intrarenally infused PAF caused renal vasoconstriction leading to a reduction in renal blood flow in anaesthetized dogs (13). When administered by the femoral vein, PAF also reduced renal plasma flow in dogs (14). PAF stimulates the release of other mediators such as leukotrienes and prostaglandins from various cell types and organs. Indeed, Weisman et al. (15) showed that isolated perfused rabbit kidney stimulated with PAF, generated PGE$_2$ and TxB$_2$. In cultured mesangial cells, PAF also caused the release of PGE$_2$ concomitant with cellular contraction (16). These observations suggest that the reduction of C$_{Cr}$ during glomerular injury may result from a sequential generation of various inflammatory mediators. Although there is evidence to suggest that CsA increases renal thromboxane production, the precise interaction between PAF and CsA remains to be defined. Such results could be linked to those obtained in this study concerning the increased generation of TxB$_2$ induced by CsA and the presence of inflammatory cells. A number of studies performed in the dog and rat indicate that PAF antagonists possess a glomerular protective effect in renal diseases.

In the dog, the PAF antagonist BN 52021 inhibited the decrease of C$_{Cr}$ and urinary sodium excretion induced by PAF injection (13). Using the same antagonist, we were able to block the acute renal failure induced by PAF in the rat (17). BN 52021 has also been shown to protect against proteinuria and glomerular damage in adriamycin nephrosis (18).

The histologic alterations of CsA (25 mg/kg/day) were completely prevented by BN 52063. These results suggest that PAF may be generated by renal cells and/or by macrophages during CsA treatment. Therefore, the mechanism by which BN 52063 exerts its protective effect on CsA nephrotoxicity may be explained by the various renal actions of the mediator (12). In fact, PAF could be included among the various mediators which participate in the side effects induced by the drug.

In conclusion, CSA-induced nephrotoxicity in the rat is effectively inhibited by BN 52063. Although this study revealed a strong relationship between PAF, TxB$_2$, cellular infiltrates and CsA toxicity, the pathogenetic mechanism is still unclear.

ACKNOWLEDGEMENTS

The authors would like to thank Nadia Khirat for her secretarial assistance during the preparation of this manuscript.

REFERENCES

1. Thiel G: Nephrotoxicity of ciclosporin. TIPS 7:167-169, 1986.

2. Perico N, Benigni A, Zoja C, Remuzzi G: Functional significance of the increased renal thromboxane synthesis induced by chronic administration of cyclosporine. Clin Res 34:405-408, 1986.

3. Benveniste J, Henson PM, Cochrane CG: Leukocyte-dependent histamine release from rabbit platelets. The role of IgE, basophils and a platelet- activating factor. J Exp Med 136:1356-1377, 1972.

4. Pirotzky E, Page C, Morley J, Bidault J, Benveniste J: Vascular permeability induced by PAF-acether (platelet-activating factor) in the isolated perfused rat kidney. Agents Actions 16:17-18, 1985.

5. Pirotzky E, Bidault J, Burtin T, Gubler MC, Benveniste J: Release of platelet-activating factor, slow-reacting substance and vasoactive amines from isolated rat kidneys. Kidney Int 25:404-410, 1984.

6. Pirotzky E, Ninio E, Bidault J, Pfister A, Benveniste J: Biosynthesis of platelet-activating factor. VI. Precursor of platelet-activating factor and acetyltransferase activity in isolated rat kidney cells. Lab Invest 51:567-572, 1984.

7. Paller MS, Murray BM, Ferris FF: Decreased renal blood flow after cyclosporine infusion. Kidney Int (abst.) 27:346, 1985.

8. Mihatsch MJ, Thiel G, Spichtin HP, Oberholzer M, Brunner FP, Harder F, Olivieri V, Bremet R, Ryffel B, Stocklin E, Torshorst J, Gudat F, Zollinger HU, Lörstcher R: Morphological findings in kidney transplants after treatment with cyclosporin. Transplant Proc 15:2821-2835, 1983.

9. Egido J, Mampaso F, Rodriguez HJ, Martinez JC, Mendiluce A, Hernando P, Hernando L: Papel de las antagonistas del factor activador de las plaquettas (PAF) en la nefrotoxicidad inducida por la ciclosporina en ratas. Nefrologia 8:30-37, 1988.

10. Platt JL, Ferguson RM, Sibley RK, Gajl-Peczalska KS, Michael AF: Renal interstitial cell populations in ciclosporine nephrotoxicity. Transplantation 36:343-346, 1983.

11. Koniecskowki M, Dunn JM, Stork JE, Hassid A: Glomerular synthesis of prostaglandins and thromboxane in spontaneously hypertensive rats. Hypertension 5:446-452, 1983.

12. Pirotzky E, Braquet P: Paf-acether and kidney pathology. Prog Biochem Pharmacol 22:168-180, 1987.

13. Plante GE, Hebert RL, Lamoureux C, Braquet P, Sirois P: Hemodynamic effects of PAF-acether. Pharmacol Res Commun 18:173-179, 1986.

14. Bessin P, Bonnet J, Thibaudeau D, Agier B, Beaudet Y, Gilet F: Pathophysiology of shock states caused by PAF-acether in dogs and rats. INSERM Symp. Platelet-Activating Factor Structurally Related Ether-Lipids, (Elsevier, Amsterdam), 23:343-356, 1983.

15. Weisman SM, Felsen D, Darracott Vaughan E: Platelet-activating factor is a potent stimulus for renal prostaglandin synthesis. Possible significance in unilateral uretral obstruction. J Pharmacol Exp Ther 235:10-15, 1985.

16. Schlondorff D, Goldwasser P, Neuwirth R, Satriano JA, Clay RL: Production of platelet-activating factor in glomeruli and cultured glomerular mesangial cells. Am J Physiol 250:1123-1127, 1986.

17. Pirotzky E, Colliez Ph, Guilmard C, Schaeverbeke J, Mencia-Huerta JM, Braquet P: Protection of platelet-activating factor-induced acute renal failure by BN 52021. Br J Exp Path 69:291-299, 1987.

18. Egido J, Robles A, Ortiz A, Ramirez F, Gonzalez E, Mampaso F, Sanchez-Crespo M, Braquet P, Hernando F: Role of platelet-activating factor in adriamycin-induced nephropathy in rats. Eur J Pharmacol 138:119-123, 1987.

31

PREVENTION AND REVERSAL OF ACUTE CYCLOSPORIN A NEPHROTOXICITY USING THROMBOXANE A$_2$ SYNTHETASE INHIBITION

E.M. Grieve (1,2,3), G.M. Hawksworth (1,2), P.H. Whiting (3)

Department of Medicine & Therapeutics (1), Department of Pharmacology (2), and Clinical Biochemistry (3), University of Aberdeen, Foresterhill, Aberdeen, U.K.

INTRODUCTION

Cyclosporin A (CsA) is the immunosuppressant of choice for organ transplantation but its use is limited by a variety of side effects, the most serious of which is nephrotoxicity (1,2). The goal of current research is therefore to develop a treatment protocol which maintains the immunosuppressant qualities of the peptide whilst limiting or removing the damaging side effects.

The problem has been addressed in two main ways: firstly, by attempts to alter the molecular structure of CsA, as in cyclosporin G (3) or by influencing the pharmacokinetics and cellular distribution of the drug (4). Another strategy involves inhibition of the pathogenic mechanisms responsible for the development of nephrotoxicity. Among these, altered eicosanoid metabolism, in particular increased production of thromboxane A$_2$ (TxA$_2$) without synergistic elevation of vasodilator prostanoids, appears to be an important factor (5,6).

The therapeutic value of thromboxane synthetase inhibitors (TSI) in CsA treated animals has previously been documented (7-9). We have extended these studies by assessing the ability of CGS 12970 to reverse acute drug toxicity in the rat.

MATERIALS AND METHODS

Animals: Adult male Sprague-Dawley rats (245-310 g) obtained from Charles River U.K.

Ltd., Margate, Kent, were allowed free access to food and water throughout the experimental period.

Drugs: A stock solution of CsA (100 mg/ml; Sandimmun, Sandoz Ltd, Basle) was diluted with equal parts olive oil (Boots Company Ltd, Nottingham, U.K.) and administered to the conscious animal by gastric intubation using a No.4 gauge cannula (Portex Ltd, Hythe, Kent, U.K.). Thromboxane synthetase inhibitor (CGS 12970; Ciba Geigy, Horsham, Sussex, U.K.) was suspended in NaCl (0.9%, pH9) to give a 2 mg/ml solution which was administered as above.

Experimental Protocol: Four groups of 6 rats received CsA (50 mg/kg) once daily for 14 days, either alone (Group A) or with CGS 12970 (10 mg/kg) from day 0 (Group B) or from day 7 (Group C) onwards. Group D additionally received saline (0.9%, pH9) from day 7. Renal function, enzymuria and body weight were measured on days 0, 4, 7, 10 and 14.

Blood and Urine Sampling: Animals were placed in individual metabolic cages overnight (18 hours) and urine free from faecal contamination was collected at ambient temperature. Blood samples were obtained by tail clipping under light anaesthesia and were placed in tubes containing lithium heparin as an anticoagulant. Samples were centrifuged at 4000 rpm for 10 min and the plasma expressed immediately separated.

Biochemical Determinations: Plasma and urine concentrations of creatinine were estimated using an Astra Discrete Analyser (Beckman RIIC Ltd, Glenrothes, Scotland, U.K.) and an RA Technicon 1000 respectively. Urinary N-acetyl-β-D-glucosaminidase (NAG) activity was measured as previously described (10) and was expressed as nmol reaction product/hr/mmol of urinary creatinine, a measure independent of urine flow rate (UFR).

Measurement of CsA: Trough concentrations of CsA after 14 days treatment were measured in whole blood by radioimmunoassay using kits supplied by Sandoz Ltd, Basle, Switzerland. The antibody does not differentiate between the parent CsA molecule and certain of its metabolites.

Statistics: Results were compared by one way ANOVA with significances assigned using Dunnett's test.

RESULTS AND DISCUSSION

While there are currently divergent views and observations relating to the nature and extent of CsA toxicity, it is generally agreed that the most important functional event is a reduction in glomerular filtration rate (GFR) caused by increased renal vasoconstriction (11). In this study, creatinine clearance (CCR) was significantly lower by day 14 in animals treated with CsA only or CsA plus saline than in those groups additionally receiving TSI (Table 1). The absence of any TSI effect on the circulating level of CsA (Fig. 1), confirms its protective role (12) and further implicates inappropriate TxA_2 production as a factor responsible for altered renal haemodynamics. Inhibition of TxA_2 did not, however, provide complete protection against CsA toxicity, suggesting the involvement of additional pathogenic factors.

The level of urinary NAG which has been used to indicate proximal tubule damage in both man (13) and animals (10) was also increased by CsA treatment. As with CCR, a significant degree of protection was mediated by inhibition of thromboxane A_2 (Table 2). Although it has been argued that CsA is directly toxic to the renal epithelium (14), an alternative hypothesis is that degenerative changes in tubules are secondary to vascular changes, particularly to hyalinisation affecting the afferent arterioles (15). Therefore, the apparent cytoprotective ability of TSI, may simply be a secondary expression of the ability of the drug to prevent vasoconstriction.

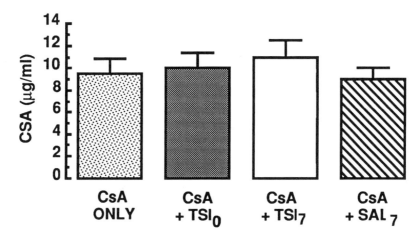

Figure 1. Whole blood CsA levels after 14 days drug treatment. No significant differences were observed between groups.

Table 1. The effect on creatinine clearance of administering CGS 12970 on days 0 and 7 to CsA treated animals.

| GROUP | Creatinine clearance (ml/hr/kg) | | | | |
| | DAY | | | | |
	0	4	7	10	14
A. CsA only	362±5	272±6	247±10	208±25*	153±55*#
B. CsA + TSI0	369±76	325±133	297±95	280±40	277±71
C. CsA + TSI7	317±64	304±73	255±40	283±54	285±80
D. CsA + Sal7	376±125	284±84	266±82	178±58^'	160±50^'

Values are given as means±S.D. Significant differences between groups are denoted as * for A vs B (p<0.05 on day 10 and 14); # for A vs C (p<0.05 on day 10: p<0.01 on day 14); ^ for D vs B (p<0.01 on day 10: p<0.05 on day 14); ' for D vs C (p<0.01 on day 10: p<0.05 on day 14).

Table 2. The effect on NAG enzymuria of administering CGS 12970 on days 0 and 7 to CsA treated animals.

| GROUP | NAG (nmol 4MU/hr/mmol creatinine) | | | | |
| | DAYS | | | | |
	0	4	7	10	14
A. CsA only	57±1	124±4	195±6	228±25	180±59#
B. CSA + TSI0	61±19	146±34	170±37	165±75	133±50
C. CSA + TSI7	78±18	148±41	224±61	131±18	124±43
D. CSA + Sal7	71±23	154±52	175±55	231±88'	165±34

Significant differences between groups are denoted # for A vs C (p<0.05 on day 10 and 14); ' for D vs C (p<0.05 on day 10).

Another manifestation of CsA toxicity is weight loss; whereas untreated rats gain approximately 12 g/day (data not shown), CsA treated animals showed only small fluctuations in body weight. Inhibition of TxA2 had no effect on weight loss, suggesting that the protective effect of TSI was selective for the kidney (Fig. 2). This corresponds with the findings of Smees-ters et al. (9); using the unilaterally nephrectomised rat as a model to examine CsA toxicity, this group showed that CGS 12970 significantly reduced serum creatinine without improving body weight.

Of novel interest is the finding that inhibition of thromboxane in the last 7 days of CsA treatment was as effective at preventing CsA

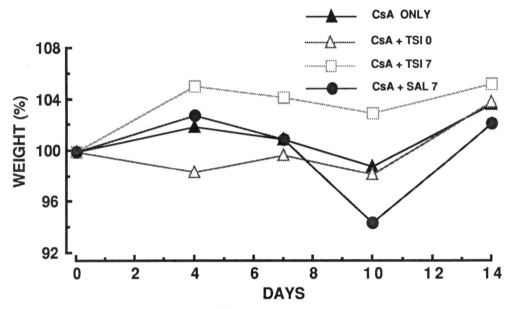

Figure 2. Change in body weight in CsA and TSI treated animals. No significant differences were observed between treatment groups.

induced nephrotoxicity as co-administration of the inhibitor. This is true for both CCR and NAG and suggests that concomitant administration of the inhibitor is not essential to achieve protection. CGS 12970 also partially reversed nephrotoxicity as is evidenced by the improvement in CCR in group C, and particularly by the reduction in NAG levels on day 10 compared with the corresponding values on day 7. Whereas CsA nephrotoxicity is progressive in nature, at least over the short term, the protective effect of TSI administration in group C was realised over a single measurement period, on day 10, with no further improvement in renal function observed on day 14.

The ability of TSI to reverse the adverse effects of CsA on renal haemodynamics has been previously demonstrated. Perico et al. (8), treated animals with 50 mg/kg CsA for 7 weeks; UK-38,485 was administered during the final week causing a significant increase in GFR. Urinary thromboxane B_2 excretion was also significantly decreased. Therefore inhibition of

thromboxane synthetase can reverse both chronic and acute CsA induced decreases in GFR.

Although this study has focused on the involvement of TxA_2 as the causative agent in CsA induced vasoconstriction, the possible involvement of other factors has been investigated. These include suppression of the synthesis of vasodilator prostaglandins (16), increased tone in renal sympathetic nerves (17), activation of the renin angiotensin system (18,19) and interference with renal Ca^{2+} metabolism leading ultimately to vascular smooth muscle contraction (20). In accordance with these alternative theories, Paller (21) has shown recently that administration of misoprostol - an analogue of the vasodilator prostanoid PGE_1 - can also reverse the reduction in GFR in CsA treated animals. However, as reported in this study, a return to normal GFR was not achieved. The ability of misoprostol to reverse CsA-induced vasoconstriction suggests that either CsA inhibits synthesis of vasodilatory prostanoids or that the drug is merely a potent vasodilator capable of reversing vasoconstriction produced by another mechanism, for example, TxA$_2$. These observations, therefore, do not contradict the findings reported in this study.

In conclusion, we have confirmed the ability of TSI to protect against renal damage when the inhibitor is given concomitantly with CsA. Treatment with TSI for the last 7 days of the experimental period showed that this protocol was equally protective against CsA-induced vasoconstriction. The capacity of TSI to reverse CsA damage partially was also observed and supports the previous finding that CsA toxicity is not permanent and can be alleviated by drug withdrawal or dose reduction (22,23). Studies using TSI which aim at reversing pre-existent CsA induced renal functional impairment pharmacologically will both improve our understanding of the lesion and offer an obvious clinical benefit.

REFERENCES

1. Flechner SM, Buren CV, Kerman RH, Kahan BD: The nephrotoxicity of cyslosporine in renal transplant recipients. Trans Proc 15: 2689-2694, 1983.

2. Mihatsch MJ, Thiel G, Basler V, Ryffel B, Landmann J, von Overbeck J, Zollinger HU: Morphological patterns in cyclosporine-treated renal transplant recipients. Trans Proc 17 (Suppl.1): 101-116, 1985.

3. White DJG, Calne RY, Collier StJ, Rolles K, Winter S, Drakopoulos S: Is cyclosporine G more or less immunosuppressive than cyclosporine A? Trans Proc 18: 1244-1245, 1986.

4. Hsieh HH, Schreiber M, Stowe N: Preliminary report: the use of liposome-encapsulated cyclosporine in a rat model. Trans Proc 17: 1397-1400, 1985.

5. Perico N, Benigni A, Zoja C, Delaini F, Remuzzi G: Functional significance of exaggerated renal thromboxane A$_2$ synthesis induced by cyclosporin A. Amer J Physiol 251: F581-587, 1986.

6. Kawaguchi A, Goldman HM, Shapiro R, Foegh ML, Ramwell PW, Lower RR: Increase in urinary thromboxane B$_2$ in rats by cyclosporine. Transplantation 40: 214-216, 1985.

7. Whiting PH, Burke MD, Thomson AW: Drug interactions from animal studies. Trans Proc 18 (Suppl.5): 56-70, 1986.

8. Perico N, Zoja C, Benigni A, Ghilardi F, Gualandris L, Remuzzi G: Effect of short term cyclosporine administration in rats on renin-angiotensin and thromboxane A$_2$: possible relevance to the reduction in glomerular filtration rate. J Pharmacol Exp Ther 239: 229-235, 1986.

9. Smeesters C, Chaland P, Giroux L, Mountquin JM, Etienne P, Douglas F, Corman JM, St Louis G, Daloze P: Prevention of acute cyclosporine A neprotoxicity by a thromboxane synthetase inhibitor. Trans Proc 20: 663-669, 1988.

10. Whiting PH, Thomson AW, Blair JT, Simpson JG: Experimental cyclosporin A nephrotoxicity. Br J Exp Pathol 63: 88-94, 1982.

11. English J, Evan A, Houghton DC, Bennett WM: Cyclosporine induced acute renal dysfunction in the rat. Transplantation 44: 135-141, 1987.

12. Grieve EM, Hawksworth GM, Whiting PH: Protection mediated by inhibition of thromboxane synthesis is not enhanced by ACE inhibition in cyclosporin A treated animals. Br J Pharmacol 96: 173P, 1989.

13. Whiting PH, Ross IS, Borthwick L: Serum and urine N-acetyl-beta-D- glucosaminidase in diabetics on diagnosis and subsequent treatment and stable insulin-dependent diabetics. Clin Chim Acta 92: 459-463, 1979.

14. von Willebrand E, Hayry P: Cyclosporin A deposit in renal allografts. Lancet ii: 189-192, 1983.

15. Schachter M: Cyclosporine A and hypertension. J Hyper 6: 511-516, 1988.

16. Fan TP, Lewis GP: Mechanisms of cyslosporine A-induced inhibition of prostacyclin

synthesis by macrophages. Prostaglandins 30: 735-747, 1985.

17. Kone BC, Racussen LC, Whelton A, Solez K: Cyclosporine nephrotoxicity in rats: vehicle and ischaemic effects. Kidney Int 29: 304, 1986.

18. Baxter CR, Duggin CG, Hall BM, Horval JS, Tiller DJ: Stimulation of renin release from rat cortical slices by cyclosporine A. Res Commun Chem Pathol Pharmacol 43: 417-423, 1984.

19. Siegl H, Ryffel B, Petrie R: Cyclosporine, the renin-angiotensin- aldosterone system and renal adverse reactions. Trans Proc 15 (Suppl.1): 2719-2725, 1983.

20. Sumpio BE, Chaudry IH, Baue AE: Alleviation of cyclosporine nephrotoxicity with verapamil and adenosine triophosphate-magnesium chloride treatment. Surg Forum: 336-341, 1985.

21. Paller MS: The prostaglandin E_1 analog misoprostol reverses acute cyclosporine nephrotoxicity. Trans Proc 20 (Suppl 3): 634-637, 1988.

22. Thomson AW, Whiting PH, Blair JT, Davidson RJL, Simpson JG: Pathological changes developing in the rat during a 3 week course of high dosage cyclosporin A and their reversal following drug withdrawal. Transplantation 32: 271-277, 1981.

23. Cohen DJ, Loertscher R, Rubin MF: Cyclosporine: a new immunosuppressive agent for organ transplantation. Ann Intern Med 101: 667-682, 1984.

32
REVERSIBLE CHANGES IN N-ACETYL-BETA-D-GLUCOSAMINIDASE ACTIVITY ALONG THE PROXIMAL RENAL TUBULES OF CYCLOSPORINE-A TREATED RATS

H. Schmid, I. Lindmeier, H. Schmitt, R. Eissele, G. Neuhaus and M. Wehrmann

Institute of Pathology, University of Tübingen, Liebermeisterstrasse 8, D-7400 Tübingen, Germany

INTRODUCTION

Cyclosporine A (CyA) is known to induce lysosomal changes in the proximal tubules (1). We have recently found that the specific catalytic activity of N-acetyl-beta-D-glucosaminidase (2- acetamido- 2- deoxy-beta-D-glucoside acetamidodeoxyglucohydrolase (EC 3.2.1.30, NAG)), a lysosomal enzyme, that appears to be evenly distributed in the lysosomes along the rat nephron (2), changes heterogeneously in the proximal tubules of rats treated for 12 days with CyA (3). In the present study we examined the effect of CyA administration for a longer period and of discontinuation of the drug on the intranephronal activity of NAG.

METHODS

Cyclosporine A (Sandimmune[R], Sandoz AG, Nürnberg, Germany) (15, 30 or 50 mg/ kg/day) or olive oil (30 mg/kg/day) was administered by gavage to 25 male Sprague-Dawley rats (Ivanovas, Kisslegg, FRG) (mean body weight: 271 ± 19 g) for 24 days. The rats were fed with standard diet (Alma Diät, Friedrich Botzenhardt KG, Kempten, FRG) and had free access to drinking water. Nineteen animals were then killed and 6, which had been treated with 15 or 50 mg/kg/day CyA, remained untreated for a further 24 days. The kidneys were prepared for microdissection (4): 16 μm serial cryostat sections were stained by the periodic acid-Schiff (PAS) reaction, lyophilized, and stained for succinate dehydrogenase (SDH) activity (5). Nephron segments were microdissected from the lyophilized sections after identification in the two parallel stained sections, and were classified according to their SDH activity. The catalytic activity of NAG (expressed in μmol/min/g tissue dry weight) was determined fluorometrically in single nephron segments using 4-methylumbelliferyl-N-acetyl-beta-D-glucosaminide as substrate (4).

RESULTS

After 24 days of CyA administration, intrarenal SDH activity was normal in some areas and reduced in others (Fig. 1). The sites of reduced SDH activity, indicating damage to mitochondrial inner membranes, were identical to those of histological alterations seen in the sections stained by the PAS reaction. At these sites, the borders of the tubules, normally clear-cut in lyophilized sections, were hardly discernible because of loss of cell mass or interstitial cell infiltration. SDH activity was reduced in both proximal and distal tubules in circumscribed subcapsular areas of the cortical labyrinth, the medullary rays, and the outer stripe of the outer medulla. The number of tubules with reduced SDH activity appeared to depend on the CyA dosage. These changes in SDH activity were not present after discontinuation of CyA (Fig. 2).

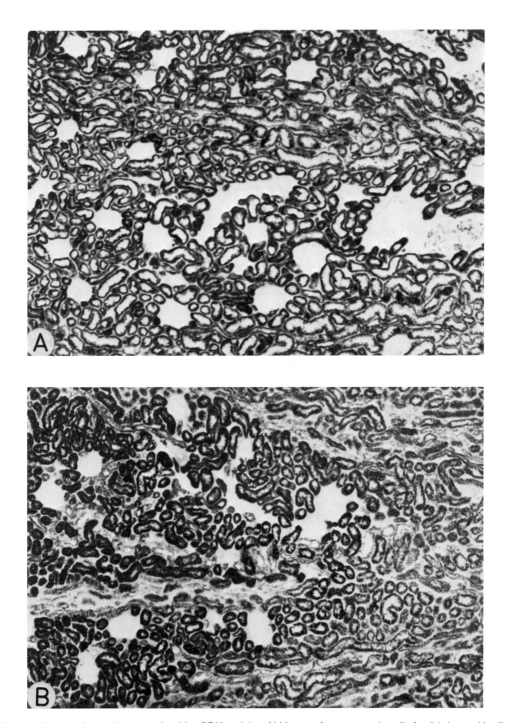

Figure 1. Cryosections (16 μm) stained for SDH activity of kidneys of rats treated orally for 24 days with olive oil (30 mg/kg/day) (A) or with CyA (50 mg/kg/day) (B).

In contrast to SDH activity, NAG activity appeared to be unchanged in distal tubules with normal and reduced SDH activity, in the collecting ducts (Fig. 3B) and in the glomeruli (Fig. 3A) after CyA administration. NAG activity in proximal convoluted tubules (PCT) with normal SDH activity was increased to 140-163% of the control value, but was almost unchanged in proximal straight tubules (PST) with normal SDH activity. In the PST with reduced SDH activity, the increase in NAG activity compared to controls gradually enlarged from the upper part of the medullary rays to the outer medulla. NAG activity was decreased to 66-70% in the PCT with reduced SDH activity. These effects appeared to be independent of the dosage of CyA (Fig. 3A). Fig. 4 shows that after discontinuation of CyA, intranephronal NAG activities were no different from the control values. However, in the PCT, the mean activities are derived from individual values belonging to two groups

clustered around 60 and around 80 µmol/min/g dry weight.

DISCUSSION

This study demonstrates that CyA-induced alterations in renal epithelial cells are markedly heterogeneous and reversible. The intrarenal distribution of areas of normal and altered histological appearance after 24 days' CyA administration resembles that observed after 12 days of treatment with the drug (3). However, at the later stage, the changes show greater variability, which may be due to the cyclical nature of CyA nephrotoxicity described by several authors (6,7).

The changes in specific catalytic activity of NAG after 24 days' CyA administration are similar to those seen after 12 days' treatment. The finding that they are detectable only in the proximal tubules is consistent with the fact that

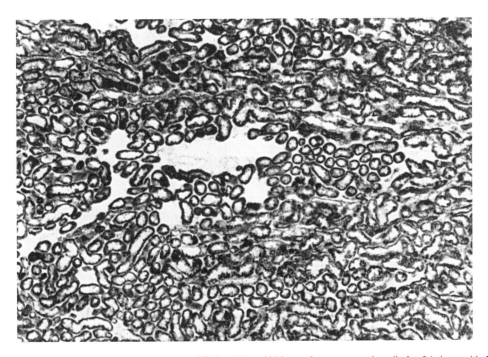

Figure 2. Cryosection (16 µm) stained for SDH activity of kidney of a rat treated orally for 24 days with CyA (50 mg/kg/day) and then left untreated for 24 days.

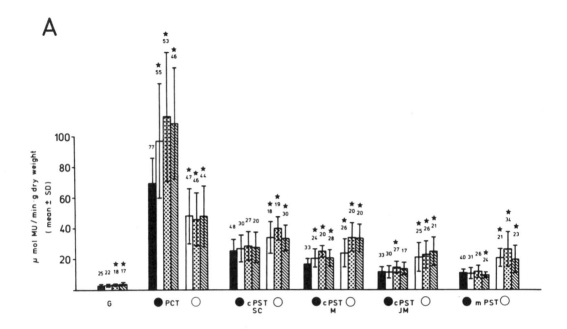

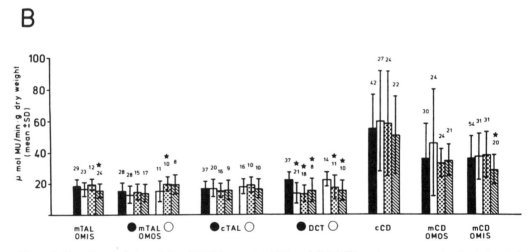

Figure 3. Specific catalytic activity of NAG in proximal (A) and distal (B) nephron segments of rats treated for 24 days with CyA (mean ± SD, number of determinations).

MU = 4-methylumbelliferone, G = glomerulus, PCT = proximal convoluted tubule, PST = proximal straight tubule (**c** = cortical, m = medullary; SC = subcapsular, M = midcortical, JM = juxtamedullary), TAL = thick ascending limb of Henle's loop (OMOS = outer stripe of outer medulla, OMIS = inner stripe of outer medulla), DCT = distal convoluted tubule, CD = collecting duct. ● Segments with normal SDH activity, o segments with reduced SDH activity. ■ Controls: 30 mg/kg/day olive oil (4 rats), □ 15 mg/kg/day CyA (5 rats), ▨ 30 mg/kg/day CyA (5 rats), ◩ 50 mg/kg/day CyA (5 rats); statistically significant difference compared with control values (p<0.05).

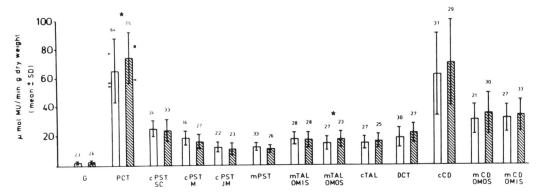

Figure 4. Specific catalytic activity of NAG in the nephron of rats treated for 24 days with CyA. □ 15 mg/kg/day, (3 rats), ▧ 50 mg/kg/day, (3 rats) and then left untreated for 24 days (mean ±SD, number of determinations). Abbreviations as in Fig. 3. ★ statistically significant difference between the two groups (p<0.05). I mean value for each animal.

changes in lysosomal ultrastructure are confined to the proximal tubules after CyA treatment (1). The changes in specific catalytic activity of NAG may be due to changes both in catalytic enzyme activity and in cell mass.

Since in the lyophilized sections all the tubules with reduced SDH activity appeared to have undergone a substantial loss of cell mass, the various changes in catalytic activity of NAG per tissue dry weight along the proximal tubules with reduced SDH activity imply differing changes in enzyme activity. The variable increases in specific NAG activity along the PST with reduced SDH activity do not necessarily reflect true changes in catalytic enzyme activity or enzyme content. This is especially evident in the medullary PST with reduced SDH activity, where the flat epithelial cells show signs of regeneration at the ultrastructural level (1). On the other hand, the reduced specific activity of NAG in PCT with reduced SDH activity may indicate an imbalance of their NAG content due to slightly increased urinary excretion (6) and insufficient supply of active NAG after CyA administration. Our earlier finding of reduced NAG activity in the PCT of a human kidney allograft with normal function and the same allograft during subsequent acute rejection (4), and the recent finding of Pfaller et al. (8) of highly elevated NAGuria and slightly diminished lysosomal volume in cortical proximal tubules after maleate administration to rats support this

hypothesis. In contrast, the increased NAG activity in PCT with normal SDH activity may represent a true increase in enzyme activity corresponding to the ultrastructural finding of a CyA-induced increase in the number and volume of lysosomes in these tubules, together with the signs of autophagocytosis (1). Because of the normal appearance of the tubules, this phenomenon may be considered to represent lysosomal adaptation rather than damage. Interestingly, although no signs of damage are detectable in the recovery phase after CyA administration, persistence of increased NAG activity in these segments was seen in some animals. This process may reflect the normalization of function of secondarily altered lysosomes and seems to depend on the dosage of CyA.

This variety of effects indicates metabolic heterogeneity of the nephron. The specific intrarenal distribution of these effects suggests direct tubulotoxicity of CyA. It is possible that the renal cells take up this lipophilic drug, via passive diffusion (9), in differing amounts according to their position along the post-glomerular capillaries and that the reverse process occurs after withdrawal of the drug. The volume of distribution of CyA may be determined by blood levels as well as by the reduced renal blood flow induced by this drug (10).

ACKNOWLEDGEMENTS

This study was supported by the Deutsche Forschungsgemeinschaft (Schm 418/2-1 and Schm 418/2-2). We thank Dr. Margaret Ruck and Martina Fausel for help in preparation of the manuscript.

REFERENCES

1. Fasel J, Kaissling B, Ludwig KS, Ryffel B, Mihatsch MJ: Light and electron microscopic changes in the kidney of Wistar rats following treatment with cyclosporine A. Ultrastruct Pathol 11: 435-448, 1987.

2. Guder WG, Ross BD: Enzyme distribution along the nephron. Kidney Int 26: 101-111, 1984.

3. Schmid H, Lindmeier I, Schmitt H, Eissele R, Neuhaus G, Wehrmann M: N-Acetyl-beta-D-glucosaminidase activities in the rat nephron after cyclosporine-A treatment. Pflügers Arch 412, Suppl 1: R50, 1988.

4. Schmid H, Mall A, Bockhorn H: Catalytic activities of alkaline phosphatase and N-acetyl-beta-D-glucosaminidase in human cortical nephron segments: Heterogeneous changes in acute renal failure and acute rejection following kidney allotransplantation. J Clin Chem Clin Biochem 24: 961-970, 1986.

5. Schmid H: Quantitative microphotometric succinate dehydrogenase histochemistry in human nephron. Basic Appl Histochem 28: 221-231, 1984.

6. Whiting PH, Thomson AW, Simpson JG: Cyclosporine and renal enzyme excretion. Clin Nephrol 25, Suppl 1: S100-S104, 1986.

7. Pfaller W, Kotanko P, Bazzanella A: Morphological and biochemical observations in rat nephron epithelia following cyclosporine A (CsA) treatment. Clin Nephrol 25, Suppl 1: S105-S110, 1986.

8. Pfaller W, Joannidis M, Gstraunthaler G, Kotanko P: Quantitative morphologic changes of nephron structures and urinary enzyme activity pattern in sodium-maleate-induced renal injury. Renal Physiol Biochem 12: 56-64, 1989.

9. Nagineni CN, Lee DBN, Misra BC, Yanagawa N: Cyclosporine-A transport in isolated renal proximal tubular cells: Inhibition by calcium channel blockers. Biochem Biophys Res Commun 157: 1226-1230, 1988.

10. Murray BM, Paller MS, Ferris TF: Effect of cyclosporine administration on renal hemodynamics in conscious rats. Kidney Int 28: 767-774, 1985.

33

CYCLOSPORINE NEPHROTOXICITY: EFFECTS OF RENAL DENERVATION IN THE NON-TRANSPLANTED AND TRANSPLANTED RAT KIDNEY

S.D. Heys (1), M. Stephen (3), J.I. Duncan (2,3), J.G. Simpson (3) and P.H. Whiting (2)

Departments of Surgery (1), Clinical Biochemistry (2) and Pathology (3), University of Aberdeen
Medical Buildings, Foresterhill, Aberdeen, AB9 2ZD, UK

INTRODUCTION

The increasing use of Cyclosporine (CsA) has been a major factor in the prevention of organ allograft rejection following transplantation. However, a major side-effect of such therapy which may limit its clinical use, has been an induced nephrotoxicity (1-3). This is manifested by a reduction in glomerular filtration rate, elevated serum urea and creatinine levels, increased enzymuria, and structural damage to the renal proximal tubules (4-6).

The pathogenesis of this nephrotoxicity has not been fully elucidated, but the sympathetic nervous system has been implicated by Murray and Paller (7). Sympathetic denervation of the rat kidney, in vivo, abolished the CsA induced fall in glomerular filtration rate that occurred in innervated kidneys. Furthermore, administration of the adrenoreceptor antagonist, Prazosin, prevented the rise in serum creatinine and fall in renal blood flow observed after seven days of CsA therapy.

The aim of this study was, therefore, to determine whether renal denervation influenced CsA nephrotoxicity in both the transplanted and non-transplanted rat kidney.

METHODS

Animals

Adult male Sprague-Dawley rats were housed under conditions of constant temperature with a 12hr lighting cycle, fed Oxoid pasteurised breeding diet and water ad libitum.

Cyclosporine (CsA)

CsA was administered daily to conscious animals by gavage at a dose of 50 and 40mg/kg body weight to non-transplanted and transplanted animals, respectively.

Nephrectomy and Renal Denervation

The rats were premedicated with 200 units of atropine injected subcutaneously, and anaesthesia induced with 1ml of chloral hydrate (5% w/v) injected intraperitoneally. Anaesthesia was maintained by a combination of intraperitoneal chloral hydrate and diethyl ether by inhalation. The abdomen was opened by a mid-line incision and the right kidney removed. Denervation of the contralateral kidney was achieved by dissecting its vasculature free from the retroperitoneal fat and then "painting" the renal artery and vein with a 20% solution of phenol.

After allowing five minutes, the phenol was then washed off these structures with normal saline. The abdominal wound was then closed with a continuous 3/0 vicryl suture (Ethicon Ltd.).

Renal transplantation

The animals were premedicated and anaesthesia induced as described above. Kidneys from male Lewis rats were then transplanted into the recipient Lewis rat by a modification of the method of Fabre et al (8), using an end to end anastomosis for both vessels and ureter. All transplants were orthotopic and the contralateral, "native", kidney was left in situ.

Experimental protocol

(a) Non-transplanted rat kidney: groups of animals which had undergone either unilateral nephrectomy or unilateral nephrectomy plus sympathetic denervation of the remaining kidney, received CsA daily for 7 days. Blood samples were taken under ether anaesthesia before surgery and at days 4 and 7. Urine was collected prior to blood sampling during an overnight stay in metabolic cages. Animals were sacrificed on day 7 and the kidney removed for histological examination.

(b) Transplanted rat kidney: a group of 4 animals which had undergone orthotopic, syngeneic renal transplantation were given CsA 2 hr later and then daily for 28 days. Blood samples were obtained before transplantation and at days 3, 7, 14, 21, 28. Urine samples were obtained before transplantation and at days 7, 14, 21, 28.

Biochemical determinations

Serum urea and creatinine were measured using a SMAC analyser (Technicon Ltd., Basingstoke, UK). Urine creatinine concentrations, creatinine clearance rates and urinary N-acetyl-beta-D-glucosaminidase activity (NAG) were measured as previously described (4).

Histology

The rats were killed on day 28, both kidneys removed, fixed in neutral buffered formalin and sections examined by an experienced renal histopathologist.

Statistics

Differences between group means were assessed using Students t-test, with a p<0.05 accepted as being statistically significant.

RESULTS

Effect of renal denervation on CsA nephrotoxicity

The results in Table 1 show that there were no significant differences between serum urea and creatinine, creatinine clearance rates and NAG enzymuria between animals which had been nephrectomized and those which had undergone nephrectomy and denervation.

Histological examination of the kidneys for evidence of acute and chronic CsA toxicity revealed no significant differences in these changes between either the nephrectomy or the denervation and nephrectomy groups.

Effect of renal transplantation on CsA nephrotoxicity

The results for serum urea and creatinine concentrations and urinary NAG activities are shown in Table 2. The serum urea concentration was significantly elevated by day 3 and remained so throughout the experiment. The serum creatinine concentration was also elevated, but did not achieve statistical significance. A cyclical pattern was observed in the urinary NAG activities, also becoming significantly elevated by day 3 and throughout the experiment.

Histology

Both kidneys from the group of allografted rats were examined for evidence of acute and

Table 1. The effect of renal denervation on CsA nephrotoxicity

Group	Day	Creatinine μmol/l	Creatinine clearance ml/hr/kg	NAG IU/mmol creatinine
	0	47 ± 5	340 ± 79	53 ± 16
Nephrectomy	4	$65 \pm 7^{**}$	$152 \pm 36^{**}$	53 ± 18
(n=6)	7	55 ± 8	273 ± 58	53 ± 19
Nephrectomy	0	39 ± 4	472 ± 85	50 ± 9
& denervation	4	$66 \pm 16^{*}$	$177 \pm 17^{**}$	68 ± 16
(n=5)	7	52 ± 5	$235 \pm 27^{**}$	74 ± 22

(Values are mean±SD, *p<0.01, **p<0.001 compared with day 0 values)

Table 2. The effect of renal transplantation on CsA nephrotoxicity

	Days					
	0	3	7	14	21	28
serum urea (mmol/l)	8±1	13±11[*]	12±3[*]	14±4[*]	12±1[*]	17±3[*]
serum creatinine (umol/l)	56±38	83±38	79±13	80±12	84±13	81±15
urinary NAG (IU/mg creatinine)	313±56	---	581±220[*]	307±139[*]	563±87[*]	448±331[*]

(Values shown are means±SD, [*]p<0.05 compared to day 0 levels)

chronic CsA-induced damage and the findings are shown in Table 3. There was no acute toxicity, which is characterized by vacuolation of proximal tubules, in any of the transplanted kidneys.

In contrast the "native" kidneys were found to have 10-50% of their proximal tubules affected. Chronic toxicity, characterized by tubular dilation and collapse in association with interstitial fibrosis, was observed in all kidneys and was graded from "minimal" to "severe". There was no difference in chronic toxicity between the native and transplanted kidneys.

DISCUSSION

The results from this study indicate that acute histological damage in renal ultrastructure can be prevented in rats receiving high doses of CsA by denervation of the kidney. This effect was demonstrated in renal allografted animals, and is believed to be attributable to denervation of the sympathetic nervous system, since it was shown that the remaining innervated kidney exhibited proximal tubular vacuolation.

Murray and Paller (7) have already shown that sympathetic denervation prevented a reduction in the glomerular filtration rate in normal rats following one intravenous infusion of CsA. In contrast, however, when rats were nephrectomized and denervated in the first part of our study there was a significant deterioration in renal function following seven days of CsA treatment compared with animals whose kidneys were innervated. Furthermore, the degree of acute and chronic ultrastructural damage in the kidney was similar in both groups. One reason for our failure to show an improvement in renal function and architecture may be that renal denervation was incomplete. This was suggested by a subsequent group of rats whose kidneys were removed four days after denervation. Tissue sections revealed not only damaged fascicles but also some regenerating nerve tissue. It is possible that the phenol treatment was insufficient because significant neural re-growth had occured by seven days.

As a consequence of the above findings, renal transplantation was performed which provided a surgical model of complete renal denervation. The observation that chronic nephrotoxicity was not prevented in the denervated transplanted kidney suggests that this feature of CsA-mediated toxicity is without sympathetic nervous control. Although several vasoconstrictive mediators may be responsible for inducing the chronic damage demonstrated, it

TABLE 3. Histological assessment of renal damage (see text)

Rat	"Native kidney"		Transplanted kidney	
	acute	chronic	acute	chronic
1	25-50%	mild	0	minimal
2	10%	moderate	0	mild
3	10%	moderate	0	severe
4	10%	mild	0	moderate

has been shown that in hypertensive renal transplant patients receiving CsA, vasopressin levels remained consistently raised and it has been suggested that vasopressin stimulation might act as a vasoconstrictor in the denervated kidney (9).

CONCLUSIONS

1. Renal denervation following unilateral nephrectomy and nephrectomy did not prevent nephrotoxicity in rats receiving high dose CsA for 7 days.

2. After 1 month of high dose CsA, transplanted kidneys, although displaying chronic renal damage, had no evidence of acute nephrotoxicity in contrast to the remaining intact kidney which showed both acute and chronic damage.

3. Complete denervation, as achieved by renal transplantation, prevents acute proximal vacuolation, suggesting that normally the sympathetic nervous system is implicated in the induction of this toxicity possibly via the renin-angiotensin system.

4. It is unlikely that chronic renal damage is perpetuated by the sympathetic nervous system but instead may be induced by vasopresssin.

REFERENCES

1. Klintmalm GBG, Iwatsuki S, Starzl TE: Nephrotoxicity of cyclosporin A in liver and kidney transplant patients. Lancet 1: 470-471, 1981.

2. Thomson AW, Whiting PH, Blair JT, Davidson RJL, Simpson JG: Pathological changes developing in the rat during a 3-week course of high dosage cyclosporin A and their reversal following drug withdrawal. Transplantation 32: 271-277, 1981.

3. Whiting PH, Thomson AW, Blair JT, Simpson JG: Experimental cyclosporin A nephrotoxicity. Br J Exp Pathol 63: 88-99, 1982.

4. Blair JT, Thomson AW, Whiting PH, Davidosn RJL, Simpson JG: Toxicity of the immune suppressant cyclosporin A in the rat. J Path 135: 163-178, 1982.

5. Mihatsch MJ, Thiel G, Basler V, Ryffel B, Landmann J, von Overbeck J, Zollinger HU: Morphological patterns in cyclosporine-treated renal transplant patients. Transplant Proc 17(suppl 1): 101-116, 1985.

6. Thomson AW, Whiting PH, Simpson JG: Cyclosporine: immunology, toxicity and pharmacology in experimental animals. Agents Actions 15: 306-327, 1984.

7. Murray BM, Paller MS: Beneficial effects of renal denervation and prazosin on GFR and renal blood flow after cyclosporine in rats: Clin Nephrol 25 (Suppl 1): 37-49, 1986.

8. Fabre JW, Lim SH, Morris PJ: Renal transplantation in the rat: details of a technique. Aust N Z J Surg 41: 69-75, 1971.

9. Stanek B., Kovarik J., Rasoul-Rockenschaubs S., Silberbauerk K. Renin- angiotensin-aldosterone system and vasopressin in cyclosporin-treated renal allografted recipients. Clin Nephrol 28: 186-189, 1987.

PART VII
RADIOCONTRAST MEDIA

34

PREVENTION OF RADIOCONTRAST-INDUCED NEPHROTOXICITY BY THE CALCIUM CHANNEL BLOCKER NITRENDIPINE - A PROSPECTIVE RANDOMIZED CLINICAL TRIAL

H.-H. Neumayer[*], *W. Junge, A. Küfner, A. Wenning*

Department of Internal Medicine and Nephrology, Klinikum Steglitz, Free University of Berlin, Germany

INTRODUCTION

The widespread use of radio-opaque contrast media (CM) continues to be a common cause of renal injury in patients admitted to hospitals. Renal damage after application of intravascular CM is clinically seen as an acute reduction of the glomerular filtration rate (GFR) varying between a more transient, and asymptomatic course and the development of oliguric acute renal failure. Pre-existing renal insufficiency and/or other risk factors such as diabetes mellitus, dehydration, paraproteinaemia, hyperuricaema, hypalbuminaemia and congestive heart failure may increase the risk of nephrotoxicity and enhance renal damage. The reported incidence of CM-induced nephrotoxicity varies considerably in the literature, ranging between less than 1% to over 70%; this might be due to differences in patient selection, the type of radiographic investigation, the source and amount of CM used and the definitions of renal injury. It has been claimed, particularly by data in animal studies (1), that the newly developed and much more expensive non-ionic, low osmolality contrast agents are much safer and may reduce the incidence of nephrotoxicity. However, some recently published investigations failed to demonstrate a significant benefit of these new and more costly

drugs (2-4). The exact mechanisms of CM-induced renal injury have not yet been fully explained. Besides direct toxic effects on renal tubular cells and an accelerated protein precipitation, distinct alterations of renal haemodynamics with prolonged renal vasoconstriction following an initial vasodilatation seem to be a major cause of the impaired glomerular filtration rate. It has been demonstrated in various animal studies (5) and in recent clinical studies (6,7) that calcium channel blockers do antagonize renal vasoconstriction and may inhibit intracellular calcium overload, thus ameliorating postischaemic acute tubular necrosis. In addition, calcium antagonists are also thought to be of substantial value in preventing different types of toxic renal injury, such as gentamycin nephrotoxicity (8) or cyclosporine nephrotoxicity (9). It was therefore the purpose of the present study to investigate the effects of the calcium channel blocker nitrendipine on CM-induced renal injury in humans.

PATIENTS AND METHODS

The studies were approved by the ethics committee of our clinic according to the principles of the WHO declaration of Helsinki. After informed consent, 35 patients were included in the prospectively randomized and double-blind study. All patients were submitted to an X-ray examination, including computed tomography (24), phlebography (1), renal arteriography (8), angiography of the legs (2) with intravenous or

[*] New address: Transplantationszentrum der Universität Erlangen-Nürnberg 4 Medizinisch Klinik Kontumazgarte 14-18 850 Nürnberg Germany

intraarterial application of non-ionic contrast media (138±10 ml) (Iopamidol, Solutrast[R] 370, or Iopromid, Ultravist[R] 370, Schering Co., Berlin, F.R.G.). In contrast to control group C (placebo) (n=19, 14 males, 5 females, mean age 57±3 years, mean plasma creatinine levels: 88±21 μmol/L, contrast medium: 130±17 ml), the investigational group N (n=16, 8 males, 8 females, mean age 61±2 years, mean plasma creatinine levels: 109±45 μmol/L, contrast medium: 142±13 ml) received an oral dose of 20 mg nitrendipine (Bayotensin[R], Bayropharm Co., Leverkusen, FRG) starting one day prior to the X-ray investigation and continuing for two days thereafter.

Contra-indications There were no contraindications for the oral application of nitrendipine, and no adverse effects were observed during the 3 day treatment period. Accepted contraindications were: no consent, anamnestic allergy against dihydroperidines, preexisting hypotension (systolic blood pressure   90 mm Hg), tachycardia (HR   100/min).

Exclusion criteria All patients treated with any types of calcium channel blockers, nonsteroidal anti-inflammatory drugs or other possibly nephrotoxic drugs, e.g. antibiotics, were excluded from the study. No other preventive regimens, such as hydration or application of furosemide, were allowed.

Kidney function Kidney function was monitored by determining the GFR on the day before, on the day of X-ray examination and two days later using a single-shot method with inulin. In addition, the urinary excretion of total protein and of the urinary enzymes alanine aminopeptidase (AAP), gamma-glutamyl-transpeptidase (GGT) and n-acetyl-beta-glucosamidase (beta-NAG) was measured on the same days according to accepted methods.

Statistics Statistical evaluation for comparison of the two groups was performed using the Mann-Whitney-Wilcoxon test (U-test). A probability (two-tailed) of 0.95 was regarded as significant ($p<0.05$, $p<0.01$). The data are given as means ± SEM.

RESULTS

The results are summarized in Table 1 and Figures 1 and 2. The two groups of patients were comparable with respect to age, sex, the X-ray examinations performed and the amounts of radio-contrast media applied (group C: 130±17 ml, group N: 142±13 ml). The GFR (64±7 vs 82±10 ml/min) and urinary protein excretion (252±62 vs 100±13 mg/24h) indicated that baseline renal function was clearly reduced in the treatment group N as compared to control group C. Baseline urinary excretion of enzymes (AAP, NAG, GGT), however, did not differ between the two groups.

Though the patients in the investigational group N were at higher risk for radiocontrast-induced renal injury due to their restricted renal function, they displayed no further deterioration of the GFR until day 2 after application of CM (64±6 vs 64±7 ml/min). In contrast, the GFR was significantly reduced, i.e. 26±7% ($p<0.01$), in the control group C on day 2 (62±10 vs 82±10 ml/min). In addition, urinary protein excretion increased significantly by 51±13% ($p<0.01$) (157±25 vs 100±13 mg/24h) in control group C as compared to group N (279±75 vs 252±62 mg/24h) on day 1 after the X-ray investigation. Urinary excretion of the brush-border enzymes of the proximal tubulus GGT and AAP was also more enhanced in group A and significantly differed for AAP on day 2 ($p<0.05$). Though only moderate in the two groups, the increase of NAG, predominantly found in lysosomes, was likewise more pronounced in control group C.

DISCUSSION

Based on GFR, proteinuria and enzymuria, our data clearly demonstrate that oral administration of the calcium channel blocker nitrendipine abolished or ameliorated the nephrotoxic effects of intravascularly admininistered CM. The observed beneficial effect could be demonstrated despite the fact that baseline renal function was clearly more compromised in the treatment group than in the placebo-treated patients.

Table 1: Parameters of renal function before and after CM

		before CM	CM	day 1	day 2
GFR (ml/min)	C	82±10	66±8	-	62±10[**]
	N	64±7	58±7	-	64±6
(%)	C		-12±12	-	-26±7
	N		- 9±5	-	+ 2±4[++]
Protein (mg/24h)	C	100±13	145±21[**]	157±25[**]	141±24[**]
	N	252±62	266±56	279±75	298±92
(%)	C		54±15	51±13	39±12
	N		18±11	20±11[++]	10±8
Albumin (mg/24h)	C	11±2	13±3	20±9	14±4
	N	49±18	46±16	52±22	57±19
(%)	C		29±18	168±140	14±18
	N		24±15	35±25	18±17
AAP (U/24h)	C	4±1	9±2[***]	10±2[**]	7±1[**]
	N	7±1	9±1	10±2	6±1
(%)	C		134±26	120±25	101±52
	N		73±29	77±26	2±18[+]
a-NAG (U/24h)	C	3±1	5±1[*]	5±1[*]	4±1
	N	5±1	7±1	5±1	4±1
(%)	C		70±24	62±29	18±16
	N		54±27	7±10	1±15
GGT (U/24h)	C	19±3	45±8[**]	37±9[*]	27±6
	N	24±6	37±9	31±4	19±3
(%)	C		174±64	158±75	53±24
	N		115±46	86±32	24±20

C = control patients, N = patients treated with nitrendipine.[*]p<0.05, [**]p<0.01, [***]p<0.001 versus control, [+] control versus

Two aspects of the present study seem to be of particular interest. First of all, the so-called non-ionic contrast agents like iopamidol with lower osmolarity (796 mOsm per litre) have been recommended to reduce side effects on systemic and renal haemodynamics as well as direct nephrotoxic effects (10,11). Nevertheless, non-ionic contrast agents may also cause renal injury (12), and two recently published studies have failed to detect any differences in the incidence of radiocontrast-induced nephropathy with the newer low-osmolality materials (3,4). This is confirmed by the present study, which demonstrates a profound 27% reduction of the GFR, despite the exclusive application of these newer agents. Since nearly all the previously published studies have examined only plasma creatinine levels and, more rarely, endogenous creatinine clearances for a short period of only two days, as parameters for the detection of functional renal impairment, they may have overlooked the decrease in GFR, which, in the present study, is measured by a more sensitive method, using exogenous inulin clearance.

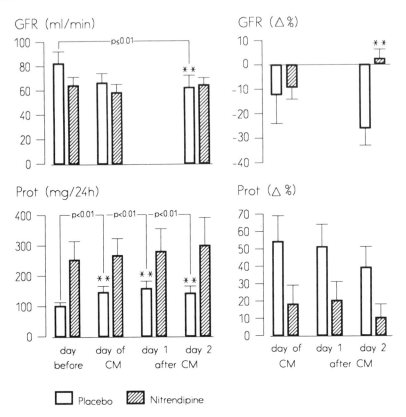

Figure 1. Course of glomerular filtration rate before and after application of radiocontrast-media.

Measurements of changes in the excretion rates of urinary enzymes are presumed to be very sensitive indicators of early renal impairment following a variety of noxious stimuli, particularly nephrotoxic drugs. However, conflicting data are available, and human enzymuria has not as yet been very well standardized either in the physiological state or during pathological conditions (13). In the present study, we assessed the excretion of three different enzymes, GGT and AAP, both restricted to the brush border of the proximal tubule, and NAG, predominantly of lysosomal origin. Due to their high molecular weight of between 130,000 and 160,000, they usually cannot be filtered through the glomerulus, thus representing tubular cell turnover or tubular damage. Urinary enzyme excretion reached its maximum peak on the day of contrast media application and declined on the two days thereafter, though still remaining above baseline values. The increase of GGT and AAP was more pronounced than that of NAG, suggesting a moderate injury of cell integrity. Conflicting data have been published with regard to differences in urinary enzyme excretion after ionic and non-ionic CM application. Some authors (14) noted significantly different excretion patterns of enzymuria in patients receiving high-osmolality CM as compared to low-osmolality CM, while others failed to detect any differences at all (15). Our data are in good agreement with the findings of Hartmann et al. (16) and Jevnikar et al. (2), who also found a significant increase of a panel of urinary enzymes with a peak excretion rate after 20 hours or on the first day after CM application, confirming a nephrotoxic effect even with the non-ionic CM. At the same time a distinct increase in urinary excretion of protein was

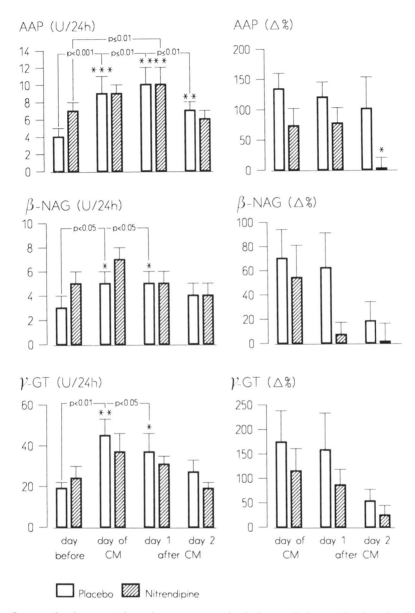

Figure 2. Course of urinary protein and enzyme excretion before and after application of radiocontrast-media.

observed in the control group, suggesting impaired glomerular permeability. Since renal albumin excretion, however, was only moderately enhanced, most of the eliminated protein was probably of tubular origin.

The second major aspect of the study is the fact that the calcium channel blocker nitrendipine clearly prevented the drop in GFR and also ameliorated the increase in urinary enzyme and protein excretion. This effect could be demonstrated despite the fact that preexisting renal function was worse in the treatment group than among control patients. The mechanisms of CM-induced nephropathy are not clearly understood. A prolonged vasoconstrictive response leading to a reduction of GFR, however, is one generally accepted effect of CM application. Calcium channel blockers may counterbalance renal vasoconstriction and preserve renal function during administration of vasoconstrictor stimuli (17). In addition, they have an inhibiting influence on contractile elements accompanied by an increase in RBF and enlargement of glomerular surface area, which explains their antagonism of the reduction of RBF and the ultrafiltration coefficient (K_f) by angiotensin II (18). Since simple renal vasodilators such as alpha-adrenoreceptor antagonists (19) or angiotensin-converting enzyme inhibitors (20) have failed to prevent CM-induced renal impairment, an additional beneficial effect of calcium antagonists has to be considered. This means that these compounds can be expected to produce so-called cytoprotective effects: an improvement of mitochondrial respiration by pharmacological blockade of cytosolic and mitochondrial calcium accumulation and a reduced generation of superoxides and other free radicals by inhibition of Ca-dependent and calmodulin-regulated enzymes. The latter may indirectly support the cellular free radical scavenger mechanisms. Thus calcium antagonists have been proven to be of substantial value in preventing various forms of experimental acute renal failure (5,21) and delayed graft function after cadaveric kidney transplantation in humans (22). Ischemic or toxic cell death in the liver (23), myocardium (24) and brain is characterized by an intracellular calcium overload and can be ameliorated by application of calcium channel blockers (25-27). In the dog, Bakris and Burnett (28) demonstrated that calcium antagonists like verapamil or diltiazem significantly attenuated the magnitude and duration of CM-induced intrarenal vasoconstriction, thus preserving a normal GFR. Finally, the evidence of a reduced urinary protein excretion under nitrendipine treatment in the present study requires a short comment, particularly with respect to the very actual and crucial discussion on the capacity of either calcium antagonists or ACE-inhibitors to influence the progression of renal failure (29,30). Our data confirm the theory that, in the presence of renal and glomerular hypoperfusion, calcium antagonists, due to their combined vasodilating effects on both the afferent and efferent arterioles, are ideal substances for maintaining kidney function without increasing protein excretion through augmentation of intraglomerular pressure.

In summary, as in connection with ischaemic or toxic injuries to various tissues, calcium antagonists have been demonstrated by the present study to be of substantial beneficial value in preventing contrast-media-induced nephrotoxicity. Their mechanisms of action might be explained by their haemodynamic and cytoprotective effects on kidney function. In the light of the controversial discussion on the benefit of non-ionic versus ionic CM, they may offer an easy, valuable and economic approach for organ preservation. More clinical data are necessary, particularly in high-risk patients, (e.g. those with diabetes or other pre-existing renal diseases), to confirm our results.

REFERENCES

1. Humes HD, Creslinski DA, Messana JM: Pathogenesis of radiocontrast- induced renal failure: comparative nephrotoxicity of diatrizoate and iopamidol. Diagn Imaging 9: S12-18, 1987.

2. Jevnikar AM, Finnie KJC, Dennis B, Plummer DT, Avila A, Linton AL: Nephrotoxicity of high and low-osmolality contrast media. Nephron 48: 300-305, 1988.

3. Parfrey PS, Griffiths SM, Barett BJ, Paul MD, Genge M, Withers J, Farid N, McManamon PJ: Contrast material-induced renal failure in patients with diabetes mellitus, renal insufficiency, or both N Engl J Med 320: 143-149, 1989.

4. Schwab ST, Hlatky MA, Pieper KS, Davidson CJ, Morris KG, Skelton TN, Bashore TM: Contrast nephrotoxicity: a randomized controlled trial of non-ionic and an ionic radiographic contrast agent. N Engl J Med 320: 149-153, 1989.

5. Neumayer HH, Wagner K, Rafelt M, Achenbach V, Molzahn M: Do calcium antagonists improve the course of postischemic acute renal failure in conscious dogs? In: Y Nose, C Kjellstrand, P Ivanovich (eds); Progress in Artificial Organs - 1985. ISAO-Press, 1986, pp. 861-864.

6. Neumayer HH, Wagner K: Prevention of delayed graft function in cadaver kidney transplants by diltiazem: Outcome of two prospective, randomized clinical trials. J Cardiovasc Pharmacol 10: S170-S177, 1987.

7. Frei U, Markreiter R, Harms A, Bsmller C, Neumann KH, Viebahn R, Gubernatis G, Wonigeit K, Pichlmayr R: Preoperative graft reperfusion with a calcium antagonist improves initial function; preliminary results of a prospective randomized trial in 110 kidney recipients. Transplant Proc 19: 3539-3541, 1987.

8. Lee SM, Pattison ME, Michael UF: Nitrendipine protects against aminoglycoside nephrotoxicity in the rat. J Cardiovasc Pharmacol 9: S65-S69, 1987.

9. Sumpio BE, Baue AE, Chaudry IH: Alleviation of cyclosporine nephro toxicity with verapamil and ATP-MgCl2. Ann Surg 206: 655-660, 1987.

10. Wolf GL: Safer, more expensive iodinated contrast agents: How do we decide? Radiology 159: 557-558, 1986.

11. Katzberg RW: New and old contrast agents: Physiology and nephrotoxicity. Urol Radiol 10: 6-11, 1988.

12. Gomes AT, Lois JF, Baker JD, McGlade CT, Bunnell DH, Hartzmann S: Acute renal dysfunction in high risk patients after angiography: Comparison of ionic and non-ionic contrast media. Radiology 17: 65-68, 1989.

13. Plummer DT, Noorazar S, Obatomi DH, Haslam JD: Assessment of renal injury by urinary enzymes. Uremia Invest 9: 97-102, 1986.

14. Cavaliere G, Arrigo G, D'Amico G, Bernasconi P, Schiavina G, Dellafiore L, Vergnaghi D: Tubular nephrotoxicity after intravenous urography with ionic high-osmolal and non-ionic low-osmolal contrast media in patients with chronic renal insufficiency. Nephron 46: 128-133, 1987.

15. Gale ME, Robbins AH, Hamburger RJ, Widrich WC: Renal toxicity of contrast agents: iopamidol, iothalamate, and diatrizoate. Am J Roentg 142: 333-335, 1984.

16. Hartmann HG, Braedel HE, Jutzler GA: Detection of renal tubular lesions after abdominal aortography and selective renal arteriography by quantitative measurements of brush-border enzymes in the urine. Nephron 39: 95-101, 1985).

17. Loutzenhuiser R, Epstein M: Effects of calcium antagonists on renal haemodynamics. Am J Physiol 249: F619-F629, 1985.

18. Ichikawa I, Miele JF, Brenner BM: Reversal of renal cortical actions of angiotensin II by verapamil and manganese. Kidney Int 16: 137-147, 1979.

19. Caldicott WJH, Hollenberg NK, Abrams HL: Characteristics of response of renal vascular bed to contrast media. Evidence of vasoconstriction induced by reninangiotensin system. Invest Radiol 5: 539-547, 1970.

20. Larson TS, Hudson K, Mertz JI, Romero JC, Knox FG: Renal vasoconstrictive response to contrast medium. The role of sodium balance and the renin-angiotensin system. J Lab Clin Med 101: 385-391, 1983.

21. Malis CHD, Cheung JY, Leaf A, Bonventre JV: Effects of verapamil in models of

ischemic acute renal failure in the rat. Am J Physiol 245: F735-F742, 1983.

22. Neumayer HH, Wagner K: Prevention of delayed graft function in cadaveric kidney transplants by diltiazem: Outcome of two prospective, randomized clinical trials. J Cardiovasc Pharamcol 10: S170-S177, 1987.

23. Farber JL, Mofty EL: The biochemical pathology in liver cell necrosis. Am J Pathol 79: 237-250, 1975.

24. Chien KR, Pfau RG, Farber J: Ischemic myocardial cell injury. Am J Pathol 97:505-522, 1979.

25. Landon EJ, Jaiswal RK, Naukam RJ, Sastry BVR: Effects of calcium channel blocking agents on membrane microviscosity and calcium in the liver of the carbon tetrachloride treated rat. Biochem Pharmacol 35: 679-705, 1986.

26. Urquhart J, Patterson RE, Bacharach SL, Green MV, Speir EH, Aamodt R, Epstein SE: Comparative effects of verapamil, diltiazem and nifedipine on haemodynamics and left ventricular function during acute myocardial ischaemia in dogs. Circulation 69: 382-390, 1984.

27. Gelmers HJ: Effect of nimodipine on the clinical course of patients with acute ischemic stroke. Acta Scand 64: 232-239, 1984.

28. Bakris GL, Burnett JC: A role for calcium in radiocontrast-induced reductions in renal haemodynamcis. Kidney Int 27: 465-468, 1985.

29. Anderson S, Meyer TW, Rennke HG, Brenner BM: Control of glomerular hypertension limits glomerular injury with reduced renal mass. J Clin Invest 76: 612, 1985.

30. Reisch C, Mann J, Ritz E: Konversionshemmer in der antihypertensiven Behandlung niereninsuffizienter Patienten. Dtsch Med Wochenschr 112: 1249, 1987.

35

EFFECT OF CONTRAST MEDIA ON RENAL HANDLING OF ALPHA-2μ-GLOBULIN IN RAT

C. Donadio (1), G. Tramonti (1), I. Auner (1), G. Deleide (2), F. Lunghi (2), C. Bianchi (1)

Nefrologia Medica, Istituto di Clinica Medica 2, University of Pisa, 56100 Pisa, Italy (1), SORIN Biomedica, Saluggia VC, Italy (2)

INTRODUCTION

The kidney plays an important role in the handling of low molecular weight (mw) proteins (1). In particular, the kidney (probably the proximal tubule) is the organ of highest accumulation of many low mw proteins such as: alpha-1-microglobulin, beta-2-microglobulin, lysozyme, retinol binding protein, alpha-2a-interferon, aprotinin, cytochrome C and alpha-2u-globulin (2, 3). Alpha-2u-globulin (alpha-2UG), a protein unique to the adult male rat and mouse, is accumulated by the rat kidney more than the other proteins cited above (3). The proximal tubule is the main target of nephrotoxicity of iodinated contrast media (CM), as indicated by the increase of enzymuria after CM administration.

The aim of this study is the evaluation of the effect of two different CM, diatrizoate meglumine (an ionic, high-osmolar CM) and iopamidol (a nonionic, low-osmolar CM), on renal handling of alpha-2UG in rat. The basic assumption is that alpha-2UG is accumulated in the same part of the nephron which is affected by CM.

MATERIALS AND METHODS

Animals. Male Sprague-Dawley rats (n=33, body weight 180-310 g, mean 223) were used. They were anesthetized with pentothal sodium (50 mg/kg body weight intraperitoneally).

Contrast media. The main characteristics of diatrizoate meglumine (Angiografin 65 - Schering SpA, Milano, Italy) and of iopamidol (Iopamiro 300 - Bracco Industria Chimica SpA, Milano, Italy) are reported in Table I.

Alpha-2u-globulin, pI ca. 4.9, mw 19,000, was kindly provided by Dr. O.W. Neuhaus, who extensively studied this protein (4,5). Alpha-2UG was labelled with I^{131} using the iodogen method (6). The iodination efficiency was 95% and the specific activity was 14 mCi/mg of protein. Alpha-2UG was purified by anion-exchange chromatography prior to administration; after purification free iodine was <2%.

Experimental protocol. Eleven rats were treated with saline (5 ml/kg bw iv), 11 with diatrizoate (5 ml/kg bw, corresponding to 3.3 g of CM/kg bw) and 11 with iopamidol (5 ml/kg bw, corresponding to 3.1 g of CM/kg bw). The duration of iv injection was approximately 30 seconds. A dose of about 20 μCi of alpha-2UG-I^{131} was injected immediately after saline or CM. After 11 min from alpha-2UG-I^{131} the animals were sacrificed. The kidneys were removed and weighed. The radioactivity of the

Table 1. Contrast media

	Diatrizoate	Iopamidol
Osmolality (mOsm/kg of water)	1500	616
CM concentration (g/100 ml)	65	61.2
Iodine concentration (g/100 ml)	30.6	30

injected dose and that of kidneys, urine and plasma was measured using the same scintillation counter (Italelettronica, Italy).

RESULTS

The administration of CM produced a macroscopically evident effect on the kidneys. After both CM the kidneys appeared pale and enlarged.

The quantitative results of this study are reported in Table II.

The kidney weight resulted higher in rats treated with CM than in the group of saline. This effect was more evident in the animals treated with diatrizoate.

Both diatrizoate and iopamidol induced a moderate, but statistically significant, decrease of kidney uptake of labelled alpha-2UG, expressed as kidney radioactivity percent of the injected dose. This effect was more marked in rats treated with diatrizoate, but the difference with iopamidol was not statistically significant.

Urinary excretion of radioactivity was lower after CM, mainly with diatrizoate. Plasma concentration of radioactivity was slightly higher after CM.

DISCUSSION

It is known that CM induces a functional disturbance of the renal proximal tubule, as demonstrated by the increase of enzymuria. Furthermore, CM interferes with important functions of the proximal tubular cell, such as the renal extraction of para-aminohippurate (7). Diatrizoate and, to a lesser extent, iopamidol have also a direct toxic effect on different metabolic functions of tubule cells (8,9).

The results of this study indicate that both diatrizoate and iopamidol decrease the kidney uptake of alpha-2UG in rat. This effect suggests an influence of CM on renal handling of low mw proteins, which is another important metabolic function of the proximal tubule. Glomerular filtration and proximal tubular reabsorption is the main pathway of renal accumulation of small proteins. Some proteins are taken up also

Table II. Effects of contrast media (mean±SD)

	Saline	Diatrizoate	Iopamidol
RATS			
n	11	11	11
body weight (g)	220±42	227±35	222±41
KIDNEYS			
weight (g)	1.62±0.24	2.12±0.26***	1.99±0.38*
radioactivity (% of dose)	50.90±2.88	43.12±3.39***	45.61±4.48**
URINE			
radioactivity (% of dose)	3.36±2.58	1.49±0.90*	1.66±1.45
PLASMA			
radioactivity/g (% of dose)	1.39±0.33	1.94±0.32***	1.69±0.50

*$p<0.05$; **$p<0.01$; ***$p<0.001$.

from the peritubular circulation. The observed effect of CM on renal uptake of alpha-2UG could be due to a decrease of glomerular filtration and/or of peritubular uptake of alpha-2UG, while luminal reabsorption does not seem to be affected. In fact, the reduced renal uptake of labelled alpha-2UG was not accompanied by an increase of urinary excretion of radioactivity. Further investigation is necessary to clarify the mechanism of the effect of CM on renal handling of alpha-2UG. Nevertheless, kidney uptake of alpha-2u-globulin could be a useful tool to evaluate the effects of contrast media and of other drugs or chemicals on renal handling of low mw proteins.

ACKNOWLEDGEMENTS

This research has been supported in part by a research fund from Ministero Pubblica Istruzione, Italy. Mr. Joseph Franceschina is gratefully acknowledged for his valuable help in the preparation of this paper.

REFERENCES

1. Maack T, Hyung Park C, Camargo MJC: Renal filtration, transport, and metabolism of proteins. In: Seldin DW, Giebisch G (eds); The kidney: Physiology and pathophysiology. New York, Raven Press, 1985, pp. 1773-1803.

2. Bianchi C, Donadio C, Tramonti G, Auner I, Lorusso P, Deleide G, Lunghi F, Salvadori P: Renal handling of cationic and anionic small proteins: Experiments in intact rats. Contr Nephrol 68: 37-44, 1988.

3. Bianchi C, Donadio C, Tramonti G, Auner I, Lorusso P, Deleide G, Lunghi F, Vannucci C, Vitali S: High and preferential accumulation in the kidneys of low mw proteins. Abstracts of the Sixth International Symposium of Nephrology at Montecatini - Kidney, Proteins and Drugs, 1989, p. 32.

4. Neuhaus OW: Renal reabsorption of low-molecular weight proteins: alpha-2u-globulin. Proc Soc Exp Biol Med 182: 531-539, 1986.

5. Neuhaus OW: Alpha-2u-globulin: a model protein for studies of the renal reabsorption of low molecular weight proteins. Contr Nephrol 68: 32-36, 1988.

6. Knight L, Budzynski AZ, Olexa SA: Radiolabelling of fibrinogen using the iodogen technique. Thromb Haemost 46: 593-596, 1981.

7. Dibona GF: Effect of anionic and nonionic contrast media on renal extraction of para-aminohippurate in the dog. Proc Soc Exp Biol Med 157: 453-455, 1978.

8. Humes HD, Hunt DA, White MD: Direct toxic effect of the radiocontrast agent diatrizoate on renal proximal tubular cells. Am J Physiol 21: F246-F255, 1987.

9. Messana JM, Cieslinski DA, Nguyen VD, Humes HD: Comparison of the toxicity of the radiocontrast agents, iopamidol and diatrizoate, to rabbit renal proximal tubule cells in vitro. J Pharmacol Exp Ther 244: 1139-1144, 1988.

PART VIII
HALOGENATED COMPOUNDS

36

TOXICITY OF THE S-CONJUGATES OF FOUR STRUCTURALLY RELATED DIFLUOROETHYLENES IN FRESHLY ISOLATED AND CULTURED PROXIMAL TUBULAR CELLS FROM RAT KIDNEY

P.J. Boogaard (1), J.N.M. Commandeur (2), G.J. Mulder (1), N.P.E. Vermeulen (2) and J.F. Nagelkerke (1)

Division of Toxicology, Center for Bio-Pharmaceutical Sciences, Leiden University, P.O.Box 9503, 2300 RA LEIDEN, The Netherlands (1) and Department of Pharmacochemistry (Molecular Toxicology), Free University, De Boelelaan 1083, 1081 HV Amsterdam, The Netherlands (2)

INTRODUCTION

A major pathway in the elimination of electrophilic compounds is excretion as mercapturic acid (R-NAc) in urine. The first step in the biosynthesis of R-NAc is conjugation with glutathione (GSH). The GS-conjugate is degraded to the corresponding cysteine-S- conjugate (R-Cys), which can be taken up by the proximal tubular cell (PTC), and subsequently be N-acetylated to R-NAc and excreted in the urine. Alternatively, R-Cys can be N-acetylated before it reaches the kidney. R-NAc can be taken up by the PTC and be excreted, or may eventually be deacetylated back to R-Cys by renal N-acylase (1,2). The GSH conjugation of certain halogenated, unsaturated hydrocarbons, does not lead to detoxification. Cleavage of the thioether bond, catalyzed by the renal cysteine-S-conjugate β-lyase, results in the formation of highly reactive intermediates, which cause severe nephrotoxicity (2-4).

In the present work, we report investigations on the uptake and bio- activation of R-Cys and corresponding R-NAc of four structurally related difluoroethylenes (Fig.1). These S-conjugates were studied in freshly isolated rat PTC and in a primary cell culture of rat PTC.

	X	Y
Tetrafluoroethylene (TFE)	F	F
Chlorotrifluoroethylene (CTFE)	Cl	F
Dichlorodifluoroethylene (DCDFE)	Cl	Cl
Dibromodifluoroethylene (DBDFE)	B	B

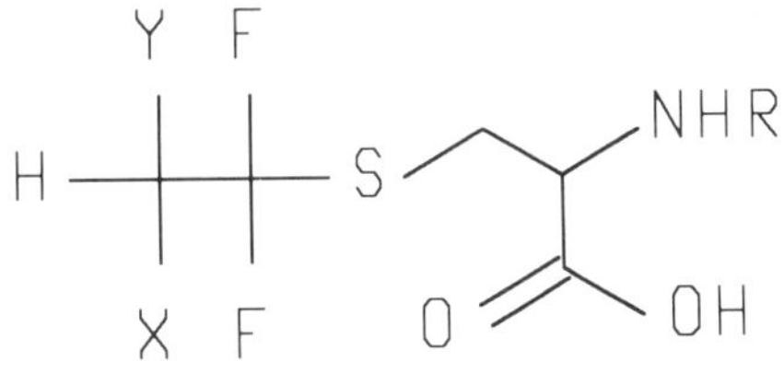

Figure1. Structures of the cysteine-S-conjugates (R = H) and mercapturic acids (R = CO-CH3) of the four 2,2-difluoroethylenes.

METHODS

Animals

In all experiments male Wistar rats (150-200 g) were used, that had free access to a commercial diet and tap water. PTC were isolated by collagenase perfusion and purified by isopycnic centrifugation as described previously (5,6). Cytosol was prepared from kidneys homogenized in 3 volumes 50 mM potassium phosphate buffer (pH 7.40). The homogenate was centrifuged at 11,000 g (20 min, 4°C). The supernatant was centrifuged at 100,000 g for 60 min to prepare the cytosolic fraction (S_{100} fraction).

Incubations

Isolated PTC (3.5×10^6 PTC/ml) were incubated in Hanks'-buffer (pH 7.40) supplemented with 0.25 mM HEPES and 2.5% w/v BSA. Cytosol (4 mg protein/ml) was incubated in 50 mM potassium phosphate buffer pH 7.40. Incubations were carried out at 37°C under 95% O_2/5% CO_2 on a rotary shaker.

Cultures

Isolated PTC were grown on plastic culture plates or rat tail collagen-coated filters in a modified DMEM-Ham F_{12} medium, at 37°C in a humidified atmosphere of 95% air/5% CO_2. The medium contained D-valine and L-ornithine instead of L-valine and L-arginine respectively, in order to prevent fibroblast growth (7), and was supplemented with 0.1% w/v BSA, 10% w/v FCS, amphotericin B (2.5 mg/l), penicillin G (10^5 U/l), and ciprofloxacine (4 mg/l).

Cytotoxicity

Functional integrity of the PTC was assessed by their ability to transport alpha-methylglucose (α-MG), as described previously (5-8).

Analyses

R-NAc was quantified by GC/MS. Reactions were stopped by addition of 38% w/v HCl; N-acetyl-S-benzyl-L-cysteine was added as internal standard. R-NAc was methylated after extraction with ethyl acetate. The methylated samples were analyzed using a CP-Sil SE-30 capillary column and detected by selected ion monitoring of ions at w/z 117, 144 and 176 (9). R-Cys were derivatized with o-phthaldialdehyde and 2-mercaptoethanol and analyzed by RP-HPLC on a Lichrosorb 5RP18 column by fluorimetric detection. TFE-Cys, CTFE-Cys and DCDFE-Cys were eluted isocratically (60% MeOH/40% 12.5 mM potassium phosphate buffer, pH 7.2); DBDFE-Cys was separated from cytosolic amines by gradient elution, starting from 30% CH_3CN/70% potassium phosphate buffer to 50%/50% (9). β-Lyase activity was measured by the formation rate of pyruvate. Pyruvate was determined as its 2,4-dinitrophenylhydrazone by RP-HPLC using a Lichrosorb 5RP18 column and 55% MeOH/44% 50 mM TEA iodide/1% HAc as eluent (9).

RESULTS

Cytotoxicity of R-Cys and R-NAc in freshly isolated and cultured PTC

Both freshly isolated and cultured PTC were incubated with R-Cys and R-NAc. R-Cys was cytotoxic in both systems; this toxicity could completely be blocked by preincubation of the cells with aminooxyacetic acid (AOA), an inhibitor of β-lyase (Fig. 2).

Toxicity of R-Cys decreased in the order TFE ~ CTFE > DCDFE > DBDFE. In isolated PTC the toxicities of TFE-Cys, TFE-NAc, CTFE-Cys and CTFE-NAc were similar, but DCDFE-Cys and DBDFE-Cys were more toxic than DCDFE-NAc and DBDFE-NAc respectively. However, DCDFE-NAc and DBDFE-NAc caused the same extent of toxicity as DCDFE-Cys and DBDFE-Cys respectively if the cells were exposed for a longer period.

R-NAc, in contrast to R-Cys, was not cytotoxic when incubated with PTC cultured on plastic. However, when the PTC were cultured on collagen-coated filter membranes, R-NAc showed toxicity comparable with that in isolated PTC (Fig. 3).

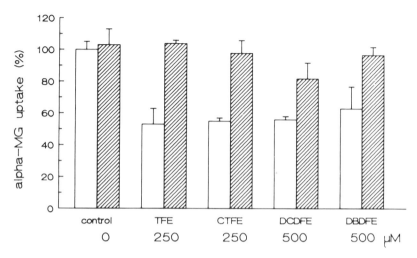

Figure 2. Toxicity in cultured PTC of R-Cys (2 hr incubation). Dashed bars cell preincubate wit 100µM AOA

Transport of R-Cys and R-NAc in isolated and cultured PTC

As previously reported (6,8), PTC actively transport organic anions. Preincubation of the cells with probenecid inhibits this transport. The differences in toxicity between the S-conjugates might be attributable to dissimilar transport mechanisms into the PTC. Hence, we studied the effect of probenecid on the toxicity of the R-Cys and R-NAc in both in vitro systems. Probenecid had no effect on the toxicity of R-Cys in isolated nor cultured PTC (Fig. 3). R-NAc toxicity was reduced by preincubation with probenecid both in isolated PTC as well as in PTC cultured on filters (Fig. 3)

Metabolism of the S-conjugates by freshly isolated PTC

The differences in toxicity observed might also be explained by different rates of activation. R-NAc has to be deacetylated in order to become substrate for β-lyase; R-Cys, on the other hand, can be N-acetylated by renal N-acetyltransferases and thus escape metabolic activation by β-lyase (1,2,4). To prevent extracellular metabolism by enzymes which have leaked from the cells due to toxicity, the freshly isolated PTC were incubated for only 15 min with R-Cys and for 30 min with R-NAc. TFE-

and CTFE-conjugates were incubated at 0.5 mM, and DCDFE- and DBDFE-conjugates at 2.0 mM. Within the 15 min incubation of R-Cys no or small amounts of R-NAc were formed (Table 1). Even in the presence of AOA (1.0 mM), no TFE-NAc could be detected upon incubation of PTC with TFE-Cys. CTFE-Cys yielded only traces of CTFE-NAc. In contrast, much higher concentrations of DCDFE-NAc and DBDFE-NAc were formed from DCDFE-Cys and DBDFE-Cys. Large decreases in concentration of R-NAc, and concomitant formation of R-Cys, were detected upon incubation with isolated PTC (Table 1). TFE-NAC and CTFE-NAc were deacetylated for over 90% in 30 min, indicating very efficient uptake and high N-acylase activity. However DCDFE-NAc and DBDFE-NAc were converted to their corresponding R-Cys for only 5-20%. This might be due to either a rate limiting uptake or a low deacetylation activity.

β-Lyase activity towards R-Cys

Apart from the balance between acetylation and deacetylation, differences in β-lyase activity towards the various R-Cys might explain the differences in toxicity observed. Activity of β-lyase decreased in the order TFE-Cys> CTFE-Cys > DCDFE-Cys > DBDFE-Cys, which

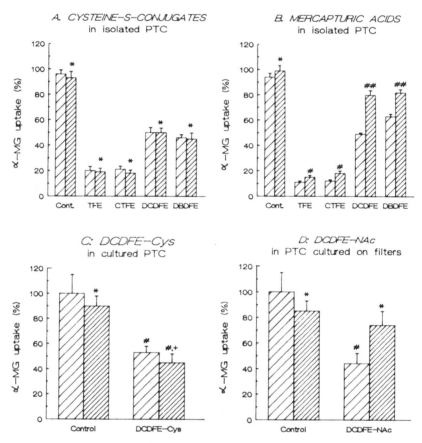

Figure 3. Effect of 0.5 mM probenecid (double dashed bars) on the toxicity of 100 μm M R-Cys and R-NAc (dashed bars) in freshly isolated and cultured PTC. * not different from control/treated group, + not different from non treated group, # p<0.05, ## p<0.02
(Student t, one-tailed, unpaired)

Table 1. <u>N</u>-acetylation of R-Cys to R-NAc and deacetylation of R-NAc to the corresponding R-Cys by isolated PTC. PTC were incubated with and without AOA.

Compound	R-Cys formed mmoles (%)		Compound	R-NAc formed μmoles	
	- AOA	+ AOA		-AOA	+AOA
TFE-NAc	0.45 (89)	0.46 (92)	TFE-Cys	N.D	N.D.
CTFE-NAc	0.47 (94)	0.48 (96)	CTFE-Cys	11	N.D.
DCDFE-NAc	0.092 (5)	0.55 (28)	DCDFE-Cys	36	53
DBDFE-NAc	0.55 (27)	0.26 (13)	DCDFE-Cys	32	38

N.D.: not detectable. Values have an analytical variance < 5%.

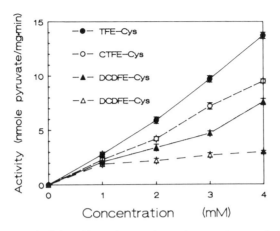

Figure 4. Activity of beta-lyase of renal cytosol towards R-Cys.

DISCUSSION

The extent of toxicity exerted by the S-conjugates of the four difluoroethylenes differs in vivo (3,10). We investigated in two in vitro systems of rat PTC whether these differences may be explained by differences in transport and/or differences in metabolism by (de)activating enzymes.

The toxicity of all conjugates in both systems was blocked by preincubation with AOA, which indicates that the bioactivating β-lyase pathway is involved (2,3). Moreover, the toxicity of the four cysteine-S-conjugates ranked in the same order as their activity towards β-lyase.

In order to be a substrate for β-lyase R-NAc has to be deacetylated to the corresponding R-Cys. However, the kidney has a (detoxifying) capacity to N-acetylate as well, which competes with the (toxifying) β-lyase for R-Cys. It was found that isolated PTC converted TFE-NAc and CTFE-NAc to TFE-Cys and CTFE-Cys for 90-95% within 30 min, whereas

DCDFE-NAc and DCDFE-NAc were deacetylated for only 5-30% in the same period. TFE-Cys and CTFE-Cys were not N-acetylated during a 15 min incubation, while DCDFE-Cys and DBDFE-Cys were. It appears that the ratio acetylation/deacetylation is more directed towards R-Cys for TFE and CTFE than DCDFE and DBDFE. This is in agreement with the greater toxicity of the former in PTC.

However, interconversion between R-Cys and R-NAc and cleavage of R-Cys can only occur intracellularly. Therefore, the uptake of the conjugates was studied. One of the advantages of cultured PTC over freshly isolated PTC is that they retain their polarity (7). PTC cultured on plastic only expose the apical membrane to the medium; the basolateral membrane is inaccessible. R-NAc was not toxic in PTC cultured on plastic, but R-Cys was. The basolateral membrane is exposed when the PTC are cultured on filters. Under these conditions, toxicity of R-NAc was observed. This toxicity was prevented by probenecid as in isolated cells. In contrast, both in isolated and cultured PTC, probenecid had no effect on toxicity due to R-Cys. This suggests that R-NAc, but not R-Cys, is transported *via the organic anion carrier* in the basolateral membrane (Fig. 5).

is similar to the decrease in toxicity (Fig. 4). No pyruvate formation could be detected when the incubations were carried out in the presence of 0.5 mM AOA.

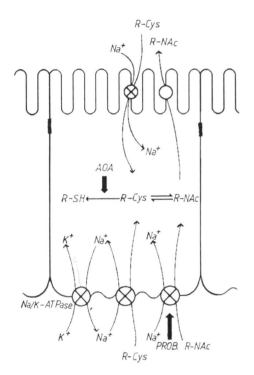

Figure 5. Proximal tubular handling of the difluo-roethylene-S-conjugates. Both types of conjugates accumulate intracellularly via carrier-mediated transport systems (O/X), which depend on the Na^+ gradient provided by the basolateral Na^+/K^+ AT-Pase. Only the mercapturates (R-NAc) are taken up by a process that is inhibited by probenecid (PROB), and can leave the cell by facilitated diffusion (O). Big black arrows indicate inhibition of the process.

In conclusion, the observed differences in toxicity of the halogenated difluoroethylenes in PTC may be explained by differences in:

1. conversion rate of R-Cys to toxic metabolites by renal β-lyase,

2. balance between acetylation and deacetylation by the PTC, and

3. transport into the PTC, as illustrated in figure 5.

As we recently reported for subcellular systems (9), in which transport is not relevant, the interconversion between R-Cys and R-NAc is very rapid. In freshly isolated PTC about the same balance between R-Cys and R-NAc was

found as in subcellular fractions. Therefore, although transport into the PTC is very important for the toxicity per se, it does not explain the differences in toxicity between the S-conjugates. These differences are due rather to the equilibrium between R-NAc and R-Cys, and the differences in activity of β-lyase towards R-Cys.

REFERENCES

1. Jakoby WB, Stevens J, Duffel MW, Weisiger RA: The terminal enzymes of mercapturate formation and the thiomethyl shunt. Rev Biochem Toxicol 6:97-115, 1984

2. Lock EA: Studies on the mechanism of nephrotoxicity and nephrocarcinogenicity of halogenated alkenes. CRC Crit Rev Toxicol 19:23-42, 1988

3. Dekant W, Vamvakas S, Anders MW: Bioactivation of nephrotoxic haloalkenes by glutathione conjugation: Formation of toxic and mutagenic intermediates by cysteine conjugate β-lyase. Drug Met Rev 20:43-83, 1989

4. Monks TJ, Lau SS: Renal transport processes and glutathione conjugate- mediated nephrotoxicity. Drug Met Disp 15: 437-441, 1987

5. Boogaard PJ, Mulder GJ, Nagelkerke JF: Alpha-methylglucose uptake by isolated rat kidney proximal tubular cells as a parameter for cell integrity in vitro. In: Nephrotoxicity: extrapolation from in vitro to in vivo and animals to man. London (U.K.), Plenum Press, 1989, pp. 337-342

6. Boogaard PJ, Mulder GJ, Nagelkerke JF: Isolated proximal tubular cells from rat kidney as in vitro model for studies on nephrotoxicity. I. An improved method for preparation of proximal tubular cells and their functional characterization by alpha-methylglucose uptake. Toxicol Appl Pharmacol 101:135-143, 1989

7. Boogaard PJ, Zoeteweij JP, Van Berkel TJC, Van't Noordende JM, Mulder GJ, Nagelkerke JF. Primary culture of proximal tubular cells from normal rat kidney as an in vitro model

to study mechanism of nephrotoxicity. Toxicity of nephrotoxicants at low concentrations during prolonged exposure. Biochem Pharmacol 39:1335-1345, 1990

8. Boogaard PJ, Mulder GJ, Nagelkerke JF: Isolated proximal tubular cells from rat kidney as in vitro model for studies on nephrotoxicity. II. Alpha-methylglucose uptake as a sensitive parameter for mechanistic studies of acute toxicity by xenobiotics. Toxicol Appl Pharmacol 101:144-157, 1989

9. Boogaard PJ, Commandeur JNM, Mulder GJ, Vermeulen NPE, Nagelkerke JF: Toxicity of the cysteine-S-conjugates and mercapturic acids of four structurally related difluoroethylenes in isolated proximal tubular cells from rat kidney. Uptake of the conjugates and activation to toxic metabolites. Biochem Pharmacol 38:3731-3741, 1989

10. Commandeur JNM, Brakenhoff JPG, De Kanter FJJ, Vermeulen NPE: Nephrotoxicity of mercapturic acids of three structurally related 2,2 difluoroethylenes in the rat. Biochem Pharmacol 37: 4495-4505, 1988

37

BIOCHEMICAL CHANGES INDUCED BY DICHLOROVINYLCYSTEINE IN MICE RENAL CORTEX

C. Cojocel

Hoechst Aktiengesellschaft, Postfach 80 03 20, D-6230 Frankfurt am Main 80, Germany

INTRODUCTION

Results of recent studies (1) provide evidence indicating that dichlorovinylcysteine (DCVC) may be formed in vivo during the metabolism of trichloroethylene (TCE). DCVC was shown to be a potent nephrotoxin (2). Following glutathione conjugation of TCE, the glutathione S-conjugates are degraded to S-cysteine conjugates such as DCVC (1). The necrosis of the pars recta of the proximal tubule could be due to accumulation of the S-cysteine conjugates and their subsequent activation by the kidney, via renal beta-lyase (3). Cleavage of these S-cysteine conjugates by beta-lyase could lead to formation of reactive electrophilic species (4). Treatment of rats with TCE induced destruction of liver cytochrome P-450 and altered the activity of drug metabolizing enzymes (5). Both TCE and DCVC were shown to cause a dose-dependent formation of lipid peroxidation products such as ethane in vivo and MDA in the kidney cortex of mice (6,7). These results suggest that DCVC and/or its reactive metabolites, in addition to inducing peroxidative damage, could destroy and/or inactivate cytosolic and membrane-bound proteins. The aim of the present study was to investigate the effects of DCVC on the contents of liver and renal cortical cytochromes P-450 and b5 and on the activities of drug metabolizing enzymes and the inhibition of these effects by aminooxyacetic acid (AOAA).

METHODS

Male NMRI mice (25 - 30 g) were treated i.p. with DCVC in a dosage from 20 to 500 mg/kg. Control mice were given saline. After 0, 1, 2, and 3 hr mice were killed and liver and renal cortical microsomes were prepared as described previously (8). In a series of experiments, mice were pretreated i.p. with 40 mg/kg AOAA 1 hr prior to i.p.-administration of 40 mg/kg DCVC. Freshly prepared microsomes (300-400 μg) were homogenized in 5 ml of thiobarbituric acid containing reagent mixture (9) and incubated for 15 min at 100°C. Subsequently MDA concentration was measured spectrophotometrically as described previously (8).

Cytochromes P-450 and b5 were measured as described by Omura and Sato (10). The fluorometric assay of 7-hydroxycoumarin was used to measure the O-deethylation of 7-ethoxycoumarin (11). The N-demethylation of aminopyrine was estimated by measuring the formaldehyde released by the method of Nash (12). The hydroxylation of aniline was determined by measuring the p-aminophenol release (13). NADPH-cytochrome-c- reductase activity was determined according to the method of Pederson et al. (14) using the extinction coefficient of $21 \times mM^{-1} \times cm^{-1}$ (15). Glutathione-S-transferase activity was measured as described by Habig et al. (16) with 1-chloro-2,4-dinitrobenzene (CNDB) as substrate. Protein was assayed by the method of Schacterle and Pollack (17) using bovine serum albumin as standard.

Mean value x, standard deviation (SD) and one-way analysis of variance were used for the statistical analysis of the data. The 0.05 level of probability was used as the criterion of significance.

RESULTS

Three hours after exposure of male mice to DCVC, a dose-dependent increase of MDA content was found in the renal cortical microsomes but not in the liver microsomes. MDA content increased in the renal cortical microsomes from a control value of 0.240 ± 0.083 to 1.440 ± 0.167 nmol/mg protein after treatment of mice with 200 mg/kg DCVC.

Treatment of mice with DCVC caused a time- and dose-dependent decrease in the contents of cytochromes P-450 and b5 in renal cortical microsomes but not in liver microsomes. The decrease in cytochrome P-450 content was greater than that of cytochrome b5 (Table 1).

Treatment of mice with DCVC induced slight or no changes in the activity of liver drug metabolizing enzymes. DCVC treatment induced differential changes in the activity of drug me-

Table 1: Effects of dichlorovinylcysteine (DCVC) on the content of cytochromes P-450 and b5 from mice renal cortex

	Control mice	DCVC treated mice	
		20 mg/kg	40 mg/kg
Cytochrome P-450 (nmoles/mg protein)	0.482 ± 0.041	$0.150 \pm 0.083^{*}$	N.D.
Cytochrome b5 (nmoles/mg protein)	0.268 ± 0.057	$0.168 \pm 0.041^{*}$	$0.127 \pm 0.018^{*}$

Results are x ± S.D of measurements from 5 different preparations 3 hr after i.p.-administration of DCVC. *, Values are significant at P< 0.05. N.D. not detectable

Table 2: Effects of dichlorovinylcysteine (DCVC) on the activity of some drug metabolizing enzymes from mice renal cortex

	Control mice	DCVC treated mice	% of control
NADPH-cytochrome-c-reductase (nmoles/mg protein/min)	47.950 ± 3.14	$17.160 \pm 1.09^{*}$	37.79
Aminopyrine-N-demethylase (nmoles/mg protein/min)	1.890 ± 0.09	$0.470 \pm 0.07^{*}$	24.87
Aniline hydroxylase (nmoles/mg protein/min)	0.350 ± 0.01	$0.180 \pm 0.02^{*}$	51.43
7-ethoxycoumarin-O-deethylase (nmoles/mg protein/min)	0.315 ± 0.02	0.321 ± 0.02	101.90
Cytosolic glutathione-S-transferase (nmoles/mg protein/min)	340.600 ± 12.9	$215.240 \pm 11.1^{*}$	63.18

.Results are x ± SD of measurements from 5 different preparations 3 hr after i.p.-administration of DCVC* (40 mg/kg). , Values are significant at P< 0.05.

tabolizing enzymes in mice renal cortex. A time- and concentration-dependent decrease in the activity of NADPH-cytochrome-c-reductase, aminopyrine-N-demethylase and aniline hydroxylase occurred while no changes in the activity of 7-ethoxycoumarin-O-deethylase was measured. DCVC had a weaker effect on the enzymatic activity of the cytosolic glutathione-S-transferase (Table 2).

With the exception of a slight decrease in the enzymatic activity of the cytosolic glutathione-S-transferase, no changes occurred in the activity of liver drug metabolizing enzymes after DCVC treatment.

After pretreatment of mice with 40 mg/kg AOAA 1 hr prior administration of 40 mg/kg DCVC, cytochrome P450 was depleted in the renal cortex only to 56% of control. When mice were given 40 mg/kg DCVC alone, renal cortical cytochrome P450 was depleted to about 43% of control.

DISCUSSION

Carbon tetrachloride (18), trichloroethylene (5) or cadmium (19) have been shown to destroy cytochrome P-450, and/or to inhibit the activity of various drug metabolizing enzymes. Similarly, treatment of mice with DCVC, in the present study, caused a time- and dose-dependent decrease in the content of cytochromes P-450 and b5 from the renal cortical microsomes. The decrease in cytochrome P-450 content was greater than that of cytochrome b5. Additionally DCVC induced slight or no changes in the activity of liver drug metabolizing enzymes. However, DCVC treatment induced differential changes in the activity of drug metabolizing enzymes in mice renal cortex. Enzymatic and nonenzymatic degradation of DCVC can result in the formation of reactive species that can bind to protein (20) and/or react with unsaturated fatty acids of microsomal membrane lipids to cause the peroxidative injury (6). The significant stimulation of lipid peroxidation by DCVC in mice maintained under hypoxic conditions (6) suggests that a reductive metabolic pathway may be important for the generation of DCVC free radicals which

cause peroxidation of unsaturated fatty acids in the kidney but not in the liver. It is possible that under hypoxic conditions, DCVC could be metabolized by renal cortical cytochrome P-450 via a reductive pathway to (presently unknown) electrophilic intermediates. Thus, the specific loss in the contents of cytochromes P-450 and b5 and inactivation of drug metabolizing enzymes in the renal cortex induced by DCVC may be due either to a direct attack of radicals on proteins or to initiation of the peroxidation of microsomal lipids. These primary biochemical lesions could result in the DCVC-induced damage to the cytochrome P-450 and inactivation of drug metabolizing enzymes.

Alternatively, DCVC reactive species could be formed after conjugation of DCVC with glutathione in the liver and in the kidney, subsequent processing of these conjugates by renal dipeptidase and activation of DCVC by renal beta-lyase. Cysteine S-conjugates of several halogenated alkenes such as hexachloro-1,3-butadiene (21,22), tetrafluoroethylene (23) and trichloroethylene (1) are potent nephrotoxins which require enzymatic activation by a-lyase to produce cytotoxicity. The identification of S-1,2-dichlorovinyl-N-acetyl-cysteine in the urine of TCE-treated rats (24) supports the hypothesis that the glutathione conjugates of TCE are further processed by peptidases to DCVC which could be cleaved by the renal beta-lyase to toxic reactive intermediates (25). Pretreatment of mice in the present study with the beta-lyase inhibitor AOAA prior to DCVC administration provided a partial protection against depletion of cytochrome P-450 and inhibition of drug metabolizing enzymes caused by the treatment of mice with DCVC.

In conclusion, the reactive intermediates formed via cytochrome P-450 and/or beta-lyase activation pathways could cause nephrotoxicity after inducing peroxidation of membrane lipids (6) and/or mitochondrial injury (25).

ACKNOWLEDGEMENTS

The author thanks Dr. B. Seuering, Hoechst AG, for the synthesis of S-(1,2-dichlorovinyl)-L-cysteine. The excellent technical assistance of B. Alka, B. Knauf and A. Stricker is appreciated.

REFERENCES

1. Dekant W, Metzler M, Henschler D: Identification of S-1,2-dichlorovinyl-N-acetyl-cysteine as a urinary metabolite of trichloroethylene: a possible explanation for its nephrocarcinogenicity in male rats. Biochem Pharmacol 35: 2455-2458, 1986.

2. Gandolfi AJ, Nagle RB, Soltis JJ, Plescia FH: Nephrotoxicity of halogenated vinyl cysteine compounds. Res Commun Chem Pathol Pharmacol 33: 249, 1981.

3. Elfarra AA, Anders MW: Renal processing of glutathione conjugates. Role of nephrotoxicity. Biochem Pharmacol 33: 3729-3732, 1984.

4. Anders MW, Elfarra AA, Lash LH: Cellular effects of reactive intermediates: nephrotoxicity of S-conjugates of amino acids. Arch Toxicol 60: 103-108, 1987.

5. Pessayre D, Allemand H, Wandscheer JC, Descartoire V, Artigou J-Y, Benhamou J-P: Inhibition, activation, destruction, and induction of drug-metabolizing enzymes by trichloroethylene. Toxicol Appl Pharmacol 49: 355-363, 1979.

6. Beuter W, Cojocel C, Müller W, Donaubauer HH, Mayer D: Peroxidative damage and nephrotoxicity of dichlorovinylcysteine in mice. J Appl Toxicol 9: 181-186, 1989.

7. Cojocel C, Beuter W, Müller W, Mayer D: Lipid peroxidation: A possible mechanism of trichloroethylene-induced nephrotoxicity. Toxicology 55: 131-134, 1989.

8. Cojocel C, Hannemann J, Baumann K: Cephaloridine-induced lipid peroxidation initiated by reactive oxygen species as a possible mechanism of cephaloridine nephrotoxicity. Biochim Biophys Acta 834: 432-410, 1985.

9. Buege JA, Aust SD: Microsomal lipid peroxidation. Methods Enzymol 52: 302-310, 1978.

10. Omura T, Sato R: The carbon monoxide-binding pigment of liver microsomes. I. Evidence for its hemoprotein nature. J Biol Chem 239: 2370-2378, 1964.

11. Greenlee WF, Poland A: An improved assay of 7-ethoxycoumarin-O-deethylase activity: induction of hepatic activity in C 57BL/6J and DBA/2J mice by phenobarbital, 3-methylcholanthrene and 2,3,7,8-tetrachlordibenzo-p-dioxin. J Pharmacol Exp Ther 205: 596-605, 1978.

12. Nash T: The colorimetric estimation of formaldehyde by means of the Hantzsch reaction. J Biol Chem 55: 416-422, 1953.

13. Schenkman B, Remmer H, Estabrook RW: Spectral studies of drug interaction with hepatic microsomal cytochrome. Mol Pharmacol 3: 113-121, 1967.

14. Pederson TL, Buege TA, Aust SD: Microsomal electron transport. The role of reduced nicotinamide adenine dinucleotide phosphate-cytochrome-c- reductase in liver microsomal lipid peroxidation. J Biol Chem 25: 7134-7141, 1973.

15. Massey V: The microestimation of succinate and the extinction coefficient of cytochrome c. Biochim Biophys Acta 34: 255-256, 1959.

16. Habig WH, Pabst MJ, Jakoby WB: Glutathione-S-transferases. The first enzymatic step in mercapturic acid formation. J Biol Chem 249: 7130-7139, 1974.

17. Schacterle GR, Pollack RL: A simplified method for quantitative assay of all amounts of protein in biological material. Anal Biochem 51: 654-655, 1973.

18. Noguchi T, Fong K-L, Lai EK, Alexander SS, King MM, Olson L, Poyer JL, McCay PB: Specificity of phenobarbital-induced cytochrome P-450 for metabolism of carbon tetrachloride to the trichloromethyl radical. Biochem Pharmacol 31: 615-624, 1982.

19. Yoshida T, Suzuki Y, Hashimoto Y: Sex-related effect of cadmium on hepatic

cytochrome P-450 drug-metabolizing enzymes and delta-aminolevulinic acid synthetase and heme oxygenase in the rat. Toxicol Lett 4: 97-102, 1979.

20. Schaeffer VH, Stevens JL: Mechanism of transport for toxic cysteine conjugates in rat kidney cortex membrane vesicles. Mol Pharmacol 32: 293-298, 1987.

21. Lock EA, Ishmael J: The acute toxic effects of hexachloro-1,3- butadiene on the rat kidney. Arch Toxicol 43: 47-57, 1979.

22. MacFarlane M, Foster JR, Gibson GG, King LJ, Lock EA: Cysteine conjugate beta-lyase of rat kidney cytosol: characterization,

immunocytochemical localization, and correlation with hexachlorobutadiene nephrotoxicity. Toxicol Appl Pharmacol 98: 185-197, 1989.

23. Odum J, Green T: The metabolism and nephrotoxicity of tetrafluoroethylene in the rat. Toxicol Appl Pharmacol 76: 306-318, 1984.

24. Dekant W, Metzler M, Henschler D: Novel metabolites of trichloroethylene through dechlorination reactions in rats, mice and humans. Biochem Pharmacol 33: 2021, 1984.

25. Lash LH, Anders MW: Cytotoxicity of S-(1,2-dichlorovinyl)glutathione and S-(1,2-dichlorovinyl)-L-cysteine in isolated rat kidney cells. J Biol Chem 261: 13076-13081, 1986.

38

GLUTATHIONE S-TRANSFERASE CATALYZED CONJUGATION OF HEXAFLUOROPROPENE WITH GLUTATHIONE

M. Koob, A. Köchling and W. Dekant

Institut für Toxikologie, Universität Würzburg, Versbacher Str. 9, D-8700 Würzburg, Germany

INTRODUCTION

Fluoroalkenes are a group of commercially important monomers and have been manufactured in quantity for 30 years. Hexafluoropropene (HFP) is used as a monomer for the production of heat stable polymers and formed during pyrolysis of polytetrafluoroethene. HFP is selectively nephrotoxic in rats (1). This nephrotoxicity is not caused by inorganic fluoride formed during metabolism (2). The organ-specific toxicity of the structurally related alkenes tetrafluoroethene and chlorotrifluoroethene may be due to a conjugation reaction with glutathione (GSH), processing of the GSH S-conjugates to cysteine S-conjugates followed by formation of reactive intermediates catalyzed by renal cysteine conjugate beta-lyase (3).

Experimental evidence for the formation of GSH S-conjugates of HFP has not been presented. Since GSH S-conjugate formation may be involved in the HFP-nephrotoxicity, the experiments reported here were designed to investigate the metabolism of HFP in rats and to identify and quantify any metabolites formed by GSH conjugation reactions.

MATERIALS AND METHODS

Animals and treatment

Female Wistar rats (weighing 220-260 g) from the Institut für Versuchstierkunde (Hannover, FRG) were used for the studies. Immediately after application of HFP, the animals were transferred to an all-glass metabolic cage. Urine was collected for 24 hr in a cooled (4°C)

flask. Standard diet (Altromin[R]) and tap water were supplied ad libidum.

Preparation of subcellular fractions and their analysis

Rat liver and kidney microsomes and cytosol were prepared as described (4). All enzymatic assay incubations with HFP (4mM) were performed in airtight vials as described previously (5). Separation and quantification of S-conjugates were performed as described for other haloalkene derived GSH S-conjugates (6,7).

Chemicals

Hexafluoropropene was obtained from Aldrich-Chemie (Steinheim, Germany). Purity was 99% as determined by GC/MS. HFP-derived GSH S-conjugates and mercapturic acids were prepared from HFP by methods described previously for the synthesis of haloalkene-derived GSH S-conjugates and mercapturic acids (5). Purity of S-conjugates after HPLC-purification was greater than 99% as checked by HPLC and TLC.

RESULTS

Metabolism of hexafluoropropene by rat liver and kidney subcellular fractions.

Incubations of HFP with liver and kidney subcellular fractions in the presence of glutathione resulted in the time and protein concentration dependent formation of 2 metabolites. One of these metabolites showed a UV-spectrum with an absorption maximum at 246 nm (extinction coefficient = 3800), whereas the other metabolite did not show any absorption above 225 nm. Formation of these two compounds was not observed in incubations with denaturated microsomal and cytosolic protein and could be inhibited completely by the competitive GSH S-transferase inhibitor dinitrochlorobenzene (2mM). The metabolites were isolated by semi-preparative HPLC for structure elucidation. The thermospray mass spectrum of one isolated metabolite (UV_{max}=246nm) recorded after esterification showed an intensive fragment with m/z 466 and 3 minor fragments with m/z 488, 452 and 323 (Fig. 1). The molecular weight of a possible GSH conjugate (as dimethylester) formed from HFP, S-(1,2,3,3,3-penta-fluoro-propenyl)glutathione (PFPG) is 465 u; therefore, m/z 466 most likely represents $(M+H)^+$ and m/z 488 $(M+Na)^+$. M/z 452 represents the loss of a methylene group (14u) and m/z 323 the loss of glutamine methyl ester (143u) from $(M+H)^+$.

The second metabolite (Fig. 2) showed an intensive fragment with m/z 486 $(M+H)^+$ and also the fragments indicating a loss of a methylene group and glutamine methyl ester respectively, addition of sodium. The spectrum therefore suggests that this metabolite represents S- (1,1,2,3,3,3-hexafluoropropyl) glutathione (HFPG).

Further support for the suggested structures can be derived from the ^{1}H-NMR-spectra of the metabolites, showing signals attributable to the 10 non-exchangeable protons of glutathione, although some signals were shifted downfield. Metabolite B showed an additional doublet of multiplets at delta = 5.32 (J^1_{HF} = 44Hz). This is consistent with a proton and a fluorine on carbon atom b of the hexafluoropropyl residue.

Table 1 shows the reaction rates for the formation of S-(1,1,2,3,3,3-hexafluoropropyl) glutathione (HFPG) and S-(1,2,3,3,3- pentafluoropropenyl)glutathione (PFPG) from hexafluoropropene.

Table 1. Formation rates of HFP-derived GSH S-conjugates as determined by HPLC.

	HFPG (nmol/min/mg)	PFPG (nmol/min/mg)
liver cytosol	136	nd*
liver microsomes	36	240
renal cytosol	46	nd
renal microsomes	nd	nd

*nd=not detected
HFP (1mM) was incubated with different rat subcellular fractions in the presence of glutathione (10 mM). Protein concentrations used were between 0.1 and 0.5 mg/ml for microsomal protein and 0.25 and 1 mg/ml for cytosolic protein.

Metabolism of hexafluoropropene in rats in vivo.

For exposure to HFP, two rats were transferred into the closed exposure system and HFP-gas introduced with an airtight syringe through an airtight septum to give a final concentration of 800 ppm. Within 40 min after the start of the exposure, all HFP was consumed as indicated by monitoring HFP in the exposure atmosphere by gas chromatography. After 1 hr, the rats were transferred to an all-glass metabolic cage and urine was collected for 6 hr, extracted with ether and the extract was analyzed by GC/MS after methylation. The chromatogram showed a peak with identical retention time and mass spectrum as the synthetic mercapturic acid N-acetyl-S-(1,1,2,3,3,3- hexafluoropropyl)-L-cysteine (N-Ac-HFPC) methyl ester. The fragment with m/z 268 is formed by the loss of the methyl ester group (59u) from the molecular ion (calculated as m/z 327). M/z 144 and 88 are fragments typical for methyl esters of mercapturic acids. No evidence for the formation of N-acetyl-S-(1,2,3,3,3-pentafluoro- propenyl)-L-cysteine (N-Ac-PFPC) could be obtained.

The selective identification of N-Ac-HFPC in rat urine, accounting to 10% of HFP dose, suggested that the corresponding GSH S-conjugate might be exclusively formed in rats. To investigate the hepatic metabolism of HFP in vivo and to determine the structure of con-

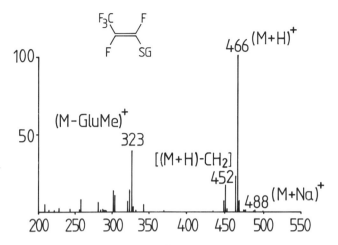

Figure 1.   Thermospray mass spectrum of S-(1,2,3,3,3-pentafluoropropenyl)glutathione (PFPG).

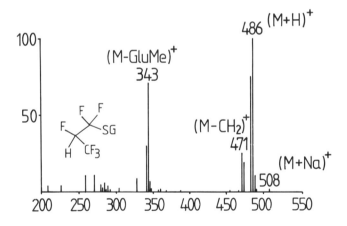

Figure 2. Thermospray mass spectrum of S-(1,1,2,3,3,3-hexafluoropropyl)glutathione (HFPG).

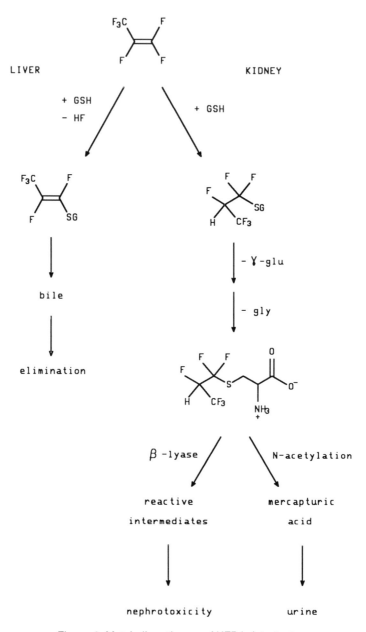

Figure. 3. Metabolic pathways of HFP in intact rats.

jugates formed in the liver, rats were fitted with a bile cannula before HFP- exposure. The thermospray mass spectrum of the bile fraction obtained after HPLC separation presumably containing the GSH S-conjugates showed that only PFPG was present in this bile fraction; the formation and excretion of HFPG in bile amounted to less than 0.1% of PFPG (=detection limit). Nevertheless, in urine of the rats fitted with a bile cannula, N-Ac-HFPG amounted to 10% of HFP dose.

DISCUSSION

Hexafluoropropene, a selective nephrotoxin, undergoes metabolism via GSH-conjugation. Studies with other halogenated alkenes have elucidated this metabolic pathway as a possible route for the formation of toxic and mutagenic intermediates (8). Two GSH S-conjugates can be formed by the glutathione S-transferase catalyzed step. In the first step, GSH adds to the double bound of HFP, forming a carbanion with a definite lifetime. This intermediate can be transformed to S-(1,1,2,3,3,3-hexafluoropropyl)glutathione (HFPG) by addition of a proton or alternatively to S-(1,2,3,3,3- pentafluoropropenyl)glutathione (PFPG) by elimination of F⁻. The presence of protons might thus control the structure of the product formed. In microsomal membranes, the concentration of water is very low, thus the intermediate carbanion is transformed to PFPG by F⁻ elimination. With soluble S-transferases, the carbanion reacts more likely with a proton to give HFPG. These considerations may explain the different structures of HFP-derived S-conjugates formed by soluble and membrane bound GSH S-transferases.

In in vivo experiments with rats exposed to HFP by inhalation, only one mercapturic acid N-acetyl-S- (1,1,2,3,3,3- hexafluoropropyl)-L-cysteine (N-Ac-HFPC) was detected in urine (about 10% of HFP dose). This observation might suggest that HFPG is selectively formed in rats. To investigate further the formation of S-conjugates in vivo and the hepatic metabolism of HFP, we identified the GSH-dependent biliary metabolites.

In rats fitted with a bile cannula we could demonstrate that PFPG is the exclusive GSH-dependent bile metabolite after HFP exposure. The formation of PFPG in the liver can be rationalized since membrane bound GSH S-transferases account for the majority of hepatic GSH- dependent metabolism of haloalkenes, such as hexachlorobutadiene and chlorotrifluoroethene. HFPG concentration in bile fluid was lower than the detection limit for this assay. In urine of the cannulated rats the mercapturic acid N-Ac-PFPC, corresponding to the GSH conjugate PFPG was not detectable. In contrast, N-Ac-HFPC amounted to 10% of the HFP dose.

These data suggest that PFPG formed in the liver was not translocated to the kidney and transformed to N-Ac-PFPC. Furthermore, the detection of the saturated mercapturic acid N-Ac-HFPC seems to indicate that HFP could be conjugated with GSH in the kidney forming HFPG and subsequent metabolism of the conjugate leads to the urine excretion of the corresponding mercapturic acid. Fig. 3 shows the proposed metabolic pathways of HFP in rats in vivo.

Therefore, we propose that intrarenal glutathione conjugation reaction may be an important step in the bioactivation of nephrotoxic alkenes and liver metabolism by GSH S-transferases is not absolutely necessary, at least in the bioactivation of HFP.

ACKNOWLEDGEMENT

This work was supported by the Deutsche Forschungsgemeinschaft, Bonn (SFB-172) and the Doktor-Robert-Pfleger-Stiftung, Bamberg.

REFERENCES

1. Potter CL, Gandolfi AJ, Nagle R, Clayton JW: Effects of inhaled chlorotrifluoroethylene and hexafluoropropene on the rat kidney. Toxicol Appl Pharmacol 59:431-440, 1981.

2. Dilley JV, Carter VL Jr, Harris ES: Fluoride ion excretion by male rats after inhalation of one of several fluoroethylenes or hexafluoropropene. Toxicol Appl Pharmacol 27: 582-590, 1974.

3. Dohn DR, Anders MW: The enzymatic reaction of chlorotrifluoroethylene with

glutathione. Biochem Biophys Res Commun 109:1339-1345, 1982.

4. Wolf CR, Berry PN, Nash JA, Green T, Lock EA: Role of microsomal and cytosolic gluta-thione S-transferases in the conjugation of hexachloro-1:3-butadiene and its possible re-levance to toxicity. J Pharmacol Exp Therap 228:202-208, 1984.

5. Dekant W, Martens G, Vamvakas S, Met-zler M, Henschler D: Bioactivation of tetrachloroethylene - Role of glutathione S-transferase-catalyzed conjugation versus cytochrome P-450-dependent phospholipid al-kylation. Drug Metab Dispos 15:702-709, 1987.

6. Vamvakas S, Dekant W, Berthold K, Schmidt S, Wild D, Henschler D: Enzymatic transformation of mercapturic acids derived from halogenated alkenes to reactive and mut-agenic intermediates. Biochem Pharmacol 36:2741-2748, 1987.

7. Dekant W, Metzler M, Henschler D: Identi-fication of S-1,2,2-trichlorovinyl-N-acetyl cysteineasa urinary metabolite of tetrachlo-roethylene: Bioactivation through glutathione conjugation as a possible explanation of its nephrocarcinogenicity. J Biochem Toxicol 1:57-72, 1986.

8. Anders MW, Lash LH, Dekant W, Elfarra AA, Dohn DR: Biosynthesis and biotransforma-tion of glutathione S-conjugates to toxic metabolites. CRC Crit Rev Toxicol 18:311-342, 1988.

39

SPECIES DIFFERENCES IN RENAL BINDING AND TOXICITY OF PENTACHLOROBUTADIENYL CYSTEINE AND DICHLOROVINYL CYSTEINE

P.O. Darnerud (1), L. Olsson (1) and A. Wallin (2)

Dept. of Toxicology, Uppsala University, BMC, Box 594, S-751 24 Uppsala, Sweden (1) and W. Alton Jones Cell Science Center, Lake Placid NY, USA (2)

INTRODUCTION

The nephrotoxin dichlorovinyl cysteine (DCVC) was first identified in trichloroethylene-extracted animal feed, where it had been formed in vitro (1,2). DCVC was originally considered to be a unique example of an amino acid conjugate with toxic properties after beta-lyase activation. However, a number of nephrotoxic cysteine conjugates, transformed in vivo from various halogenated alkenes and suggested to share the same bioactivation mechanism as DCVC, have since been found (3,4). One of these is pentachlorobutadienyl cysteine (PCBC), formed in considerable amounts in vivo (5) from the industrial chemical hexachlorobutadiene (HCBD). There are similarities between DCVC and PCBC regarding the site of lesion in the rat kidney - the cortico-medullary junction (6,7) - which support the hypothesis of a similar renal handling of these two conjugates. Furthermore, the radiolabel is also bound to the same region of the rat kidney after ^{14}C-HCBD (precursor to ^{14}C-PCBC) administration (5).

However, the similarities between DCVC and PCBC distribution and toxicity are less clear in the mouse. The earlier observed specific binding of ^{14}C-DCVC in the cortico-medullary region (8) cannot be found for ^{35}S-PCBC. Indeed, earlier toxicity data (9) on HCBD in mice indicate a more cortical lesion. The present paper will concentrate on the difference between the two conjugates regarding toxicity and binding in the mouse, and the lack of difference in the rat. Species differences in the kidney binding of ^{14}C-DCVC will be further discussed referring to results on avian and fish species.

METHODS

Labelled ^{14}C-DCVC, ^{35}S-DCVC, ^{35}S-PCBC and unlabelled DCVC and PCBC were synthesized according to (1). Mice (C57BL) and rats (Sprague-Dawley) were purchased from Alab, Sollentuna, Sweden. Japanese quails and rainbow trout were obtained from local breeders.

Parts of the ^{14}C-DCVC results have been presented separately (8) and this paper can be used for further details on the methods. Briefly, the labelled compounds were given intravenously or orally (5-25 mg/kg b.w.) and the administered animals were killed after 1 hr - 12 days. Whole-body autoradiography was then performed using standard procedures (see ref. 8). In addition, some animals were used for autoradiography at the light microscope level on 4 µm paraffin sections of the kidney.

The toxicity studies were performed on mice given compounds in doses of 5-25 mg/kg b.w. The animals were killed 24 hr after oral administration of the nephrotoxin. The kidneys were excised, formalin-fixed, paraffin-embedded, sectioned and stained before microscopic evaluation.

RESULTS

The whole-body distribution of ^{35}S-PCBC-derived radioactivity in the mouse is given in Fig. 1. The kidney was the main target of ^{35}S-accumulation and binding. The label within the kidney was fairly homogenously distributed in the cortex, suggesting convoluted proximal tubule localization. In contrast, the kidney distribution of ^{35}S-DCVC was specifically localized to the cortico-medullary region (Fig. 2, right). This distribution pattern, together with those from the micro-autoradiograms (not shown), defines the straight proximal tubules as the target for DCVC attack. The binding of ^{14}C-DCVC in the kidney (Fig. 2, left; ref. 8) is identical with the ^{35}S-labelled compound, giving evidence for participation of both the vinyl and the sulphur groups in the reactive, tissue-binding metabolite. For both PCBC and DCVC,

the site of lesion corresponds to the initial site of binding of the radioactive counterparts. Thus, the PCBC lesion is most marked in the cortical region of the kidney, whereas the DCVC effects are seen deeper in the kidney, i.e. in the straight segments of the proximal tubules (Fig. 3).

In Fig. 4, the kidney distribution of ^{14}C-DCVC and ^{35}S-PCBC in the rat is shown. The patterns of the two compounds are identical (cortico-medullary localization) in the rat kidney, which was not the case seen in the mouse kidney (see above).

Other species have also been studied for renal ^{14}C-DCVC accumulation and binding. Both the Japanese quail and the rainbow trout show specific and firm binding of radiolabel, but the distribution patterns differ: in the quail, the label seems to be accumulated all along the

PCBC 1 hr

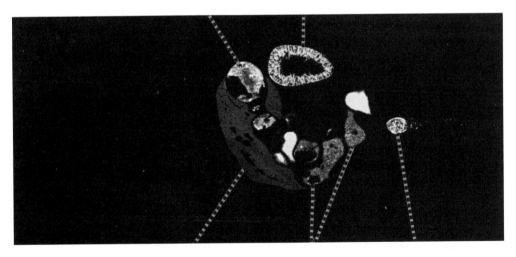

Figure 1. Whole-body autoradiogram of a C57BL mouse killed 1 hr after i.v. injection of ^{35}S-pentachlorobutadienyl cysteine (ca. 5 mg/kg b.w.). Note the strong and evenly distributed labelling in the kidney cortex. (Adjacent, extracted section gives rise to similar accumulation of radioactivity in the kidney; not shown.)

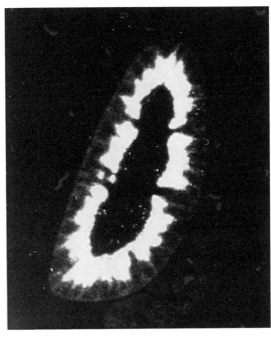

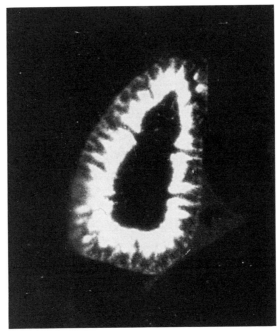

Figure 2. Details of whole-body autoradiograms from C57BL mice 24 hr after i.v. injections of ^{14}C- and ^{35}S-dichlorovinyl cysteine, respectively (ca. 5 mg/kg b.w.). The prominent cortico-medullary binding of radioactivity in the kidney is seen for both the differently labelled DCVC forms.

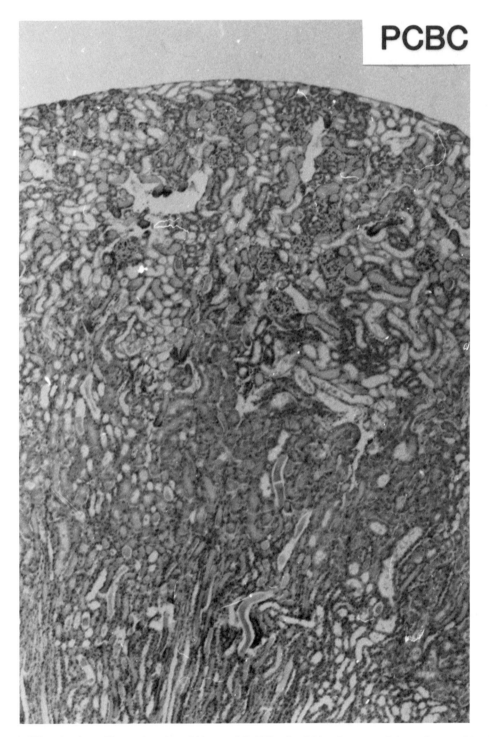

Figure 3. HE-stained paraffin sections from kidneys of C57BL mice 24 hr after an oral dose of pentachlorobu-tadienyl cysteine or dichlorovinyl cysteine (10 and 5 mg/kg b.w., respectively; near-equimolar doses). Note the broader and more superficial lesion after PCBC as compared to the specific, deeper DCVC-lesion.

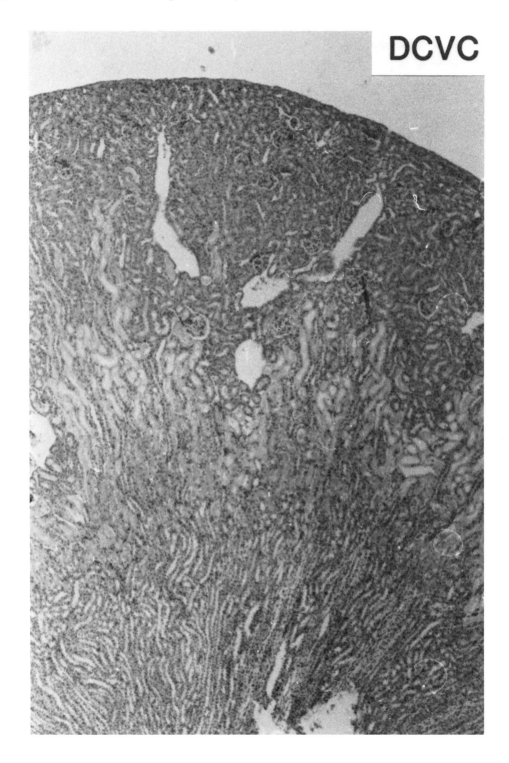

S–D rat

35S–PCBC

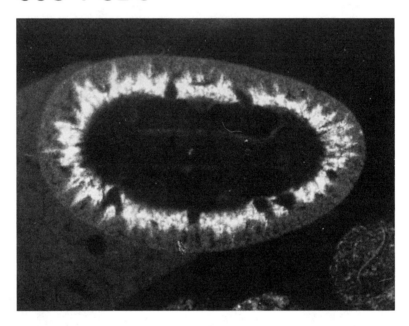

14C–DCVC

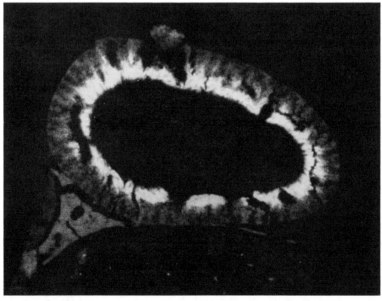

Figure 4. Details of whole-body autoradiograms of juvenile S-D rats 24 hr after oral administration of ^{35}S-pentachlorobutadienyl cysteine and ^{14}C-dichlorovinyl cysteine, respectively (ca. 25 mg/kg b.w.). As observed, the cortico-medullary binding of radioactivity is identical for the two conjugates.

proximal tubules, while in the trout, the label is concentrated to a defined (proximal?) segment of the tubules (not shown).

DISCUSSION

The specificity in the binding and toxicity of nephrotoxic cysteine conjugates to the S_3-region of the proximal tubule have been the object of many studies. The different hypotheses discuss whether the site of kidney lesion may be regulated by the distribution of a) beta-lyase (the primary activating enzyme), b) other enzymes of importance, e.g. deacetylase, and c) specific transport proteins within the kidney. If beta-lyase is a prerequisite for the binding of the toxic cysteine conjugates, the distribution of PCBC in the mouse implies that the entire cortex contains beta-lyase activity, at least in this strain. However, the differences in PCBC and DCVC distribution in mice do not favour the hypothesis of beta-lyase being the determinant for the specific distribution of bound radiolabel. In support of this, Jones et al. (10) have identified beta-lyase (glutamine transaminase K) immunohistochemically in the entire kidney cortex of the rat. Possibly, transport mechanisms are more likely to cause the specificity in conjugate metabolite binding to kidney tissues, and there are several transport shunts working on both the luminal and the basolateral side of the epithelial cells (11). The big difference in lipophilicity between PCBC and DCVC could influence the transmembral transport and lead to the observed differences in sites of renal binding in the mouse.

The studies on the metabolism of the cysteine conjugates to the subsequently-formed toxic species have revealed a whole sequence of metabolic steps (12). It means that the toxic end products could include thionoacyl derivates, haloacetic acids and inorganic chloride/fluoride. Our results show that both the vinyl and the sulphur groups are members of the bound metabolite, which suggests that the first of the above possible toxins might be responsible for renal tissue binding. However, comparative, quantitative studies of the ^{14}C-

and ^{35}S-labelled DCVC have not been performed.

The difference in distribution pattern of ^{35}S-PCBC, but not of ^{14}C-DCVC, between the mouse and the rat is notable. Furthermore, the DCVC studies in Japanese quail and rainbow trout shows that the enzymes activating this nephrotoxic cysteine conjugate seem to be widely distributed among the animal species but that there are differences in sites of radiolabel binding within the kidney. These interspecies differences, probably reflecting differences in the distribution and activity of bioactivation and/or transport mechanisms, could be used as tools for the further understanding of cysteine conjugate nephrotoxicity.

To conclude: a) A difference between PCBC and DCVC in the distribution of bound radiolabel is found in the mouse but not in the rat. b) Using conjugates labelled in different positions the nature of the tissue-bound metabolite can be better understood. c) Interspecies comparisons of disposition and toxicity may help in answering questions regarding cysteine conjugate nephrotoxicity.

REFERENCES

1. McKinney LL, Weahley FB, Eldridge AC, Campbell RE, Cowan JC, Picken Jr, JC, Biester, HE: S-(dichlorovinyl)-L-cysteine: An agent causing total aplastic anemia in calves. J Amer Chem Soc 79: 3932-3933, 1957.

2. Schultze MO, Klubes P, Perman V, Mizuno NS, Bates FW, Sautter JH: Blood dyscrasia in calves induced by S-(dichlorovinyl)-L-cysteine. Blood 14: 519-529, 1959.

3. Anders MW, Lash LH, Dekant W, Elfarra AA, Dohn DR: Biosynthesis and metabolism of glutathione S-conjugates to toxic forms. CRC Crit Rev Toxicol 18: 311-341, 1988.

4. Lock EA: Studies on the mechanism of nephrotoxicity and nephrocarcinogenicity of halogenated alkenes. CRC Crit Rev Toxicol 19: 23-42, 1988.

5. Nash JA, King LJ, Lock EA, Green T: The metabolism and disposition of hexachloro-1,3-butadiene in the rat and its relevance to nephrotoxicity. Toxicol Appl Pharmacol 73: 124-137, 1984.

6. Terracini B, Parker, VH: A pathological study on the toxicity of S-dichlorovinyl-L-cysteine. Food Cosmet Toxicol 3: 67-74, 1965.

7. Jaffe DR, Brendel K, Gandolfi AJ: In vivo and in vitro nephrotoxicity of the cysteine conjugate of hexachlorobutadiene. J Toxicol Environ Health 11: 857-867, 1983.

8. Darnerud PO, Brandt I, Feil VJ, Bakke, JE: S-(1,2-dichloro[^{14}C]vinyl)-L- cysteine (DCVC) in the mouse kidney: Correlation between tissue-binding and toxicity. Toxicol Appl Pharmacol 95: 423-434, 1988.

9. Lock EA, Ishmael J, Hook JB: Nephrotoxicity of hexachloro-1,3-butadiene in the mouse: The effect of age, sex, monooxygenase modifiers, and the role of glutathione. Toxicol Appl Pharmacol 72: 484-494, 1984.

10. Jones TW, Qin C, Schaeffer VH, Stevens JL: Immunohistochemical localization of glutamine transaminase K, a rat kidney cysteine conjugate -lyase, and the relationship to the segment specificity of cysteine conjugate nephrotoxicity. Mol Pharmacol 34: 621-627, 1988.

11. Monks TJ, Lau SS: Commentary: Renal transport processes and glutathione conjugate-mediated nephrotoxicity. Drug Metab Dispos 15: 437-441, 1987.

12. Dekant W, Lash LH, Anders MW: Bioactivation mechanism of the cytotoxic and nephrotoxic S-conjugate S-(2-chloro-1,1,2-trifluoroethyl)-L-cysteine. Proc Natl Acad Sci 84: 7443-7447, 1987.

40

EXTRACELLULAR ACIDOSIS INHIBITS 2-BROMOHYDROQUINONE INDUCED TOXICITY TO RABBIT RENAL PROXIMAL TUBULES

D.P. Rodeheaver and R.G. Schnellmann

Department of Physiology and Pharmacology, College of Veterinary Medicine, University of Georgia, Athens, GA, 30602 USA

INTRODUCTION

Metabolic acidosis has been shown to both ameliorate and potentiate cell injury and death induced by several chemical and physical agents in a number of cell systems. Evidence of cytoprotection from ischemic cell death has been reported when extracellular pH (pH_e) was decreased below 7 with membrane integrity, oxygen consumption, ion homeostasis and ATP levels being maintained (1,2). Acidosis has also been demonstrated to reduce cell injury induced by potassium cyanide and iodoacetate (2), p-chloromercuribenzoate (3) and amphotericin B (4). In contrast, low pH_e potentiates tobramycin (5) and bleomycin-induced cell death (6). The basis for pH-induced amelioration or potentiation of cell death has not been determined.

The function of the kidney is the reabsorption and secretion of solutes and the maintenance of plasma acid-base balance, thereby potentially exposing the renal tubules to high concentrations of toxicants in an environment of varying pH. Previous studies have shown that the model toxic hydroquinone, bromohydroquinone (BHQ), is a potent toxicant to rabbit renal proximal tubules, causing glutathione depletion, mitochondrial dysfunction and ultimately cell death (7). To determine the role of pH in toxicant-induced renal cell death, we examined the effect of pH_e acidification on the toxicity of BHQ to rabbit renal proximal tubules. Specifically, BHQ-induced decreases in glutathione, mitochondrial function and viability of tubules in pH_e 6.4 and 7.4 buffers were compared.

METHODS

Renal Proximal Tubule Suspensions (RPT). RPT were isolated from female New Zealand White rabbits (2-3 kg) by the method of Vinay et al. (8) as modified by Weinberg et al. (9). The isolation media contained DME/F-12 media, 15 mM $NaHCO_3$, 2mM heptanoate and 100 units penicillin G/ml, pH 7.55 (295 mOsm). The minced cortex was digested in 25 ml media containing 2% bovine serum albumin, 1800 units DNase (Type I), 2800 units collagenase (Type I), and 1 mM deferoxamine. RPT were purified on an unformed 50% Percoll gradient, washed and resuspended in isolation media at 1 mg protein/ml.

Incubation of RPT. RPT were incubated at 37°C under 95% air/5% CO_2 for 15 min, then washed and resuspended in pH 6.4 or 7.4 incubation buffer. The incubation buffer contained (mM): alanine, 1; dextrose, 5; heptanoate, 2; lactate, 4; malate, 5; NaCl, 115; $NaHCO_3$, 15; KCl, 5; NaH_2PO_4, 2; $MgSO_4$, 1; $CaCl_2$, 1; and either MES, 10 (pH 6.4) or HEPES, 10 (pH 7.4). RPT were incubated an additional 15 min prior to addition of 0.2 mM BHQ.

Oxygen Consumption (QO_2). The QO_2 of RPT suspensions was monitored using a Clark-type oxygen electrode and an oxymeter. The chamber (1.5 ml) was warmed to 37°C and

253

stirred magnetically. After obtaining the basal QO_2, the monovalent ionophore, nystatin (1400 units), was added to the chamber. The addition of nystatin to proximal tubules leads to a rapid increase in QO_2 caused by the entry of sodium ions from the extracellular medium and consequently the stimulation of the Na,K-ATPase. The QO_2 obtained with nystatin addition has been shown to equal the mitochondrial state 3 respiratory rate under normal conditions (10).

Biochemical Assays. To separate RPT from the medium, aliquots of RPT suspensions were placed on a layer of dibutylphthalate:dioctylphthalate (2:1) and centrifuged. Glutathione (oxidized + reduced) concentrations were determined by the method of Griffith (11). Lactate dehydrogenase (LDH) activity was determined by the method of Bergmeyer (12). Protein content was measured by the biuret method of Gornall et al. (13).

Statistics. The data are presented as the mean ± SEM. Each proximal tubule isolation represents N = 1. Data were assessed by analysis of variance and multiple means tested for significance using Fisher's protected least significant difference test. P<0.05 was considered significant.

RESULTS

To determine the effect of pH_e on BHQ-induced toxicity to RPT, 0.2 mM BHQ was added to RPT incubated in pH_e 6.4 or 7.4 buffer. LDH release was used as a marker of irreversible cell death. RPT incubated at pH_e 7.4 and exposed to BHQ underwent a time-dependent increase in LDH release over the 6 hr experimental period (Fig. 1). The initial increase in LDH release occurred at 4 hr. In contrast, RPT incubated at pH_e 6.4 and exposed to BHQ did not exhibit any increase in LDH release compared to vehicle-treated incubations (4%). The equivalent low degree of LDH release from

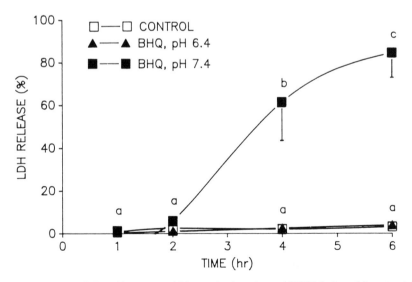

Figure 1. Effect of extracellular pH on 0.2 mM bromohydroquinone (BHQ)-induced lactate dehydrogenase (LDH) release from rabbit renal proximal tubules (RPT). Values are mean ± SEM, N=4. Control values of vehicle-treated RPT suspensions incubated in pHe 6.4 and 7.4 were equivalent. Datum points with different superscripts within a given treatment or at a given time point are significantly different from one another (P<0.05).

RPT incubated at pH_e 6.4 and 7.4 established the sustained viability of this preparation under both conditions.

We have previously identified the mitochondrion of RPT as an early target of BHQ and that NYS-QO_2 is an indicator of BHQ-induced mitochondrial dysfunction (7). A 1 hr exposure of RPT incubated at pH_e 7.4 to BHQ resulted in a 31% decrease in NYS-QO_2 (Fig. 2). Longer exposures produced time-dependent decreases in NYS-QO_2 with a maximum of 94% at 6 hr. In contrast, NYS-QO_2 of RPT incubated at pH_e was unaffected by BHQ over the 6 hr experimental period.

NYS-QO_2 of RPT incubated at pH_e 6.4 or 7.4 did not change over the experimental period (Fig. 2). However, RPT incubated at pH_e had a NYS-QO_2 rate of 65% of those RPT incubated at pH_e 7.4.

BHQ produces a marked depletion of glutathione in RPT (7). Schnellmann et al. (14) demonstrated that the glutathione depletion in RPT that accompanied BHQ exposure resulted from the conjugation of glutathione to the BHQ metabolites bromoquinone or bromosemiquinone. A reduction in RPT glutathione, then, is an index of the oxidation of BHQ to these compounds. BHQ decreased RPT glutathione in a time-dependent manner when RPT were incubated at pH_e 7.4 (Fig. 3). RPT incubated at pH_e 6.4 and exposed to BHQ also underwent a time-dependent decrease in RPT glutathione (Fig. 4).

However, the rate of glutathione depletion was markedly slower. Glutathione contents of RPT incubated at pH_e 6.4 were consistently 61% of glutathione contents of RPT incubated at pH_e 7.4. RPT glutathione increased over time in both preparations.

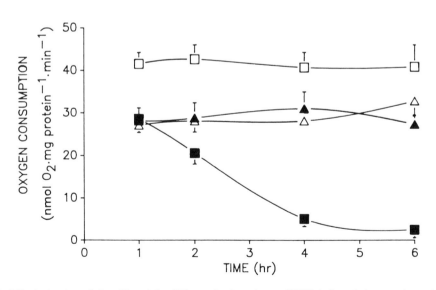

Figure 2. Effect of extracellular pH on 0.2 mM bromohydroquinone (BHQ)-induced changes in nystatin-stimulated oxygen consumption of rabbit renal proximal tubules (RPT). Values are Mean ± SEM, N=4. Open and filled symbols are control and BHQ-treated RPT suspensions, respectively. Triangles and squares are RPT suspensions incubated at pH_e 6.4 and 7.4, respectively.

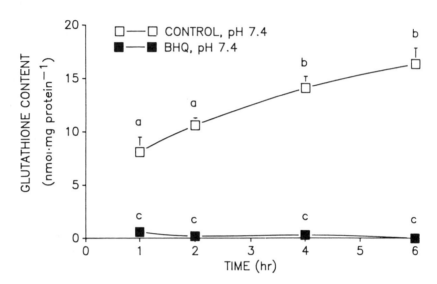

Figure 3. The effect of 0.2 mM bromohydroquinone (BHQ) on intracellular glutathione content of rabbit renal proximal tubules incubated in pHe 7.4 buffer. Values are Mean ± SEM, N=4. Datum points with different superscripts within a given treatment or a given time point are significantly different from one another (P<0.05).

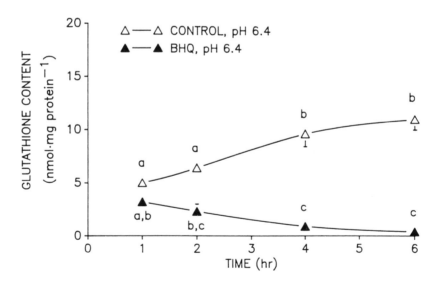

Figure 4. The effect of 0.2 mM bromohydroquinone (BHQ) on intracellular glutathione content of rabbit renal proximal tubules incubated in pHe 6.4 buffer. Values are Mean ± SEM, N=4. Datum points with different superscripts within a given treatment or a given time point are significantly different from one another (P< 0.05).

DISCUSSION

BHQ-induced RPT cell death was ameliorated when RPT were incubated at pH_e 6.4. In concert with this observation, a pH_e of 6.4 blocked BHQ-induced mitochondrial dysfunction and decreased the rate of glutathione depletion. RPT must oxidize BHQ to the reactive compounds bromoquinone or bromosemiquinone for glutathione depletion, mitochondrial dysfunction and cell death to occur (14). RPT glutathione depletion results from the conjugation of glutathione to bromoquinone or bromosemiquinone, while the mitochondrial dysfunction is thought to result from the covalent binding of bromoquinone or bromosemiquinone to mitochondrial proteins (14). The results from this study suggest that a pH_e of 6.4 decreases the amount of bromoquinone or bromosemiquinone formed and consequently, the resultant mitochondrial dysfunction and cell death.

Decreasing pH_e to 6.4 did not alter RPT viability or stability of mitochondrial function over the 6 hr experimental period. However, RPT incubated at pH_e 6.4 had a 35% decrease in NYS-QO2 and 39% decrease in glutathione content compared to RPT incubated at pH_e 7.4. The decreases in NYS-QO2 and glutathione content may result from a generalized decrease in RPT metabolism.

REFERENCES

1. Bonventre JV, Cheung JY: Effects of metabolic acidosis on viability of cells exposed to anoxia. Am J Physiol 249: C149-C159, 1985.

2. Lemasters JJ, DiGuiseppi J, Nieminen AL, Herman B: Blebbing, free Ca^{2+} and mitochondrial membrane potential preceding cell death in hepatocytes. Nature 325: 78-81, 1987.

3. Penttila A, Trump BF: Studies on the modification of the cellular response to injury. Virchows Arch B Cell Path 18: 17-34, 1975.

4. Shanley PF, Shapiro JI, Chan L, Burke TJ, Johnson GC: Acidosis and hypoxic medullary injury in the isolated perfused kidney. Kidney Int 34: 791-796, 1988.

5. Peterson, LN: Inhibition of tobramycin reabsorption in proximal and distal nephron segments by alkalinization: A micropuncture study. Kidney Int 35: 416, 1988.

6. Urano M, Khan J, Kenton LA: Effect of bleomycin on murine tumor cells at elevated temperatures and two different pH values. Cancer Res 48: 615-619, 1988.

7. Schnellmann RG, Ewell FPQ, Sgambati M, Mandel LJ: Mitochondrial Toxicity of 2-bromohydroquinone in rabbit renal proximal tubules. Toxicol Appl Pharmacol 90: 420-426, 1987.

8. Vinay P, Gougoux A, Lemieux G: Isolation of a pure suspension of rat proximal tubules. Am J Physiol 241: F403-F411, 1981.

9. Weinberg JM, Davis JA, Abarzua M, Rajan M: Cytoprotective effect of glycine and glutathione against hypoxic injury to renal tubules. J Clin Invest 80: 1446-1454, 1987.

10. Harris SI, Balaban RS, Barrett L, Mandel LJ: Mitochondrial respiratory capacity and Na- and K- dependent adenosine triphosphatase-mediated ion transport in the intact renal cell. J Biol Chem 256: 10319-10328, 1981.

11. Griffith, OW: Determination of glutathione and glutathione disulfide using glutathione reductase and 2-vinylpyridine. Anal Biochem 106: 207-212, 1980.

12. Bergmeyer H-U, Bernt E, Hess B: Lactic dehydrogenase. In: H-U Bergmeyer (ed); Methods of Enzymatic Analysis. New York, Academic Press, 1963, pp. 736-743.

13. Gornall AC, Bardwill CJ, David MM: Determination of serum proteins by means of the biuret reaction. J Biol Chem 177: 751-766, 1949.

14. Schnellmann RG, Monks TJ, Mandel LJ, Lau SS: 2-Bromohydroquimome- induced toxicity to rabbit renal proximal tubules: The role of biotransformation, glutathione, and covalent binding. Toxicol Appl Pharmacol 99: 19-27, 1989.

PART IX
ORGANIC SOLVENTS

41

CHRONIC RENAL DISEASE RISK ASSOCIATED WITH EMPLOYMENT IN INDUSTRIES WITH POTENTIAL SOLVENT EXPOSURE

D.P. Sandler and J.C. Smith

Epidemiology Branch, National Institute of Environmental Health Sciences, Research Triangle Park, NC, USA

INTRODUCTION

More than $3 billion a year is spent in the United States on treatment of end stage renal disease. Despite the large number of individuals receiving dialysis or transplant, little is known about the causes of renal disease. There is some indication that occupational and environmental exposures play a role in the etiology of renal disease, but few epidemiologic studies have been carried out (1,2).

Glomerulonephritis, which has been linked with several environmental exposures, accounts for about 20-30% of end stage renal disease, and about 10-20% of all renal dysfunction (3,4). A causal association between exposure to hydrocarbon solvents and the development of chronic glomerulonephritis has been proposed, with most of the human evidence coming from case reports and case-control studies of patients with specific forms of glomerulonephritis (1,2,5,6).

Studies of occupational groups with known exposure to solvents provide little information about the existence of a causal relationship - largely because the incidence of primary chronic renal disease is low and few studies are large enough to identify more than a handful of renal disease deaths (2).

Altogether about 9 or 10 case-control studies have been carried out. Many (7-11), but not all (12), have suggested a risk associated with solvent exposure. These studies have been critically reviewed and most have been found to have serious methodological problems (2,5,13). Yet, the consistency of the findings in these different studies, together with what is known about acute effects of solvents in animals and man, makes it difficult to dismiss the likelihood of a causal association.

We evaluated chronic renal disease risk associated with exposure to solvents and other potential hazards at home and in the workplace in a multi-center case control study. We conducted our study in North Carolina, in the southeastern United States, a region where mortality from chronic renal disease tends to be higher than elsewhere in the USA.

METHODS

Cases were North Carolina residents aged 30-79 who were hospitalized between September 1, 1980 and August 31, 1982 at one of four local medical centers with a first diagnosis of chronic renal disease. Patients who had a renal problem mentioned somewhere on their discharge summary and had a sustained elevation in serum creatinine greater than or equal to 1.5 mg/dl (130 µmol/l) were eligible for inclusion. Cases were excluded if they had certain hereditary or systemic conditions with known renal manifestations or if renal dysfunction was due to nonrenal causes. Patients with hypertension and diabetes were not excluded.

The charts of over 4000 patients were reviewed to identify approximately 700 qualifying patients with newly diagnosed disease. Cases ranged in severity from minor renal insufficiency to end stage disease at diagnosis.

Controls under age 65 were chosen by random digit dialing in North Carolina. Controls over age 65 were selected randomly from Social Security/Medicare records. In all, we identified approximately 700 potential controls who were North Carolina residents and were frequency matched to cases on age, race, sex and whether or not they lived near study hospitals.

About 15% of eligible cases and controls were lost, but we obtained telephone interviews for 90% of the cases and 85% of the controls we located, which gave us an overall response rate of 75%. In all, we obtained data for 554 cases and 516 controls. The interviewed cases and controls were similar on the study matching factors of age, race, sex and residence. However, renal disease patients were less well educated and had lower incomes.

In the USA, renal biopsies are infrequently performed and are usually done for very selected subsets of patients. In order to include a representative sample of newly diagnosed patients with primary renal disease, patients were selected into the study on the basis of renal function. Only 7% of identified patients had a biopsy - and even other less invasive diagnostic evaluations were not uniformly carried out. Using available clinical and laboratory data, nephrologists were able to classify about 70% of the patients.

About 14% of patients were considered to have glomerulonephritis. More than a third of this group was classified on the basis of a biopsy. For the present analysis, the patients with glomerulonephritis are compared to controls and patients with disease that was not glomerulonephritis - nephrosclerosis (19%), diabetic nephropathy (20%) and interstitial nephritis (19%) combined are also compared with controls. Patients whose disease could not be subclassified beyond insufficiency or end-stage disease (28%), who may or may not have glomerulonephritis, will be ignored.

We obtained information about solvents and other hazardous exposures in several ways. We first obtained a chronologic job history for all jobs held two or more years. As part of this, for each job, we asked if the subject was exposed at least 5 times to solvents, degreasers or cleaning agents.

The history was followed by an occupational checklist that was used both as a reminder for jobs of interest as well as to obtain information about jobs that may not have been held for two consecutive years. We also asked about specific exposures, including compounds that contain solvents, such as glues or paints, as well as specific individual chemicals and solvents that may have been used at home or at work.

Because persons with solvent exposure may not recognize that they have been exposed, we classified the likelihood of exposure to solvents in each reported job according to an exposure matrix. This matrix used industrial hygiene data to rank both the likelihood and intensity of solvent exposure for specific job titles within specified industries. By combining these rankings, we were able to classify jobs as unexposed, possibly exposed and probably exposed. Jobs where both the likelihood of exposure and the intensity of exposure were high were classified as "probably exposed" and given a ranking of 2. Those for which either the likelihood or the intensity was high were scored "possibly" exposed with a ranking of 1, and the remainder were classified as unexposed jobs. A cumulative score for each subject was calculated by multiplying the number of years in any job times the exposure score for that job, and summing across jobs.

The risk of disease in the presence of solvent exposure was estimated using odds ratios (OR) and 95% confidence intervals (CI). Adjusted odds ratios were calculated using Mantel Haenszel estimation and logistic regression. In general, overall unadjusted results are presented because results were not altered by taking into account sex, race, age, income, or other potential confounding factors, including analgesic use, through stratification or adjustment.

An association between analgesic use and renal disease risk has previously been reported in this population (14). However, adjustment for analgesic use did not alter the present results.

RESULTS

Starting with the checklist, we identified individuals who had ever been employed in industries where exposure to solvents can occur. For employment in these industries, most odds ratios were close to 1 for the non-glomerular renal diseases indicating no risk, whereas potential risks were suggested for glomerulonephritis, including employment in furniture manufacturing, lumbering, plumbing trades, and commercial painting (Table 1).

Most of the subjects reporting employment in these industries were men. Women with industrial employment tended to be in dry cleaning, the textile industry or the tobacco industry. Even for these, the proportion of exposed women was small, and confidence intervals for risk estimates were wide. Nonetheless, there is the suggestion of an association with employment of women in dry cleaning (OR=1.8, 95% CI=0.02-9.8) or in textile manufacturing (OR=2.0, 95% CI=0.7-5.6).

For self-reported exposures that occurred at home or on the job, the overall odds ratios were all close to one for the non-glomerular disease group. For glomerulonephritis, there appeared to be associations with certain exposures that are again consistent with an effect of solvents on disease risk (Table 2). Odds ratios were increased for exposure to any named solvent, for self-reported exposure to professional glues, stains and varnishes, paint, and other materials. These apparent risks were seen for women as well as for men.

Self-reported exposures are subject to potential reporting biases as individuals might not be aware of hazardous exposures or might mistakenly report use of harmless household products as solvent exposure. The chronologic job histories allow independent assessment of exposures. Using these, there were no differences between non-glomerular disease patients and controls in the frequency with which they reported occupations with likely solvent exposure. For glomerulonephritis, on the other hand, while none of the odds ratios reached statistical significance, there was a suggestion of increased risk for persons with at least 2 years of employment in construction (OR=1.8), tobacco manufacturing (OR=1.9), furniture manufacturing (OR=2.1), transportation (OR=2.1), and wholesale trades (OR=2.2). Overall, patients with glomerulonephritis were twice as likely as controls to directly report solvent exposure on one or more jobs (OR=2.1, 95% CI=1.2-3.5), whereas there was no association for the other patients (OR=0.9, 95%CI=0.6-1.2).

Using industrial hygiene data to infer solvent exposure from the job titles reported by subjects, 85% of study subjects were classified as having no exposure. Too few women were classified as exposed according to this matrix to allow for analysis. Even for men, the numbers exposed were too small for statistically significant results. Nonetheless, patients with glomerulonephritis were 60% more likely than controls to have held at least one job with any level of solvent exposure, and twice as many held at least one job that involved probable or definite solvent exposure (Table 3). Odds ratios were similar using the cumulative solvent score, but no dose-response was apparent.

COMMENT

The results of this analysis point to an association between solvents and risk of glomerulonephritis, but the data are limited in a number of ways. Most seriously, the number of patients with glomerulonephritis - even though twice as large as in previous studies, was too small to identify statistically significant associations - especially for relatively uncommon exposures.

Compared with other studies that focused on otherwise healthy young men with biopsy-diag-

Table 1. Employment in Selected Industries and Risk of Chronic Renal Disease.

Industry	Glomerulonephritis OR	(95% CI)	Other Renal Disease OR	(95% CI)
Furniture Manufacturing	1.7	(0.7-3.7)	1.3	(0.8-2.2)
Lumbering	1.5	(0.7-3.3)	1.0	(0.6-1.7)
Textile Industry	1.2	(0.7-2.1)	1.1	(0.8-1.4)
Auto Mechanics	1.5	(0.5-4.3)	0.9	(0.4-1.9)
Plumbing	3.5	(1.0-11.7)	1.1	(0.4-3.3)
Commercial Painting	2.6	(0.4-11.2)	1.6	(0.5-4.8)

Table 2. Self-reported Exposures and Risk of Chronic Renal Disease.

Exposure	Glomerulonephritis OR	(95% CI)	Other Renal Disease OR	(95% CI)
Any Named Solvent	1.7	(1.0-2.9)	1.0	(0.7-1.4)
Cutting/Cooling Oils	1.0	(0.5-1.9)	0.5	(0.3-0.8)
Epoxy Glues	2.0	(1.0-3.8)	0.8	(0.5-1.3)
Stains, Varnish, etc.	1.6	(0.8-3.1)	0.8	(0.5-1.3)
Paint	2.2	(0.9-5.2)	1.1	(0.5-2.0)
Alcohols	1.7	(0.8-3.4)	1.0	(0.6-1.5)
Glazes	2.0	(0.6-6.0)	1.0	(0.4-2.3)

Table 3. Cumulative Solvent Exposure and Risk of Chronic Renal Disease among Men.

	Glomerulonephritis OR	(95% CI)	Other Renal Disease OR	(95% CI)
Highest Exposure Level				
No Exposure	1.0	(----------)	1.0	(----------)
Any Exposure	1.6	(0.8-3.1)	0.9	(0.5-1.5)
Possible	1.4	(0.6-3.0)	0.6	(0.3-1.2)
Probable/Definite	2.2	(0.7-6.4)	1.6	(0.7-3.6)
Solvent Exposure Score				
No Exposure	1.0	(----------)	1.0	(----------)
95th to 90th percentile	1.8	(0.5-4.9)	0.7	(0.3-1.7)
> 90th percentile	1.7	(0.7-3.8)	1.1	(0.6-1.9)

nosed glomerulonephritis, the broader age range and inclusion of women in our study decreased the likelihood that subjects would have occupational solvent exposure. Because the study was not occupationally based, it was necessary to rely on long lists of occupations or activities that may involve solvents to identify exposures. As a result, increased odds ratios could be due to chance and it is not possible to identify with any certainty that the common factor for all of these jobs is solvent exposure.

Data were retrospectively gathered from subjects who were often old and quite sick, or from next-of-kin. Inaccurate or biased reporting may have occurred. The limitation of findings to glomerulonephritis is somewhat reassuring in this regard, since any resulting biases could be expected to have affected all subgroups equally.

The finding of a potential risk for glomerulonephritis and not other forms of renal disease is consistent with past studies, but the nearly 2-fold risk we observed is somewhat lower than the 4-5 fold risks reported by others (6). This could be due, in part to our use of healthy population controls rather than controls chosen from hospitalized patients, or could reflect the decreased ability of our study to discriminate between subgroups of renal disease patients. Without biopsy data for almost 2/3 of the patients we classified as having glomerulonephritis, it is possible that some of these patients had other diagnoses.

While the results of this study suggest a potential role for solvent exposure in the etiology of chronic renal disease, such an association is far from proven. It is clear from the difficulties encountered in this and past studies, that other study designs will be needed to clarify the risk associated with solvent exposure.

REFERENCES

1. Landrigan PJ, Goyer RA, Clarkson TW, Sandler DP, Smith JH, Thun MJ, Wedeen RP: The work-relatedness of renal disease. Arch Environ Health 39: 225-230, 1984.

2. Sandler DP: Epidemiology in the assessment of nephrotoxicity. In: Bach PH, Lock EA, (eds); Nephrotoxicity in the experimental and clinical situation. Part 2. Lancaster, Martinus Nijhoff Publishers, 1987, pp. 847-883.

3. Sugimoto T, Rosansky, SJ: The incidence of treated end stage renal disease in the eastern United States: 1973-1979. Am J Publ Health 74: 14-17, 1984.

4. McGeown MG: Chronic renal failure in Northern Ireland, 1968-70. A prospective survey. Lancet 1: 307-310, 1972.

5. Churchill DN, Fine A, Gault MH: Association between hydrocarbon exposure and glomerulonephritis. An appraisal of the evidence. Nephron 33: 169-172, 1983.

6. Daniell WE, Couser WG, Rosenstock L: Occupational solvent exposure and glomerulonephritis. JAMA 259: 2280-2283, 1988.

7. Bell GM, Gordon ACH, Lee P, Doig A, MacDonald MK, Thomson D, Anderton JL, Robson JS: Proliferative glomerulonephritis and exposure to organic solvents. Nephron 40: 161-165, 1985.

8. Zimmerman SW, Groehler K, Beirne GJ: Hydrocarbon exposure and chronic glomerulonephritis. Lancet 2: 199-201, 1975.

9. Ravnskov U, Forsberg B, Skerfving S: Glomerulonephritis and exposure to organic solvents: A case-control study. Acta Med Scand 205: 575-579, 1979.

10. Ravnskov U, Lundstrom S, Norden A: Hydrocarbon exposure and glomerulonephritis: Evidence from patients' occupations. Lancet 2: 1214-1216, 1983.

11. Finn R, Fennerty AG, Ahmad R: Hydrocarbon exposure and glomerulonephritis. Clin Nephrol 14: 173-175, 1980.

12. Van der Laan G: Chronic glomerulonephritis and organic solvents. Int Arch Occup Environ Health 47: 1-8, 1980.

13. Lauwerys R, Bernard A, Viau C, Buchet JP: Kidney disorders and haemotoxicity from

organic solvent exposure. Scand J Work Environ Health 11 (suppl 1): 83-90, 1985.

14. Sandler DP, Smith JC, Weinberg CR, Buckalew VM, Dennis VW, Blythe WB, Burgess WP: Analgesic use and chronic renal disease. N Engl J Med 320: 1238-1243, 1989.

42

NEPHROTOXICITY OF AVIATION GASOLINE IN THE RAT

M. Gérin(1), C. Viau(1), D. Talbot(1) and E. Greselin(2)

Département de médecine du travail et d'hygiène du milieu, Université de Montréal, C.P. 6128, succ. A, Montréal, Québec, Canada, H3C 3J7 (1) and Département de pharmacologie, Université de Montréal, Montréal (2)

INTRODUCTION

Renal tubular changes associated with hydrocarbon-induced nephropathy (HIN) have been shown to occur in male rats following exposure to various hydrocarbons or hydrocarbon-containing mixtures (1). Among them, unleaded automotive gasoline (ULG) was shown not only to induce HIN but also to be associated with the development of renal tumours in male rats (2). Human exposure to aviation gasoline (AVG) has been shown to be associated with a significant increase in the incidence of renal cancers in a Montreal epidemiological study (3). This fact, and the high reported content of strongly nephrotoxic branched alkanes in AVG (4), prompted us to study, as a first step, the nephrotoxicity of AVG in vivo.

In a previous report (5) we presented the results of a 2-week study comparing various nephrotoxicity parameters in groups of rats exposed to ULG, 2,2,4-trimethylpentane (TMP) and AVG. These results established the increased nephrotoxicity of AVG compared to ULG and indicated that AVG could be even more nephrotoxic than TMP. We report here a more comprehensive 4-week study covering 2 doses of the same substances and including the measurement of urinary parameters at three different time points.

METHODS

Treatment of Animals

Male Fischer-344 rats weighing 205-245 g were purchased from Charles River Canada, St-Constant, Quebec. They received water and food (Purina Laboratory Chow) ad libitum. Animals (10 per group) were randomly assigned to either control or 6 experimental groups. All groups were treated by gavage once daily, 5 days a week for 4 weeks for a total of 20 administrations. The control group received 2.0 g/kg of saline solution. The experimental groups received 0.125 g/kg or 0.5 g/kg of regular unleaded gasoline (ULG), grade 100 aviation gasoline (AVG) or 2,2,4-trimethylpentane (TMP). Gasoline samples were obtained from the Shell refinery in Montreal-Est, Quebec. TMP was obtained from BDH Chemicals (Montreal, Quebec) Omnisolv grade. 24 hr urine samples were collected, by placing animals in metabolic cages, at three different time points during the 4-week experiment: immediately after the first treatment (day 1), after the fifth treatment (day 5), and at the end of the experiment after the twentieth treatment (day 26). At the end of that last urine collection period, blood was withdrawn and the animals were sacrificed and the kidneys removed. These were weighed, one lobe was fixed in Bouin's solution and the other frozen.

Biochemical Determinations

Immediately after each 24 hr urine collection period, an aliquot of each sample was dialysed for 16 hr against running tap water. The dialysed sample was used for the measurement of lactate dehydrogenase (LDH, EC 1.1.1.27) activity from the decrease of NADH absorbance upon addition of pyruvate (6). Small aliquots of undialysed urine were used for the measurement of activity of beta-N-acetyl-D-glucosa-minidase (NAG, EC 3.2.1.30) using the fluorometric assay of Leaback and Walker (7). Urinary glucose was determined with Sigma kit No. 115-A (Sigma Chemicals, St. Louis, MO). Total urinary proteins were determined from the dialysed urine using a method previously described (6). Urinary creatinine was measured using the alkaline picrate assay kit No. 557-A from Sigma. Blood urea nitrogen (BUN) was measured with Sigma kit No. 535-B. Kidney content in alpha$_{2U}$-globulin (alpha$_{2U}$-G) was determined on whole kidney homogenates using an immunoassay based on latex particles agglutination.

Histopathologic Evaluations

Optical microscopic examination of the kidneys was performed from paraffin sections after staining with Haematoxylin and Eosin (H&E) and Azocarmine B. Histopathology was assessed with a knowledge of the group distribution of the individual kidney samples, but not the treatment corresponding to each group. The criteria used in this evaluation were: presence of hyaline droplets in the cytoplasm of proximal cells (Azocarmine stain), presence of granular casts within the lumen of the tubules (H&E) and evidence of tubular cell regeneration (H&E). Results were reported using a semi-quantitative scale comparable to that used by Halder et al (1). The mean score obtained for each group was multiplied by 10 and reported thus.

Statistical Analysis

Data on biochemical parameters and kidney relative weights were analysed by applying the Tukey B multiple comparison procedure with a level of significance set at alpha = 0.05. Histopathologic scores were compared using a distribution-free multiple comparison procedure based on Kruskal-Wallis rank sums with Dunn's approximation (alpha = 0.05).

RESULTS

Gavaging errors resulted in the early death and rejection of two rats from the group treated with TMP at the 0.5 g/kg dose. Values for the

various parameters of nephrotoxicity are presented in Figs. 1 and 2.

Treatment with either of the 3 substances generally resulted in significant increases in urinary excretion of LDH, NAG, glucose and total proteins for the higher dose at days 5 and 26 and the lower dose at day 26. For the lower dose at day 5, only treatment with TMP and AVG resulted in significant increases in all urinary parameters. Only a few significant changes in urinary parameters were observed in treated groups versus controls at day 1.

When comparing treated groups within one another, urinary parameter values in ULG treated groups were usually significantly lower than for TMP or AVG groups at days 5 and 26. When comparing urinary parameters between the TMP and AVG groups there were several time-dose combinations in which LDH and occasionally another urinary parameter was significantly higher in the TMP treated animals.

Observation of histograms revealed few apparent time trends in urinary parameters, at either dose. LDH, NAG and protein values were higher in the TMP and AVG groups at days 5 and 26 compared to day 1, but with no apparent or systematic increase between days 5 and 26. At day 26 a slight but significant increase in BUN was observed for the AVG groups compared to the other treated groups. Exposure to ULG resulted in a near 2-fold increase in renal alpha$_{2U}$-G whereas AVG and TMP induced an accumulation 3- to 4-fold higher than that observed in controls, with TMP being significantly higher than AVG at the higher dose.

Hyaline droplet accumulation was observed in all groups. It was minimal in controls, minimal to slight in ULG groups and slight to severe in TMP and AVG groups. Minimal to slight regenerative epithelium lesions were found in controls and ULG treated groups, whereas they were slight to severe in TMP and AVG groups.

Only in the TMP and AVG groups did one observe tubular cast formation, which were minimal to slight, except in the high dose AVG group where moderate to severe formations

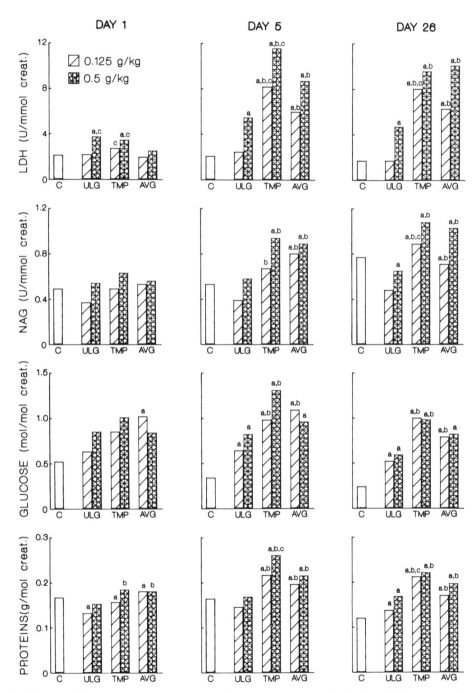

Figure 1. Influence of subchronic treatment (4 weeks, 5 days a week, 0.125 and 0.5 g/kg, p.o.) with regular unleaded automobile gasoline (ULG), 2,2,4-trimethylpentane (TMP) and aviation gasoline (grade 100) (AVG) on various urinary parameters of nephrotoxicity in rats at various times during the treatment. LDH: Lactate dehydrogenase; NAG: beta-N-acetyl-D-glucosaminidase. Bars represent means (n= 8 to 10). [a] significantly different from control group (C) (alpha = 0.05); [b] significantly different from ULG-treated group at the same dose (alpha=0.05); [c] significantly different from AVG-treated group at the same dose (alpha = 0.05).

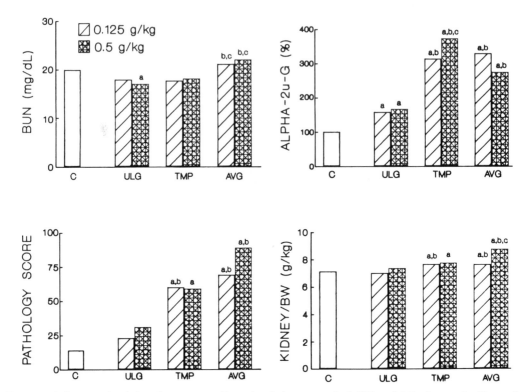

Figure 2. Influence of subchronic treatment (4 weeks, 5 days a week, 0.125 and 0.5 g/kg, p.o.) with regular unleaded automobile gasoline (ULG), 2,2,4-trimethylpentane (TMP) and aviation gasoline (grade 100) (AVG) on various parameters of nephrotoxicity in rats. BUN: Blood urea nitrogen; Alpha-2U-G: alpha-2u-globulin; Kidney/BW: Kidney relative weight. Bars represent means (n = 8 to 10). [a] significantly different from control group (C) (alpha = 0.05); [b] significantly different from ULG-treated group at the same dose (alpha = 0.05); [c] significantly different from either TMP or AVG-treated groups at the same dose (alpha = 0.05).

were observed. The overall nephropathy scores were 4 to 6 times higher in the AVG and TMP groups compared to controls and 2 to 3 times higher compared to ULG treated rats.

Relative kidney weights were significantly increased in TMP and AVG groups, with AVG being significantly higher than both TMP and ULG at the higher dose. For the 3 substances the 4-fold dose difference generally resulted in small changes in all studied parameter values.

DISCUSSION

The present findings support our hypothesis that AVG is a strong nephrotoxin in the male rat. They are in line with results presented in our

first report (5), establishing the increased toxicity of AVG and TMP compared to ULG. When considering all the parameters evaluated at all time periods, in the present study, it appears difficult, however, to rank the toxicity of AVG and TMP. Some parameters such as BUN, histopathology and relative kidney weight being generally higher in the AVG vs TMP groups whereas the reverse was true for LDH excretion and alpha$_{2U}$-G accumulation in the kidney.

These results support the role played by branched alkanes in the development of this type of nephrotoxicity (1), but no data were available on the composition of the gasoline samples. Furthermore, it is not known how representative our one-batch gasoline samples are. The presence of low concentrations of organolead additives in our AVG sample (8), however, is unlikely to have played a role in this nephrotoxicity (9).

The early onset and plateauing of the urinary excretion of NAG, LDH and proteins suggest that, within the time frame and the doses used in this study, the evolution of HIN towards renal cancer might not be accompanied by a parallel evolution in those nephrotoxicity parameters.

Only small increases were apparent with a 4-fold increase in dose in any of the eight nephrotoxicity parameters studied. Results, not presented here, on a group of rats treated with 2.0 g/kg of AVGAS, are consistent with this statement. This plateauing suggests a saturation phenomenon in the mechanism of nephrotoxicity. As expected, the hyalin droplet score was highly correlated to the renal concentration of alpha$_{2u}$-G($r=0.943$, $p<0.01$) when group averages were used. Total histopathology score, glucose excretion and total proteins excretion were also statistically correlated to renal alpha$_{2u}$-G concentration. Overall, these results are compatible with the postulated role of alpha$_{2u}$-G in the pathogenic mechanism of nephrotoxicity in this model.

If there is a link between nephrotoxicity and renal carcinogenicity in male rats exposed to ULG (2), our results point out to AVG as a possible potent carcinogen in this model. Two samples of aviation gasoline have been reported to induce mutations in mouse lymphoma cells but did not increase the frequency of sister chromatic exchange in cultured Chinese hamster ovary cells nor were they active in the Ames test (10). Furthermore, even though there is only inadequate evidence on the human carcinogenicity of any type of gasoline (11), results of the Montreal epidemiological study (3) did generate the hypothesis that exposure to AVG may cause renal cancer in humans. A number of jet fuels, which, as a general category, were strong confounders in that study, have also been found to be nephrotoxic in the male rat (12). A next step in our study of AVG, is to study the human nephrotoxicity of AVG in groups of workers.

ACKNOWLEDGEMENTS

This work was supported by the CAFIR fund of the Université de Montréal and by the Canadian Medical Research Council (MA 10058). We would like to thank Shell Canada Ltd for providing us with gasoline samples.

REFERENCES

1. Halder CA, Holdsworth CE, Cockrell BY, Piccirillo VJ: Hydrocarbon nephropathy in male rats: identification of the nephrotoxic components of unleaded gasoline. Toxicol Ind Health 1: 67-87, 1985.

2. MacFarland HN, Ulrich CE, Holdsworth CE, Kitchen DN, Halliwell WH, Blum SC: A chronic inhalation study with unleaded gasoline vapor. J Am Coll Toxicol 3: 231-248, 1984.

3. Siemiatycki J, Dewar R, Nadon L, Gérin M, Richardson L, Wacholder S: Associations between several sites of cancer and twelve petroleum-derived liquids. Results from a case-control study in Montreal. Scand J Work Environ Health 13: 493-504, 1987.

4. Concawe: Health Aspects of Petroleum Fuels. Potential Hazards and Precautions for Individual Classes of Fuel (Concawe Report No. 85/51), Concawe, The Hague, 1985, p. 7.

5. Gérin M, Viau C, Talbot D, Greselin E: Aviation gasoline: comparative subchronic nephrotoxicity study in the male rat. Toxicol Lett 44: 13-19, 1988.

6. Bernard A, Buchet JP, Roels H, Masson P, Lauwerys R: Renal excretion of proteins and enzymes in workers exposed to cadmium. Eur J Clin Invest 9: 11-22, 1979.

7. Leaback DH, Walker PG: Studies on glucosaminidase. 4. The fluorimetric assay of N-acetyl-beta-D-glucosaminidase. Biochem J 78, 151-156, 1961.

8. Shell Canada Ltd.: Material Safety Data Sheet, Code 101-100. Shell Avgas 100, Shell Canada Ltd., Montreal, 1984.

9. Wedeen RP: Occupational renal disease: Am J Kidney Dis 3: 241-257, 1984.

10. Farrow MG, McCarroll N, Cortina T, Draus M, Munson A, Steinberg M, Kirwin C, Thomas W. In vitro mutagenicity and genotoxicity of fuels and paraffinic hydrocarbons in the Ames, sister chromatid exchange, and mouse lymphoma assays. Toxicologist 3: 36, 1983.

11. International Agency for Research on Cancer: Occupational exposures in petroleum refining; crude oil and major petroleum fuels. IARC Monographs on the evaluation of carcinogenic risks to humans, Vol 45, IARC, Lyon, 1989, pp. 159-201.

12. MacNaughton MG, Uddin DE: Toxicology of mixed distillate and high-energy synthetic fuels. In: Mehlman MA (Ed.); Advances in Modern Environmental Toxicology, Vol 7, Princeton Scientific Publisher, Princeton, 1984, pp. 121-132.

43

SCREENING OF AROMATIC COMPOUNDS FOR THEIR POTENCY OF INDUCING HYALINE DROPLET ACCUMULATION IN MALE RAT KIDNEY

E. Bomhard (1), M. Marsmann (2), Ch. Rühl-Fehlert (1), R. Schade-Lehn (1) and G. Schüürmann (3)

(1) Department of Toxicology, Bayer AG, Friedrich-Ebert-Strasse 217-333, 5600 Wuppertal 1, (2) Environmental Protection/Product Safety, Bayer AG, 5090 Leverkusen, and (3) Central Research, Bayer AG, 5090 Leverkusen, Germany

INTRODUCTION

Induction of hyaline droplet accumulation (HDA) in renal cortex of adult male rats with-subsequent nephrotoxicity and nephrocarcinogenicity has been reported for a rapidly growing list of chemicals, principally of aliphatic and cycloaliphatic hydrocarbons. This HDA is considered to be a consequence of $alpha_2$-microglobulin binding to a specific stereochemical moiety of certain hydrocarbons or their metabolites (1). This complex could exhibit elevated resistance to normal protein catabolism by renal lysosomes (2-4). Only a limited number of aromatic hydrocarbons has been investigated in this respect (5-8). In addition, attempts to correlate the structure and activity of aromatic compounds have not been published so far. This study evaluated HDA-inducing potency of 18 halogenated and/or alkylated benzenes or toluenes both by histological assessment and electrophoretic measurements. Furthermore, the first results of an analysis of the HDA with respect to quantitative structure-activity relationships (QSAR) are presented.

METHODS

The test substances (Table 1) were administered at a dose level of 250 mg/kg body weight to 5 adult male Wistar rats each (weight range 220-240 g, age 10-12 weeks) once daily for 5 days by gavage. The compounds 1,2,4-trihy-droxybenzene, 1,4-diiodobenzene, 1,4-dibromobenzene and 1,3,5-tribromobenzene were dissolved in peanut oil (application volume 2 ml/kg body weight). The other compounds were administered undiluted. A group of 5 adult male rats receiving the vehicle served as controls. Necropsy was performed 2-3 hours after the 5th administration. Gross sections of the kidneys were stained with H&E, and Azan. For semi-quantitative grading of the occurrence of the hyaline droplets the following scale was applied: 0 = no droplets; 1 = occasional droplets in some proximal tubules; 2 = mild response in a large number of proximal tubules; 3 = moderate response with an increase of droplets in cells and a more wide-spread cortical distribution and 4 = extensive response with marked increase and widespread distribution.

Frozen parts of the kidneys were separated into medulla and cortex. Transverse slices of 3 to 4 mm thickness were taken from the middle of the cortex and placed in a TRIS buffer solution (50 µl/10 mg tissue), homogenized and centrifuged, 50 µl aliquots of the diluted solutions (approx. 40 µg protein) were subjected and one-dimensional electrophoresis was carried out at 30 mA/gel for at least 4 hr on a 12% SDS-polyacrylamide using a vertical slab gel (Protean II Slab Cell, BIO-RAD, Munich). Separated proteins were stained with Coomassie brillant blue and evaluated by densitometry.

Following the general hypothesis that the interaction between the xenobiotics and the protein alpha2-microglobulin is determined to a large degree by specific structural features of the compounds a number of molecular parameters were calculated and analyzed with respect to possible correlations with the HDA variation among the test compounds. In particular, the octanol/water partition coefficient K_{ow} and the molar refractivity (MR) were calculated using the Medchem software (9), and geometric as well as electronic descriptors (for details see 10) were derived from the three-dimensional structure as calculated within the semiempirical quantum chemical MNDO model (11) using the AMPAC computer package (12).

RESULTS

Results of the semiquantitative grading of hyaline droplets from Azan stained kidney

Table 1. Amount of HDA and renal marker protein after application of aromatic hydrocarbons to male rats

Test compound	HDA (mean score)	Protein amount (μg $\pm$ SD)
Control	2.0	2.45 $\pm$ 0.39
1,2,4-trihydroxybenzene	1.5	2.22 $\pm$ 0.66
2-ethyltoluene	1.3	2.24 $\pm$ 0.89
1,3,5-trifluorobenzene	2.0	2.49 $\pm$ 0.18
4-chlorotoluene	2.0	2.69 $\pm$ 0.71
2,5-dichlorotoluene	1.8	2.83 $\pm$ 0.47
1,2-diethylbenzene	1.8	2.88 $\pm$ 1.25
4-chloro-o-xylene	2.2	2.89 $\pm$ 0.91
4-chlorofluorobenzene	2.4	3.11 $\pm$ 0.71
1,3-diethylbenzene	2.2	3.15 $\pm$ 0.70
2-chloro-p-xylene	1.8	3.30 $\pm$ 0.63
3-chlorotoluene	3.0	3.42 $\pm$ 1.12
1,4-diiodobenzene	3.6	3.63 $\pm$ 0.55
1,4-difluorobenzene	3.6	3.92 $\pm$ 0.96
1-ethyl-2-bromobenzene	3.4	3.98 $\pm$ 1.03
2-bromotoluene	3.4	4.35 $\pm$ 1.10
1,4-dibromobenzene	4.0	4.93 $\pm$ 1.22
2-chlorotoluene	3.4	4.88 $\pm$ 0.79
1,3,5-tribromobenzene	3.8	5.44 $\pm$ 0.91

slices are presented as mean scores together with the protein amounts (means $\pm$ standard deviation) obtained from the densitometric evaluation of gels in Table 1.

The data are largely in agreement, showing 1,4-diiodobenzene, 1,4-difluorobenzene, 1-ethyl-2-bromobenzene, 2-bromotoluene, 1,4-dibromobenzene, 2-chlorotoluene, and 1,3,5-tribromobenzene as the most active compounds. The compounds 1,2,4-trihydroxy- benzene, 2-ethyltoluene, 1,3,5-trifluorobenzene and 4-chlorotoluene are judged as inactive based on both densitometric and histopathologic evaluation. Some compounds like 2,5-dichlorotoluene, 1,2-diethylbenzene, 4-chloro-o-xylene, 1,3-diethylbenzene and 2-chloro-para-xylene do not differ significantly with regard to their mean HDA score. Taking into account the higher than normal level of hyaline droplets in 1 or 2 of the test animals as well as their amount of marker protein they might be classified as weakly or questionably active. 4-chlorofluorobenzene and 3-chlorotoluene were clearly above normal in the histopathologic as well as densitometric evaluation but with slight to moderate activity only.

The typical protein band to be seen after treatment with compounds binding to alpha2-microglobulin like pentachlorethane or 2,3,3-trimethylpentane is also present after treatment with the active aromatic compounds (Fig. 1).

Typical densitograms of aromatic as well as those of aliphatic compounds used for comparison are shown in Figs. 2 and 3.

Inspection of the benzene derivatives together with their HDA values does not reveal a simple structural dependence of the biological effects. Among the highly active compounds are three 1,4-dihalogenated benzenes and one 1,3,5-trihalogenated congener, but similar structural patterns also occur with very little HDA potency. The plot of HDA versus log K_{ow} as shown in Fig. 4 reveals that for this set of compounds the lipophilicity as quantified by log K_{ow} does not have any significant influence on

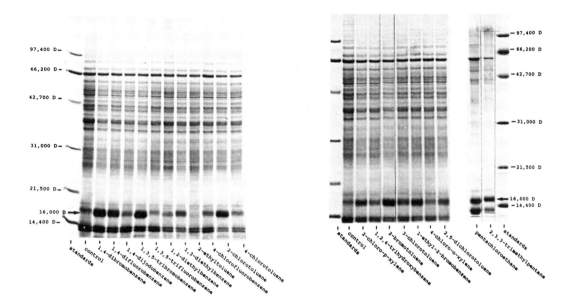

Figure 1. SDS-PAGE of renal cortical tissue.

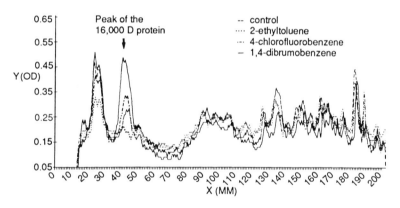

Figure 2. Densitogram of three typical aromatic hydrocarbons.

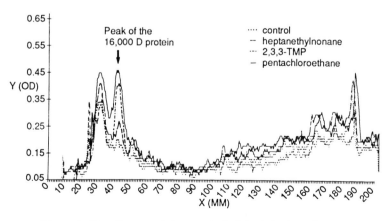

Figure 3. Densitogram of three typical aliphatic hydrocarbons.

the chemicals' HDA activity. Thereby the almost random-like data distribution is somewhat surprising, as for chemically-related sets of compounds distinct influences of log k_{ow} on in vivo effects are often found (13, 14).

The highest one-parameter correlation coefficient was achieved with the simple molecular weight (MW, r=0.60); the corresponding plot is shown in Fig. 5. Application of multilinear regression analysis revealed that the variation of HDA could be described by three-parameter equations the best of which included MW, DE (electrophilic delocalizability) and the Hardness

(see 10). The data distribution of HDA versus both MW and DE is shown in Fig. 6. Fig. 7 contains the plot of calculated versus experimental HDA values using the three descriptors as mentioned above (r=0.82, s=0.56, $F_{3,14}$=9.37).

The current QSAR model is a first attempt to account for the HDA variation in a quantitative way. However, it is planned to extend the QSAR analysis by including other molecular descriptors and by performing a distinct shape analysis of the three-dimensional molecular structures.

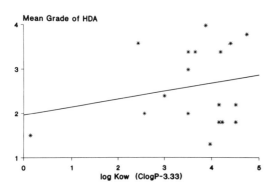

Fig. 4. HDA vs log Kow.

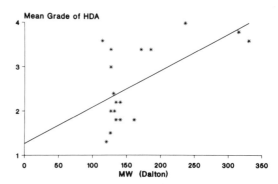

Fig. 5. HDA vs Molecular Weight.

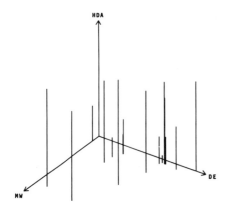

Fig. 6. HDA vs MW and DE.

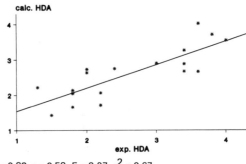

r = 0.82, s = 0.58, F = 9.37, r^2 = 0.67
MW = Molecular Weight, DE and Hardness = MNDO Paramters

Fig. 7. HDA; calculated vs experimental values.

CONCLUSIONS

1. There are many aromatic compounds with the potential to induce "light hydrocarbon nephropathy".

2. One-dimensional SDS-PAGE with homogenates from cortical slices and subsequent densitometric evaluation allows a quantitative measurement of the degree of a specific marker protein (16,000D).

3. The amount of this protein correlates well to the degree of typical HDA after administration of aliphatic and aromatic light hydrocarbons.

4. Results from a first attempt to quantify the relationships between structure and activity of aromatic hydrocarbons are provided which indicate some differences to criteria which have been identified for aliphatic compounds.

REFERENCES

1. Kanerva RL, Ridder GM, Stone LC, Alden CL: Characterization of spontaneous and decalin-induced hyaline droplets in kidneys of adult male rats. Fd Chem Toxicol 25:63-82, 1987

2. Alden CL: A review of unique male rat nephropathy. Toxicol Pathol 14:109-111, 1986

3. Garg BD, Olson MJ, Demyan WF, Roy AK: Rapid postexposure decay of alpha$_2$-microglobulin and hyaline droplets in the kidneys of gasoline-treated male rats. J Toxicol Environ Health 24: 145-160, 1988

4. Lock EA, Charbonneau M, Strasser J, Swenberg JA, Bus JS: 2,2,4-Trimethylpentane-induced nephropathy II. The reversible binding of a TMP metabolite to a renal protein fraction containing alpha$_2$-microglobulin. Toxicol Appl Pharmacol 91: 182-192, 1987

5. Bomhard E, Luckhaus G, Voigt WH, Loeser E: Induction of light hydrocarbon nephropathy by p-dichlorobenzene. Arch Toxicol 61: 433-439, 1988

6. Bomhard E, Luckhaus G, Marsmann M, Zywietz A: Induction of hyaline droplet accumulation in renal cortex of male rats by aromatic compounds. In: Bach PH, Lock EA (eds) Nephrotoxicity: Extrapolation from in vitro to in vivo and from animals to man. Plenum Press, London, 1989, pp 551-556

7. Charbonneau M, Strasser J, Lock EA, Turner MJ, Swenberg JA: Involvement of reversible binding to alpha$_2$-microglobulin in 1,4-dichlorobenzene-induced nephrotoxicity. Toxicol and Appl Pharmacol 99: 122-132, 1989

8. Halder CH, Holdsworth CE, Cockrell BY, Piccirillo VJ: Hydrocarbon nephropathy in male rats. Identification of the nephrotoxic components of gasoline. Toxicol Ind Health 1: 67-87, 1985

9. Leo A: CLOGP-3.33 MedChem Software, Medicinal Chemistry Project, Pomona College, Claremont, CA, 1985

10. Schüürmann, G: QSAR analysis of the acute fish-toxicity of organic phosphorothionates using theoretically derived molecular descriptors. Environ Toxicol Chem (accepted for publication)

11. Dewar MLS, Thiel W: Ground states of molecules.38: The MNDO method. Approximations and parameters. J Am Chem Soc 99: 4899-4907, 1977

12. Dewar MLS, Stewart JJP: AMPAC. A general molecular orbital package. QCPE No.506, Quantum Chemistry Program Exchange Bulletin 6:24, 1986

13. Connell DW, Schüürmann G: Evaluation of various molecular parameters as predictors of bioconcentration in fish. Ecotox Environ Safety 15: 324-335, 1988

14. Schüürmann G, Klein W: Advances in bioconcentration prediction. Chemosphere 17: 1551-1574, 1988

44

STRUCTURE TOXICITY MODEL OF LIGHT HYDROCARBON NEPHROPATHY

E. Bomhard (1), M. Marsmann (2) and A. Zywietz (3)

(1) Institute of Industrial Toxicology, Bayer AG, Wuppertal, Germany, (2) Environmental Protection/Product Safety, Bayer AG, Leverkusen, Germany, (3) Central Research, Bayer AG, Leverkusen, Germany

INTRODUCTION

The interaction between alpha-2-microglobulin and a specific stereochemical moiety of certain hydrocarbons or their metabolites is followed by a pathological accumulation of hyaline droplets with subsequent development of chronic nephrosis in adult male rats (1,2). This so-called light hydrocarbon nephropathy (LHN) is still a matter of growing interest. Among others the following reasons may be responsible for this interest:

a) more compounds from other chemical classes (e.g. 3,4) have been identified which seem to act by the same mechanism; b) several proteins of similar structure as alpha-2-microglobulin have been identified in different species including man (5) so that similar proteins may interact with similar or other classes of chemical compounds in a similar manner; c) the late occurrence of renal tubular adenomas and adenocarcinomas seem to be the result of this chronic disease possibly on the basis of a chronically stimulated cell proliferation under non-physiologic conditions (6,7) which may give rise to an increase in initiated cells. The latter aspect may have several implications for the understanding of cancer development as a result of high dose treatment with non-genotoxic compounds.

Although this specific alpha-2-microglobulin-related nephropathy seems to have no relevance for humans, it is still of major importance to know which of the thousands of compounds and isomers among those aliphatic, alicyclic and aromatic hydrocarbons may interfere with alpha-2-microglobulin, and thereby have the potential for inducing LHN. This may have practical implications in that adult male rats may not be the animal model of choice with respect to kidney toxicity. Since not all compounds can be tested for their LHN potential, for reasons of time and expense, we tried to develop a structure-activity model for this effect on the basis of selected literature data. This would enable the prediction of such interactions.

Due to the semiquantitive nature of reported activity data we based our approach on an analysis of whole molecular properties such as the partition coefficient and the molecular shape. The latter can be analyzed in great detail using molecular modelling techniques (8,9), thereby revealing spatial similarities and dissimilarities of the active and inactive compounds.

MATERIAL AND METHODS

The compounds analyzed for their potency for inducing LHN are compiled in Table 1. The data originate from studies by the American Petroleum Institute, the Wright-Patterson Airforce Base and the NTP. They were graded on an activity scale ranging from inactive to highly active (10-12). Hydrocarbons of different activity score as well as inactive representatives are included.

For all compounds in Table 1 octanol-water partition coefficients (log Kow) were calculated using the standard CLOGP incremental procedure (13). Minimum-energy molecular structures were calculated by the MM2 force-field-method starting from different conformational isomers (14). Molecular volumes for the lowest-energy conformers were calculated from tabulated van der Waal (VDW) radii and further processed using the volume comparison routines in the SYBYL molecular modelling package (15).

RESULTS

The calculated values of log Kow are shown in Table 1. These data indicate a certain degree of lipophilicity as a prerequisite for LHN-inducing activity. Only inactive compounds can be found at a calculated log Kow below about 3.5. This may tentatively be interpreted as a penetration barrier which prevents compounds which otherwise may be active from reaching the receptor site. Since log Kow alone does not allow complete discrimination between active and inactive analogs, we next focussed on identifying some common structural features of LHN-inducing hydrocarbons. Our initial working hypothesis involved the presence of an isopentyl substructure which can be identified in all highly active non-cyclic compounds. Since this substructure is also present in some of the inactive compounds we then turned to analyze molecular shape. The most active representatives of these structures - i.e. 2,3-dimethylpentane, 2,2,4-trimethylpentane, 2,3,4- trimethylpentane, 2,2,5-trimethylhexane and 2,2,4,4-tetramethyloctane - were superimposed along the common isopentyl substructure using three-dimensional computer graphics. The union VDW volume of these 5 compounds has been calculated. This parameter, commonly termed the "receptor excluded volume" defines the minimum size and shape of a cavity capable of accommodating an active compound. For the remaining compounds we calculated the "excess volume" - the volume difference between the molecular volume in each case and the "receptor excluded volume". Due to the three-dimensional nature

Table 1: Chemicals tested, nephropathy score (male rats), logarithm of n- octanol/water partition coefficient and calculated excess volumes (EV) of light hydrocarbons

Chemical	LHN score	log Kow	EV** (A3)
2-Methylpentane	+	3.7	0.1 (A)
2-Methylhexane	+	4.3	2.8 (A)
2,2,4,4-Tetramethyldecane	+	7.6	33.1 (A)
2,3-Dimethylbutane	++	3.6	0.2 (A)
2,2,3-Trimethyloctane	++	6.1	32.2 (A)
2,3-Dimethylpentane	+++	4.1	0
2,2,5-Trimethylhexane	+++	5.1	0
2,2,4-Trimethylpentane	++++	4.5	0
2,2,4,4-Tetramethyloctane	++++	6.5	0
2,3,4-Trimethylpentane	positive	4.5	0
Methylcyclohexane	positive	3.9	4.7 (C)
Decalin	positive	4.8	13.5 (C)
Tricyclodecane	positive	3.9	10.7 (C)
n-Pentane	-	3.3	-*
2-Methylbutane	-	3.2	-*
2-Methyl-2-pentene	-	3.2	-*
trans-2-Pentene	-	2.8	-*
n-Hexane	-	3.9	-*
n-Octane	-	4.9	-*
3-Methyloctane	-	5.3	15.0 (A)
2,3-Dimethyloctane	-	5.7	40.5 (B)
2,2,3-Trimethyldecane	-	7.2	65.1 (A)
n-Decane	-	6.0	-*
2-Methyldecane	-	6.4	65.1 (A)
2,3-Dimethyldecane	-	6.8	73.3 (A)
2,2,4,4,5,5,7,7-Octamethyloctane	-	8.1	97.7 (A,B)
Methylcyclopentane	-	3.3	1.9 (C)

*   not calculated because of log Kow < 3.5 or missing isopentyl fragment
** predominant region in parenthesis

of these excess volumes, their numerical volumes must be separated into contributions from different spatial regions, as shown in the schematic drawing (Figure 1).

From the analysis of the excess volumes given in Table 1, region A outside the union volume cavity was identified as most probably being responsible for reducing activity. Excess volume in this region not only discriminates

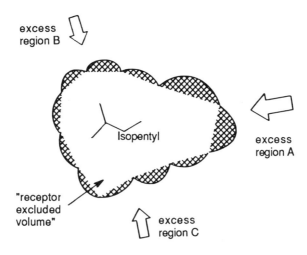

Figure 1. Schematic drawing of "excess volume" regions.

between active and inactive compounds, but also correlates with the degree of activity. The less active compounds 2,2,4,4-tetramethyldecane and 2,2,3-trimethyloctane extend by about 30 A^3 into region A. Compounds with an excess volume of about 65 or more A^3 proved to be inactive.

The contribution of region B outside the union volume with respect to the influence on activity cannot be assessed at the moment due to the lack of sufficient data.

The initial working hypothesis requiring the presence of an isopentyl substructure in active compounds was mainly useful in the superimposition procedure for acyclic hydrocarbons. In an approach to extend the receptor cavity model to include cyclic hydrocarbons, this requirement could be relaxed to a more general need for the presence of at least one tertiary carbon atom. For cyclic hydrocarbons we performed simple steric fitting of the minimum-energy conformers having maximum steric overlap with the union volume. The calculated excess volume of compounds like methylcyclohexane, decalin and tricyclode-

cane is restricted mainly to the region C which, at least up to the excess volume of decalin (13.5 A^3), does obviously not reduce activity. These compounds have been shown to be highly active.

Reduction in activity seems not to be confined to increasing excess volumes in region A. Also volumes smaller than the receptor excluded volume obviously reduce activity. This can be exemplified by such compounds like 2-methylpentane and 2-methylhexane. Despite having a log Kow above 3.5 and only negligible excess volume in region A, these compounds are only very slightly active, most probably because their molecular volume is smaller than the "ideal" receptor excluded volume.

Only a few references on the significance of metabolism on LHN exist in the literature to date (6,16-19). In addition, metabolism was studied in male and female rats of several LHN-inducing compounds without addressing the question which of the urinary metabolites found in fact were bound to alpha-2-microglobulin (20-22). In the case of 2,2,4-trimethylpentane, it has been shown that only the metabolite

2,4,4-trimethyl-2-pentanol binds reversibly to alpha-2-microglobulin (19). With regard to the suggested model, any step of metabolism necessary to form an intermediate capable of binding to alpha-2-microglobulin can be incorporated, provided it always alters the three-dimensional structure in the critical area of the molecule in practically the same way, or proceeds in an uncritical area.

On the basis of these structure-activity considerations we have started to select compounds not yet tested to assess their ability and/or potency of inducing hyaline droplet accumulation in adult male rats. For those compounds where enough related data are available (e.g. compounds with excess volume predominantly in region A) activity will be predicted, others will be selected to refine the model by clarifying e.g. the influence of increasing excess volume in region B or C of the "receptor excluded volume" cavity.

REFERENCES

1. Kanerva RL, Ridder GM, Stone LC, Alden CL: Characterization of spontaneous and decalin-induced hyaline droplets in kidneys of adult male rats. Fd Chem Toxic 25: 63-82, 1987.

2. Kanerva RL, McCracken MS, Alden CL, Stone LC: Morphogenesis of decalin-induced renal alterations in the male rat. Fd Chem Toxic 25: 53-61, 1987.

3. Evans GO, Goodwin DA, Parsons CE, Read NG: The effects of levamisole on urinary enzyme measurements and proximal tubule cell inclusions in male rats. Br J Exp Path 69: 301-308, 1988.

4. Read NG, Astbury PJ, Morgan RJI, Parsons DN, Port CJ: Induction and exacerbation of hyaline droplet formation in the proximal tubular cells of the kidneys from male rats receiving a variety of pharmacological agents. Toxicology 52: 81-101, 1988.

5. Sawyer L: One fold among many. Nature 327: 659, 1987.

6. Charbonneau M, Short BG, Lock EA, Swenberg JA: Mechanism of petroleum-induced sex-specific protein droplet nephropathy and renal cell proliferation in Fischer-344 rats: relevance to humans. In: Hemphill DD (ed); Trace Substances in Environmental Health, University of Missouri, Columbia, 1987, pp. 263-273.

7. Goldsworthy TL, Lyght O, Burnett V, Popp JA: Potential role of alpha-2-microglobulin, protein droplet accumulation, and cell replication in the renal carcinogenicity of rats exposed to trichloroethylene, perchlorethylene, and pentachloroethane. Toxicol Appl Pharmacol 96: 367-379, 1988.

8. Marshall GA: The conformational parameter in drug design: The active analog approach. In: Olson EC and Christoffersen RE (eds); Computer assisted drug design. ACS Symp Ser 112: 205-226, 1979.

9. Frühbeis H, Klein R, Wallmeier H: Computergestütztes Moleküldesign (CAMD) - ein Überblick. Angew Chem 99:413-428.

10. Craig P: Paper presented at the Toxicology Forum, Annual Summer Meeting, Aspen, Colorado, 1986.

11. Halder CH, Holdsworth CE, Cockrell BY: Hydrocarbon nephropathy in male rats. Identification of the nephrotoxic components of gasoline. In: Bach PH, Lock EA (eds); Renal heterogeneity and target cell toxicity. John Wiley & Sons, Chichester, New York, Brisbane, Toronto, Singapore, 1985, pp. 480-484.

12. Halder CH, Holdsworth CE, Cockrell BY, Piccirillo VJ: Hydrocarbon nephropathy in male rats. Identification of the nephrotoxic components of gasoline. Toxicol Ind Health 1: 67-87, 1985.

13. Leo A: CLOGP, Pomona Medical College, Claremont CA 91711.

14. Allinger NL: MM2: Quantum Chemistry Program Exchange Bloomington, Indiana, No. 395.

15. Tripos Ass, St. Louis, Missouri 63144.

16. Charbonneau M, Lock EA, Strasser J, Cox MG, Turner MJ, Bus JS: 2,2,4- Trimethylpentane-induced nephrotoxicity. I. Metabolic disposition of TMP in male and female F344 rats. Toxicol Appl Pharmacol 91: 171-181, 1987.

17. Olson CT, Yu KO, Hopson DW, Serv MP: Identification of urinary metabolites of the nephrotoxic hydrocarbon 2,2,4-trimethylpentane in male rats. Biochem Biophys Res Commun 130: 313-316, 1985.

18. Olson CT, Yu KO, Serv MP: Metabolism of nephrotoxic cis- and trans- decalin in Fischer-344 rats. J Toxicol Environ Health 18: 285-292, 1986.

19. Lock EA, Charbonneau M, Strasser J, Swenberg JA, Bus JS: 2,2,4- Trimethylpentane-induced nephropathy. II. The reversible binding of a TMP metabolite to a renal protein fraction containing alpha-2-microglobulin. Toxicol Appl Pharmacol 91: 182-192, 1987.

20. Henningsen GM, Yu KO, Salomon RA, Ferry MJ, Lopez I, Roberts J, Servé MP: The metabolism of t-butylcyclohexane in Fischer-344 male rats with hyaline droplet nephropathy. Tox Lett 39: 313-318, 1987.

21. Henningsen GM, Salomon RA, Yu KO, Lopez I, Roberts J, Servé MP: Metabolism of nephrotoxic isopropylcyclohexane in male Fischer 344 rats. J Toxicol Environ Health 24: 19-25, 1987.

22. Servé MP, Llewelyn BM, Yu KO, McDonald GM: Metabolism and nephrotoxicity of tetralin in male Fischer 344 rats. J Toxicol Environ Health 26: 267-275, 1989.

PART X
THE MECHANISM OF RENAL CANCER AND ANTI-CANCER THERAPY

45

CELLULAR AND MOLECULAR MECHANISMS OF CHEMICALLY INDUCED RENAL CARCINOGENESIS

J.C. Barrett and *J.E. Huff*

National Institute of Environmental Health Sciences, P.O. Box 12233, Research Triangle Park, North Carolina 27709

INTRODUCTION

There are approximately 18,000 to 20,000 new cases of cancer of the kidney diagnosed each year in the United States (1,2). This malignancy, which represents 2-3% of all cancers, ranks 11th in cancer incidence and results in 8,000 fatalities annually in the United States (2). White males have the highest mortality rate, equalling 4.8/100,000, whereas black females have the lowest rate (2.0/100,000). About 85 percent of the kidney cancers diagnosed are renal cell cancers, which occur with a prevalence two to three times greater in men than in women (3); for 1986 the incidence per 100,000 was 11.3 for white males, 11.9 for black males, 5.6 for white females, and 5.6 for black females (2). The trends in kidney cancers in the United States are rising; percentage age-adjusted increases (per 100,000) in mortality (and in incidence) are for whites 9.1% (21.7%), for blacks 38.2% (19.8%), for white males 7.8% (21.3%), for black males 44.0% (26.9%), for white females 13.5% (23.0%), and for black females 34.7% (11.9%) (2).

Renal cancers in humans have been associated with exposures to tobacco smoke, certain environmental and occupational factors (e.g., coke oven emissions and possibly the rubber industry byproducts), and therapeutic agents, particularly analgesic mixtures containing phenacetin (4). There is also a suspicion that arsenic may be related to cancers of the kidney (5). However, most causes of kidney cancers are unknown and these malignancies remain an important human health problem. The true incidence and mortality rates in the human population may be considerably higher than the rates now reported. As proof of this assertion, relatively few autopsies are conducted routinely in the United States and for those that are reported, over one third disclose undiagnosed cancers (6). According to Holm-Nielsen and Olsen (7), renal adenomas (minute cortical foci of proliferating tubular or papillary epithelium) occur frequently and are present in 15-22% of all adult kidneys. Whether these small tumours (2-3 mm, up to 6 mm) should be regarded as carcinomas or as benign precursors of renal cell carcinomas remains controversial (7).

A better understanding of the environmental and genetic factors involved in renal cancer and the underlying molecular mechanisms of nephrotoxicity and carcinogenicity is clearly needed. In this paper, we focus on three areas that impact on this problem. First, using the National Toxicology Program's database of two-year carcinogenesis studies in rodents (8-10), we report on (a) the frequency at which the kidney is a target site for chemical carcinogenesis relative to other cancer sites, (b) the species and sex differences and similarities in kidney carcinogenesis, (c) the types of chemicals that are kidney carcinogens, and (d) the correlation of cancer at this site with the presence of hyaline droplets, an indicator of alpha-2μ-globulin accumulation. Second, we review in general the molecular genetics of cancer with an emphasis on renal cancers, including a discussion of the possible roles of oncogenes and tumour suppressor genes in kidney cancers. Finally, we discuss two proposed mechanisms for renal carcinogens (11,12), i.e., hormonal effects of oestrogens and the induction of regenerative cell proliferation by nephrotoxins.

CHEMICALS SHOWN TO CAUSE RENAL CANCER IN TWO-YEAR RODENT BIOASSAYS

Nearly 400 chemicals have been evaluated for long-term toxicity and carcinogenicity by the National Cancer Institute and by the National Toxicology Program (9,13-15). Complete two-year studies in male and female Fischer 344 rats and B6C3F1 mice have been completed on 375 chemicals (8-10). About one-half of the chemicals studied were considered to be carcinogenic in at least one organ or tissue in at least one sex of one species (8,10).

As shown in Table 1 for the rat, the liver was the most common site for cancer induction in these bioassays (16), while the kidney was the second most common site for cancer induction (17). In 358 long-term carcinogenesis studies, 26 chemicals (approximately 7%) induced kidney cancers. Twenty-three chemicals were positive in the male rat and eight in the female rat. This 3:1 sex-related prevalence ratio compares directly with the relative incidences seen in male and female humans (2,3). In mice, however, the kidney was not among the top ten sites of tumour formation following treatment with these chemicals (Table 2). Only three chemicals increased the incidence of renal cancers in male mice and one in female mice. Clearly, species and sex differences exist in the induction of kidney cancers in long-term carcinogen bioassays. Nonetheless, the overall concordance of responses in rats and mice for cancer induction in any organs or tissues was 74% (18).

When the data for rats and mice are combined (Table 3), the kidney, along with the lung and mammary gland, is the third most common cancer site; seven percent of the chemicals (26 of 358) were positive in the kidney. Each carcinogenesis bioassay usually involved four experiments. In 1,328 total experiments with 358 chemicals, approximately 3% were positive for kidney cancers. This is relatively infrequent considering that most chemicals are excreted via the kidney. It is perhaps remarkable that this is not a more common cancer site.

Table 1. Top Ten Tumour Sites Observed in Rats in Long-Term Chemical Carcinogenesis Studies of 358 Chemicals

Male Rats		Female Rats	
Tumour site	Positive chemicals	Tumour site	Positive chemicals
Liver	34	Liver	28
KIDNEY	23	Mammary Gland	21
Forestomach	15	Thyroid Gland	13
Thyroid Gland	14	Zymbal Gland	12
Zymbal Gland	13	Forestomach	11
Skin	11	Urinary Bladder	10
Hematopoietic System	11	Hematopoietic System	9
Urinary Bladder	10	KIDNEY	8
Nasal Cavity/Turbinates	8	Uterus	8
Pancreas	7	Nasal Cavity/Turbinates	7
Spleen	7	Clitoral Gland	7

Table 2. Top Ten Tumour Sites Observed in Mice in Long-Term Carcinogenesis Studies of 358 Chemicals

Male Mice		Female Mice	
Tumour site	Positive chemicals	Tumour site	Positive chemicals
Liver	57	Liver	73
Lung	18	Lung	20
Forestomach	15	Forestomach	16
Hematopoietic System	8	Hematopoietic System	13
Circulatory System	8	Circulatory System	9
Thyroid Gland	6	Mammary Gland	9
Harderian Gland	5	Thyroid Gland	8
Adrenal Gland	4	Ovary	8
Six sites tied*	3	Uterus	7
		Harderian Gland	6
[KIDNEY]	3	[KIDNEY]	1

*Skin, Kidney, Nasal Cavity/Turbinates, Preputial Gland, Urinary Bladder, and Heart.

Table 3. Top Ten Tumour Sites Observed in Long-Term Chemical Carcinogenesis Studies of 358 Chemicals

	Positive chemicals	% Positive among 358 chemicals	No. of chemicals positive in				% Positive responses in in 1328 experiments[a]
			Male rats	Female rats	Male mice	Female mice	
1. Liver	97	27	33	28	55	71	14
2. Hematopoietic system	28	8	11	9	8	13	3
3. Kidney	26	7	23	8	3	1	3
Lung	26	7	3	4	17	19	3
Mammary gland	26	7	3	21	0	9	2
4. Forestomach	23	6	15	11	15	16	4
5. Thyroid gland	19	5	13	12	6	7	3
6. Urinary bladder	16	4	10	10	3	3	2
7. Uterus	15	4	0	8	0	7	1
Zymbal gland	15	4	13	12	1	2	2
8. Adrenal gland	13	4	5	3	4	4	1
Circulatory system	13	4	4	2	8	9	2
9. Skin	12	3	11	4	3	2	1
10. Subcutaneous tissue	9	2	6	3	0	3	1
		Totals:	150 (26%)	135 (23%)	123 (21%)	166 (29%)	42

[a]358 chemicals were tested generally in two species and both sexes. However, some were tested only in one species. Also, inadequate experiments have been deleted, resulting in 1328 experiments instead of 1432 (4 x 358).

Table 4. Chemicals Producing Neoplasms of the Kidney in 31 of 358 Long-term Carcinogenesis Studies (1976-summer 1990) [a]

	Chemical	Route	MR	FR	MM	FM
1.	1-Amino-2-methylanthraquinone	Feed	+	[+]	-	[+]
2.	2-Amino-4-nitrophenol	Gav	(+)	-	-	-
3	o-Anisidine hydrochloride	Feed	+	[+]	[+]	[+]
4	Aspirin, phenacetin, and caffeine	Feed	-	(E)	-	-
5	Benzofuran	Gav	-	(+)	[+]	[+]
6	Bromodichloromethane	Gav	+	+	(+)	[+]
7	Chlorinated paraffins: C12, 60% chlorine	Gav	+	[+]	[+]	[+]
8	Chlorothalonil	Feed	(+)	(+)	-	-
9	C.I. acid orange 3	Gav	-	(+)	-	-
10	Cinnamyl anthranilate	Feed	+	-	[+]	[+]
11	1,4-Dichlorobenzene (p-dichlorobenzene)[b]	Gav	(+)	-	[+]	[+]
12	Dimethylmethylphosphonate[b]	Gav	(+)	- I	-	
13	Furosemide	Feed	E	-	-	[+]
14	Hexachloroethane[b,c]	Gav	(+)	-	NO	NO
	Hexachloroethane[c]	Gav	-	-	[+]	[+]
15	Hydroquinone	Gav	(+)	[+]	-	[+]
16	Isophorone[b]	Gav	+	-	[E]	-
17	d-Limonene[b]	Gav	(+)	-	-	-
18	8-Methoxypsoralen	Gav	+	-	NO	NO
19	alpha-Methylbenzyl alcohol	Gav	(+)	-	-	-
20	Methyldopa sesquihydrate	Feed	-	-	(E)	-
21	Mirex	Feed	+	[+]	NO	NO
22	Monuron	Feed	+	-	-	-
23	Nitrilotriacetic acid (NTA)	Feed	+	[+]	(+)	(+)
24	Nitrilotriacetic acid trisodium monohydrate [c]	Feed	+	+	NO	NO
	Nitrilotriacetic acid trisodium monohydrate [c]	Feed	(E)[d]	[E]	-	
25	Nitrofurantoin	Feed	(+)	-	-	[+]
26	Ochratoxin A	Gav	(+)	+	NO	NO
27	Phenylbutazone	Gav	(E)	(+)	[+]	-
28	N-Phenyl-2-naphthylamine	Feed	-	-	-	(E)
29	Tetrachlorethylene[b]	Inhal	+	[+]	[+]	[+]
30	Trichloroethylene (without epichlorohydrin)	Gav	(I)	(I)	NO	NO
31	Tris(2,3-dibromopropyl)phosphate	Feed	(±)	(±)	±	[±]
	Experiment Totals: + or (+) = 35		23	8	3	1
	E, (E), or (I) = 7		3	2	1	1

[a]Tris(2-chloroethyl)phosphate has since been shown to cause benign tumors (adenomas) of the kidney tubular cell in both sexes of rats (+)(+). [b]Presence of hyaline droplets. [c]Considered to be a single chemical study. [d]Not counted in totals because positive response in companion study.
+ : Positive in kidney and other sites.
(+): Kidney is the only positive site in this sex/species experiment.
[+]: Sites other than kidney were positive in this sex/species experiment.
E : Equivocal for kidney and another site.
(E): Equivocal increases in kidney cancers.
[E]: Tumor sites other than kidney showed equivocal increases.
I : Experiment considered inadequate for evaluation.
(I): Experiment considered inadequate for evaluation; yet, tubular cell neoplasms of the kidney were observed in exposed rats.
- : No increases in tumor response.
NO: Not studied in that particular species.

Table 4 lists the individual chemicals for which a positive or equivocal response in the kidney was observed in these studies. The 14 chemicals that induced tumours in the kidney and other sites are indicated as +, the 12 chemicals that induced tumours only in the kidney are indicated as (+), and chemicals that were positive in the bioassay, but induced tumours at sites other than the kidney, are indicated as [+]. Equivocal (or inadequate) increases of kidney tumours occurred with three chemicals in male rats, two in male rats, one in male mice, and one in female mice.

Most of the tumours induced were tubular cell kidney cancers. The incidence of only this type of kidney neoplasm was increased in 29 of 35 experiments. Transitional cell renal cancers were observed with two chemicals (ortho-anisidine hydrochloride and C.I. acid orange 3), and both types of cancer were seen with three other chemicals (dimethylmethylphosphonate, nitrilotriacetic acid, and phenylbutazone) and one mixture (aspirin-phenacetin-caffeine).

In these studies with rats and mice, pronounced sex differences existed in chemically induced kidney tumours. Approximately three times as many chemicals induced tumours in male animals compared to female animals. Because the incidence of renal cancers in humans is also consistently higher in males than females (2,3), the basis for the sex differences is a key question in kidney carcinogenesis. Interestingly, three chemicals uniquely induced kidney tumours in female rats only. One proposed sex-related difference in rats is the greater concentration of alpha-2μ-globulin in male rats than in female rats (19-20). We will return later to the possible role of this protein in kidney carcinogenesis, but we have noted with an asterisk the chemically exposed animals in the bioassays that displayed hyaline droplets, which represent accumulation of alpha-2μ-globulin protein (19-23) (Table 4). Six chemicals were considered positive for hyaline droplets: 1,4-dichlorobenzene, dimethylmethylphosphonate, hexachloroethane, isophorone, d-limonene, and tetrachloroethylene. Other chemicals (e.g., unleaded gasoline and penta-

chlorothane) not included in this study also induce kidney tumours and alpha-2μ-globulin production in male rats (19,22).

Of the six chemicals that were observed to induce hyaline droplets in the NTP bioassays, only **d**-limonene caused tubular cell neoplasms without inducing other positive responses in male or female rats or in mice (21,24). Therefore, most of these chemicals are not exclusively male rat kidney carcinogens. This is important in terms of understanding the mechanisms of carcinogenicity by these chemicals. Also, the majority of chemicals that show a sex difference in the induction of kidney cancers have not been shown to increase alpha-2μ-globulin production in the kidney. Therefore, the basis for the higher prevalence of tumours in the male is not established.

The results of the NTP/NCI carcinogen bioassays and the chemicals that are renal carcinogens are summarized in Table 5.

Interestingly, the majority of kidney tumours in rodents occur late in life, i.e., at 25-26 months of age when two-year exposure experiments are ended; yet the ability of kidney tissue homogenates to metabolically activate procarcinogens to mutagenic metabolites or to the ultimate carcinogen decreases with age by approximately 35-65%. For example, Suiter et al. (25) showed using S-9 extract from kidney homogenates that Fischer 344 male rats had substantially decreased activation capacity for aflatoxin B_1 using Salmonella typhimurium TA 98. They observed 104 revertants with kidney homogenates from animals at 4 months of age, 97 revertants with kidney homogenates from animals at 12 months, and 44 revertants with kidney homogenates from animals at 26 months.

MOLECULAR AND CELLULAR BASIS OF RENAL CARCINOGENESIS

Both anatomically and functionally, the mammalian kidney is an extremely complex organ (26). The basic unit of the kidney, and the site of most chemically associated toxicity, is the nephron (11,27) and in particular the tubular

Table 5. Summary of NTP/NCI Chemical Carcinogenesis Studies

1. Nearly 400 chemicals evaluated (375 two-species studies fully completed).

2. About 50% of the chemicals are carcinogenic in at least one sex of one species group. Approximately 30% of the individual sex-species experiments show a positive carcinogenic response in one or more organs.

3. Of the positive studies, only 31 of 358 chemicals (8.5%) showed induction of renal cancers (23 in male rat, 8 in female rat, 3 in male mice, and 1 in female mice). From 1328 experiments, 35 positive responses (2.6%) were observed.

4. Most chemicals increased tubular cell neoplasms (29 of 35 experiments), whereas transitional cell neoplasms were seen in 4 of 35 experiments (orthoanisidine hydrochloride, C.I. acid orange 3, mirex, phenylbutazone) and neoplasms of both cell types were seen in 2 of 35 experiments (dimethylmethylphosphonate, nitrilotinacetic acid trisodium monohydrate).

5. Six chemicals induced hyaline droplets (likely indicator of increases in alpha-2-microglobulin): 1,4,dichloroben-zene, dimethylmethylphosphonate, hexachloroethane, isophorone, d-limonene, and tetrachloroethylene.

6. Of these 6, only d-limonene caused tubular cell neoplasms of the kidney without inducing other positive responses in male or female rats or in mice.

cells. Renal cell tumours of the tubular parenchyma are the dominant kidney neoplasms in humans, rats, mice, and hamsters (28).

Age-related nephropathy of the renal tubule cells commonly occurs more often and with greater severity in male rats than in female rats. Despite consistent and disruptive age-related nephropathy seen in rodents (29), the spontaneous incidence of renal cancer is a rare event, less than 0.5% in Fischer rats (30). Likewise, as we reported above, relatively few chemicals induce neoplasia of the kidney. The two chemical classes that most commonly cause non-neoplastic chronic renal disease and tumours in rodents are aromatic amines and organohalides (30), especially the short chain halogenated aliphatic hydrocarbons.

The multistep process of carcinogenesis can be operationally divided into three stages: initiation, promotion, and progression (31,32). Initiation represents the first heritable alteration that predisposes a cell to neoplastic transformation. Promotion is the clonal expansion of initiated cells, and progression is the acquisition of other changes that are required for a cell to become fully malignant. Since it is now believed that more than two genetic changes are required for a neoplastic conversion of a cell

(33), additional clonal evolutions most likely occur in the later stages, making the distinction between promotion and progression sometimes difficult (31). However, it is important not to confuse these two processes. Promotion involves the multiplication of the initiated cell, whereas progression involves the acquisition of additional, heritable changes in the initiated cell. Promotion may lead to progression, although with a low frequency. Progression can occur as a direct result of the chemical on the initiated cell. Increasing the target size of the population of initiated cells by promotional mechanisms will also increase the probability of secondary spontaneous or chemically induced changes and therefore progression. The rate limiting step in malignant development is the acquisition of additional genetic changes in an initiated cell. Therefore, a weak mutagenic effect may be equally or more important than a potent tumour promoting effect for cancer development.

A better way to define the multistep process of carcinogenesis is to identify the genetic alterations in tumour cells and attempt to determine how chemical carcinogens affect the neoplastic process leading to these changes. There is now convincing evidence (33) to suggest the

Table 6. Two Classes of Genes Involved in Carcinogenesis

Proto-oncogenes	Tumor Suppressor Genes
Involved in cellular growth and differentiation	Function unknown but possibly involved in cellular growth and differentiation (negative regulators of cell growth?)
Family of genes exists.	Family of genes exists.
Must be activated (quantitatively or qualitaively) in cancers	Must be inactivated, lost and/or mutated in cancers
Mutational activation by point mutation, chromosome translocation, or gene amplification	Mutational inactivation by chromosome loss, chromosome deletion, point mutation, somatic recombination, or gene conversion
Little evidence for involvement in hereditary cancers	Clear evidence for involvement in hereditary and nonhereditary cancers

importance of two distinct classes of genes in the carcinogenic process, proto-oncogenes and tumour suppressor genes (Table 6). Proto-oncogenes are a family of cellular genes with at least 40 members, which appear to be involved in normal cellular growth and development; activation or inappropriate expression of these genes results in proliferative signals involved in neoplastic growth (34,35). On the other hand, tumour suppressor genes are less well defined, but the function of these genes may also be in the control of normal cell division and possibly differentiation (36-39). For a tumour cell to emerge, these suppressor genes must be inactivated or lost (40,41). The number of tumour suppressor genes is unknown, but multiple genes are likely to exist (36,42,43).

Oncogenes have received a great deal of attention since their discovery, and the importance of their role in carcinogenesis has been adequately demonstrated in many systems (33-35). However, considerable evidence exists that tumour suppressor genes play an equally important role in neoplastic development (36,39-45). Recent data from our laboratory have shown that in the multistep process of carcinogen-induced neoplastic transformation of Syrian hamster embryo cells in culture, the loss of a tumour suppressor gene

function is an essential step; without the loss of this gene activity, multiple oncogenes are unable to neoplastically transform the cells (45,46).

One important distinction between oncogenes and tumour suppressor genes is the difference in the mechanisms by which carcinogens act upon these genes (Table 6). Proto-oncogenes must be activated to influence carcinogenesis. This activation event may be a qualitative or quantitative alteration caused by point mutations, chromosome rearrangement, or gene amplification (Table 6). In contrast, tumour suppressor genes must be inactivated for the tumourigenic phenotype to be expressed. This inactivation may result from chromosome loss, chromosome or gene deletion, recombination, gene conversion, or point mutation. The mechanisms of action and dose responses of carcinogens in inducing the different types of genetic changes required for the activation of proto-oncogenes or inactivation of tumour suppressor genes may vary considerably.

ONCOGENE ACTIVATION AND TUMOUR SUPPRESSOR GENE INACTIVATION IN RENAL CANCERS

Although several studies have examined the alterations in expression or activation of oncogenes in adult renal carcinomas, there are no consistent findings. Fujita et al. (47) reported activated H-**ras** oncogenes in 2 out of 16 human primary kidney tumours. In a study of 51 renal carcinomas, Nanus et al. (48) found a **ras** oncogene mutation in a single tumour. Although activation of the H-**ras** oncogene is infrequent, in those few tumours where it occurs, it probably plays a role in the renal cell transformation. In fact, Nanus et al. (49) have shown that ras-containing retroviral infection can induce transformation-related alterations in human proximal tubule cells.

Reports of overexpression of different oncogenes in renal cell carcinomas, including **myc** (50-54), c-**erbB**-1 (51), **fos** (52), and **fes** (52,53) have been published. However, it is not clear whether this overexpression is simply related to alterations in cell proliferative rates in the normal versus tumour cells. Overexpressions of transforming growth factors alpha and beta have also been reported in renal adenocarcinomas (55,56).

Karyotypic analyses have shown that gains of chromosome 7 (trisomy 7 and tetrasomy 7) are frequent in renal tumours (57-61). Trisomy 7 is commonly seen in a wide variety of premalignant tumours of different tissues (57), and chromosome 7 has been associated with expression of invasive and malignant properties in mouse-human cell hybrids (62). Several genes possibly involved in growth (e.g., epidermal growth factor receptor and the alpha-chain of the platelet-derived growth factor) are located on this chromosome. Therefore, an increased dosage of this chromosome may have a significant role in the development of renal and other cancers.

The involvement of tumour suppressor genes in renal cancers is clearly established. Deletion of genes on the short arm of chromosome 3 are commonly observed in renal cell carcinomas (57) and have led to the hypothesis that a tumour suppressor gene resides in this region. Cohen et al. (63) first reported a balanced translocation involving chromosomes 3 and 8, t(3:8)(p21;q24) in the lymphocytes of individuals with familial renal cell carcinoma. Pathak

et al. (64) found a translocation between chromosomes 3 and 11, t(3;11)(p13or14;p15) in cancer cells of an individual with renal cell carcinoma. Numerous karyotypic analyses of renal cell carcinomas have shown losses of genetic material on 3p due to chromosome translocations, terminal and interstitial deletions of 3p, and loss of an entire chromosome 3 (56-58,65-72). Von Hippel-Lindau disease, an autosomal dominant disorder with inherited susceptibility to various forms of cancer including renal cell carcinoma, has also been linked to chromosome 3p (73).

Recently, Oshimura and colleagues (74) have shown that the introduction of a normal chromosome 3 into a renal cell carcinoma suppresses the tumourigenicity of these cells. This provides an elegant demonstration that chromosome 3 encodes a tumour suppressor gene for this cancer. Loss or inactivation of this gene must be a key step in the development of this malignancy.

EXAMPLES OF MECHANISTIC STUDIES OF RENAL CARCINOGENS

In this section we discuss a few possible mechanisms involved with induction of renal tumours in experimental animals by two types of carcinogenic influences.

Hormone Induced Hamster Kidney Tumours

The kidney is a primary target for the carcinogenic action of steroidal or stilbene oestrogens in Syrian hamsters. This system has been extensively studied and offers some interesting insights that may have relevance to other renal carcinogens. Renal tumours can be induced by diethylstilboestrol and other oestrogens at a high incidence (90-100%) in intact and castrated male hamsters or in ovariectomized females (75,76). Tumours arise within 6-8 months after treatment and are hormonally dependent. The hamster renal cortex has four steroid hormone receptors (oestrogen, progesterone, androgen and glucocorticoid), indicating that it is a hormone sensitive tissue (76). The oestrogen and progesterone receptors are induced by carcinogenic hormones.

However, not all oestrogens are carcinogenic in this model. Tumours are induced equally well by diethylstilboestrol (DES) and 17beta-oestradiol, but ethinyl oestradiol has weak carcinogenic activity even though it competes equally well with DES and 17beta-oestradiol for oestrogen receptor binding and has activity similar to carcinogenic oestrogens in inducing renal progesterone receptor and serum prolactin levels (77).

Similarly, 2-fluoroestradiol does not induce renal clear-cell carcinomas in hamsters despite its oestrogenic potency (78). One hypothesis to explain the weak carcinogenicity of ethinyl oestradiol and 2-fluoroestradiol is that they are poor substrates for catechol oestrogen formation (78-80). A better correlation with carcinogenic activity is observed with metabolism to catechol oestrogen than with oestrogenic activity in this tumour model (78-83). Also, catechol oestrogen formation is greater in kidneys of animals susceptible to the carcinogenic activity of oestrogens (79), and agents that inhibit catechol formation in the kidney, such as alpha-naphthoflavone and ascorbic acid, inhibit oestrogen-induced renal tumours (79,83). Taken together, these data support the hypothesis that metabolism of oestrogens plays a role in their carcinogenic activity, analogous to the metabolic activation requirement for other chemical carcinogens (83,84). This hypothesis also explains certain observations on oestrogen-induced hepatocellular carcinoma in Syrian hamsters. Synthetic oestrogens only induce these tumours when the animals are treated with alpha-naphthoflavone, which alters the metabolism of oestrogens in this tissue (85). Thus, in addition to effects on cell proliferation in oestrogen-dependent tissues, oestrogens may have the ability to induce heritable alterations in cells. The latter may result from reactive intermediates following metabolic activation (86,87). Further support for a mutational activity of hormones is provided from in vitro studies.

DES and 17beta-oestradiol have been reported to be inactive in several mutational assays with bacteria (87-89) and mammalian cells (90-93). However, there are some reports that indicate genotoxic effects of DES in certain test systems, which seem to conflict with the negative findings cited earlier. DES is mutagenic in mouse lymphoma cells in the presence of a rat liver postmitochondrial supernatant (94,95). Martin et al. (96) reported that DES induces unscheduled DNA synthesis (UDS) in HeLa cells treated in the presence of rat liver homogenate, while Althaus et al. (97) found no effect of DES on UDS in cultured rat hepatocytes. Rudiger et al. (89) reported that DES and some of its metabolites induce sister-chromatid exchanges in human fibroblasts in culture. Hill and Wolff (98) observed that DES induced sister chromatid exchanges in lymphocytes from pregnant and premenopausal women, but had only a small effect on lymphocytes from men and postmenopausal women. On the other hand, Abe and Sasaki (99) failed to observe an effect of DES on sister chromatid exchanges in Chinese hamster cells.

Tsutsui et al. (100) have proposed that those seemingly conflicting results can be explained on the basis of the metabolic activation systems used in the study. These authors have shown that UDS induction in Syrian hamster embryo cells, which have some endogenous metabolizing activity for DES (101), depends on an exogenous metabolizing system. Under these conditions, qualitative and quantitative differences in the metabolism of DES occur, resulting in the generation of DNA-damaging and mutagenic species (100). These results are possibly consistent with the in vivo results in the hamster kidney and liver discussed (77,79,80,102). Liehr et al. (103) have recently reported the detection of covalent DES-induced adducts in the DNA of hamster kidneys preceding DES-induced tumours in this organ. These adducts were target organ-specific, but occurred at a very low level. This possibly represents evidence for tumour initiation by DES via damage to cellular macromolecules (103). Based on the entirety of the results available to date, one has to conclude that DES has some mutagenic activity depending on metabolic activation, and this may be important in its target organ-specific carcinogenic action (82-84,103).

In addition to the DNA-damaging and mutagenic activity described earlier, DES as well as 17beta-oestradiol can induce genetic changes by another mechanism not involving direct DNA interaction. Several groups have recently shown that DES binds with microtubules and disrupts tubulin assembly in vivo and in vitro (104-106). Estrogens, including DES and 17beta-oestradiol, can cause mitotic abnormalities and numerical chromosome changes in a variety of cells (107-120). The interaction with microtubules provides a biochemical mechanism for the aneuploidy-inducing effects of oestrogens (119).

The possible importance of aneuploidy induction in hormonal carcinogenesis is suggested from cell-transformation studies. DES has been shown to induce morphological and neoplastic transformation of normal diploid Syrian hamster embryo cells in culture (121,122). Transformation is induced in the absence of measurable gene mutations (121) or DNA damage (100). However, treatment of the cells with DES does result in induction of numerical chromosome changes, which has the same cell-cycle dependence and dose-response curve as the induction of cell transformation (118). Chromosome analysis of the transformed cells also indicates that aneuploidy is a key event in this process (107,119). The aneuploid nature of in vivo dysplasias studied in DES-exposed females is also consistent with this mechanism, playing a role in the development of human tumours (123).

In conclusion, it is clear that hormones affect carcinogenesis by epigenetic mechanisms such as stimulation of cell proliferation of oestrogen-dependent target cells; in addition, significant evidence exists that certain oestrogens can also cause genetic alterations by different mechanisms. These findings indicate that hormonal carcinogenesis is most likely a result of the interplay of genetic and epigenetic factors.

Alpha-2μ-globulin and Rat Kidney Tumours

Recent observations in chemically induced experimental carcinogenesis have led to a proposal that an important mechanism in tubular cell carcinogenesis in rat kidneys involves the protein alpha-2μ-globulin. Alpha-2μ-globulin is an anionic protein of molecular weight 19,700 that is synthesized in the liver of mature male rats under hormonal control (23). Approximately 50 milligrams of protein are synthesized each day (124). It is readily filtered by the kidney because of its low molecular weight. Alpha-2μ-globulin is a member of a super family of proteins of similar molecular weight and homologous amino acid sequence. Persner et al. (125) have identified 13 members of the alpha-2μ-globulin super family of proteins from rats, mice, humans, and other species. The function of six of these proteins is unknown (including alpha-2μ-globulin), but the function of the other members involves transport of different lipids, including odorants, cholesterol, and retinol (125). Cavaggioni et al. (126) have suggested that alpha-2μ-globulin is a transport protein for rat pheromones. Alpha-2-globulin is believed to play a role in the neophrotoxicity of a number of chemicals or their metabolites that apparently bind to this protein, resulting in its retention in the kidney. It has been suggested that the conjugate of alpha-2μ-globulin and the chemical is more difficult to metabolize than alpha-2μ-globulin alone. This protein then accumulates in the P2 segment of the kidney tubule and results in the formation of hyaline droplets. This alpha-2μ-globulin overload results in increased cell death and increased regenerative cell replication. It is proposed further that this increased cell proliferation is the inductive stimulus for neoplastic transformation of the renal tubular cell (19,22,127-129).

This hypothesis is attractive because it can be used to explain the sex and species differences for the nephrotoxicity and renal carcinogenesis of a number of compounds that bind alpha-2μ-globulin including components of unleaded gasoline, **d**-limonene, and decalin (19,22,127-129). In total, over 20 chemicals have been shown to induce renal hyaline droplet formation

(19,22). Since this protein is made in the liver of male rats under testosterone control but to a much smaller degree in female rats (1/4 to 1/6 that of male rats) and not at all in male or female mice (19,23,124), this binding protein can be used to explain why many of these chemicals affect only the male rat kidney and fail to cause similar effects in female rats or in mice.

There are two aspects of this hypothesis that are important to keep in mind. First, this hypothesis only explains the effects of the chemicals in the kidney and cannot explain the carcinogenic effects of most of these chemicals at other sites. So far, only d-limonene appears to induce only tubular cell neoplasms of the male rat kidney and no other tumours in rats or mice (19,22). Secondly, the hypothesis has two parts. First is that the alpha-2μ-globulin results in accumulation of the chemical in the target organ, a pharmacokinetic effect. The second is the nature of the carcinogenic response. Every effect of the chemical that is dose-dependent should show the same alpha-2μ-globulin dependent sex and species effect. Increased cell proliferation is but one of a number of hypotheses that might explain the resultant cell transformation. Cell proliferation per se may be a carcinogenic stimulus, but there are arguments for and against this hypothesis, which are discussed in the next section.

ROLE OF CELL PROLIFERATION IN CARCINOGENESIS

The multistep/multigene model of carcinogenesis provides insights into many important features of cancer development and carcinogen risk assessment (31). The necessity for a malignant cell to acquire multiple heritable alterations at independent genetic loci explains, at least in part, the long latency period for cancer (33). This model also explains how noncarcinogenic substances can influence the carcinogenic process and why some mutagens have no detectable carcinogenic activity (132). Insults that influence the clonal proliferation of initiated or other intermediate cells in the neoplastic process may increase the risk of cancer development in exposed populations

Table 7. Mechanisms by Which a Substance Can Influence Multistep Carcinogenesis

1. By inducing heritable mutation in a critical gene.

2. By inducing heritable, epigenetic change in a critical gene.

3. By increasing clonal expansion of a cell with a heritable alteration in a critical gene, allowing for increased probability of additional events.

(130,131). Conversely, insults that are highly mutagenic but do not induce cell proliferation may be noncarcinogenic (132). The carcinogenicity of these chemicals will, however, depend on the state of proliferation of the target tissue. For example, polycyclic hydrocarbons, aromatic amines, and nitrosoamines are highly carcinogenic in the livers of neonatal mice while the same exposures are noncarcinogenic or weakly carcinogenic in the liver when given to adult mice due to a lack of cell proliferation (133).

There are three primary mechanisms by which a substance can influence the multistep, carcinogenic process (Table 7). A substance can induce a heritable alteration in one or more critical genes in the multistep process. This heritable change may have either a genetic or epigenetic basis (132). Although considerable insight into the mechanisms of genetic changes by chemicals exists, little is known about the mechanisms of carcinogen-induced epigenetic, heritable changes (132). A third mechanism by which a substance can influence multistep carcinogenesis is the facilitation of clonal expansion of an initiated or intermediate cell, which increases the probability of additional, spontaneous (mutation or epigenetic) heritable changes (130).

This third mechanism has led to the hypothesis that cell proliferation per se may be carcinogenic and carcinogens that increase cell proliferation may be operating exclusively by this mechanism (131,134). The failure to detect measurable mutagenic activity associated with nongenotoxic carcinogens indicates that these chemicals act by alternative mechanisms of action, increased cell proliferation being one. This hypothesis is supported by the fact that most, if not all, cancers arise "spontaneously" in at least some species. Normal cell division results in a low level of spontaneous errors during DNA replication, and spontaneous DNA damage can result from cytosine deamination at body temperatures, from oxidative damage associated with normal cellular physiology, and from mutagens in food (134,135). Thus, mutations occur "spontaneously" from normal cellular processes and increased cell proliferation without induction of mutations may result in a significant increase in the number of cancers in chemically exposed animals.

However, before cell proliferation per se can be accepted as the causative mechanism for certain carcinogens, several facts must be considered. First, many toxic and/or hyperplastic stimuli are noncarcinogenic (136,137). A review of the literature in this field and further studies of noncarcinogenic, toxic agents are needed. Second, cell division occurs frequently in all organisms (Table 8); therefore, it is not clear whether cell division is limiting in the carcinogenic process. This, of course, depends on the target tissue; furthermore, cell division of initiated or intermediate cells may occur at quite different rates than division of normal cells. Finally, the observation that multiple mutations are involved in the development of many neoplasms may suggest that even a weak mutagenic response, which is below the level of detection of current assays, is sufficient to influence the neoplastic process in a specific target tissue. This is a plausible explanation for certain nongenotoxic carcinogens, some of which may act by indirect mutagenic processes.

CONCLUSIONS

This article is not meant to represent a comprehensive review of renal carcinogenesis but rather reflects the authors' experimental find-

Table 8. Evidence Against Cell Proliferation per se Being Carcinogenic

1. Many toxic and/or hyperplastic stimuli are noncarcinogenic.

2. Cell division occurs frequently in all organisms[a]

    1 egg produces 10^{14} cells in adult organism
    10^{13} cells still capable of cell division
    10^7 cell divisions/sec occur in adult organism
    10^6 cell divisions/sec in intestine

3. Multiple mutations (3-4?) are required for a normal cell to evolve into a cancer cell.

[a]Reference David Prescott, personal communication.

ings and thoughts on this topic. A number of important factors of renal carcinogenesis strike us as particularly important and require additional experimental investigation. These include the following observations:

1. The kidney rarely shows neoplasia in chemically exposed animals, despite the fact that most chemicals are excreted via the kidney.

2. Although the kidney of most mammals (and in particular laboratory rodents) exhibit age-related pathology, this organ has a low incidence of "spontaneous" neoplasms.

3. Clear sex differences exist in the incidence of renal cancer in rodents and humans. This cannot be explained at present solely on the basis of alpha-2μ-globulin. Species differences in the susceptibility of malignancy also are not fully understood. Familial predisposition to this cancer exists in humans, but few animal models to study this exist (138).

A further understanding of renal carcinogenesis requires elucidation of the molecular basis for this malignancy. Given the rapid advances in defining the molecular genetics of oncogenes and tumour suppressor genes in this and other cancers, it is hoped that new insights into this field will be available in the near future. With this information in hand, it will be possible to better understand how chemicals influence this process. The mechanisms involved will undoubtedly be complicated, and it will require interaction between nephrotoxicologists and cancer biologists to fully explain the development of this disease in this important organ.

ACKNOWLEDGEMENTS

We thank Drs. Dale Sandler and Roger Wiseman, National Institute of Environmental Health Sciences, and Dr. Cheryl Walker, Chemical Institute of Toxicology, for their critical reviews and comments. We also thank Joseph Cirvello, National Institute of Environmental Health Sciences, for compiling the information used in Tables 1-4 and Sandy Sandberg for typing and editorial assistance. Participation in this symposium was supported by the UK Cancer Research Campaign.

REFERENCES

1. National Cancer Institute: Cancer Rates and Risks. NIH Publication No. 85-691, 1985, pp. 118-121.

2. National Cancer Institute: Cancer Statistics Review 1973-1986. 1989.

3. Paulson DE, Perez CA, Anderson T: Cancer of the kidney and ureter. In: DeVita VT Jr, Hellman S, Rosenberg SA (eds); Cancer: Principles & Practice of Oncology. Philadelphia, JB Lippincott, 1985, pp. 895-1007.

4. IARC. 1987. IARC monographs on the evaluation of carcinogenic risks to humans. Overall evaluations of carcinogenicity: an updating of IARC Monographs Vols 1-42, Suppl 7. International Agency for Research on Cancer, Lyon.

5. Tomatis L, Aitio A, Wilbourn J, Shuker L: Human carcinogens so far identified. Jpn J Cancer Res 80:795-807, 1989.

6. Silverberg SG: The autopsy and cancer. Arch Pathol Lab Med 108:476- 478, 1984.

7. Holm-Nielsen P, Olsen TS: Ultrastructure of renal adenoma. Ultrastruct Pathol 12:27-39, 1988.

8. Haseman JK, Huff JE, Zeiger E, McConnell EE: Comparative results of 327 chemical carcinogenicity studies. Environ Health Perspect 74:229-235, 1987.

9. Huff JE, McConnell EE, Hasemen JK, et al.: Carcinogenesis studies: results of 398 experiments on 104 chemicals from the U.S. National Toxicology Program. Ann N Y Acad Sci 534:1-30, 1988.

10. Huff JE, Eustis SL, Haseman JK: Occurrence and relevance of chemically induced benign neoplasma in long-term carcinogenicity studies. Cancer Metastasis Rev 8:1-21, 1989.

11. Bach PH, Gregg NJ: Experimentally induced renal papillary necrosis and upper urothelial carcinoma. In: Richter GW, Solez K (eds); International Review of Experimental Pathology. New York, Academic Press, 1988, pp. 1-54.

12. Lipsky MM Jr, Trump BF: Chemically induced renal epithelial neoplasia in experimental animals. In: Richter GW, Solez K (eds); International Review of Experimental Pathology. New York, Academic Press, 1988, pp. 357-383.

13. Chu KC, Cueto C Jr, Ward JM: Factors in the evaluation of 200 National Cancer Institute carcinogen bioassays. J Toxicol Environ Health 8:251-280, 1981.

14. Griesemer RA, Cueto C Jr: Toward a classification scheme for degrees of experimental evidence for the carcinogenicity of chemicals for animals. In: Montesano R, Tomatis BL (eds); Molecular and Cellular Aspects of Carcinogenic Screening Tests. IARC Scientific Pubications No. 27, Lyon, 1980, pp. 259-281.

15. Chhabra RS, Huff JE, Schwetz BS, Selkirk J: An overview of prechronic and chronic toxicity/carcinogenicity experimental study designs and criteria used by the National Toxicology Program. Environ Health Perspect, in press.

16. Maronpot RR, Haseman JK, Boorman GA, Eustis SE, Rao GN, Huff JE: Liver lesions

in B6C3F1 mice: The National Toxicology Program, experience and position. Arch Toxicol (Suppl) 10:10-26, 1987.

17. Huff JE, Bucher JR, Haseman JK, Cirvello JD: Chemicals associated with site-specific neoplasia evaluated in 1328 long-term carcinogenesis experiments in laboratory rodents. Environ Health Perspect (submitted).

18. Haseman JK, Huff JE: Species correlation in long-term carcinogenesis studies. Cancer Lett 37:125-132, 1987.

19. U.S. Environmental Protection Agency, Risk Assessment Forum: Alpha-2μ-globulin: synthesis, accumulation in hyaline droplets of the renal proximal tubule, and association with the production of renal toxicity and renal tumor formation in the male rat. In press.

20. Borghoff SJ, Short BG, Swenberg JA: Biochemical mechanisms and pathobiology of 2-globulin nephropathy. Annu Rev Pharmacol Toxicol 30:349-367, 1990.

21. NTP Technical Report on the toxicology and carcinogenesis studies of **d**-limonene (CAS No. 5989-27-5) in F344/N rats and B6C3F1 mice (gavage studies). NIH Publication No. 90-2802, January 1990.

22. Swenberg JA, Short B, Borghoff S, Strasser J, Charbonneau M: The comparative pathobiology of alpha-2μ-globulin nephropathy. Toxicol Applied Pharmacol 97:35-46, 1989.

23. Roy AK, Neuhaus OW: Androgenic control of a sex-dependent protein in the rat. Nature (London) 214:618-620, 1967.

24. Lehman-McKeeman LD, Rodriguez PA, Takigiku R, Caudill D, Fey ML: **d**-Limonene-induced male rat-specific nephrotoxicity: evaluation of the association between **d**-limonene and alpha-2μ-globulin. Toxicol Applied Pharmacol 99:250-259, 1989.

25. Suiter MA, Churnesky P, Jayaraj A, Richardson A: Metabolic activation of chemical carcinogens by kidney from rats and mice of various ages. Comp Biochem Physiol 73C:435-438, 1982.

26. Hook JB, Hewitt WR: Toxic responses of the kidney. In: Klaassen CD, Amdur MO, Doull J (eds); Casarett and Doull's Toxicology: The Basic Science of Poisons. New York, Macmillan, 1986, pp. 310-329.

27. Berndt WO, Davis ME: Renal methods for toxicology. In: Hayes AW (ed); Principles and Methods of Toxicology. New York, Raven Press, 1989, pp. 629-648.

28. Hiasa Y, Ito N: Experimental induction of renal tumors. CRC Crit Rev Toxicol 17:279-343, 1987.

29. Goldstein RS, Tarloff JB, Hook JB: Age-related nephropathy in laboratory rats. FASEB J 2:2241-2251, 1988.

30. Kluwe WM, Abdo KM, Huff J: Chronic kidney disease and organic chemical evaluations of causal relationships in humans and experimental animals. Fundam Appl Toxicol 4:889-901, 1984.

31. Boyd JA, Barrett JC: Genetic and cellular basis of multistep carcinogenesis. Pharmacol Ther 46:469-486, 1990.

32. Pitot HC, Goldsworthy T, Moran S: The natural history of carcinogenesis: implication of experimental carcinogenesis in the genesis of human cancer. J Supramol Struct Cell Biochem 17:133-146, 1981.

33. Barrett JC, Fletcher WF: Cellular and molecular mechanisms of multistep carcinogenesis in cell culture models. In: Barrett JC, (ed); Mechanisms of Environmental Carcinogenesis: Multistep Models of Carcinogenesis. Boca Raton, CRC Press, 1987, vol. II, 1987, pp. 73-116.

34. Weinberg RA: The action of oncogenes in the cytoplasm and nucleus. Science 230:770-776, 1985.

35. Bishop JM. The molecular genetics of cancer. Science 235:305-311, 1987.

36. Knudson AG Jr: Hereditary cancer, oncogenes, and antioncogenes. Cancer Res 45:1437-1443, 1985.

37. Koi M, Afshari C, Annab LA, Barrett JC: Role of a tumor suppressor gene in the negative control of anchorage-independent growth of Syrian hamster cells. Proc Natl Acad Sci USA 86:8773-8777, 1989.

38. Weissman BE: Suppression of tumorigenicity in mammalian cell hybrids. In: Barrett JC (ed); Mechanisms of Environmental Carcinogenesis. Boca Raton, CRC Press, 1987, pp. 31-45.

39. Klein G. The approaching era of the tumor suppressor genes. Science 238:1539-1545, 1987.

40. Cavanee WK, Dryja TP, Phillips RA, et al.: Expression of recessive alleles by chromosomal mechanisms in retinoblastoma. Nature 305:779-784, 1983.

41. Murphree AL, Benedict WF: Retinoblastoma: clues to human oncogenesis. Science 223:1028-1033, 1984.

42. Gateff E: Malignant neoplasms of genetic origin in **Drosophila melanogaster**. Science 200:1448-1459, 1978.

43. Vogelstein B, Fearon ER, Hamilton SR, et al.: Genetic alterations during colorectal tumor development. N Eng J Med 319:525-532, 1988.

44. Sager R: Genetic expression of tumor formation: new frontier in cancer research. Cancer Res 46:1573-1580, 1986.

45. Koi M, Barrett JC: Loss of tumor-suppressive function during chemically induced neoplastic progression of Syrian hamster embryo cells. Proc Natl Acad Sci USA 83:5992-5996, 1986.

46. Oshimura M, Gilmer TM, Barrett JC: Nonrandom loss of chromosome 15 in Syrian hamster tumours induced by v-Ha-**ras** plus v-**myc** oncogenes. Nature 316:636-639, 1985.

47. Fujita J, Kraus MH, Onoue H, et al.: Activated H-**ras** oncogenes in human kidney tumors. Cancer Res 48:5251-5255, 1988.

48. Nanus DM, Mentle IR, Motzer RJ, et al.: Infrequent **ras** oncogene point mutations in renal cell carcinoma. J Urol 143:175-178, 1990.

49. Nanus DM, Ebrahim SAD, Bander NH, et al.: Transformation of human kidney proximal tubule cells by **ras**-containing retroviruses. J Exp Med 169:953-972, 1989.

50. Kinouchi T, Saiki S, Naoe T, et al.: Correlation of c-**myc** expression with nuclear pleomorphism in human renal cell carcinoma. Cancer Res 49:3627-3630, 1989.

51. Yao M, Shuin T, Misaki H, Kubota Y: Enhanced expression of c-myc and epidermal growth factor receptor (C-**erbB**-1) genes in primary human renal cancer. Cancer Res 48:6753-6757, 1988.

52. Slamon DJ, deKernion JB, Verma IM, Cline MJ: Expression of cellular oncogenes in human malignancies. Science 224:236-262, 1984.

53. Karthaus H-FM, Schalken JA, Feitz WFJ, et al: Expression of the human fes cellular oncogene in renal cell tumors. Urol Res 14:123-127, 1986.

54. Tatosyan AG, Galetzki SA, Kisseljova NP, et al.: Oncogene expression in human tumors. Int J Cancer 35:731-736, 1985.

55. Derynck R, Goeddel DV, Ullrich A, et al.: Synthesis of messenger RNAs for transforming growth factors alpha and beta and the epidermal growth factor receptor by human tumors. Cancer Res 47:707-712, 1987.

56. Gomella LG, Sargent ER, Wade TP, et al.: Expression of transforming growth factor in normal human adult kidney and enhanced expression of transforming growth factors alpha and beta-1 in renal cell carcinoma. Cancer Res 49:6972-6975, 1989.

57. Walter TA, Berger CS, Sandberg AA: The cytogenetics of renal tumors. Where do we

stand, where do we go? Cancer Genet Cytogenet 43:15-34, 1989.

58. Weaver DJ, Michalski K, Miles J: Cytogenetic analysis in renal cell carcinoma: Correlation with tumor aggressiveness. Cancer Res 48:2887-2889, 1988.

59. Cin PD, Sandberg AA, Huben R, et al.: New cytogenetic subtype of renal tumors. Cancer Genet Cytogenet 32:313, 1988.

60. Miles J, Michalski K, Kouba M, Weaver DJ: Genomic defects in nonfamilial renal cell carcinoma. Possible specific chromosome change. Cancer Genet Cytogenet 34:135-142, 1988.

61. Vanni R, Nieddu M, Scarpa RM, et al.: Trisomy 7 in a case of transitional cell carcinoma of the kidney. Cancer Genet Cytogenet 41:149-151, 1989.

62. Collard JG, van de Poll M, Scheffer A, et al.: Location of genes involved in invasion and metastasis on human chromosome 7. Cancer Res 47:666-6670, 1987.

63. Cohen AJ, Li FP, Berg S, Marchetto DJ, et al.: Hereditary renal cell carcinoma associated with a chromosomal translocation. N Engl J Med 301:592-596, 1979.

64. Pathak S, Strong LC, Ferrell RE, Trindade A: Familial renal cell carcinoma with a 3:11 chromosome translocation limited to tumor cells. Science 217:939-941, 1982.

65. Drabkin HA, Bradley C, Hart I, et al.: Translocation of c-myc in the hereditary renal cell carcinoma associated with a t(3;8)(p14.2;q24.13) chromosomal translocation. Proc Natl Acad Sci USA 82:6980-6984, 1985.

66. Harris P, Morton CC, Guglielmi P, et al.: Mapping by chromosome sorting of several gene probes, including c-myc, to the derivative chromosomes of a 3;8 translocation associated with familial renal cancer. Cytometry 7:589-594, 1986.

67. Yoshida MA, Ohyashiki K, Ochi H, et al.: Cytogenetic studies of tumor tissue from patients with nonfamilial renal cell carcinoma. Cancer Res 46:2139-2147, 1986.

68. Teyssier JR, Henry I, Dozier C, et al.: Recurrent deletion of the short arm of chromosome 3 in human renal cell carcinoma: Shift of the c-raf 1 locus. J Natl Cancer Inst 77:1187-1195, 1986.

69. Kovacs G, Sz Gcs S, De Riese W, Baumgartel H: Specific chromosome aberration in human renal cell carcinoma. Int J Cancer 40:171-178, 1987.

70. Teyssier J-R: What is the genetic mechanism underlying the recurrent 3p rearrangement in human renal cell carcinoma? Cancer Genet Cytogenet 25:179-181, 1987.

71. van der Hout AH, Kok K, van den Berg A, et al.: Direct molecular analysis of a deletion of 3p in tumors from patients with sporadic renal cell carcinoma. Cancer Genet Cytogenet 32:281-285, 1988.

72. Kovacs G, Frisch S: Clonal chromosome abnormalities in tumor cells from patients with sporadic renal cell carcinomas. Cancer Res 49:651-659, 1989.

73. Seizinger BR, Rouleau GA, Ozelius LJ, et al.: Von Hippel-Lindau disease maps to the region of chromosome 3 associated with renal cell carcinoma. Nature 332:268-269, 1988.

74. Shimizu M, Yokota J, Mori N, et al.: Introduction of normal chromosome 3p modulates the tumorigenicity of a human renal cell line YCR. Oncogene 5:184-194, 1990.

75. Kirkman H, Bacon RL: Estrogen-induced tumors of the kidney. I. Incidence of renal tumors in intact and gonadectomized male golden hamsters treated with diethylstilbestrol. J Nat Cancer Inst 13:745-755, 1952.

76. Li JJ, Li SA, Oberley T, et al.: Estrogen carcinogenicity: hormonal, morphologic and chemical interactions. In: Politzer P, Martin FJ Jr (eds); Chemical Carcinogens. Activation Mechanisms, Structural and Electronic Factors, and Reactivity. New York, Elsevier, 1988, pp. 312-321.

77. Li JJ, Li SA, Klicka JK, et al.: Relative carcinogenic activity of various synthetic and natural estrogens in the Syrian hamster kidney. Cancer Res 43:5200-5204, 1983.

78. Liehr JG: 2-Fluoroestradiol: separation of estrogenicity from carcinogencity. Mol Pharmacol 23:278-281, 1983.

79. Li SA, Klicka JK, Li JJ: Estrogen 2-and 4-hydroxylase activity, catechol estrogen formation, and implication for estrogen carcinogenesis in the hamster kidney. Cancer Res 45:181-185, 1985.

80. Liehr JG: Modulation of estrogen-induced carcinogenesis by chemical modifications. Arch Toxicol 55:119-122, 1983.

81. McLachlan JA, Wong A, Degen GH, Barrett JC: Morphological and neoplastic transformation of Syrian hamster embryo cells by diethylstilbestrol and its analogs. Cancer Res 42:3040-3045, 1982.

82. Purdy RH: Carcinogenic potential of estrogen in some mammalian model system. Prog Cancer Res Ther 31:401-415, 1984.

83. Metzler M, McLachlan JA: Is diethylstilbestrol bioactivated through peroxidase-mediated oxidation? J Environ Pathol Toxicol 1:531-533, 1978.

84. Metzler M, McLachlan JA: The metabolism of diethylstilbestrol. CRC Crit Rev Biochem 10:171-212, 1981.

85. Li JJ, Li SA: High incidence of hepatocellular carcinomas after synthetic estrogen administration in Syrian golden hamsters fed - alpha-naphthoflavone: a new tumor model. J Natl Cancer Inst 73:543-547, 1984.

86. Metzler M: Diethylstilbestrol: reactive metabolites derived from a hormonally active compound. In: Greim H, Jung K, Karmer M, et al. (eds); Biopchemical Basis of Chemical Carcinogenesis. New York, Raven Press, 1984, pp. 69-75.

87. Glatt HR, Metzler M, Oesch F: Diethylstilbestrol and 11 derivatives: a mutagenicity study with **Salmonella typhimurium**. Mutat Res 67:113-121, 1979.

88. Lang R, Redmann U: Non-mutagenicity of some sex hormones in the Ames **Salmonella**/microsome mutagenicity test. Mutat Res 67:361-365, 1979.

89. Rudiger HW, Haenisch F, Metzler M, et al.: Metabolites of diethylstil- bestrol induce sister chromatid exchanges in human cultured fibroblasts. Nature 281:392-394, 1979.

90. Barrett JC, McLachlan JA, Elmore E: Inability of diethylstilbestrol to induce 6-thioguanine-resistant mutants and to inhibit metabolic cooperation of V79 Chinese hamster cells. Mutat Res 107:427-432, 1982.

91. Barrett JC, Wong A, McLachlan JA: Diethylstilbestrol induces neoplastic transformation without measurable gene mutation at two loci. Science 212:1402-1404, 1981.

92. Drevon C, Piccoli C, Montesano R: Mutagenicity assays of estrogenic hormones in mammalian cells. Mutat Res 89:83-90, 1981.

93. Kinsella AR: Elimination of metabolic cooperation and the induction of sister chromatid exchanges are not properties common to all promoting or co-carcinogenic agents. Carcinogenesis 3:499-503, 1982.

94. Myhr B, Bowers L, Caspary WJ: Assays for the induction of gene mutations at the thymidine kinase locus in L5178Y mouse lymphoma cells in culture. In: Ashby J, deSerres FJ (eds); Progress in Mutation Research, Amsterdam, Elsevier, 1985, pp. 555-568.

95. Clive D, Johnson KO, Spector JFS, et al.: Validation and characterization of the L5178Y TK+/- mouse lymphoma mutagen assay system. Mutat Res 59:61-108, 1979.

96. Martin CN, McDermid AC, Garner RC: Testing of known carcinogens and non-carcinogens for their ability to induce unscheduled DNA synthesis in HeLa cells. Cancer Res 38:2621-2627, 1978.

97. Althaus FR, Lawrence SD, Sattler GL, et al.: Chemical quantification of unscheduled

DNA synthesis in cultured hepatocytes as an assay for the rapid screening of potential chemical carcinogens. Cancer Res 42:3010-3015, 1982.

98. Hill A, Wolff S: Increased induction of sister chromatid exchange by diethylstilbestrol in lymphocytes from pregnant and premenopausal women. Cancer Res 42:893-896, 1982.

99. Abe S, Sasaki M: Chromosome aberrations and sister chromatid exchanges in Chinese hamster cells exposed to various chemicals. J Natl Cancer Inst 58:1635-1641, 1977.

100. Tsutsui T, Degen GH, Schiffman D, et al.: Dependence of exogenous metabolic activation for induction of unscheduled DNA synthesis in Syrian hamster embryo cells by diethylstilbestrol and related compounds. Cancer Res 44:184-189, 1984.

101. Degen GH, Wong A, Eling TE, et al.: Involvement of prostaglandin synthetase in the peroxidative metabolism of diethylstilbestrol in Syrian hamster embryo fibroblast cell cultures. Cancer Res 43:992-996, 1983.

102. Naylor PH, Rabinder NK, Loring JM, Villee CA: The estrogen- induced/dependent renal adenocarcinoma of the Syrian hamster. In: McKerns KW (ed); Regulation of Gene Expression by Hormones. New York, Plenum Press, 1983, pp. 39-50.

103. Liehr JG, Randerath K, Randerath E: Target organ-specific covalent DNA damage preceding diethylstilbestrol-induced carcinogenesis. Carcinogenesis 6:1067-1069, 1985.

104. Sato Y, Murai T, Tsumuraya M, et al.: Disruptive effects of diethylstilbestrol on microtubules. Gann 75:1046-1048, 1984.

105. Sharp DC, Parry JM: Diethylstilbestrol: the binding and effects of diethylstilbestrol upon the polymerisation of purified microtubule protein in vitro. Carcinogenesis 6:865-872, 1985.

106. Tucker RW, Barrett JC: Decreased numbers of spindle and cytoplasmic microtubules in hamster embryo cells treated with a carcinogen, diethylstilbestrol. Cancer Res 42:2088-2095, 1986.

107. Oshimura M, Barrett JC: Chemically induced aneuploidy in mammalian cells: Mechanisms and biological significance in cancer. Environ Mutagen 8:129-159, 1986.

108. Kuchler RJ, Graver RC: Effects of natural estrogens on L strain fibroblasts in tissue culture. Proc Soc Exp Biol Med 110:287-292, 1982.

109. Rao PN, Engelberg J: Structural specificity of estrogens in the induction of mitotic chromatid non-disjunction in Hela cells. Exp Cell Res 48:71-81, 1967.

110. Lycette RR, Whyte S, Chapman CJ: Aneuploid effects of oestradiol on cultured human synovial cells. N Z Med J 72:114-117, 1970.

111. Chrisman CL: Aneuploidy in mouse embryos induced by diethylstilbestrol diphosphate. Teratology 9:229-232, 1974.

112. Chrisman CL, Hinkle LL: Induction of aneuploidy in mouse bone marrow cells with diethylstilbestrol-diphosphate. Can J Genet Cytol 16:831-835, 1974.

113. Chrisman CL, Lasley JF: Effects of diethylstilbestrol diphosphate on mitotic activity in bovine lymphocyte cultures. Cytologia 40:817-821, 1975.

114. McGaughey RW: The culture of pig oocytes in minimal medium, and the influence of progesterone and estradiol-17beta on meiotic maturation. Endocrinology 100:39-45, 1977.

115. Sawada M, Ishidate M Jr: Colchicine-like effect of diethylstilbestrol (DES) on mammalian cells in vitro. Mutat Res 57:175-182, 1978.

116. Parry JM, Parry EM, Barrett JC: Tumour promoters induce mitotic aneuploidy in yeast. Nature 294:263-265, 1981.

117. Danford N, Parry JM: Abnormal cell division in cultured human fibroblasts after ex-

posure to diethylstilbestrol. Mutat Res 103:379-383, 1982.

118. Tsutsui T, Maizumi H, McLachlan JA, Barrett JC: Aneuploidy induction and cell transformation by diethylstilbestrol: a possible chromosome mechanism in carcinogenesis. Cancer Res 43:3814-3821, 1983.

119. Barrett JC, Oshimura M, Tsutsui T, Tanaka N: Role of aneuploidy in early and late stages of neoplastic progression of Syrian hamster embryo cells in culture. In: Dellarco VL, Voytek RE, Hollaender A (eds); Aneuploidy: Etiology and Mechanisms. New York, Plenum Press, 1985, pp. 523-538.

120. Satya-Prakash KL, Hsu TC, Wheeler WJ: Metaphase arrest, anaphase recovery and aneuploidy induction in cultured Chinese hamster cells following exposure to mitotic arrestants. Anticancer Res 4:351-356, 1984.

121. Barrett JC, Wong A, McLachlan JA: Diethylstilbestrol induces neoplastic transformation without measurable gene mutation at two loci. Science 212:1402-1404, 1981.

122. Pienta RJ: Transformation of Syrian hamster embryo cells by diverse chemicals and correlation with their reported carcinogenic and mutagenic activities. In: deSerres FJ (ed); Chemical Mutagens. New York, Plenum Publishing Corp, 1980, pp. 175-202.

123. Fu YS, Robboy SJ, Prat J: Nuclear DNA study of vaginal and cervical squamous cell abnormalities in DES-exposed progeny. J Obstet Gynecol 52:129-137, 1978.

124. Neuhaus OW, Flory W, Biswas N, Hollerman CE: Urinary excretion of alpha-2µ-globulin and albumin by adult male rats following treatment with nephrotoxic agents. Nephron 28:133-140, 1981.

125. Pevsner J, Reed RR, Feinstein PG, Synder SH: Molecular cloning of odorant-binding protein: member of a ligand carrier family. Science 241:336-339, 1988.

126. Cavaggioni A, Sorbl RT, Heen JN, Pappin DJC, Findlay CBC: Homology between the pyrazine-binding protein from nasal mucosa and major urinary proteins. FEBS Lett 212:225-226, 1987.

127. Halder CA, Holdsworth CE, Cockrell BY, Piccirillo VJ: Hydrocarbon nephropathy in male rats: identification of the nephrotoxic components of unleaded gasoline. Toxicol Indust Health 1:67-87, 1985.

128. HEI: An update on gasoline vapor exposure and human cancer. An evaluation of scientific information published between 1985 and 1987. Health Effects Institute, Report of the Institute's Health Review Committee, January 6, 1988.

129. Goldsworthy TL, Lyght O, Burnett VL, Popp JA: Potential role of alpha-2µ-globulin, protein droplet accumulation, and cell replication in the renal carcinogenicity of rats exposed to trichloroethylene, perchloroethylene, and pentachloroethane. Toxicol Appl Pharmacol 96:367-379, 1988.

130. Moolgavkar SH, Knudson AG Jr: Mutation and cancer: A model for human carcinogenesis. J Natl Cancer Inst 66:1037-1052, 1981.

131. Clayson DB, Nera EA, Lok E: The potential for the use of cell proliferation studies in carcinogen risk assessment. Regul Toxicol Pharmacol 9:284-295, 1989.

132. Barrett JC: A multistep model for neoplastic development: role of genetic and epigenetic changes. In: Barrett JC (ed); Mechanisms of Environmental Carcinogenesis: Multistep Models of Carcinogenesis. Boca Raton, CRC Press, 1987, vol. II, pp. 117-126.

133. Vesselinovitch SD, Rao KVN, Mihailovich N: Neoplastic response of mouse tissue during perinatal age periods and its significance in chemical carcinogenesis. J Natl Cancer Inst 51:239-245, 1979.

134. Ames BN: Endogenous oxidative DNA damage, aging, and cancer. Free Rad Res Comms 7:121-128, 1989.

135. Loeb LA: Endogenous carcinogenesis: Molecular oncology into the twenty-first century. Presidential Address. Cancer Res 49, 5489-5496, 1989.

136. Hoel DG, Haseman JK, Hogan MD, et al.: The impact of toxicity on carcinogenicity studies: implications for risk assessment. Carcinogenesis 9:2045-2052, 1988.

137. Ledda-Columbano GM, Columbano A, Curto M, et al.: Further evidence that mitogen-induced proliferation does not support the formation of enzyme-altered islands in rat liver by carcinogens. Carcinogenesis 10:847-850, 1989.

138. Eker R, Mossige J, Johannessen JV, Aars H: Hereditary renal adenomas and adenocarcinomas in rats. Diagnostic Histopathology 4:99-110, 1981.

46

PATHOGENESIS OF RADIATION NEPHROPATHY: A FUNCTIONAL AND MORPHOLOGICAL ASSESSMENT

M. Wooldridge (1), D. Campling (2), M.E.C. Robbins (2) and J.W. Hopewell (2)

MRC Radiobiology Unit, Chilton, Didcot, Oxon OX11 0RD UK (1), CRC Normal Tissue Radiobiology Research Group, Research Institute (University of Oxford), Churchill Hospital, Oxford OX3 7LJ UK (2)

INTRODUCTION

In the radiotherapeutic treatment of pelvic and abdominal tumours the dose that can be safely administered to the patient is limited by the response of the normal tissues included in the treatment area. The kidney is one of the most radiosensitive of these organs, a total dose of 20Gy being considered to be the upper limit of tolerance (1). Acute radiation nephritis, or to give it its more correct terminology radiation nephropathy, usually presents after a latent period of some 6 to 12 months. The clinical picture is one of oedema, dypsnoea, headaches, moderate hypertension and anaemia. The latter has been characterised as a normochromic normocytic anaemia (2). Experimental studies have shown reductions in GFR and ERPF within several weeks of irradiation (3,4); an early decrease in GFR and ERPF has also been noted in patients, both during and after radiotherapy (5). Thus the latent period represents the period during which renal damage remains sub-clinical. This appears to be followed by a chronic progressive reduction in function, which, if the radiation dose is great enough, can be life-threatening.

The precise pathophysiologic mechanisms responsible for the development of radiation nephropathy are ill-defined. Studies of changes in renal morphology should, ideally, help ascertain the cell type(s) at risk and, in conjuction with functional data, provide a basis for understanding the pathogenesis of radiation nephropathy and developing rational protocols for treating and preventing the development of radiation nephropathy. This study describes the functional and morphological changes seen in irradiated pig kidneys. Since the pig and man have essentially identical kidneys (6), experimental observations in the pig may be of direct clinical application.

METHODS

A total of 23 Large White female pigs, approximately 45 weeks old, were entered into the functional arm of the study. Both kidneys were irradiated in 19 animals, the remaining 4 pigs acted as unirradiated age-matched controls. Groups of 3-7 animals were irradiated with single doses of either 7.8, 9.8, 11.9 or 14.0Gy of ^{60}Co gamma rays. All experimental studies were performed with the animals anaesthetized using a gas mixture of 2-3% halothane, ~70% oxygen and ~30% nitrous oxide.

Prior to, and at intervals of 2,4,6,8,12,16,20 and 24 weeks after irradiation, individual kidney GFR and ERPF were measured using 99mTc-DTPA and ^{131}I-hippuran renography (7). Blood samples were also taken at these times to determine the red blood cell count (RBC), the white blood cell count (WBC), the haemoglobin concentration (Hb), the haematocrit (Hct), the mean corpuscular volume (MCV), the mean corpuscular haemoglobin concentration (MCHC) and the platelet number.

Both kidneys of a further 13 age-matched Large White pigs were irradiated with 9.8Gy gamma rays. Groups of these pigs were serially killed at periods up to 24 weeks after irradiation. The kidneys were perfusion-fixed in formol acetic and paraffin-wax embedded. Histological evaluation was performed on 5μm thick sections stained with H&E, PAS, Martius Scarlet Blue (MSB), van Gieson's, and Mallory's.

RESULTS

The time-related changes in individual kidney GFR and ERPF following renal irradiation with 7.8-11.9Gy gamma rays are shown in Figure 1. At 2 weeks after irradiation there was a general increase in GFR, particularly after 11.9Gy. This was followed by a dose-dependent decline in GFR with minimal levels being noted between 8 and 12 weeks after irradiation. From ~12-16 weeks after irradiation there was an apparent recovery, such that by 20-24 weeks after treatment with 7.8Gy gamma rays GFR values were similar or greater than those found in the unirradiated age-matched controls. With higher doses the GFR remained below control values. Since only 1/3 of the pigs irradiated with 14.0Gy gamma rays survived up to 24 weeks after irradiation the results for this group are not shown. The remaining 2 animals died as a consequence of renal failure ~8 weeks after irradiation.

The radiation-induced changes in RBC count, Hb and Hct are shown in Figure 2. All three parameters exhibited a similar pattern of changes i.e. a significant reduction to values less than those of unirradiated age-matched controls within 6-8 weeks of irradiation (p<0.002). There was a dose-dependent decline between 6 and 16 weeks after irradiation; values then plateaued. There was little change in the number of circulating WBCs or platelets following renal irradiation.

Morphological changes

Non-glomerular changes: There was little change evident in the medulla during the experimental period. In the cortex, two weeks after irradiation minimal changes were observed, consisting of focal areas of interstitial fibrosis or tubular atrophy. By 4 weeks these areas were more extensive, and were more apparent in the corticomedullary region, or along the path of the medullary rays. Maximal damage was seen 6 weeks after irradiation. This consisted of severe interstitial fibrosis, tubular atrophy and inflammatory cell infiltrate of both mild diffuse and dense focal patterns. Interstitial fibrosis was seen to involve a complete band of subcapsular tissue of varying depth, with "fingers" of fibrotic tissue which extended deep into the cortex. The damaged area appeared to consist of more than 50% of the cortex. At later times, up to 24 weeks after irradiation, similar but less severe non-glomerular changes were seen.

Glomerular changes: These consisted of progressive increases in PAS positive staining mesangial matrix, glomerular cellularity with clumping of cells and the occasional polymorph, a thickening of the capillary basement membrane and a decrease in the capillary lumina. Thus within 2 weeks of irradiation mild changes in the form of cell clumping and a slight increase in the mesangial matrix were evident. By 4-6 weeks the glomeruli appeared moderately damaged; there was a continuing increase in mesangial matrix and cellularity resulting in a marked lobular pattern. Some capillaries in these lobules were almost completely obliterated, whilst others were only mildly affected. There was some evidence of capillary basement membrane thickening. Between 12-24 weeks glomerular damage became progressively more severe, ranging from pronounced mesangial matrix with little patent capillary lumina, to completely sclerotic end-stage glomeruli. In general the most severely damaged glomeruli were subcapsular in location, although occasionally these were also located in the juxtamedullary region. In these kidneys, where there was a high proportion of severely damaged and sclerotic subcapsular glomeruli, the mildly affected glomeruli appeared to have increased in size relative to glomeruli seen in unirradiated controls.

Vascular changes: Other than those changes in glomerular capillaries described previously little vascular change was apparent.

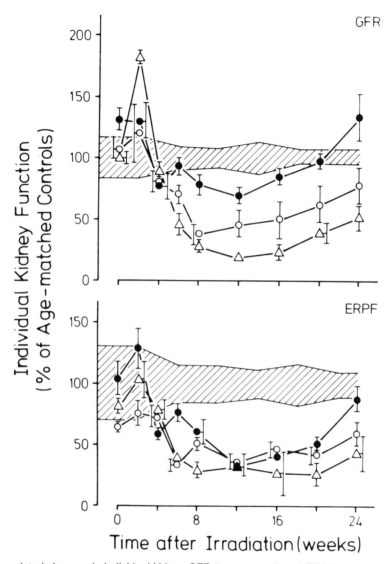

Figure 1. Time-related changes in individual kidney GFR (upper panel) and ERPF (lower panel) after renal irradiation in 45-week-old pigs. 7.8Gy; 9.8Gy; 10.7Gy. The hatched area represents the 95% confidence limits for unirradiated age-matched controls. Error bars represent ± SE.

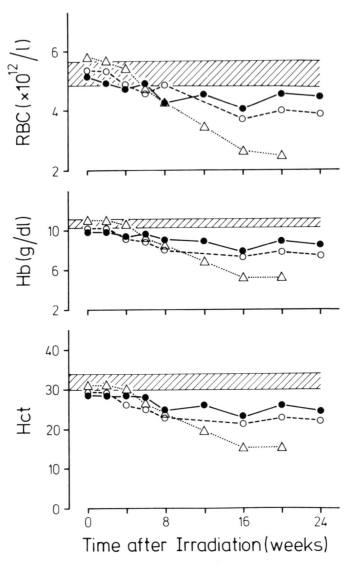

Figure 2. Time-related changes in RBC, Hb and Hct after renal irradiation in 45-week-old pigs. The errors on the mean values were all smaller than the symbols. See Fig. 1 for legend.

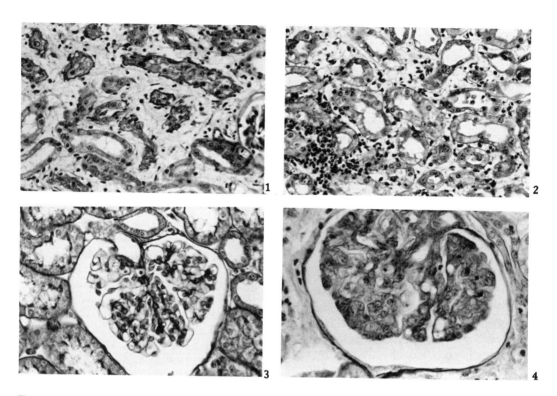

Figure 3. Non-glomerular damage. 1) Severe tubular atrophy, interstitial fibrosis and diffuse lymphocyte infiltration, 6 weeks post-irradiation, PAS, x170. 2) Dense focal infiltration, mainly lymphocytes, and some tubular damage, PAS x170. Glomerular damage: 3) Glomerulus from 9 month old unirradiated control, PAS x270. 4) Glomerulus 20 weeks post-irradiation, with increase in PAS positive material and loss of capillary lumina, PAS x270.

DISCUSSION

These findings indicate that the irradiation of both kidneys, in pigs, with single doses of 7.8-14Gy of gamma rays results in a pronounced dose-dependent decline in both GFR and ERPF within 4-6 weeks of treatment. Associated with these radiation-induced reductions in renal haemodynamics there was a dose-dependent reduction in RBCs, Hb and Hct, such that within 6-8 weeks of irradiation all animals were anaemic. Whereas there was an apparent recovery in renal function between 16-24 weeks, the extent of which depended on the initial radiation dose, the blood parameters remained at the levels seen earlier.

There were also marked morphological changes seen within weeks of irradiation. Interstitial fibrosis and tubular atrophy, first evident 2 weeks after irradiation, increased in severity until maximum damage was observed 6 weeks after irradiation. Although these lesions persisted up until the end of the study i.e. 24 weeks after irradiation, they did not appear to be as severe as those seen at week 6. In contrast to this biphasic response, the glomerular lesions progressively increased with time with respect to their severity. Thus the initial lesions seen 2 weeks after irradiation, which were an increased cellularity and mesangial matrix, had by 24 weeks after irradiation developed into severely damaged glomeruli with extensive mesangial involvement and loss of capillary lumina; sclerotic end-stage glomeruli were also evident.

Similar radiation-induced reductions in renal function, occurring within weeks of irradiation, have been reported in rodents (7,8). However, these have also shown that radiation nephropathy is characterised by a progressive decline in renal function. The current findings of a marked recovery in GFR and ERPF between 12-24 weeks after irradiation would appear at first glance to contradict these earlier data. It should be pointed out, however, that this recovery may be more apparent than real in the sense that GFR and ERPF may increase as a result of hypertrophy of relatively undamaged nephrons. Thus the finding of relatively normal values of renal function 24 weeks after irradiation does not necessarily infer the presence of a repaired organ, but may reflect an organ in which the total number of functioning nephrons has been reduced, with a compensatory response by the remaining nephrons. The present findings of chronic progressive glomerular lesions accompanied by an apparent hypertrophy of mildly damaged glomeruli would seem to support this hypothesis.

Since neither the MCHC or the MCV changed during the study, the anaemia currently observed was characterized as a normochromic normocytic anaemia, similar to that seen clinically (2). It is generally believed that this anaemia reflects a radiation-induced reduction in renal production of erythropoietin (Epo), which leads to a decrease in RBC production. If the site of renal production of Epo could be identified then this might indicate particular areas of the kidney that showed early evidence of radiation-induced damage. Although the identity of these kidney cells remains controversial, recent evidence would seem to favour the tubular epithelium as the site of Epo synthesis (9). It is interesting to note that the maximal tubular damage occurred at the same time as that when the number of RBCs, Hct and Hb

values were significantly decreased below control levels i.e. 6 weeks after irradiation. This may well help substantiate the claims of the tubular epithelium as the site of Epo synthesis. However, it is also worth noting that whereas the morphological data implied some recovery of tubular integrity at later times, this was not associated with any recovery in the blood parameters.

The histological studies show that there are early changes in both the tubules and the glomeruli; the tubular changes seem to peak at 6 weeks after irradiation and then resolve somewhat, while the glomerular changes are progressive and do not exhibit any recovery. Thus it is the glomerular changes which may well be important in the development of radiation nephropathy. Similar glomerular changes to those currently described have been seen clinically (10,11,12), and this has lead to speculation that the glomerular endothelial cell may be the critical target cell. Whilst the present study cannot provide evidence to support this hypothesis, the marked similarities between the functional and morphological findings seen in the pig kidney following irradiation compared with those seen in patients after radiotherapy would suggest that the pig is a useful model for evaluating the pathogenic mechanisms responsible for the development of radiation nephropathy.

ACKNOWLEDGEMENTS

The authors would like to thank Mrs E Whitehouse and Miss S Luckett for the preparation of the histological material.

REFERENCES

1. Greenberger JS, Weichselbaum RR, Carsady JR: Radiation nephropathy. In: Cancer and the kidney. Recelback RE and Garnick MO (eds); Philadelphia, Lea and Febiger, 1982, pp.814-823.

2. Luxton RW: Effects of irradiation on the kidney. In: Diseases of the Kidney, Vol 2. Strauss MB and Walt CG (eds); Boston, Little Brown & Co, 2nd Edition, 1971, pp.1049-1070.

3. Jongejan HTM, van der Kogel A, Provoost AP, et al.: Radiation nephropathy in young and adult rats. Int J Radiat Oncol Biol Phys 13: 225-232, 1987.

4. Hoopes PJ, Gillette EL, Cloran JA, et al.: Radiation nephropathy in the dog. Brit J Cancer 53: Suppl VII, 273--276, 1986.

5. Avioli LV, Lazor MZ, Cotlove E, et al.: Early effects of radiation on renal function in man. Amer J Med 34: 329-337, 1963.

6. Terris JM: Swine as a model in renal physiology and nephrology; an overview. In: Tumbleson ME (ed); Swine in Biomedical Research. New York, Plenum Press, pp. 1673-1693, 1986.

7. Lebesque JV, Stewart FA, Hart G: Analysis of the rate of expression of radiation-induced renal damage and the effects of hyperfractionation. Radio ther Oncol 5: 147-157, 1986.

8. Moulder JE, Holcenberg JS, Kamen BA, et al.: Renal irradiation and the pharmacology and toxicity of methotrexate and cisplatinum. Int J Radiat Oncol Biol Phys 12: 1415-1418, 1986.

9. Caro J, Erslev AJ: Biologic and immunologic erythropoietin in extracts from hypoxic whole rat kidneys and in their glomerular and tubular fractions. J Lab Clin Med 103: 922-931, 1984.

10. Rosen S, Swerdlow MA, Muehrcke RC, et al.: Radiation nephritis: light and electron microscopic observations. Amer J Clin Path 41: 487-502, 1964.

11. Kapur S, Chandra R, Antonvych T: Acute radiation nephritis: light and electron microscopic observations. Arch Pathol Lab Med 101: 469-473, 1977.

12. Bergstein J, Andreoli SP, Provisor AJ, et al.: Radiation nephritis following total-body irradiation and cyclophosphamide in preparation for bone marrow transplantation. Transplantation 41: 63-66, 1986.

47

ENHANCEMENT BY GLUTATHIONE DEPLETION OF CISPLATIN-INDUCED NEPHROTOXICITY IN RATS: EFFECT OF ANTIOXIDANT PRETREATMENT

M. Gemba, T. Matsushita, C. Fujisawa, T. Yamaguchi and Y. Kameyama

Division of Pharmacology, Osaka University of Pharmaceutical Sciences, Kawai, Matsubara, Osaka 580, Japan

INTRODUCTION

Superoxide dismutase and antioxidants have been reported to ameliorate nephrotoxicity caused by the antineoplastic drug cisplatin in experimental animals (1-3). Cisplatin has been shown to increase lipid peroxidation in renal slices in vitro, and the enhanced formation of lipid peroxides is prevented by antioxidants (4,5). It thus has seemed reasonable to expect that free radicals or peroxides participate in the genesis of cisplatin nephrotoxicity. Cellular glutathione (GSH) is important in the protection of cells from free radicals and peroxides (6-8). Depletion of the tissue level of GSH by pretreatment of rats with diethylmaleate (DEM), a GSH depletor that conjugates with GSH (9), results in an increase in the nephrotoxicity of cisplatin as monitored by the level of blood urea nitrogen (BUN) (10). However, pretreatment with another GSH depletor, DL-buthionine-(S,R)-sulfoximine (BSO), which inhibits γ-glutamylcysteine synthetase in the GSH synthetic pathway (11), diminishes the rise in BUN caused by cisplatin (12). The experiments reported here were designed to investigate whether GSH depletion following the use of both DEM and BSO affects cisplatin-induced nephrotoxicity assessed by the measurement of the urinary excretion of certain enzymes, another index of nephrotoxicity. We also wanted to find out whether pretreatment of rats with a radical scavenger alters urinary enzyme excretion induced by cisplatin when the rats have been treated with DEM and BSO.

METHODS

Male Sprague-Dawley rats (mean weight, 200g) received cisplatin intraperitoneally (i.p.) in the dose of 5 mg/kg. A GSH depletor, BSO (50 mg/kg) plus DEM (0.25 ml/kg), was injected i.p. 2 hr before and 6 hr after the single injection of cisplatin. Rats were pretreated i.p. with di-methylthiourea (DMTU), a radical scavenger (13), at the dose of 250 mg/kg/day for 3 consecutive days (at 49, 25, and 1 hr before the cisplatin injection). The animals were kept individually in stainless steel metabolic cages and urine was collected in small test tubes surrounded by ice for 6 hr on days 1, 2, and 3 after the cisplatin injection. Blood, tissues, and urine of rats were used for assays of BUN, GSH, and enzyme activities, respectively. Values are expressed as means ± s.e.

RESULTS

Changes after the injection of cisplatin and GSH depletors in the GSH level in tissues and in the BUN are shown in Tables 1 and 2, respectively. Renal GSH had risen 8 hr after cisplatin injection and remained elevated until 48 hr, but liver GSH was not affected at 48 hr after the injection. Cisplatin and GSH depletors had decreased the renal GSH level at 8 hr, but the level was higher than with cisplatin alone 24 and 48 hr after cisplatin injection. Cisplatin alone did not cause nephrotoxicity, as seen in the BUN, for up to 2 days after the injection. However, nephrotoxicity was induced by cisplatin together with the two GSH depletors.

Table 1. Effect of cisplatin and the GSH depletors BSO and DEM on the GSH level in kidney cortex and liver after injection of cisplatin or its vehicle

	GSH (mmoles/kg tissue)			
	Kidney cortex			Liver
	8 hr	24 hr	48 hr	48 hr
Control	2.59±0.21	2.57±0.18	2.75±0.16	7.11±0.33
Cisplatin	3.83±0.27*	4.22±0.15**	3.72±0.25**	7.02±0.29
Cisplatin with BSO plus DEM	0.56±0.08**,#	5.19±0.31**,#	4.97±0.57**,#	6.18±0.56
BSO plus DEM	1.09±0.10**	3.13±0.17	4.21±0.36**	7.34±0.34

BSO = DL-buthionine-(S,R)-sulfoximine; DEM = diethylmaleate. Results are from at least three experiments. Significantly different from the control value on that time, *$P<0.01$, **$P<0.005$. Significantly different from the group given cisplatin alone, #$P<0.05$.

Table 2. Changes in BUN following the injection of cisplatin in rats treated with the GSH depletors BSO and DEM

	BUN (mg/dl)	
	Day 1	Day 2
Control	15.6±1.3 (9)	15.6±1.0 (7)
Cisplatin	13.5±0.4 (8)	18.6±1.7 (8)
Cisplatin with BSO plus DEM	19.7±2.3 (4)	55.4±19* (5)
BSO plus DEM	18.5±2.3 (4)	15.8±1.6 (5)

The values in parentheses are the number of experiments. Significantly different from the control value on that day, * $p<0.05$.

Figure 1 shows the effect of cisplatin and the GSH depletors on the activity of the excretion of lactate dehydrogenase (LDH) into the urine.

The urinary excretion of LDH had risen 1 day after the injection of cisplatin, and the elevation lasted for the 3 days of the experiment. The increase in the activity of urinary LDH by cisplatin was further enhanced by BSO and DEM. Cisplatin had also increased urine volume and the urinary excretion of both N-acetyl-beta-D-glucosaminidase (NAG) and gamma-glutamyltranspeptidase (GGT) at 2 days after the injection of cisplatin (Table 3). Of these different increases caused by cisplatin, the urinary excretion of NAG was further enhanced by the GSH depletors. The increase in the urinary excretion of LDH and NAG by cisplatin was changed little by the doses used here of BSO or DEM alone, except for the effect of DEM together with cisplatin on the urinary excretion of LDH (Figure 2). The results shown in Figure 3 indicate that treatment of rats with the radical scavenger DMTU tended to overcome the increase in the urinary excretion of LDH and NAG caused by the injection of cisplatin together with the GSH depletors.

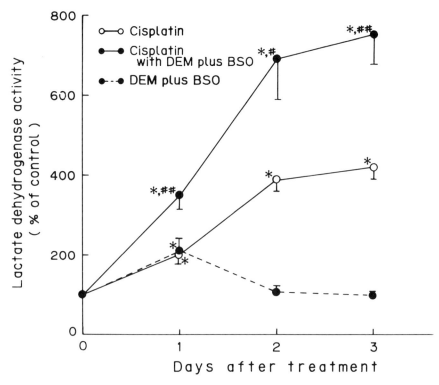

Figure 1. Changes in the excretion of lactate dehydrogenase in urine following an injection of cisplatin in rats treated with the GSH depletors BSO and DEM. Results are from at least six experiments. Significantly different from the control period (days before treatment), *P<0.001. Significantly different from the group given cisplatin alone, #P<0.002, ##P<0.001.

Table 3. Effect of cisplatin and GSH depletors on urine volume and excretion of urinary enzymes 2 days after cisplatin treatment

	Number of rats	Urine and urinary enzymes (% of control)		
		Urine volume	NAG	GGT
Cisplatin	13	163 ± 28*	151 ± 10***	174 ± 32*
Cisplatin with BSO plus DEM	6	162 ± 15***	217 ± 22***,#	175 ± 23**
BSO plus DEM	6	132 ± 26	115 ± 13	183 ± 30**

NAG = N-acetyl-beta-D-glucosaminidase; GGT = gamma-glutamyltranspeptidase; Significantly different from the control period (days before treat ment), *P<0.05, **P<0.02 and ***P<0.005. Significantly different from the group given cisplatin alone, #P<0.01.

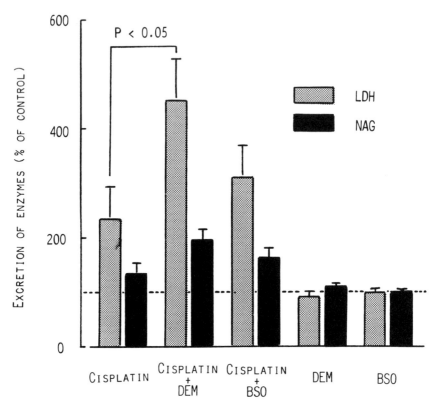

Figure 2. Effect of treatment of rats with BSO or DEM together with cisplatin on the excretion of lactate dehydrogenase (LDH) and N-acetyl-beta-D-glucosaminidase (NAG) in urine two days after cisplatin injection. Results are from six experiments.

DISCUSSION

The increase in the urinary excretion of enzymes by cisplatin is an early event in rats that occurs before the increase in BUN, suggesting that urinary enzyme measurements are a more sensitive index of cisplatin nephrotoxicity than BUN. The administration of cisplatin to rats increased renal GSH. Our results are in agreement with those of other studies (14-16). It has been reported that a GSH depletor DEM enhances the cisplatin-induced increase in BUN (10) but another GSH depletor, BSO, diminishes such increases in BUN induced by cisplatin (12). Here, GSH depletion by BSO and DEM strongly enhanced cisplatin-induced nephrotoxicity when monitored by the urinary excretion of enzymes. Even BSO given by itself

did not diminish the increases in LDH and NAG excretion in urine caused by cisplatin. The discrepancy between the results of the study by Mayer et al. (12) and ours in terms of the effect of BSO on cisplatin nephrotoxicity may be due to the different doses of BSO used. The higher dose of BSO used in the previous study (12) probably diminishes cisplatin-induced nephrotoxicity by a mechanism other than GSH depletion. Such enhancement of urinary enzyme excretion caused by the combination of cisplatin and GSH depletors was reduced by the radical scavenger DMTU. This showed indirectly that the easy generation of free radicals by cisplatin under conditions of GSH depletion may be involved at least in part in cisplatin nephrotoxicity.

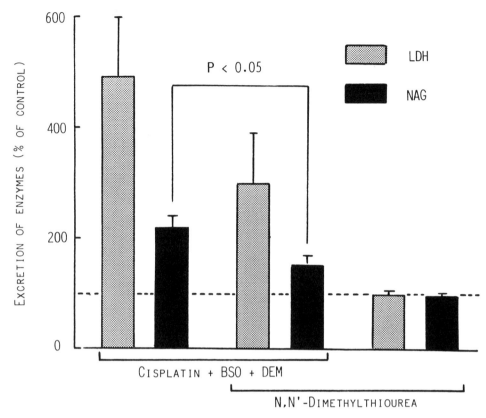

Figure 3. Effect of pretreatment with the radical scavenger N,N'-dimethylthiourea on the excretion of LDH and NAG in urine in rats treated with cisplatin and GSH depletors (BSO + DEM) two days after injection of cisplatin. Results are from at least five experiments.

ACKNOWLEDGEMENTS

We thank Ms. Caroline Latta for help in preparing the manuscript.

REFERENCES

1. McGinness JE, Proctor PH, Demopoulos HB, Hokanson JA, Kirkpatrick DS: Amelioration of cis-platinum nephrotoxicity by Orgotein (superoxide dismutase). Physiol Chem Physics 10: 267-277, 1978.

2. Dobyan DC, Bull JM, Strebel FR, Sunderland BA, Bulger, RE: Protective effects of O-(β-hydroxyethyl)-rutoside on cis-platinum-induced acute renal failure in the rat. Lab Invest 55: 557-563, 1986.

3. Sugihara K, Gemba M: Modification of cisplatin toxicity by antioxidants. Jap J Pharmacol 40: 353-355, 1986.

4. Sugihara K, Nakano S, Gemba M: Effect of cisplatin on in vitro production of lipid peroxides in rat kidney cortex. Jap J Pharmacol 44: 71-76, 1987.

5. Hannemann J, Baumann K: Cisplatin-induced lipid peroxidation and decrease of gluconeogenesis in rat kidney cortex: Different effects of anti-oxidants and radical scavengers. Toxicology 51: 119-132, 1988.

6. Christophersen BO, Formation of monohydroxypolyenic fatty acids from lipid peroxides by a glutathione peroxidase. Biochim Biophys Acta 164: 35-46, 1968.

7. Little C, O'Brien PJ: An intracellular GSH-peroxidase with a lipid peroxide substrate. Biochem Biophys Res Commun 31: 145-150, 1968.

8. Younes M, Siegers C.-P: Lipid peroxidation as a consequence of glutathione depletion in rat and mouse liver. Res Commun Chem Pathol Pharmacol 27: 119-128, 1980.

9. Boyland E, Chasseaud LF: Enzyme-catalysed conjugations of glutathione with unsaturated compounds. Biochem J 104: 95-102, 1967.

10. Litterst CL, Bertolero F, Uozumi J: The role of glutathione and metallothionein in the toxicity and subcellular binding of cisplatin. In: McBrien DCH, Slater TF (eds); Biochemical Mechanisms of Platinum Antitumour Drugs. Oxford, IRL Press, 1986, pp.227-254.

11. Sekura R, Meister A: γ-Glutamylcysteine synthetase. J Biol Chem 252: 2599-2605, 1977.

12. Mayer RD, Lee K, Cockett ATK: Inhibition of cisplatin-induced nephrotoxicity in rats by buthionine sulfoximine, a glutathione synthesis inhibitor. Cancer Chemother Pharmacol 20: 207-210, 1987.

13. Paller MS, Hoidal JR, Ferris TF: Oxygen free radicals in ischemic acute renal failure in the rat. J Clin Invest 74: 1156-1164, 1984.

14. Levi J, Jacobs C, Kalman SM, McTigue M, Weiner MW: Mechanism of cis-platinum nephrotoxicity: I. Effects of sulfhydryl groups in rat kidneys. J Pharmacol Exp Ther 213: 545-550, 1980.

15. Litterst CL, Tong S, Hirokata Y, Siddik ZH: Alterations in hepatic and renal levels of glutathione and activities of glutathione S-transferases from rats treated with cis-dichlorodiammineplatinum-II. Cancer Chemother Pharmacol 8: 67-71, 1982.

16. Leyland-Jones B, Morrow C, Tate S, Urmacher C, Gordon C, Young CW: Cis-diamminedichloroplatinum (II) nephrotoxicity and its relationship to renal gamma-glutamyltranspeptidase and glutathione. Cancer Res 43: 6072-6076, 1983.

48
LIPID PEROXIDATION IN RENAL MICROSOMES OF CISPLATIN-TREATED RATS

J. Hannemann, J. Duwe and K. Baumann

Department of Cell Physiology, Institute of Physiology, University of Hamburg, Grindelallee 117, D-2000 Hamburg 13, FRG

INTRODUCTION

Nephrotoxicity is the major side effect of the anticancer drug cisplatin (cis-dichlorodiammine platinum II - CP) (1). Increased generation of lipid peroxidation-products, like malondialdehyde (MDA), in vivo (2) and in vitro (3), after CP-treatment has been shown. In vivo, MDA-content, determined in the whole kidney of CP-injected rats, rose by day 3 (2). In vitro the renal cortical slices, incubated in CP-media, exhibited a 2-fold elevation in MDA-content (3). Thus, lipid peroxidation and the nephrotoxic effect of CP seem to be associated. But subcellular fractions, which might be target organelles for lipid peroxidation have not been investigated. Microsomes contain the long-chain polyunsaturated fatty acids, arachidonic and linoleic acid in their phospholipid components which are susceptible to peroxidation (4). In the present study, the vulnerability to peroxidation of renal microsomes, isolated from CP-injected rats on day 3, was investigated. Since different incubation conditions alter the stimulation of lipid peroxidation (5), non-enzymatically induced lipid peroxidation, measured as MDA-production, was investigated in two different buffer-systems, phosphate buffer and Tris-HCl-buffer. In addition the effect of different medium-pH- values was investigated. Fe^{2+} or ascorbic acid, or a combination of both were used in various concentrations as pro-oxidants.

METHODS

Male Wistar rats (Winkelmann, Kirchborchen, F.R.G.), weighing 240 - 280 g, received a single intraperitoneal dose of CP (6 mg/kg body weight). Control and CP-injected rats were sacrificed on day 3 (72 hr) by cervical dislocation, and kidneys were removed immediately. The nephrotoxic effect of CP was verified by the determination of kidney weight (day 3) and body weight (day 0, day 3) as well as concentration of plasma-creatinine and blood urea nitrogen (BUN) (day 3, Test-Combinations, Boehringer Mannheim, F.R.G.). Microsomal fractions of kidneys of control and CP-injected rats were prepared according to Albro et al. (6), washed, frozen in liquid nitrogen and stored at -80°C. Microsomal suspensions were assayed for protein content (7).

Renal microsomes were incubated at 37°C under 100%-O_2 atmosphere in sodium phosphate buffer (100 mM, pH 7.2 - 7.8) or Tris-HCl buffer (30 mM, pH 7.4, and 100 mM KCl) for different periods of time (0 - 120 min) in media containing various concentrations of either ascorbic acid (1 mM) or ferric(II)chloride (0.1, 0.4 mM) or both pro-oxidants (1 mM ascorbic acid and 0.1 mM Fe^{2+}). Lipid peroxidation was monitored, after termination of the incubation, by estimating the formation of malondialdehyde (MDA) using the thiobarbituric acid assay (8). The extinction coefficient of $1.56 \times 10^5 .M^{-1}.cm^{-1}$ was used to calculate the MDA concentration of the sample. Statistical analysis were carried out using Student's t test.

RESULTS

A single i.p. injection of 6 mg CP per kg rat body weight resulted in a decrease in body weight and an increase in kidney weight as measured on day 3. Plasma concentration of creatinine and BUN were significantly elevated after 72 hr in CP-injected rats compared to control rats (Table 1).

In an incubation medium containing phosphate buffer (pH 7.8), the addition of 0.1 mM Fe^{2+} showed only a very small stimulatory effect on MDA production in rat renal microsomes (Fig. 1). Ascorbic acid at a concentration of 1 mM induced a time-dependent generation of MDA, which was higher in microsomes isolated from CP-injected rats than in microsomes of control rats (Fig. 1). The highest stimulation was reached by the simultaneous addition of both pro-oxidants (0.1 mM Fe^{2+} and 1 mM ascorbic acid) to the incubation medium (Fig. 1). The MDA-production in microsomes of CP-injected rats was up to 25% higher than in control microsomes. Data from a single experiment are shown on figure 1.

No significant differences in MDA-generation were observed after changing the pH-value of the medium to 7.2, 7.4 or 7.6 (data not shown). Using an incubation medium containing Tris-HCl buffer (pH 7.4), the combination of both pro-oxidants (0.1 mM Fe^{2+} and 1 mM ascorbic acid) showed a similar effect on MDA-production compared to experiments in phosphate

buffer (data not shown). A high rate of MDA-production in renal microsomes was noted, in contrast to experiments in phosphate buffer, after adding Fe^{2+} to an incubation medium containing Tris-HCl buffer (Fig. 2). After stimulation by 1 mM ascorbic acid, generation of MDA in Tris-HCl buffer was significantly lower, when compared to phosphate buffer (Fig. 2). Without stimulation by pro-oxidants, renal microsomes isolated from either CP-injected or control rats, revealed no significant MDA-production in an incubation medium containing Tris-HCl buffer or phosphate buffer (data not shown).

DISCUSSION

In order to characterize the condition of the rats after a single injection of CP, alterations of body weight and kidney weight, and concentrations of plasma-creatinine and BUN were determined. The known depression in body weight after CP-treatment is primarily a consequence of decreased food intake (9). Increase in kidney weight and elevation of concentrations of plasma-creatinine and BUN are results of CP-induced nephrotoxicity and the present findings are consistent with other reports (9).

Ascorbic acid and ferrous ions have been described as important initiators of non-enzy-

Table 1. Effect of a single CP-injection (6 mg/kg body weight) on body and kidney weight, plasma concentration of creatinine and blood urea nitrogen (BUN).

	Day	Control rats	CP-injected rats
% of initial	0	100.000 ± 1.970	100.000 ± 1.750
body weight	3	105.380 ± 1.600[#]	88.460 ± 2.090[*,#]
Kidney weight (g)	3	0.886 ± 0.014	0.991 ± 0.017[*]
Creatinine (mg/dl)	3	0.980 ± 0.200	1.720 ± 0.130[*]
BUN (mg/dl)	3	47.500 ± 2.960	110.500 ± 8.430[*]

The table contains data (x $\pm$ SEM) obtained from 4 groups of rats used for microsomal preparations. * (P<0.05), as compared to corresponding control values on day 3, [#](P<0.05) as compared to corresponding values on day 0.

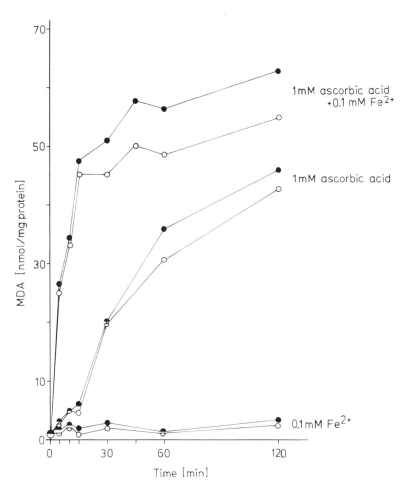

Figure 1. Effect of a single CP-injection (6 mg/kg body weight) on MDA- production of rat renal microsomes in phosphate buffer. Microsomes were incubated in phosphate buffer (100 mM, pH 7.8) containing the pro-oxidants Fe^{2+} or ascorbic acid or a combination of both. Data from a selected single experiment are shown. open circles, microsomes from control rats;   closed circles, microsomes from CP-injected rats

matic tissue peroxidation (10,11) and it has been suggested, that, compared to Fe^{3+}, Fe^{2+} is the active peroxidant species, maintained in the reduced form by ascorbic acid (11). Other findings (12,13) suggest, that an optimal Fe^{3+}:Fe^{2+} ratio, initiated by combination of iron with oxidizing or reducing agents, is an effective promoter of initiation of lipid peroxidation reactions. Minotti proposed a Fe^{2+}-dioxygen-Fe^{3+} complex as initiator of lipid peroxidation (14). In our experiments the combination of Fe^{2+} and

ascorbic acid in a molar ratio of 1:10 was the most effective promotor of lipid peroxidation, compared to Fe^{2+} or ascorbic acid alone. In phosphate buffer, Fe^{2+} without ascorbic acid had only a marginal stimulatory effect on lipid peroxidation. Loss of Fe^{2+} in phosphate buffer occurs via complexing of Fe^{3+} by phosphate with rapid shift of the equilibrium between Fe^{2+} and Fe^{3+} in favor of Fe^{3+} (5). In the presence of ascorbic acid or Tris-HCl buffer under our

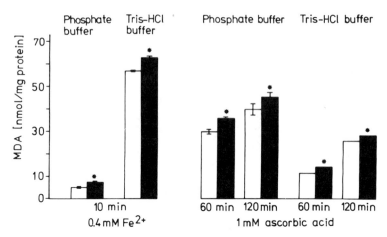

Figure 2. Effect of a single CP-injection (6 mg/kg body weight) on MDA- production of rat renal microsomes in phosphate buffer and Tris-HCl buffer. Microsomes were incubated in phosphate buffer (100 mM) or Tris-HCl buffer (30 mM) containing the pro-oxidants Fe^{2+} or ascorbic acid. Symbols represent $x \pm SD$ * ($p < 0.05$) as compared to corresponding control values. open squares, microsomes from control rats; closed squares, microsomes from CP-injected rats

experimental conditions, ferrous ions seem to be effective in initiating MDA-production.

Ascorbic acid alone, perhaps in combination with traces of endogeneous ferrous ions, increased the formation of MDA in microsomes of control and CP-injected rats. Ascorbic acid has been described as a pro-oxidant in microsomes, but also reveals antioxidative properties as long as vitamin E in a sufficient amount is present (15). Increased vulnerability of microsomes of CP-injected rats might be the consequence of CP-induced alterations in endogenous ferrous ion and/or vitamin E-content. These alterations have been shown for hepatic microsomes, isolated from rats exposed to chronic ethanol consumption (16).

The reactivity of iron, oxidants and reductants (14) are known to be effected by pH values. We observed no influence on lipid peroxidation in microsomes from control and CP-injected rats, changing the pH-values in the range of 7.2 to 7.8.

The MDA-production in rat renal microsomes of CP-injected rats was up to 25% higher than in control microsomes. The percentage difference in MDA-generation between microsomes from control and CP-injected rats

is smaller than observed in experiments with renal cortical slices or whole kidneys (3,4). Not only microsomes, but other subcellular fractions might be susceptible for peroxidative attack induced by CP. Damage of mitochondrial membranes may occur simultaneously. Preliminary results from experiments in our laboratory showed enhanced susceptibility to enzymatically induced lipid peroxidation of rat renal microsomes isolated from CP-injected rats.

In conclusion, after a single injection of CP, rat renal microsomal lipids are more vulnerable for peroxidation. Thus, renal microsomes might be target organelles of CP-induced lipid peroxidation. In addition, the composition of the incubation medium and concentrations of pro-oxidants are important to gain optimal conditions for stimulation of lipid peroxidation.

ACKNOWLEDGEMENTS

We thank Mrs. G. Hacklaender for valuable technical assistance.

REFERENCES

1. Goldstein RS, Mayor GH: Minireview: The nephrotoxicity of cisplatin. Life Sci 32: 685-690, 1983.

2. Sugihara K, Nakano S, Koda M, Tanaka K, Fukuishi N, Gemba M: Stimulatory effect of cisplatin on production of lipid peroxidation in renal tissues. Japan J Pharmacol 43: 247-252, 1987.

3. Hannemann J, Baumann K: Cisplatin-induced lipid peroxidation and decrease of gluconeogenesis in rat kidney cortex: Different effects of antioxidants and radical scavengers. Toxicology 51: 119-132, 1988.

4. Pederson TC, Aust SD: NADPH-dependent lipid peroxidation catalyzed by purified NADPH-cytochrome C reductase from rat liver microsomes. Biochem Biophys Res Commun 48: 789-795, 1972.

5. Braughler JM, Burton PS, Chase RL, Pregenzer JF, Jacobsen EJ, VanDoornik FJ, Tustin JM, Ayer DE, Bundy GL: Novel membrane localized iron chelators as inhibitors of iron-dependent lipid peroxidation. Biochem Pharmacol 37: 3853-3860, 1988.

6. Albro PW, Corbett JT, Schroeder JL: Rapid isolation of microsomes for studies of lipid peroxidation. Lipids 22: 751-756, 1987.

7. Schacterle GR, Pollack RL: A simplified method for the quantitative assay of small amounts of protein in biologic material. Anal Biochem 51: 654-655, 1973.

8. Buege JA, Aust SD: Microsomal lipid peroxidation. Methods Enzymol 52: 302-310, 1978.

9. Goldstein RS, Noordewier B, Bond JT, Hook JB, Mayor GH: cis-dichlorodiammineplatinum nephrotoxicity: Time course and dose response of renal functional impairment. Toxicol Appl Pharmacol 60: 163-175, 1981.

10. Ernster L, Nordenbrand K: Microsomal lipid peroxidation. Methods Enzymol 10: 574-580, 1967.

11. Fujimoto Y, Fujita T: Effect of lipid peroxidation on p-aminohippurate transport by rat kidney cortical slices. Br J Pharmac 76: 373-379, 1982.

12. Beckmann JK, Borowitz SM, Greene HL, Burr IM: Promotion of iron-induced rat liver microsomal lipid peroxidation by copper. Lipids 23: 559-563, 1988.

13. Braughler JM, Duncan LA, Chase RL: The involvement of iron in lipid peroxidation. J Biol Chem 261: 10282-10289, 1986.

14. Minotti G, Aust SD: The role of iron in the initiation of lipid peroxidation. Chem Phys Lip 44: 191-208, 1987.

15. Wefers H, Sies H: The protection by ascorbate and glutathione against microsomal lipid peroxidation is dependent on vitamin E. Eur J Biochem 174: 353-357, 1988.

16. Krikun G, Cederbaum AI: Effect of chronic ethanol consumption on microsomal lipid peroxidation. FEBS Lett 208: 292-296, 1986.

49

EFFECT OF CISPLATIN ON ISOLATED RAT KIDNEY PROXIMAL TUBULE FRAGMENTS: AN IN VITRO MODEL FOR NEPHROTOXICITY STUDIES

S. McGuinness, I. Pratt and M.P. Ryan

Department of Pharmacology, University College Dublin, Dublin 4, Ireland

INTRODUCTION

The study of the mechanism of drug-induced nephrotoxicity presents difficulties due to the structural and functional complexity of the kidney. A variety of in vitro systems are being developed for use in such studies, ranging from the isolated perfused kidney to membrane preparations such as brush border membrane vesicles. In vitro systems are of particular relevance to mechanistic studies of target organ and target cell toxicity. We have used rat renal proximal tubular fragments as an in vitro model for the study of the mechanisms of action of nephrotoxic agents such as the anticancer drug cisplatin.

Cisplatin (CP) is a widely used drug in the treatment of a variety of solid tumours, for example in lung, testicular and ovarian cancers. The chief dose-limiting side effect of CP is its pronounced nephrotoxicity which is cumulative and is characterised by necrosis of the S3 segment of the proximal tubule (1).

The chief objectives of the study were to develop and characterise isolated rat renal proximal tubular fragments as a model for nephrotoxicity studies and to investigate the biochemical and morphological changes in isolated rat renal proximal tubular fragments with the anticancer drug cisplatin.

MATERIAL AND METHODS

Isolation of tubules

Proximal tubules were isolated from male Wistar rats (200-250g) using collagenase digestion followed by mechanical sieving and differential centrifugation in 45% Percoll. The kidneys were perfused in situ and then removed. The cortices were dissected out and finely chopped. The cortex was digested in 0.15% collagenase for 20 min at 37 $^{\circ}$C in 95% O_2 / 5% CO_2. The digest was spray washed through a T-strainer, 140 μm and 64 μm nylon mesh. The tissue remaining on the 64 μm nylon mesh was subjected to differential centrifugation with iso-osmotic Percoll for 10 min at 10000 RPM. Two distinct fractions were obtained - fraction 1 (F1) consisted primarily of glomeruli whilst fraction 2 (F2) consisted of proximal tubules. Fraction 2 was removed, washed and resuspended in modified Krebs-Henseleit buffer, pH 7.4.

Biochemical Studies

The following enzymes were assayed on sonicated fractions of proximal tubules: alkaline phosphatase (AP, 2), gamma-glutamyltranspeptidase (gamma-GT, 3) and hexokinase (Hexo, 4).

Transport Studies

The Na^+/hexose cotransport system was assessed using the non-metabolizable, actively transported analogue [^{14}C] alpha-methyl D-pyranoside.

Electron Microscopy Studies

For transmission microscopy, tubules were pelleted and fixed in 2.5% buffered glutaraldehyde, postfixed in 1% osmium tetroxide and dehydrated in graded ethanol solutions. Following treatment with propylene oxide, the samples were embedded in Epon. Ultrathin sections (40-60 nm) were cut with a glass knife on an LKB Ultramicotome No.3. After staining with uranyl acetate and lead citrate they were examined in a Philips 201 electron microscope at 80Kv. For scanning electron microscopy, tubules were fixed in 2.5% buffered glutaraldehyde, postfixed in 1% osmium tetroxide and dehydrated in graded acetone solutions. Samples were critical point dried for 2-3 hr and then visualised in a Jeol 35 scanning electron microscope.

Viability Studies

Viability was assessed by a double fluorescence technique using acridine orange and ethidium bromide. Acridine orange passes through the cell membrane of viable tubules and is metabolised by cytoplasmic esterases to a compound which fluoresces green on activation by blue light. Ethidium bromide will only pass through damaged or non-viable cell membranes. Once in the cell it intercalates with cDNA and RNA to produce an orange fluorescence.

Cisplatin Studies

Tubules were treated with a range of CP concentrations 1 μM - 3 mM over 3 hr. The release of the lysosomal enzyme N-acetyl-beta-D-glucosaminidase (NAG, 5) or the uptake of [^{14}C] alpha-methyl D pyranoside was then assessed.

Statistics

All experiments were carried out in triplicate and values were given as means ± s.e.m. Statistical significance was assessed using the unpaired Students t-test and $p < 0.05$ was taken as significant.

RESULTS

Tubule viability was found to be between 80-90% as assessed by the acridine orange and ethidium bromide fluorescent technique. Levels of AP and gamma-GT, brush border marker enzymes for the proximal tubule were enriched in F2 over the cortical digest; ($p < 0.05$; Table 1). Fraction 1 showed reduced levels of AP ($p < 0.025$) and gamma-GT ($p < 0.05$) over the pool. Levels of hexokinase, a distal tubule enzyme, were not increased in F1 or F2. This confirmed the extensive removal of contaminating distal tubules at the 64μm nylon mesh.

In the absence of Na^+ from the modified medium, Na^+ / hexose cotransport was significantly reduced at all time points over the 3 hr period. Maximum uptake occurred at 20 min. In Na^+-containing medium, uptake at this

Table 1: Marker enzyme activities in rat cortical digests.

Sample	AlkalinePhosphatase μmol/mg protein/min	gamma-Glutamyltranspeptidase I.U./mg protein/min	Hexokinase μmol/mg protein/min
Cortical digest (A)	4.3 ± 0.04 (n=6)	9.0 ± 1.4 (n=6)	0.09 ± 0.05 (n=4)
Fraction 1 (B)	2.7 ± 0.5 (n=6)	4.0 ± 0.9 (n=5)	0.06 ± 0.03 (n=4)
Fraction 2 (c)	8.0 ± 0.2 (n=4)	20.0 ± 6.0 (n=4)	0.05 ± .004 (n=4)
	A versus B: p<0.025.	A versus B: p<0.01.	
	A versus C: p<0.05.	A versus C: p<0.05.	N.S.
	B versus C: p<0.025.	B versus C: p<0.025	

point was 27.03 $\pm$ 2.86 pmoles alpha-MG/mg protein as compared to 6.76 $\pm$ 3.03 pmoles alpha-MG/mg protein in Na^+-free medium; $p <$ 0.0005. This suggested that the tubules were proximal in origin as Na^+ / hexose cotransport is a characteristic of proximal tubules in vivo. Phloridzin, an inhibitor of Na^+ / hexose cotransport produced a dose-related decrease in alpha-methyl-D-pyranoside uptake into the isolated proximal tubules with increasing concentrations of phloridzin from 1 μm - 1 mM.

Transmission electron microscopy showed tubules with well-defined brush border and basolateral infoldings characteristic of the proximal tubule in vivo. The tubules had intact basement membranes as shown by scanning microscopy.

The effects of CP on the release of the lysosomal enzyme NAG were investigated following a three hour incubation. Increasing concentrations of CP stimulated NAG release from the isolated rat kidney proximal tubules. There was a dose related increase in NAG release with CP. At 1.5 and 3.0 mM cisplatin NAG release was significantly increased over control ($p < 0.025$: Table 3). Cisplatin was also found to inhibit alpha-MG uptake into the isolated tubules with increasing concentrations. At 0.1mM cisplatin uptake of alpha-MG was reduced from control ($p < 0.025$). With 1.0 and 3.0 mM cisplatin, uptake of alpha-MG was more significantly reduced from control, ($p < 0.0005$; Table 3).

Transmission electron micrographs of tubules treated with 3.0 mM cisplatin showed swollen mitochondria and distorted cristae. Furthermore cytoplasmic blebbing at the basement membrane level may be indicative of an acute toxic insult.

DISCUSSION

A relatively pure preparation of rat proximal tubular fragments has been prepared with good viability and transport capabilities. CP has been shown to cause a dose-related increase in N-acetyl- β-D-glucosaminidase release and to reduce alpha-methyl-D-pyranoside uptake.

Table 2: Alpha-methyl-D-pyranoside uptake into isolated rat kidney tubules over a 20 min period expressed as % of control in the presence of 118mM NaCl.

Medium	% of Control
NaMEDIUM	100
NaFREE	25.0
1μM PLZ	25.8
10μM PLZ	14.3
25μM PLZ	12.1
100μM PLZ	11.8
200μM PLZ	10.7
1000μM PLZ	8.9

$Na_{\pm}$-free medium consisted of 118 mM choline chloride. Phloridzin (PLZ) was added in concentrations ranging from 1 mM to 1000 mM in 118 mM NaCl medium.

Table 3: The effect of cisplatin on N-Acetyl-beta-D-glucosaminidase (NAG) release and alpha-methylglucose (alpha-MG) uptake into isolated rat kidney tubules.

Cisplatin mM	NAG release (Fold increase over control)	alpha-MG uptake (pmoles /mg protein)
Control	1.0	19.93 $\pm$ 1.18
0.005	1.17	16.68 $\pm$ 1.52
0.05	1.18	17.35 $\pm$ 1.11
0.1	1.34	13.99 $\pm$ 1.9
1.0	1.54	2.28 $\pm$ 0.2
1.5	1.95	-
3.0	2.16	2.6 $\pm$ 0.6

In addition, transmission electron microscopy showed tubules with swollen mitochondria and blebbing of the basement membrane. We suggest that this preparation has potential in mechanistic studies of iatrogenic nephrotoxicity.

ACKNOWLEDGEMENTS

This work was supported by the Health Research Board of Ireland.

REFERENCES

1. Dobyan DC, Levi J, Jacobs C, Kosek J, Weiner MW: Mechanism of cis-Platinum nephrotoxicity: II. Morphological observations. J Pharmacol Exp Ther 213: 551-556, 1980.

2. Lansing Al, Belkhode ML, Lynch WE, Lieberman I: Enzymes of plasma membranes of liver. J Biol Chem 94: 721-734, 1965.

3. Tate SS, Meister A: Interaction of gamma-glutamyltranspeptidase with amino acids, peptides, and derivatives and analogues of glutathione. J Biol Chem 249: 7593-7602, 1974.

4. Mira DJ, Jagannathan V: Hexokinase. Methods Enzymol 9: 371-375, 1970.

5. Jones BR, Bhalla RB, Mladek J, Kaleya RN, Gralla RJ, Alcock NW, Schwartz MK, Young CW, Reidenberg MM: Comparison of methods of evaluating the nephrotoxicity of cisplatin. Clin Pharmacol Ther 27: 557-562, 1980.

50

CISPLATIN-INDUCED REDUCTIONS IN RENAL RESERVE FOLLOWING UNILATERAL NEPHRECTOMY IN THE PIG

M.E.C. Robbins(1), D. Campling(1), J.W. Hopewell(1) and A. Michalowski(2)

CRC Normal Tissue Radiobiology Research Group, Research Institute (University of Oxford), Churchill Hospital, Oxford OX3 7LJ UK(1), MRC Cyclotron Unit, Hammersmith Hospital London UK(2)

INTRODUCTION

Cis-diamminedichloroplatinum II, or cisplatin (c-DDP), has become the agent of choice in the chemotherapeutic treatment of several solid tumours, particularly testicular and ovarian cancers. Its dose is limited by nephrotoxicity; despite the use of optimal methods for administering cisplatin, such as active hydration or sodium chloride as the vehicle (1,2), approximately 30% of patients will manifest nephrotoxicity as defined by a creatinine clearance of less than 50ml/min.

Initial clinical (3) and experimental studies (4) showed an acute reversible reduction in renal function. However, more recent findings suggest that cisplatin may cause a permanent reduction in GFR (5), which may indeed be progressive in nature (6).

It is thus likely that patients treated primarily with cisplatin may be at risk if treated subsequently with a further nephrotoxic insult. There appears to be little information available with regard to this potentially deleterious consequence of cisplatin treatment.

The present study addresses this question by studying the effect of asecond renal insult, i.e. unilateralnephrectomy (UN), on the functional status of the pig kidney previously treated with cisplatin. The pig and man are unique among mammals in possessing a multipyrimidal multipapillate kidney (7). It is likely therefore that the experimental findings of cisplatin nephrotoxicity in the pig may be of direct clinical significance.

METHODS

Sixteen mature Large White female pigs, approximately 10 months of age, were used. Twelve received single doses of 1.5, 2.0 and 2.5mg/kg cisplatin (n = 4, 5 and 3 respectively) infused intravenously. Prior to infusion of cisplatin, each pig was hydrated with 2 litres of saline administered via an ear vein. Cisplatin was then infused in a further litre of saline to which an anti-emetic agent (Maxolon, 200-350mg) had been added. A further litre of saline was subsequently infused.

Prior to, and 4 weeks after cisplatin administration, individual kidney GFR and ERPF were measured using ^{99m}Tc-DTPA and ^{131}I-hippuran renography (8). Measurements of renal haemodynamics were also carried out in 4 age-matched control animals.

After this period the left kidney of each cisplatin-treated animal, and also of the age-matched untreated controls, was removed surgically. All procedures were carried out under anaesthesia, maintained using an anaesthetic mixture of 2-3% halothane, ~30% nitrous oxide and ~70% oxygen. After UN, pigs received analgesics (Temgesic, Reckitt and Coleman) administered intramuscularly twice daily for 4 days. All the animals appeared to recover well from the surgical procedure. The left kidney was fixed in formal acetic and paraffin-wax embedded. Histological evaluation was performed on 5μm thick sections stained with Periodic-acid Schiff's reagent. GFR and ERPF were measured in the remaining kidney at 4-weekly intervals for periods up to 24 weeks after UN. At the completion of this follow-up period, the cisplatin-treated pigs were killed. The right kidney of each animal was perfusion-fixed with formal acetic, and evaluated as described previously.

RESULTS

The percentage change in GFR, observed 4 weeks after the infusion of 1.5-2.5mg/kg cisplatin, is compared with pre-treatment values in Figure 1. Although there was considerable inter-animal variation within each treatment group, an increased cisplatin dose was clearly associated with an increase in the overall incidence of animals exhibiting a reduction in GFR. There was no consistent change in ERPF 4 weeks after treatment with cisplatin.

Effect of UN on renal haemodynamics

The time-related changes in GFR and ERPF following UN are shown in Figure 2. Within 4 weeks of UN, the GFR in the remaining kidney of age-matched control animals increased markedly, reaching levels approximately 2.5 times greater than those found in individual kidneys

of intact age-matched control pigs. The GFR remained at this value throughout the period of investigation (Fig. 2a). A similar pattern of changes was evident in the remaining kidney of pigs which had been previously treated with 1.5mg/kg cisplatin. However, animals previously treated with higher doses of cisplatin exhibited a dose-related reduction in the extent of the increase in GFR seen following UN. In animals previously treated with 2.0mg/kg cisplatin, GFR did increase within 4 weeks of UN to values ~1.8 times those seen in individual kidneys of intact age-matched control pigs. This increase, however, was not statistically significant when compared with the pre-UN values in this group of animals (p>0.10). By 24 weeks after UN the GFR appeared to be declining. In pigs treated with 2.5mg/kg cisplatin, the GFR prior to UN was less than that observed in individual kidneys of intact age-matched controls. Although there appeared to be a slight increase in GFR following UN, this was not statistically significant (p>0.10), and the GFR in these kidneys reached values only slightly greater than those found in individual kidneys of intact age-matched controls.

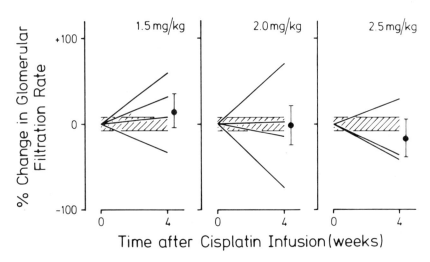

Figure 1. Percentage change in GFR seen 4 weeks after the infusion of a single dose of cisplatin in pigs. The hatched area represents the 95% confidence limits for age-matched control animals. Closed circle represents the mean percentage change ± SE.

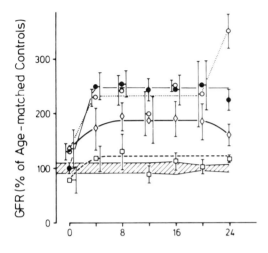

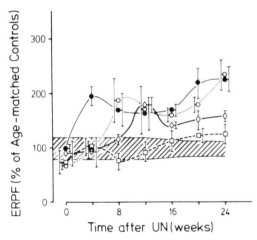

Time after UN (weeks)

Figure 2. Time-related changes in a) GFR and b) ERPF of the right kidney of mature pigs following UN performed 4 weeks after infusion of cisplatin (closed circle) 1.5mg/kg; (open triangle) 2.0mg/kg; (open square) 2.5mg/kg.   Open circle represents age-matched animals which did not receive cisplatin. The hatched area represents the 95% confidence limits for an individual kidney in intact age-matched control animals. Error bars represent ± SE.

The changes in ERPF following UN were similar to those described for GFR.

Morphological changes

a) Four weeks after cisplatin infusion, two types of tubular lesions were evident. Dilated proximal, and to a lesser extent distal tubules,

in which the brush border had been lost were present throughout the cortex. The epithelial cells appeared flattened and lined the periphery of the lumen. Dilated collecting ducts were also seen in the medulla. In addition, focal areas of atrophic tubules, often associated with stromal fibrosis and inflammatory infiltrate, were seen. These lesions appeared to extend from the corticomedullary area outwards to the subcapsular cortex. Glomerular changes were also seen. There was thickening of the basement membrane together with a proliferation of capsular epithelial cells (Figure 3a). This lesion appeared in some cases to involve the S_1 portion of the proximal convoluted tubule (Figure 3b). The incidence of all these morphological changes was dose-related.

b) Twenty-four weeks after UN, tubular changes consisted of focal areas of dilated tubules, often containing flocculent proteinaceous material. In animals treated with 1.5mg/kg cisplatin the damage was focal and moderate; with increasing dose the dilation became more pronounced and widespread. There were also pronounced glomerular changes, with lesions similar to those encountered in progressive focal glomerulosclerosis (PGF), particularly in the 2.5mg/kg group. Thus a range of glomerular damage, from focal and segmental glomerulosclerosis to completely sclerotic obsolesent glomeruli was seen; the sclerotic glomeruli appeared to be from mainly juxtamedullary nephrous. Associated with these glomerular lesions were areas of atrophic tubules and interstitial fibrosis.

DISCUSSION

The present results indicate that pigs treated with a range of single doses of cisplatin exhibited a dose-dependent increase in the incidence of animals showing a reduction in GFR 4 weeks after treatment with cisplatin. The extent of this reduction showed a marked inter-animal variation, and was not correlated with the dose of cisplatin infused. Following UN, however, a clear and consistent dose-dependent reduction in the hypertrophic response of

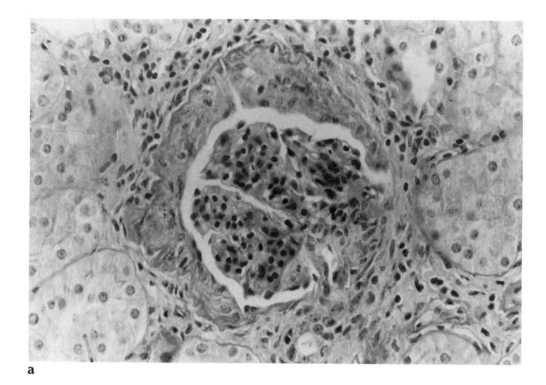

a

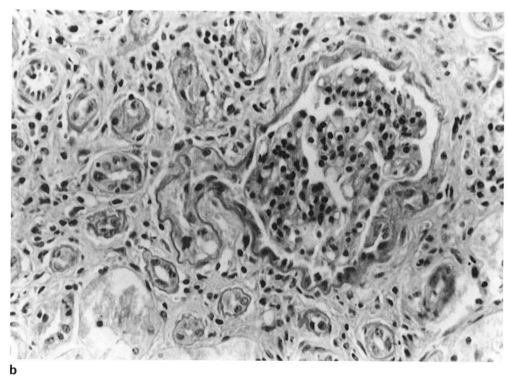

b

Figure 3. Glomerular changes seen 4 weeks after treatment with 2.5mg/kg cisplatin; a. Parietal crescent with periglomerular fibrosis and chronic inflammation, PAS x340, b. Glomerulus in which the basement membrane thickening extends to the S_1 portion of the proximal tubule. The glomerulus is surrounded by atrophic tubules with stromal fibrosis and inflammatory cells, PAS x340.

the remaining kidney was observed. Thus the increase in renal function in pigs initially treated with 2.5mg/kg cisplatin was >50% of that seen in age-matched UN controls. Prior treatment with cisplatin appears to result in a permanent reduction in renal functional status which may be clinically "silent" until a second nephrotoxic insult occurs.

Initial studies of cisplatin nephrotoxicity appeared to indicate that cisplatin produced an acute but reversible reduction in renal function. Minimal levels were observed within several days of treatment, followed by a recovery (3,4). These early studies, however, were limited by their use of relatively insensitive parameters such as serum creatinine and blood urea nitrogen (BUN) to measure decrements in renal function.

Recent clinical reports, using more sensitive measurements of renal function, indicate that cisplatin causes a permanent reduction in GFR (5) which in some cases appears progessive in nature (6). The pathophysiology of this reduction in GFR remains ill-defined. It is known that cisplatin produces an acute, mainly proximal tubular functional impairment within hours of administration. Groth et al. (6) thus attributed the chronic reduction in GFR observed in patients following cisplatin treatment to increased intratubular pressure within the damaged tubules.

Histological studies in the rat appear to support this hypothesis. Acute cisplatin-induced damage is largely confined to the proximal convoluted tubules, in particular the S_3 segment. Clinical observations, in contrast, showed that it was the distal tubules and collecting ducts which were primarily affected, and to a greater degree than the proximal convoluted tubules (9), while the glomeruli appeared to be uninvolved. These findings support the hypothesis that the reduction in GFR results from the primary action of cisplatin on the renal tubules.

In contrast to previous studies, the current findings indicate pronounced glomerular changes following cisplatin infusion. These consisted of basement membrane thickening together with a proliferation of the capsular epithelial cells. In some cases the S_1 portion of the proximal tubule was involved, as evidenced by a thickened and wrinkled appearance to the basement membrane. These observations imply that cisplatin may act not only at the tubular but also at the glomerular level. It is not possible to determine whether these lesions are responsible, in whole or in part, for the observed reduction in GFR. As discussed above, it is generally believed that the glomerulus is not directly affected by cisplatin. However, Daugaard et al. (10) reported a proteinuria, glomerular in origin, in patients treated with cisplatin. Thus cisplatin does indeed appear to cause specific glomerular damage.

The glomerular lesions presented here may explain the continued reduction in GFR observed following cisplatin treatment. Although it is unlikely that the clinically observed reductions in renal function are themselves life-threatening, the progressive nature of this reduction would appear to indicate that further treatment with nephrotoxic agents could be potentially harmful. This question was specifically addressed in the present study by performing UN 4 weeks after cisplatin infusion. Despite the fact that following UN all kidneys exhibited a compensatory increase in renal function, this increase was dose-dependently reduced in the cisplatin-treated pigs. Thus the increase in GFR and ERPF in UN pigs initially treated with 2.5mg/kg cisplatin was 2% of that seen in age-matched UN controls. It should be noted that in these animals renal function remained at or slightly above values normally seen in individual kidneys of age-matched intact control animals, and it is unlikely that such a reduction in renal function would be evident from monitoring serum creatinine levels.

This dose-dependent reduction in renal functional status was noted even in animals which prior to UN had "normal" levels of renal function. These findings indicate that these levels of renal function seen after cisplatin treatment reflect hyperfiltration by relatively undamaged nephrons rather than an essentially undamaged organ. Thus the finding of relatively normal values of renal function 4 weeks after cisplatin treatment does not necessarily imply the presence of a normal kidney, but may reflect an organ in which the total number of functioning nephrons has been reduced, with a compensatory hypertrophic response by the remaining nephrons.

Histological evaluation of these kidneys 24 weeks after UN revealed that the glomerular lesions had progressed into lesions which appeared to be similar to those encountered in PGF, with the characteristic tendency for the juxtamedullary glomeruli to be preferentially involved. There have been experimental studies in which the long term consequences of cisplatin treatment in the rat have been studied (11). These have shown that between 6 and 15 months after treatment there are some observable sclerotic glomeruli, but by far the major change is the development of cystic tubules, predominantly in the outer stripe of the outer medulla. These cysts have not been seen clinically, and do not appear in the cisplatin-treated kidneys. This may represent species differences in the cisplatin-induced lesions; in view of the morphological and functional similarities between the kidneys of the pig and man (7), it may well be the case that the current changes in porcine renal morphology are more likely to mirror those seen clinically.

These findings appear to confirm the reservations previously expressed concerning the susceptibility of patients previously treated with cisplatin to a further nephrotoxic insult. The renal status of patients needs to be accurately defined before embarking on such a course of action, to prevent the possible development of chronic renal failure.

ACKNOWLEDGEMENTS

The authors would like to thank Mrs E. Whitehouse for the histological preparations. This study was wholly supported by the Cancer Research Campaign.

REFERENCES

1. Cvitkovic E, Spaulding J, Bethune V, et al.: Improvement of cis-dichlorodiammineplatinum (NSC-119875): Therapeutic index in an animal model. Cancer 39: 1357, 1977.

2. Ozols RF, Corden BJ, Jacob J, et al.: High dose cisplatin in hypertonic saline. Ann Intern Med 100: 19, 1984.

3. Hayes DM, Cvitkovic E, Golberg RB, et al.: High dose cis-platinum diammine chloride. Cancer 39: 1372, 1977.

4. Ward JM, Fauvie KA: The nephrotoxic effects of cis-diammine-dichloroplatinum (II)(NSC-119875) in male F344 rats. Toxicol Appl Pharmacol 38: 535, 1976.

5. Fjeldborg P, Sorensen J, Helkjaer PE: The long-term effect of cisplatin on renal function. Cancer 58: 2214, 1986.

6. Groth S, Wielsen H, Sorensen JB, et al.: Acute and long-term nephrotoxicity of cisplatinum in man. Cancer Chemother Pharmacol 17: 191, 1986.

7. Terris JM: Swine as a model in renal physiology and nephrology; an overview. In: Tumbleson ME (ed); Swine in Biomedical Research. New York, Plenum Press, 1986, pp.1673.

8. Robbins MEC, Soper M, Gunn Y: Techniques for the quantitative measurement of individual kidney function in the pig. Int J Appl Radiat Isot 35: 853, 1984.

9. Dentino M, Luft FC, Yum MW, et al.: Long term effect of cis-diamminedichloride platinum (CDDP) on renal function and structure in man. Cancer 41: 1274, 1978.

10. Daugaard G, Rossing N, Rorth M: Effects of cisplatin on different measures of glomerular function in the human kidney with special emphasis on high-dose. Cancer Chemother Pharmacol 21: 163, 1988.

11. Dobyan DC, Hill D, Lewis T, et al.: Cyst formation in rat kidney induced by cis-platinum administration. Lab Invest 45: 260, 1981.

51
PHARMACOLOGICAL MODULATION OF ADRIAMYCIN-INDUCED NEPHROPATHY IN RATS

J. Egido, A. Ortiz, A. Robles, M. Gómez-Chiarri, J.L. Lerma, C. Gómez, L. Hernando, E. González

Laboratory of Nephrology, Fundación Jiménez Díaz, Universidad Autónoma, Madrid, Spain

INTRODUCTION

Rats injected with a single intravenous injection of adriamycin develop marked proteinuria and glomerular morphologic changes similar to those seen in minimal change disease in humans (1,2). The mechanisms of proteinuria in both human minimal change nephropathy and adriamycin nephropathy in rats are not completely understood. Various studies have demonstrated that the toxic effect of adriamycin on the kidney glomerular structures requires only a few minutes exposure to the drug (3), suggesting the release of some mediators by glomerular cells which could alter the permeability of the capillary basement membrane.

The aim of our study was to examine the effect of several drugs which could alter such a response. Steroids and cyclosporin are currently used in the treatment of nephrotic syndrome due to minimal change disease in humans. Heparin has been shown to increase the negative electric potential of the vascular wall, which seems altered in adriamycin nephropathy (2,4). Allopurinol has been shown to reduce proteinuria and glomerular injury in puromycin treated rats (5). Also, since several lipid mediators can be produced in this model (6,7) we have also employed various platelet-activating-factor (PAF) receptor antagonists and a 5-lipoxygenase inhibitor.

MATERIAL AND METHODS

Adriamycin (Adriablastin) was purchased from Farmitalia Carlo Erba (Milan, Italy). Steroids (6-methyl-prednisolone) from Pfizer Co. (Madrid, Spain), BN-52021, an extract of ginkgobiloba tree and BN-52726 were prepared and given to us by Institut Henri Beaufour (France). Triazolam (Upjohn Co., Kalamazoo, MI, USA), cyclosporin (Sandoz Co., Basel, Switzerland), allopurinol (Gayoso-Wellcome, Madrid, Spain) and L-656,224, Merck Frost Canada) were kindly donated.

Experimental design Male Sprague-Dawley rats weighing 200-225 g were injected through the tail vein with a single dose of adriamycin (7.5 mg/kg body weight) and were then allocated randomly to 9 groups.

In group I, 30 rats did not receive any treatment. In group II, 16 rats received daily 6-methyl-prednisolone, 2.5 mg/kg daily. In group III, 11 rats received cyclosporin 10 mg/kg daily. In group IV, 13 rats received calcium heparinate 500 U/day per kg twice daily. In group V, 14 rats received allopurinol in a single dose of 100 mg/kg. In group VI, 15 rats received BN-52021, 5 mg/kg twice daily. In group VII, 15 rats received triazolam, 6.5 mg/kg per day in a single dose. In group VIII, 15 rats BN-52726 1 mg/kg per day in a single dose. In group IX, 5 rats received L-656.224, 5 mg/kg per day in a single dose.

In all groups, drugs were given i.p. from day 0 (the day of administration of adriamycin) up to 14 days except in the group which was given a single dose of allopurinol 4 hr prior to adriamycin (5). All animals were allowed unlimited access to both water and conventional rat chow throughout the study. On day 12, each rat was placed in a metabolic cage for 2 days prior to the collection of urine for 24 hr.

Clinical biochemistry Blood was collected by intracardiac puncture from ether-anesthetized animals. Serum creatinine total serum proteins and cholesterol were determined by the standard Coulter method. Urine protein was determined by the sulfosalicylic acid method.

Kidney tissue processing On day 14, rats from each group were anesthetized with 5 mg/100 g of sodium pentobarbital. Their kidneys were perfused in situ via the abdominal aorta with 100 ml of normal saline at 4°C, removed and further processed for histological and electron microscopy studies as published (8).

Incubation of isolated glomeruli and PAF assay Renal glomeruli were isolated based on the ability of glomeruli to pass through a 105 μm sieve and to be retained in a 75 μm sieve (9). The production of PAF by glomerular cells was based upon the ability of incorporating ^{3}H-acetate substrate for lyso-PAF:acetyl-CoA acetyltransferase, into phospholipids including PAF (10). Samples were subjected to thin-layer chromatography on analytical silica gel plates of 2 mm thickness (Merck, Darmstadt, Germany) as previously described (10). The area of the plates migrating with a standard of synthetic PAF were scraped off and counted for radioactivity.

Statistical analysis The results are expressed as the mean ± SD. Significance was established using Student's t-test.

RESULTS

After 7 days animals administered adriamycin alone began to show a marked increase in 24 hr urinary protein excretion. After 14 days all animals were heavily proteinuric (Table I).

Animals treated with steroids, cyclosporin, heparin and allopurinol had a reduction in the protein excretion, but were still heavily proteinuric. Only rats receiving the three PAF receptor antagonists had very mild or no proteinuria (p<0.001). There was also a very

TABLE I. Urinary protein excretion rate in experimental animals

Group	Adriamycin (7.5 mg/kg) (+)	Proteinuria (mg/24 hr)
I		162 ± 91
II	Steroids (n=16)	125 ± 79
III	Cyclosporin (n=11)	114 ± 39
IV	Heparin (n=13)	118 ± 51
V	Allopurinol (n=14)	139 ± 16
VI, VII, VIII	PAF receptor antagonists* (n=45)	10 ± 8
IX	5-lipoxygenase inhibitor (n=5)	54 ± 2

Proteinuria in 3 months old control 7.1±3 mg/24hr (mean ± SD). For doses, see text. *It includes, BN-52021, Triazolam and BN-52726. Since the results obtained were very similar they are grouped for convenience.

striking diminution of proteinuria in animals treated with the 5-lipoxygenase inhibitor, L-656.224 (p<0.001).

Serum creatinine, determined on day 14 following injection, was only significantly elevated for the cyclosporin group (not shown). Animals injected only with adriamycin (group I) presented a significant (p<0.025) decrease in the total serum proteins (5.1±0.2 g/dl) and an increase in the blood cholesterol (201±48 mg/dl) in relation to the control group (6.6±0.7 and 49±5, respectively). Animals from groups VI, VII, VIII showed values in the normal range (6.1±0.8 and 60±11 respectively).

Striking lesions were noted on the electron microscopic level. Non-treated groups exhibited glomerular epithelium with marked loss of foot processes and epithelial cell spreading along the glomerular basement membrane, cytoplasmic vacuoles and protein reabsorption droplets (Fig. 1).

Kidneys from treated animals, except from those treated with PAF antagonists, could not be distinguished by electron microscopy from animals injected only with adriamycin. In con-

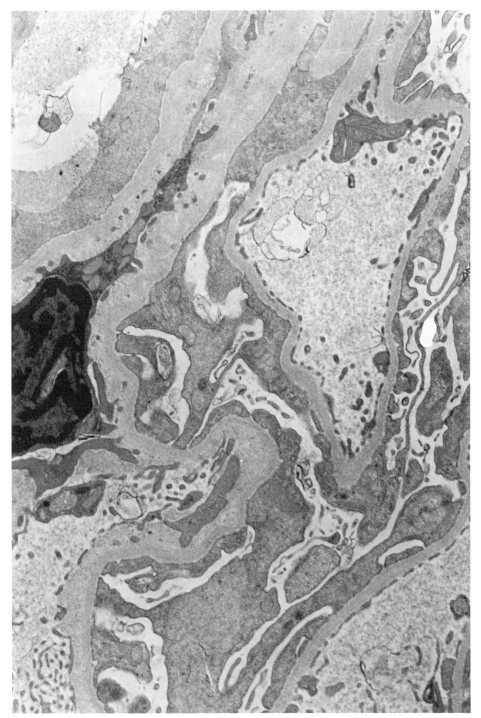

Figure 1. Electron micrograph of a glomerulus of a rat with adriamycin nephrosis not treated. Note the extensive fusion of foot processes.

trast, in animals treated with BN-52021, Triazolam or BN-52726 for 2 weeks (Groups VI, VII and VIII), no alterations in epithelial cells were observed (Fig. 2).

Animals treated with L-656.224 (group IX) had fewer lesions than those of group I, but still presented focal effacement of the podocytes, some vacuoles and a certain increased number of organelles (not shown).

Glomeruli from rats injected with adriamycin (Group I) incorporated, on days 7 and 14, ^{3}H-acetate into a polar lipid that comigrated with authentic PAF on thin layer chromatography. Maximal incorporation was seen at 14 days, corresponding to a percentage increase of 85% of that achieved by normal glomeruli.

DISCUSSION

In a model of toxic nephropathy induced by a single injection of adriamycin, characterized by epithelial cell damage and nephrotic syndrome, we have evaluated various drugs, some of them currently employed in the treatment of minimal change disease in humans. Our results show that these two entities, although with a similar clinico-pathological picture, must have different pathogenetic mechanisms on the damage of the glomerular capillary wall, since the response to some of the treatments employed were dissimilar.

The results of this paper confirm and extend the beneficial effects afforded by three different PAF antagonists on the clinical and histological lesions induced by adriamycin (8). In contrast, steroids and cyclosporin, usually employed in the treatment of minimal change nephropathy in humans, had no important effect on the proteinuria. A possible explanation for this finding is that these two substances could play a role in human nephrosis by decreasing lymphokine production from circulating cells, while in the toxic rat model, adriamycin seems to exert its effect directly on the glomerular structures. The decrease in proteinuria noted with cyclosporin might be due to the decrease in the glomerular filtration rate.

Previous studies have shown that sialoproteins, as evaluated by light microscopy, were markedly reduced in this experimental model (2). Data from Bertolatus and Hunsicker (4), using the fractional clearances of labeled proteins, also suggest a loss of the charge dependent permselectivity. However, other investigators found that the charge barrier is intact in adriamycin nephrosis (11). With that rationale in mind, heparin was used in this model. The mechanisms by which heparin decreases proteinuria in adriamycin treated rats, is unclear but the polyanionic nature of this molecule could contribute, as is the case in the rat model of renal mass reduction (12).

Recently, Diamond et al (5) reported that superoxide dismutase and allopurinol reduced proteinuria and glomerular injury in puromycin treated rats, a model of nephrosis very similar to adriamycin nephropathy. These data suggested a possible pathogenetic role for reactive oxygen products in that situation. This interpretation has been supported by recent works showing that polyethylene glycol coupled catalase (13), two hydroxyl radical scavengers and an iron chelator (14), provided marked protection against glomerular injury. Although similar studies to our knowledge have not been performed in adriamycin nephropathy, the cardiac toxicity of this drug seems to be due, at least in part, to the generation of hydroxyl radicals (15). However, in our model the treatment with allopurinol, with the same schedule employed in puromycin nephrosis (5) did not induce any important changes on proteinuria and renal histology.

We have recently hypothesized that adriamycin, by itself, or through the release of some mediators from resident glomerular cells, could provoke a damage to epithelial glomerular cells. One of these mediators is platelet activating factor (PAF), a phospholipid defined as 1-o-alkyl-2-acetyl-sn- glycero-3-phosphocholine (16). The potential role of PAF as a mediator capable of provoking proteinuria is supported by the following data: PAF induces an enhancement of vascular permeability and proteinuria when injected into the abdominal

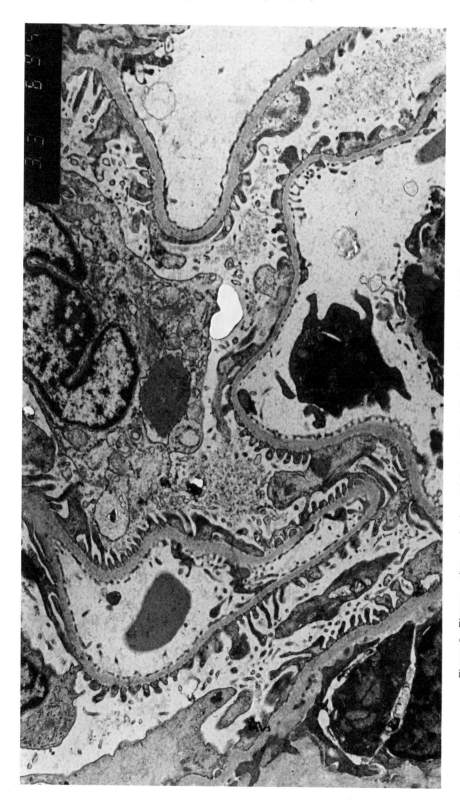

Figure 2. Electron micrograph of a rat injected with adriamycin and treated with BN-52021 for 15 days. Note the normal morphological appearance of capillary wall with well-preserved foot processes.

aorta of rabbits, as well as into isolated perfused rat kidneys (17). In this sense, glomerular cells and particularly the mesangial cells, can release PAF upon appropriate stimulation (17). We have recently observed that PAF is produced by isolated glomeruli from normal rats after incubation with adriamycin for various periods of time (7). Furthermore, as shown in this paper, an in vivo release of PAF by isolated glomeruli occurs in rats injected with adriamycin.

The striking reduction in proteinuria of animals treated with the 5-lipoxygenase inhibitor is of interest. It has been shown that PAF stimulates the synthesis and release of leukotrienes from neutrophils (16). PAF-induced degranulation of these cells and hyperalgesic response to PAF was found to be dependent on leukotrienes as evidenced by selective inhibition by agents that inhibit the lipoxygenase pathway (16,18). These data and the results observed in our model suggest that some of the in vitro and in vivo effects of PAF may be mediated by stimulation of leukotrienes synthesis.

In conclusion, the present data further extend the evidence (8) that PAF plays an important role in the pathogenesis of experimental nephrotic syndrome induced by adriamycin in rats.

ACKNOWLEDGMENTS

This paper was supported in part by grants from FISs, CICYT and Fundación Iñigo Alvarez de Toledo. Marta Gómez Chiarri is a fellow of Ministerio de Educación y Ciencia and A. Robles of the Fundación Iñigo Alvarez de Toledo. We thank Liselotte Gulliksen for secretarial assistance.

REFERENCES

1. Fajardo LF, Elhingham JK, Stewart JR and Klauber MK: Adriamycin nephrotoxicity. Lab Invest 43: 242-253, 1980.

2. Bertani T, Poggi A, Pozzoni R, Delaini F, Sacchi G, Thona Y Mecca G, Remuzzi G, Donati MB: Adriamycin-induced nephrotic syndrome in rats: sequence of pathologic events. Lab Invest 46: 16-23, 1982.

3. Remuzzi G, Zoja C, Remuzzi A, Rossini M, Battaglia C, Broggini M, Bertani T: Low-protein diet prevents glomerular damage in adriamycin-treated rats. Kidney Int 28: 21-37, 1985.

4. Bertolatus JA, Hunsicker LG: Glomerular sieving of anionic and neutral bovine albumins (BSA) in proteinuria due to Hexadimethrine (HDM) or adriamycin (Adria). (Abstract) XVth Ann Mtg Am Soc Nephrol Chicago, December 12-14, 1982.

5. Diamond JR, Bonventre JV, Karnovsky MJ: A role for oxygen free radicals in aminonucleoside nephrosis. Kidney Int 29: 478-483, 1986.

6. Remuzzi G, Imberti L, Rossini M, Morelli C, Carminati C, Cattaneo GM, Bertani T: Increased glomerular thromboxane synthesis as a possible cause of proteinuria in experimental nephrosis. J Clin Invest 75: 94-101, 1985.

7. Egido J, Ramírez F, Robles A, Ortiz A, de Arriba G, Rodríguez MJ, Mampaso F, Fierro C, Braquet P: PAF, adriamycin-induced nephropathy and ginkgolide B. In: Braquet P (ed). Ginkgolides-Chemistry, Biology, Pharmacology and Clinical Perspectives. Barcelona, JR Prous, 1988, pp. 631-640.

8. Egido J, Robles A, Ortiz A, Ramírez F, González E, Mampaso F, Sánchez Crespo M, Braquet P: Role of platelet activating factor in adriamycin-induced nephropathy in rats. Eur J Pharmacol 138:119-123, 1987.

9. Chaumet-Riffaud PH, Oudinet JP, Sraer J, Lajotte CH, Ardaillou R: Altered PGE_2 and PGF_2 production by glomeruli and papilla of sodium-depleted and sodium loaded rats. Am J Physiol 241: F517-F524, 1981.

10. Sánchez-Crespo M, Iñarrea P, Alvarez V, Alonso F, Egido J, Hernando L: Presence in normal human urine of a hypotensive and platelet activating phospholipid. Am J Physiol 244: F706-711, 1983.

11. Weening JJ, Rennke HG: Glomerular permselectivity and polyanion in adriamycin nephrosis in the rat. Kidney Int 24: 152-159, 1983.

12. Olson JL: Role of heparin as a protective agent following reduction of renal mass. Kidney Int 25: 376-381, 1984.

13. Beaman M, Birtwistle R, Howie AJ, Michael J, Adu D: The role of superoxide anion and hydrogen peroxide in glomerular injury induced by puromycin aminonucleoside in rats. Clin Sci 73: 329-332, 1987.

14. Thakur V, Walker PD, Shah SV: Evidence suggesting a role for hydroxyl radical in puromycin aminonucleoside-induced proteinuria. Kidney Int 34: 494-499, 1988.

15. Doroshow JH, Davies KJA: Redox cycling of anthracyclines by cardiac mitochondria.

II. Formation of superoxide anion, hydrogen peroxide and hydroxyl radical. J Biol Chem 261: 3068-3074, 1986.

16. Pinckard RN, Ludwig JC, McManus LM: Platelet activating factors. In: I. Gallin, I.M. Goldstein, R Snyderman (eds). Inflammation: Basic principles and clinical correlates. Raven Press, Ltd, New York, 1988, 139-167.

17. Schlondorff D, Neuwirth R: Platelet activating factor and the kidney. Am J Physiol 251: F1-F11, 1986.

18. Dallob A, Guindon Y, Goldenberg M: Pharmacological evidence for a role of lipoxygenase products in platelet-activating factor (PAF)-induced hyperalgesia. Biochem Pharmacol 36: 3201-3204, 1987.

52

MARKED NEPHROTOXICITY ASSOCIATED WITH THE ANTHRAPYRAZOLE ANTI-CANCER DRUG CI-941

D. Campling and M.E.C. Robbins

CRC Normal Tissue Radiobiology Research Group, Research Institute (University of Oxford), Churchill Hospital, Oxford OX3 7LJ, UK

INTRODUCTION

The anthracycline antibiotic Adriamycin, (Adr), is widely used in clinical oncology for the treatment of breast carcinoma, malignant lymphoma, acute lymphocytic and myelocytic leukaemia, sarcomas and other cancers (1). Its clinical use is limited by cardiotoxicity (2); additional Adr-induced lesions have been reported experimentally in the kidneys of rats (3), rabbits (4) and pigs (5). Adriamycin is indeed used in rats as a model for producing a nephrotic syndrome, characterised by a pronounced proteinuria, hypoalbuminaemia, peripheral fluid accumulation and severe hyperlipidaemia. Its effect on renal function is less well defined. Litterst and Weiss (6) reported that BUN and serum creatinine levels were either unaffected or only minimally increased. Recent reports seem to support this conclusion (7), although there have been studies in which a significant decrease in GFR has been noted (8).

Anthrapyrazoles were developed in the search for a chemotherapeutic agent with tumouricidal activity equal or superior to that of Adr, but with reduced cardiotoxicity. Reactive free-radical formation is believed to play a major role in Adr-induced cardiotoxicity (9); anthrapyrazoles, including the compound CI-941, have displayed marked anti-tumour activity, but do not undergo metabolism to form free radicals (10). Preliminary studies have shown that CI-941 appears significantly less cardiotoxic than Adr in male rats (11). However, although cardiac output remained normal throughout the 12 week follow-up period, body weight showed a severe progressive reduction, with a ~50% loss by the end of the study. In view of these findings, the potential nephrotoxicity of CI-941 was evaluated.

METHODS

A total of 30 male Sprague-Dawley rats, approximately 14 weeks old, and weighing between 360 and 470g, were used in this study. Anaesthetized rats (Chloral hydrate, 300mg/kg i.p.) received either 2 or 4mg/kg body weight CI-941 (concentration 2mg/ml), or saline, administered intravenously via the femoral vein (n=11, 11 and 8 respectively).

Immediately prior to injection, and at weekly intervals thereafter, the body weight of each rat was measured for up to 6 weeks. The experiment was stopped at this time due to the emaciated condition of the surviving rats. None of the rats treated with a dose of 4mg/kg CI-941 survived 5 weeks after injection.

GFR and ERPF were determined at 4 and 6 weeks after injection of CI-941 from the plasma clearances of ^{99m}Tc-DTPA and ^{131}I-hippuran respectively (12).

Briefly, the rats were weighed and anaesthetized. Approximately 7MBq of ^{99m}Tc-DTPA and 0.18MBq ^{131}I-hippuran in 0.2ml were injected via the sublingual vein. Thirty minutes later a blood sample was obtained by cardiac puncture. GFR (plasma clearance of ^{99m}Tc-DTPA) was determined from the formula

$$GFR = V/t. (\ln P_0/Pt)$$

where V = distribution volume of ^{99m}Tc-DTPA
P_0, Pt = plasma concentration of ^{99m}Tc-DTPA
at time zero and t (cpm/ml)

Pt is derived from the plasma sample at t minutes, P_0 is determined from $P_0 = I/V$, where I is the amount of tracer injected and V the distribution volume (ml). The latter was obtained previously, in 10 rats, from the activity in plasma samples of anephric rats after 2 hr equilibration time. To determine ERPF the ^{131}I-hippuran counts were used.

These plasma samples were subsequently used for the determination of cholesterol and albumin levels. Plasma cholesterol levels were measured enzymatically (Sigma Diagnostics Cholesterol Reagent); plasma albumin levels were determined by means of bromcresol green (Sigma Diagnostics Albumin Reagent). All results were expressed as mean ± SE.

Morphological assessment: Representative animals from each group were killed; the kidneys were perfusion fixed in formal acetic and paraffin-wax embedded. Sections 5μm thick were stained with H&E and silver methenamine.

RESULTS

Body weight: Following injection with single doses of CI-941, there was a dose-dependent progressive decline in body weight (Figure 1). Rats treated with 2mg/kg CI-941 exhibited a 15% decrease in pre-treatment body weight within 14 days; levels continued to decline,

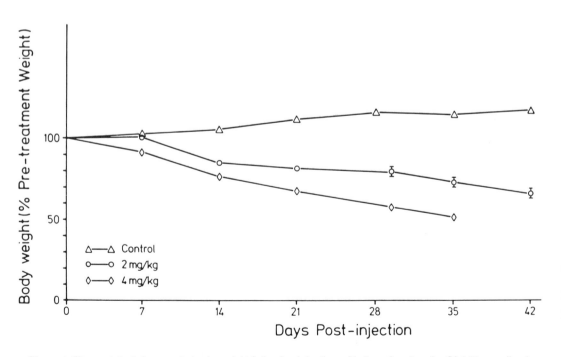

Figure 1. Time-related changes in body weight following injection with 2 mg/kg, 4mg/kg CI-941 or saline in male Sprague-Dawley rats. The data represent mean ± SE.

such that by 6 weeks the body weight was reduced by ~33%. An even more pronounced reduction was evident in rats treated with 4mg/kg CI-941. Body weight decreased by ~10% within 7 days; this was followed by a severe progressive reduction, such that by 5 weeks after injection the mean body weight was only some 50% of pre-treatment values. The

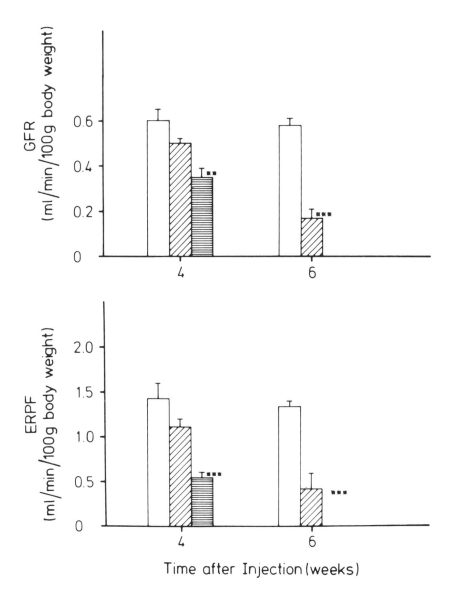

Figure 2. Effect of CI-941 on GFR and ERPF in male Sprague-Dawley rats. Results are expressed as mean ± SE; bars marked by ** and *** are significantly different from control values (p<0.01 and p<0.001 respectively).

rats were killed because of their emaciated and moribund appearance. Control rats exhibited a progressive increase in body weight over this time period.

Renal Haemodynamics: Rats treated with CI-941 exhibited dose-dependent reductions in both GFR and ERPF within 4 weeks of treatment (Figure 2). The reduction in renal function in the 2mg/kg group was not statistically significant. However, in rats treated with 4mg/kg CI-941, both the GFR and ERPF were signifi-

cantly reduced (p<0.001) by 40 and 60% respectively. By 6 weeks renal function had declined further in the 2mg/kg animals, values being only some 30% of controls.

Plasma Albumin and Plasma Cholesterol: Associated with the decline in renal function was a concomitant decrease in plasma albumin (Figure 3). By 4 weeks after injection of 2mg/kg CI-941, plasma albumin levels were significantly lower than those seen in controls (p<0.05) i.e. 1.97±0.28 vs 2.64±0.10 gm/dl. In rats treated

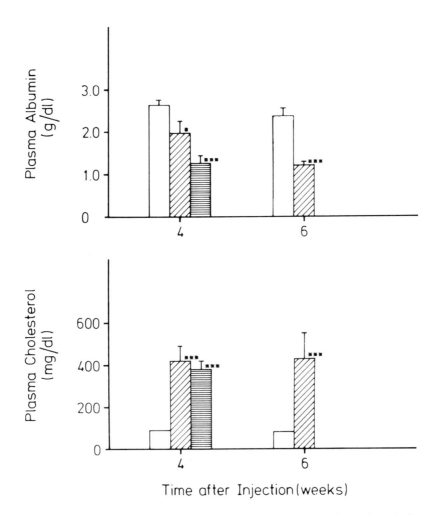

Figure 3. CI-941-induced changes in plasma albumin and plasma cholesterol levels in male Sprague-Dawley rats. Data represent mean ± SE; for key to legend see Figure 2.

with 4mg/kg CI-941, plasma albumin levels were only 1.26±0.17 gm/dl, significantly less than both the control and 2mg/kg treated rats (p<0.001 and <0.05 respectively). By 6 weeks, levels in the 2mg/kg group had declined to values similar to those seen in the 4mg/kg rats at 4 weeks.

There was a marked hyperlipidaemia following injection of CI-941 (Figure 3).

Within 4 weeks of treatment, plasma cholesterol levels in the CI-941 treated rats were some five times greater than those seen in controls; these raised levels were also evident 6 weeks after injection. The hyperlipidaemic plasma appeared "milky" in the drug treated animals.

Morphological changes: Injection of CI-941 resulted in severe progressive dose-related changes in both glomeruli and tubules. The glomerular lesions consisted of vacuolisation, thickening of the basement membrane of the Bowman's capsule, focal parietal cell proliferation and varying degrees of glomerulosclerosis (Figure 4a).

There were also severe tubular changes (Figure 4b); many tubules appeared dilated and filled with casts. These tubules had lost their brush border and the epithelial cells which lined the periphery of the lumen were flattened. These changes were particularly evident in the outer stripe of the outer medulla. Other tubules appeared atrophic, with thickened basement membranes. These were associated with areas of interstitial fibrosis. There was also an extensive inflammatory infiltrate present throughout the cortex and medulla.

DISCUSSION

These results indicate that single doses of 2 and 4mg/kg CI-941 produce a severe progressive reduction in body weight and renal function. Indeed the reduction in body weight was so severe that the experiment was stopped only 6 weeks after treatment due to the poor health and emaciated condition of the surviving animals. None of the rats dosed with 4mg/kg CI-941 survived more than 5 weeks. Associ-

ated with these functional changes there was a pronounced hypoalbuminaemia and hyperlipidaemia. Morphologically CI-941 produced severe glomerular changes, ranging from vacuolisation to focal glomerulosclerosis, whilst there were dilated tubules filled with casts, atrophic tubules, interstitial fibrosis and areas of inflammatory infiltrate. These pathologic lesions are similar to those seen following treatment with Adr (13), as are the functional and systemic changes. Thus the anthrapyrazole CI-941 appears to produce the chronic symptoms of nephrotic syndrome in rats, previously noted following treatment with the anthracycline Adr.

CI-941 appeared to cause significant reductions in both GFR and ERPF within 4 weeks of injection. Although it has been noted that Adr seemed to cause little if any reduction in GFR, this may well reflect the use of insensitive parameters such as serum creatinine to determine renal function. More recent studies of Adr-induced nephrotoxicity (14) indicate that a reduced GFR is also evident within weeks of treatment. No urine collections or urinary analyses were performed during this study; however, the CI-941 treated rats did seem to produce large amounts of urine. Polyuria was also observed after Adr injection; these findings indicate that CI-941 produces a similar progressive renal lesion to that seen after treatment with Adr.

Cardiotoxicity is the dose-limiting toxicity in the clinical use of Adr. This is believed to result from the formation of reactive free-radicals. This has led to the development of the anthrapyrazoles, including CI-941, which do not undergo reactive metabolism to form free radicals. Indeed, initial findings suggested that CI-941 is less cardiotoxic than Adr (11). However, the current findings of the marked nephrotoxicity associated with CI-941 indicate that the reduction in cardiotoxicity, by the lack of free-radical production, did not result in a concomitant decrease in nephrotoxicity. Indeed the severity of the nephrotic syndrome induced by CI-941 would appear to be more severe than that seen after treatment with Adr.

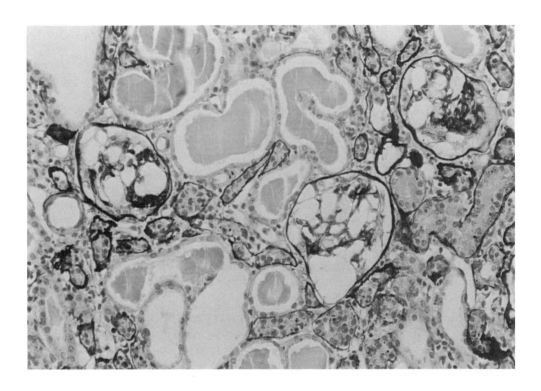

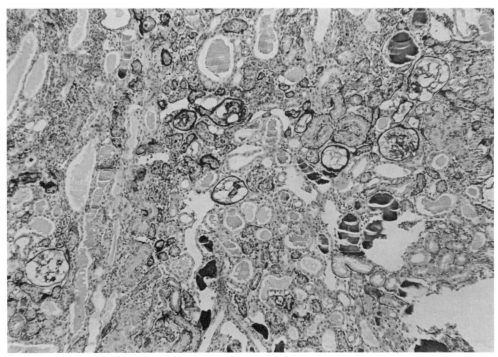

Figure 4: Morphological changes in rat kidney 5 weeks after 4mg/kg CI-941. a) Severe glomerular damage consisting of vacuolisation, thickening of Bowman's capsule and glomerular capillary basement membranes. Silver methenamine x300. b) Extensive tubular damage, including atrophy, dilatation and cast formation. Silver methenamine x125.

Hall et al. (14) reported on the progression of Adr-induced nephrotic syndrome studied over a 13 week period. Male Sprague-Dawley rats, of similar weight (and presumably age), to those currently used, received a single dose of 4mg/kg Adr. In terms of reductions in body weight and plasma albumin, the current findings following an identical dose of CI-941 appear to be more severe than those seen after Adr. The extent of the CI-941-induced reduction in body weight, plasma albumin and plasma cholesterol levels were also greater than those reported by Feehally et al. (7) following treatment with similar doses of Adr. Although these findings need to be substantiated, it would appear that CI-941 may well be more nephrotoxic than Adr.

Various pathogenic mechanisms have been proposed to explain the nephrotoxic action of Adr. These include increased glomerular basement membrane permeability due to an increased thromboxane synthesis (15) or loss of glomerular permselectivity (13). The pronounced nephrotic syndrome seen following injection of CI-941 suggests that this may be a useful compound for studying the pathophysiology of this syndrome.

The apparent increase in nephrotoxicity, associated with the production of an anti-cancer agent that has reduced cardiotoxic activity, may have clinical implications. Although Adr does not appear to be clinically nephrotoxic, it is possible that CI-941 may have a greater risk of causing clinical renal injury; further studies on this compound are required to answer these questions.

ACKNOWLEDGEMENTS

The authors would like to thank Dr. D R Newell for supplying the CI-941, and Mrs. E Whitehouse and Miss S Luckett for the histological preparations. This study was wholly supported by the Cancer Research Campaign.

REFERENCES

1. Blum RH, Carter SK: Adriamycin: a new anticancer drug with significant clinical activity. Ann. Intern. Med. 80: 249-259, 1974.

2. Lefrak EA, Pitha J, Rosenheim S, et al.: A clinicopathologic analysis of adriamycin cardiotoxicity. Cancer 32: 302-314, 1973.

3. Young DM: Pathologic effects of adriamycin in experimental system. Cancer Chemother. Rep. 6: 159-175, 1975.

4. Fajardo LF, Eltringham JR, Stewart JR, et al.: Adriamycin nephrotoxicity. Lab. Invest. 43: 242-253, 1980.

5. van Fleet JF, Greenwood LA, Ferrans FJ: Pathologic features of adriamycin toxicosis in young pigs: non skeletal lesions. Am. J. Vet. Res. 40: 1537-1552, 1979.

6. Litterst CL, Weiss RB: Clinical and experimental nephrotoxicity of cancer chemotherapeutic agents. In: Bach PH, Lock EA (eds); Nephrotoxicity in the experimental and clinical situation. Dordrecht, Martinus Nijhoff, 1987, p 771-816.

7. Feehally J, Baker F, Walls J: Dietary protein manipulation in experimental nephrotic syndrome. Nephron, 50: 247-252, 1988.

8. van Hoesel QGCM, Steerenberg PA, Dormans JAMA, et al.: Time-course study on doxorubicin-induced nephropathy and cardiomyopathy in male and female LOU/M/Wsl rats: lack of evidence for a causal relationship. J.N.C.I. 76: 299-307, 1986.

9. Kappus H: Overview of enzyme systems involved in bio-reduction of drugs and in redox cycling. Biochem. Pharmacol. 35: 1-6, 1986.

10. Graham MA, Newell DR, Butler J, et al.: The effect of the anthrapyrazole anti-tumour agent CI-941 on rat liver microsome and cytochrome P450 reductase mediated free radical processes; inhibition of doxorubicin activation in vitro. Biochem. Pharmacol. 36: 3345-3357, 1987.

11. Yeung TYK: personal communication, 1988.

12. Bryan GW, Jarchow RC, Maher JE: Measurement of glomerular filtration rate in small animals without urine collection. J. Lab. Clin. Med. 80: 845-856, 1972.

13. Bertani T, Poggi A, Pozzoni R, et al.: Adriamycin-induced nephrotic syndrome in rats. Sequence of pathologic events. Lab. Invest. 46: 16-23, 1982.

14. Hall RL, Wilke WL, Fettman MJ: The progression of adriamycin-induced nephrotic syndrome in rats and the effect of captropil. Toxicol. Appl. Pharmacol. 82: 164-174, 1986.

15. Remuzzi G, Imberti L, Rossini M, et al.: Increased glomerular thromboxane synthesis as a possible cause of proteinuria in experimental nephrosis. J. Clin. Invest. 75: 94-101, 1985.

PART XI
HEAVY METALS

53

DIFFERENTIAL HEAVY METAL CYTOTOXICITY IN HUMAN NORMAL AND TUMORAL CULTURED TUBULAR CELLS

D. Merlet (1), J.P. Merlet (2) and J. Cambar (1)

Laboratoire de Biologie Cellulaire (1); Institut de Pharmacie Industrielle (2), Faculté de Pharmacie, 3 Place de la Victoire, 33 000 Bordeaux, France

INTRODUCTION

Heavy metals (mercury, cadmium, lead) are widely used in many manufacturing industries and have been associated with occupational health problems. By contrast, cis-dichloro-diamino platinum II (CDDP) is a compound of major therapeutic interest as an anticancer drug, but one of the side effects limiting its use is nephroxicity. Heavy metal toxicity has already been described in cultured cells, and particularly in renal cell cultures (1) with dramatic changes in nuclear and membrane functions for mercury (2-4), cadmium (5), and lead (6).

Cytotoxicity tests are based on the assessment of cell viability as measured by cell membrane damage, with release of labelled substances (8), or intracellular enzymes (9). Moreover, nuclear damage can be shown with DNA breaks (11,12) or DNA synthesis inhibition (13).

The aim of the study is to compare cytoxicity induced by two heavy metals, mercuric chloride and cisplatin, in primary cultured renal epithelial tubular cells obtained from human tumoral kidneys and adjacent healthy tissues.

Cytotoxicity is determined both at membrane and nucleus level. Membrane damage was established by the release of specific proximal tubular brush border enzymes, alkaline phosphatase (ALP) and gamma-glutamyl transferase (GGT) into the culture medium. Nuclear dysfunction was assessed by DNA inhibition synthesis with the ^{3}H-thymidine incorporation test.

MATERIALS AND METHODS

Cell isolation   Healthy and tumoral cortical tissues were obtained from adult human kidneys after nephrectomy in patients with renal carcinoma. Tissue was washed with Hanks balanced salt solution (HBSS) to remove blood. Then, normal and tumoral tissues were dissected, minced with scissors and subjected to 0.02% w/v collagenase (type IV - Boehringer Chemicals) digestion in HBSS for 1 hour at $37^{o}C$ with stirring. The tubular cell mixture was then filtered through several steel sieves (450μm, 250μm, 180μm, 125μm, 63μm and 25μm). The final material was resuspended in HBSS (10ml) and used for cell culture. The viability of isolated cells was determined by the Trypan-blue exclusion test.

Cell culture   Isolated cell suspension was plated in culture flasks at a density of 10^{6} live cells/ml medium and maintained at $37^{o}C$ in an atmosphere of 95% O_2, 5% CO_2 in a humidified incubator. Cell culture medium (GIBCO) was composed of Dulbecco's modified Eagle medium plus Ham F12 (1:1) supplemented with 10% foetal calf serum, penicillin (100 Units/ml), streptomycin (100 μg/ml) and HEPES buffer (10 mM). It was changed every 3 days until confluency at 7 days for normal cells, and 14 days for malignant ones. Only primary cultures, without passage, were used.

Heavy metal intoxication At day 5-6 of primary culture, for normal cells and at day 10-12 for malignant ones, the medium was changed and an aliquot of stock $HgCl_2$ or cis-platin, prepared in sterile phosphate buffer saline (PBS), added to give a final concentration of 0.4µM; 2µM; 4µM; 40µM and 400 µM. The same amount of physiological saline was added to control cultures. Cultures were examined after 24 hrs exposure.

Enzyme assays Activities of enzymes released into the culture medium after 24 hrs of metal exposure were measured. Gamma-glutamyltransferase (GGT) activity was determined by measuring the p-nitroaniline, liberated from glutamyl-p-nitroanilide at 405 nm (13). Alkaline phosphatase (ALP) activity was determined by measuring the p-nitrophenol liberated from p-nitrophenyl phosphate (14). Enzyme activities were expressed as nmoles/min/mg total intracellular protein. Protein concentration was determined by the method of Bradford (15).

Statistical dose-dependent-cytotoxicity comparisons were obtained by using the Mann-Whitney U-test.

DNA synthesis inhibition using ^{3}H-thymidine incorporation After 24 hr of exposure to the metal, half of the culture medium was removed for enzyme assays and, ^{3}H-thymidine was added to the remaining volume of medium in each culture flask (10 µl of 0.1 mCi/ml solution). After 1 hr exposure, cells were twice washed with NaCl 0.9%, recovered with 2 ml NaCl 0.9%, then centrifuged at 3000 rev/min (5 min at 4^oC), cell pellet recovered with TCA (20%) during 3-4 hrs at 4^oC was again centrifuged. The cell pellet was dissolved for 2-3 hr at 37^oC in NaOH 1N. An aliquot (200 µl) of alkaline solution was added to 10 ml of scintillation solution (Instagel Packard). Results are expressed as percentage thymidine incorporation against control. Statistical analysis was obtained by using the Mann-Whitney U-test.

RESULTS

Characteristics of cultured cells Cultured tubular epithelial cell morphology is in accordance with previously reported observations (21). Cell proliferation in MEM D-Val culture medium indicates the absence of fibroblasts. The presence of cytokeratin, by immunofluorescence, indicates their epithelial origin and furthermore alkaline phosphatase (ALP) and gamma-glutamyltransferase (GGT) activities, demonstrated histochemically their proximal tubular origin.

Membrane damage: enzymatic measurements a) Cisplatin induces (Figure 1,2) membrane damage in normal cells with only high concentrations (40 and 400 µM), characterized by an extracellular enzymatic release increase compared to control. GGT release 378.51 nmoles/min/mg protein in normal cells and 282.53 nmoles/min/mg protein in cancerous ones, is higher than ALP release 291.27 nmoles/min/mg protein in normal cells and 256.26 nmoles/min/mg protein in tumour cells (Figure 3 and 4) suggesting lower enzymatic activities in tumoral cells than in normal ones.

b) $HgCl_2$ caused a modest enzyme release in normal and tumoral cells with 40µM; then enzymatic activities decrease, compared to control values, with 400µM.

Nuclear damage: ^{3}H-thymidine incorporation a) Cisplatin-related nuclear damage is very clear in normal cells (Figure 5), where ^{3}H-thymidine incorporation was decreased with only 0.4µM and very significantly with 40µM. In cancerous cells (Figure 6), cisplatin decreased ^{3}H-thymidine incorporation from 4 µM, but incorporation was maintained (x10 or x15) with high molarities (40µM and 400µM), compared to normal cells. b) $HgCl_2$, at low concentrations, increased ^{3}H-thymidine incorporation, particularly with 2µM in normal cells and 4µM in malignant ones; then incorporation decreases with higher concentrations compared to control (Figure 5, 6).

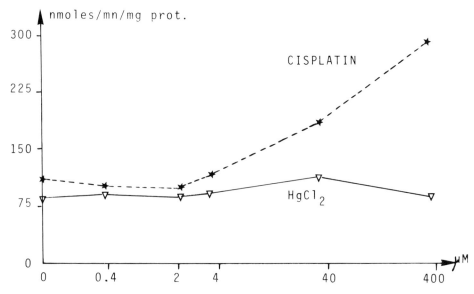

Figure 1. ALP release by normal cells after cisplatin and HgCl₂ exposure.

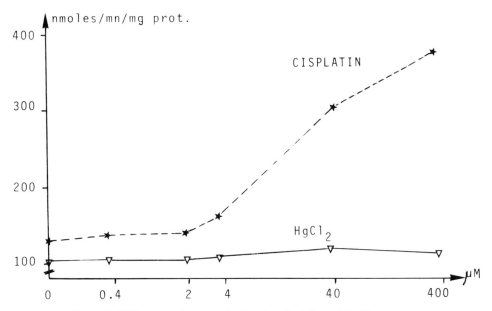

Figure 2. GGT release by normal cells after cisplatin and HgCl₂ exposure.

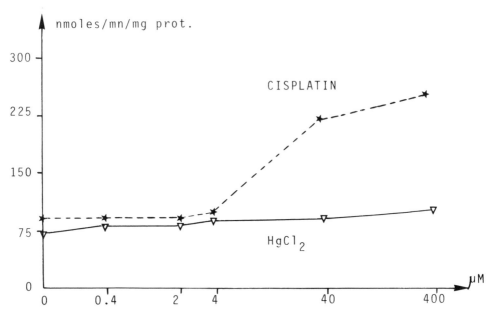

Figure 3. ALP release by tumoral cells after cisplatin and HgCl₂ exposure.

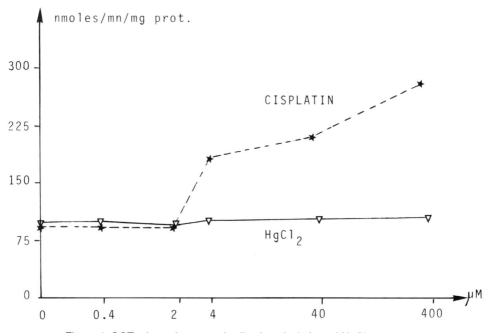

Figure 4. GGT release by tumoral cells after cisplatin and HgCl₂ exposure.

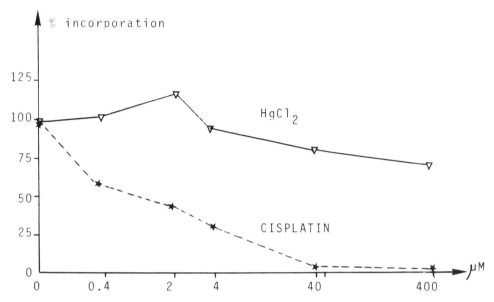

Figure 5. 3H-thymidine incorporation in normal cells after cisplatin and HgCl$_2$ exposure.

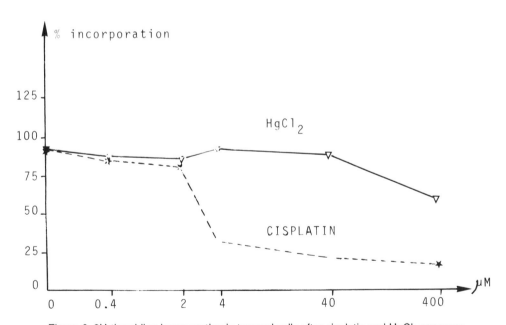

Figure 6. 3H-thymidine incorporation in tumoral cells after cisplatin and HgCl$_2$ exposure.

DISCUSSION

Numerous studies have used cultured renal cells in toxicology (1) and investigated the heavy metal toxicity of mercury, cadmium and platinum complexes (16), but not cisplatin. So far, few studies have described cultured human renal cellular material from normal kidneys (17-20) or kidneys with tumours (21).

The present study compares the cytotoxic effects of two heavy metals, cisplatin and mercuric chloride, at the membrane and nuclear level on normal and tumoral cultured tubular cells. The toxic effects of heavy metals are characterized by a proximal convoluted tubular brush border membrane fragmentation (22). After cisplatin intoxication, the compound shows a subcellular mitochondrial, microsomal and nuclear localization (23,24).

The toxic effect of mercury in cultured cells is probably due to intracellular concentration of the metal (2), mainly with $50\mu M$ of $HgCl_2$. We have shown similar membrane damages by the low enzymatic release with $400\mu M$ of $HgCl_2$. Cellular damage may be due to extracellular Ca^{2+} influx with high (100 μM) mercuric concentrations (25).

Mercury is known to affect the nuclear biochemistry by DNA breaks (26). Whereas low concentrations induce DNA synthesis, high concentrations inhibit DNA synthesis (2). We have shown toxic effects in both normal and tumoral cells.

Cisplatin targets for DNA (27) and also causes membrane damage, characterized by GGT and ALP release, particularly with high dose levels of the compound. Cytotoxic effects of cisplatin appear during all phases of the cell cycle (28). Nuclear dysfunction shown by the inhibition of DNA synthesis is greater in normal cells than in malignant ones, which can be explained by a significant difference in doubling time between normal cells (14 hr) and tumoral ones (33 hr) (21).

These results have shown that mercuric chloride damages mainly the membrane as shown by an 53.9% GGT and 36% ALP in-creased release at $40\mu M$ of $HgCl_2$. Cisplatin damages both membrane (197.7% and 75.43% increased release respectively for GGT and ALP at $40\mu M$) and the nucleus (96.19% decrease of ^3H-thymidine incorporation at $40\mu M$). Tumoral cells have a lower sensitivity to toxic compounds than normal ones (only 31% and 15% increase with $HgCl_2$ and 150% and 125.6% increase of ALP and GGT release with cisplatin, then only 65.9% decrease of ^3H-thymidine incorporation at $40\mu M$ cisplatin).

In conclusion, the present study confirms the use of human renal normal and malignant cultured cells to evaluate the nephrotoxicity of xenobiotics, by comparing cytotoxicity affecting membrane and nuclear integrity to help define subcellular targets of toxic compounds.

REFERENCES

1. Merlet D, Castaing N, Lakhdar B, Cambar J: Intérêt des cultures tubulaires en cytotoxicologie rénale. In: Adolphe M, Guillouzo A (Eds.); Méthodes in vitro en pharmaco-toxicologie, Colloque INSERM, 170, 1988, pp. 43-52

2. Bracken WM, Sharma RP: Biochemical responsiveness of a bovine kidney cell line to inorganic mercury. Arch Environ Contam Toxicol: 509, 1985

3. Rozalski M, Kuliemska E, Wierzbicki R: Content of mercuric in chromatin and level metallothionein proteins in kidney and liver of rats. Biochem Pharmacol 30: 2177, 1981

4. Rozalski M, Wierzbicki R: Effect of mercuric chloride on cultured rat fibroblasts: survival protein biosynthesis and binding of mercury to chromatin. Biochem Pharmacol 32: 2124-2126, 1983

5. Jin T, Norberg GF: Cadmium toxicity in kidney cells resistance induced by short-term pretreatment in vitro and in vivo. Acta Pharmacol Toxicol 58: 137-143, 1986

6. Peterson A, Lewne M, Walum E: Acute toxicity of organic solvents, heavy metals and DDT tested in cultures of mouse neuroblastoma cell. Toxicol Lett 9: 101-106, 1981

7. Reinhard CA, Schawalder H, Zbinden G: Cell detachment and cloning efficiency as parameters for toxicity. Toxicol 25: 47-52, 1982

8. Walum E: Membrane lesions in cultured mouse neuroblastoma cells exposed to metal compound. Toxicol Lett 25: 67-74, 1982

9. Merlet D, Mellado M, Merlet JP, Cambar J: An in vitro test for measuring cytotoxicity of mercuric chloride to human kidney epithelial cells by specific enzyme release. Cytotechnology 1: 261-266, 1988

10. Russo P, Favoni RE, Zargone D: Doxorubicine cytotoxicity to P388 lymphocytic leukemia as determined by alkaline elution and established assays. Anticancer Res 6: 1297, 1986

11. Teicher BA, Holden SA, Kelley MJ: Characterization of a human squamous carcinoma cell line resistant to cis-diamine dichlorplatinum II. Cancer Res 47: 388, 1987

12. Berhens BC, Hamilton, TC, Masuda H, Grotzinger KR: Characterization of cis-diamine dichloroplatinum II resistant human various cancer cell line and its use in evaluation of platinum analogue. Cancer Res 47: 414, 1987

13. Glossman H, Neville DMJr: Gamma-glutamyltransferase in kidney brush border membrane. Febs Lett 19: 340, 1972

14. Scholer DW, Edelman IS: Isolation of rat kidney cortical tubules enriched in proximal and distal segments. Am J Physiol 237: 350-359, 1979

15. Bradford MA: A rapid and sensitive method for the quantitation for microgram quantities of protein utilizing the principle of protein dye binding. Anal Bioch 72: 248-254, 1976

16. Batzer MA, Aggarwal SK: An in vitro screening system for the nephrotoxicity of various platinum coordination complexes. Cancer Chem Pharmacol 17: 209-217, 1986

17. Detrisac CJ, Sens MA, Garvin J, Spicer SS, Sens DA: Tissue culture of human kidney epithelial cells of proximal tubule origin. Kidney Int 25: 383-390, 1984

18. Trifillis AL, Regec AL, Trump BF: Isolation, culture and characterization of human tubular cells. J Urol 133: 324-329, 1985

19. States B, Foreman J, Lee T: Characteristics of cultured human renal cortical epithelia. Biochem Med Metab Biol 36: 151-161, 1986

20. Yang AH, Gould-Kostra DC, Oberley TD: In vitro growth and differentiation of human kidney tubular cells on a basement membrane substrate. In Vitro Cell Develop Biol 23: 34-46, 1987

21. Merlet D: Thèse Doctorat Etat ès Sci. Ph. Université Bordeaux II, no1, 1988

22. Makita T, Itagaki S, Ohokawa T: X-ray micro analysis and ultrastrutural localization of cis-platin in liver and kidney of the rat. Jpn J Cancer Res 76: 895-901, 1985

23. Makita T, Hako K, Ohokawa T: X-ray micro analysis and electron microscopy of platinum complex in the epithelium of proximal renal tubules of the cis-platin administerd rabbits. Cell Biol Int Reports 10: 447-454, 1986

24. Gordon JA, Gattone VH: Mitochondrial alterations in cisplatin-induced acute renal failure. Am J Physiol 250: F991-F998, 1986

25. Smith MW, Ambudkar IS, Phelps PC, Regec AL, Trump BF: HgCl$_2$ induced changes in cytosolic Ca^{2+} of cultured rabbit renal tubular cells. Biochem Biophys Acta 931: 130, 1987

26. Cantoni O, Christie NT, Swann A: Mechanism of HgCl$_2$ cytotoxicity in cultured mammalian cells. Molec Pharmacol 26: 360-368, 1984

27. Tourani JM: Chimiothérapie et hormonothérapie. In: Andrieu JM (ed); Traitements actuels des cancers. Paris, Medsi, 1987, pp. 38-59

28. Follezou JM, Pouillart P. In: Précis de chimiothérapie anticancéreuse. Paris, Doin, 1980, pp. 53-54

54

EFFECTS OF HEAVY METALS ON METABOLIC FUNCTIONS IN ISOLATED GLOMERULI AND PROXIMAL TUBULAR FRAGMENTS

M.F. Wilks (1), E.N. Kwizera (1,2) and P.H. Bach (1)

Nephrotoxicity Research Group, The Robens Institute, University of Surrey, Guildford, Surrey GU2 5XH, UK (1), and Dept. of Pharmacology, University of Transkei, Umtata, Transkei, Southern Africa (2)

INTRODUCTION

The kidneys are susceptible to injury caused by a number of heavy metals. The use of metallic compounds in medicine (eg cis-platinum in the chemotherapy of cancer and organic gold salts in the treatment of rheumatoid arthritis) is largely limited by their nephrotoxic potential. Acute impairment of renal function (acute renal failure) may follow exposure to other metal salts such as mercuric chloride (1), uranyl nitrate (2) and potassium dichromate (3). Progressively degenerative changes are seen after long-term exposure to cadmium and lead (4,5). Although the proximal tubule is generally regarded as the prime target for heavy metal-induced toxicity, damage to other nephron structures such as the glomerulus (the first anatomical structure in the filtration process) may contribute to the development of renal functional impairment. This, however, is difficult to assess in the intact animal.

The effects of heavy metals are modulated by extrarenal and renal factors such as uptake, transport, binding and excretion processes in vivo. Thus it is difficult to define pure nephrogenic effects. A suitable in vitro model circumvents many of these factors and may therefore help in understanding the early effects caused by heavy metals which are relevant to both acute and chronic toxicity. The use of isolated glomeruli and proximal tubular fragments (PTF) to study nephrotoxicity has been previously described (6). In order to compare the relative susceptibility of different nephron structures, we have investigated the effects of 7 heavy metal salts on de-novo protein synthesis and fatty acid oxidation in this model.

METHODS

Radiolabelled compounds: ^{3}H-Proline (specific activity 15 Ci/mM) and ^{14}C-linolenic acid (56.2 mCi/mM) were obtained from Amersham International, Aylesbury, UK.

Heavy metals: Mercuric chloride (Hg), potassium dichromate (Cr), cadmium chloride (Cd), nickel chloride (Ni), and sodium selenite (Se), were purchased from BDH, Poole, UK. Sodium meta-arsenite (AsIII) and di-sodium hydrogen arsenate (AsV) were from E. Merck, Darmstadt, Germany.

The isolation and incubation procedure has been described in detail elsewhere (7). Briefly, kidneys from 10 male Wistar rats (University of Surrey strain, 150g bw) were collected for each experiment. After decapsulation and removal of the medulla they were chopped finely and washed in Earle's balanced salt solution (EARLE'S) containing glucose (1 g/l) and buffered with HEPES (28 mM, pH 7.4). The tissue was forced through a series of stainless steel sieves (Endecotts, London, UK) starting with 250 μm mesh size. PTF were collected from a 150 μm sieve and glomeruli from a 75 μm sieve. The fragments were washed and centrifuged twice and resuspended in EARLE'S. The final preparation consisted of more than 90% glomeruli or PTF, as assessed by phase-contrast microscopy.

The incorporation of ^{3}H-labelled proline into protein was assessed by incubation over 4 hours in a shaking water bath at 37°C in the absence or presence of heavy metals at concentrations ranging from 10^{-6} to 10^{-3} molar. Protein was precipitated by addition of ice cold trichloroacetic acid (TCA) and after washing and centrifugating three times, the activity of incorporated proline was measured by liquid scintillation counting. Oxidation of ^{14}C-linolenic acid was measured by incubation in a closed system in which [14]CO_2 was trapped in filter paper impregnated with 1M NaOH. This was quantitated by liquid scintillation counting. Total protein content of the incubation mixtures was assessed using the Coomassie blue assay (8) and bovine serum albumin as a standard.

Labelled amino acid incorporation and CO_2 generation were calculated as pmoles of substrate per mg glomerular or proximal tubular protein. The effects of heavy metals are expressed as percentage of control value, relative toxicity is shown as the concentration needed to reduce amino acid incorporation or fatty acid oxidation by 50% compared to controls (IC_{50}).

RESULTS

As described elsewhere (7), incorporation of proline into TCA-precipitable macromolecules increased continuously over 4 hours. Oxidation of labelled linolenic acid to CO_2 was linear for 4 hours only in glomeruli and plateaued in PTF after 2 hours.

Protein synthesis was generally more strongly depressed by heavy metals than linolenic acid oxidation. The range of concentrations needed for 50% inhibition varied from 10^{-6} to 10^{-3} molar with Hg being the most potent glomerulotoxin at a tenth of the concentration which was effective in PTF (Fig. 1). The IC_{50} values for both parameters measured are given in Table 1.

For proline incorporation into PTF, the effect of Hg was comparable to that of Cd and AsIII and less than that of Cr (Fig. 2a). For linolenic acid oxidation, Hg was the most potent tubular toxin, but again a 10-fold higher concentration was required to cause the same effect as in glomeruli (Fig. 2b). Ni inhibited proline incorporation strongly in glomeruli (Fig. 1a), moderately in PTF (Fig. 2a) and had little effect on linolenic acid oxidation (Figs. 1b and 2b). Se showed a moderate toxicity only for PTF and

Table 1. Effects of heavy metal salts on proline incorporation and linolenic acid oxidation in isolated glomeruli and proximal tubular fragments (PTF).

| Compound | Valence | IC_{50}* (mM) | | | |
| | | Proline | | Linolenic acid | |
		Glomeruli	PTF	Glomeruli	PTF
Mercury choride	II	0.003	0.03	0.003	0.055
Potassium dichromate	VI	0.015	0.017	0.032	0.17
Nickel chloride	II	0.035	0.056	0.66	>0.5
Sodium meta-arsenite	III	0.068	0.034	0.24	0.34
Cadmium chloride	II	0.081	0.032	0.21	0.48
Sodium selenite	IV	0.28	0.065	0.67	0.30
Di-sodium-arsenate	V	1.9	1.0	>10	>5

* Concentration (mM) needed to reduce amino acid incorporation and fatty acid oxidation to 50% of control value (after incubation for 4 hrs). N = 3 to 5 separate experiments.

Glomeruli

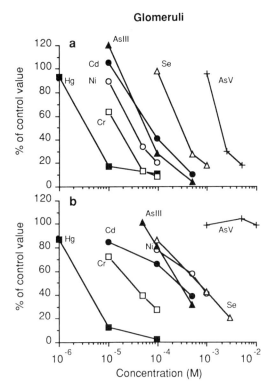

Figure 1 Effects of Heavy Metal salts on ^{3}H-proline incorporation (a) and ^{14}C-linolenic acid oxidation (b) in isolated glomeruli (for abbreviations see text).

Proximal tubular fragments

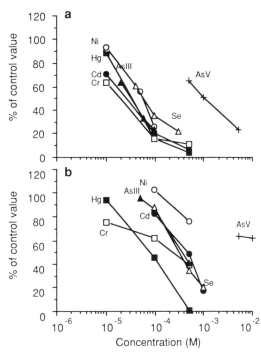

Figure 2 Effects of Heavy Metal salts on ^{3}H-proline incorporation (a) and on ^{14}C-linolenic acid oxidation (b) in proximal tubular fragments (for abbreviations see text).

AsV was the least toxic compound for both cell systems and metabolic pathways.

DISCUSSION

Heavy metal nephrotoxicity has generally been considered to affect the proximal tubule (9), but early in the development of acute metal toxicity there is a striking depression of the glomerular filtration rate (GFR), which cannot be explained by proximal tubular damage alone. Attempts to associate this fall in GFR with tubulo-glomerular feedback, vasoconstriction or tubular obstruction (10) have failed to reach a definite conclusion. Our results show that Hg and Cr, which of the metals tested, are most likely to have effects on the glomerular filtration rate in vivo, are the most potent glomerulotoxins in vitro. For Hg, a 10-fold lower concentration was effective to suppress glome-

rular metabolism compared to PTF. These data suggest that glomerular effects of metals like Hg and Cr may not manifest morphologically, but nevertheless may have profound implications on the filtration rate. The more pronounced effects of Hg may be due to its high affinity to sulphydryl groups both in the cell membrane and intracellular structures (11), while the hexavalent chromium is a strong oxidising agent (12).

Ni had a marked effect on protein synthesis in glomeruli, but not fatty acid oxidation. There is evidence that Ni binds to anionic sites in parts of the glomerular basement membrane (13). Proline, which we used to assess protein synthesis, is a major component of the glomerular basement membrane (14) and thus may be particularly affected by a compound which targets for the basement membrane. Cd and the trivial arsenite are known proximal tubular toxins after chronic exposure and are less glomerulotoxic in our in vitro system than Hg and Cr. In PTF, however, they had the same effect on proline incorporation as Hg. As in vivo, the pentavalent arsenate failed to show a strong effect.

In summary, our results suggest glomerulotoxic effects, which have not previously been recognised, of those heavy metals that cause acute renal failure. Proline incorporation is more sensitive but less specific than linolenic acid oxidation as an index of heavy metal nephrotoxicity in vitro, and the different rankings of the metals for the two parameters reflect different mechanisms of cytotoxicity. The system offers the potential to further investigate the underlying mechanisms of heavy metal nephrotoxicity.

ACKNOWLEDGEMENTS

This study was supported by the EEC Biotechnology Action Programme, and in part by the Wellcome Trust, Johns Hopkins Center for Alternatives to Animal Testing and the Dr Hadwen Trust for Humane Research. MFW was recipient of a post-doctoral fellowship by the Deutsche Forschungsgemeinschaft and ENK held a fellowship by the Association of Commonwealth Universities.

REFERENCES

1. Zalme RC, McDowell EM, Nagle RB, McNeil JS, Flamenbaum W, Trump BF: Studies on the pathophysiology of acute renal failure. I. Correlation of ultrastructure and function in the proximal tubule of the rat following administration of mercuric chloride. Virchows Arch B Cell Path 22: 197-216, 1976.

2. Blantz RC: Mechanism of acute renal failure after uranyl nitrate. J Clin Invest 55: 621-635, 1975.

3. Henry LN, Lane CE, Kashgarian M: Micropuncture studies on the pathophysiology of acute renal failure in the rat. Lab Invest 19: 309-314, 1968.

4. Bernard A, Lauwerys R: Cadmium in human population. Experientia 40: 143-152, 1984.

5. Goyer RA: The nephrotoxic effects of lead. In: Bach PH, Bonner FW, Bridges JW, Lock EA EA (eds); Nephrotoxicity, Assessment and Pathogenesis. Chichester, John Wiley & Sons, 1982. pp. 338-348.

6. Bach PH, Ketley CP, Ahmed I, Dixit M: The mechanisms of target cell injury by nephrotoxins. Fd Chem Toxicol 24: 775-779, 1986.

7. Wilks MF, Kwizera EN, Bach PH: Assessment of heavy metal nephrotoxicity in vitro using isolated rat glomeruli and proximal tubular fragments. Renal Physiol Biochem 13:275-284, 1990.

8. Bradford MM: A rapid and sensitive method for the quantitation of microgram quantities of protein, using the principle of protein-dye binding. Anal Biochem 72: 248-254, 1976.

9. Fowler BA, Mistry P, Goering PL: Mechanisms of metal-induced nephrotoxicity. In: Bach PH, Lock EA (eds); Nephrotoxicity in the experimental and clinical situation, Dordrecht, Martinus Nijhoff, 1987, pp. 659-681.

10. Stein JH, Lifschitz MD, Barnes LD: Current concepts on the pathophysiology of acute renal failure. Am J Physiol 234: F171-F181, 1978.

11. Berlin M: Mercury. In: Friberg L, Nordberg GF, Vouk VB (eds); Handbook of the Toxicology of Metals, Vol II. Amsterdam, Elsevier, 1986, pp. 387-445.

12. Langard S, Norseth T: Chromium. In: Friberg L, Nordberg GF, Vouk VB (eds); Handbook of the Toxicology of Metals, Vol II. Amsterdam, Elsevier, 1986, pp. 185-210.

13. Templeton DM: Interaction of toxic cations with the glomerulus: Binding of Ni to purified glomerular basement membrane. Toxicology 43, 1-15, 1987.

14. Kefalides VA: Basement membranes: Structure function relationships. Renal Physiology 4: 57-66, 1981.

55

CADMIUM UPTAKE BY PROXIMAL TUBULAR CELLS (LLC-PK$_1$) IN VITRO

F. Mingard, P. Hausel and J. Dièzi

Institut de Pharmacologie et Toxicologie de l'Université, CH - 1005 Lausanne, Switzerland

INTRODUCTION

Cadmium (Cd) has been found to be taken up, in vivo and in vitro, by a number of different cell species, including intestinal and renal epithelial cells. Cd uptake by the epithelial cell layer from the small intestine has been shown to constitute an initial, obligatory step of the net transfer of cadmium ions from the lumen into blood and thus to play a central role in intestinal Cd absorption. Several characteristics of this uptake mechanism have been defined in vitro by the use of everted sacs or brush border membrane vesicles (1,2). Similarly, uptake of Cd (inorganic or bound to metallothionein) by renal (proximal) tubule cells has been investigated in vivo by clearance-type and micropuncture techniques (3-5), and in vitro using an isolated kidney preparation (6), renal cell cultures (7) or brush border membrane vesicles (8).

While uptake of Cd from the apical side of renal proximal tubule cells has been well demonstrated in several of the studies mentioned above, the published evidence pointing to a significant contribution of a basolateral uptake of Cd to the intracellular accumulation of the metal ion is mostly based on the demonstration of renal uptake of Cd despite suppression of ultrafiltration, and is therefore more indirect. Similarly, the possible occurrence of a net transepithelial transfer of Cd across the tubular epithelium remains difficult to evaluate in whole kidney approaches.

The present in vitro experiments, carried out in LLC-PK$_1$ cells cultivated either on plastic dishes or on permeable filters, were therefore aimed at measuring the uptake of Cd by renal epithelial cells exposed to Cd at either the apical or the basolateral cell surface, and at estimating a possible net transepithelial transfer of Cd.

METHODS

In a first group of experiments, LLC-PK$_1$ cells were grown at confluence (9 days, 37°C, 95% air/5% CO$_2$) on plastic dishes in 3 ml of Basal Medium Eagle complemented with antibiotics (penicillin, streptomycin), glutamine, selenium, hormones (insulin, transferrin, hydrocortisone, T$_3$, prostaglandin E$_1$), and foetal calf serum. The culture was kept in a serum-free medium during the 24 hr preceding the experiments. Incubations with Cd^{2+} were carried out in serum-free medium (3 ml) containing CdCl$_2$ (1 or 5μM) and, in some experiments, ZnSO$_4$. Incubations with Cd^{2+} lasted between 60 min and 24 hr, and were carried out at 37° or 4°C. At the end, the medium was discarded and the cells washed with 2 ml phosphate buffer (PBS). After trypsinization and additional steps of washing, the cells were sonicated and the homogenate was ultracentrifuged (110,000g, 75 min, 4°C). The supernatant, corresponding to the cytosolic fraction, was analyzed for protein and Cd content (atomic absorption spectroscopy with a carbon rod atomizer).

In a second series of experiments, LLC-PK$_1$ cells were grown on permeable collagen coated filter supports (Transwell^R, Costar), allowing separate access to the basolateral and the apical sides of the cultured epithelium. The culture conditions (9) were otherwise similar to those described above. Cd^{2+} was added to either the basolateral or the apical side of the culture. Cell uptake and transepithelial transfer of Cd^{2+} were measured after incubation times varying between 1 and 6 hr.

In a third series of preliminary experiments, the apparent uptake of Cd^{2+} and Cd-metallothionein (Cd-Mt) by brush border membrane vesicles (BBMV) from rabbit kidney was measured. BBMV, prepared by standard methods (10) and a rapid filtration technique (11), were incubated with either $CdCl_2$ or Cd-Mt for periods varying between 1 and 120 min. BBMV-bound Cd was measured by AAS and expressed after correction for filter binding. Hepatic Cd-Mt was either prepared by G-75 gel filtration of liver homogenates from rats exposed to Cd, or was obtained from Sigma.

RESULTS

1. Uptake of Cd^{2+} by LLC-PK₁ cells in plastic dishes: the time-course of this uptake during 24 hr of exposure is shown in Fig.1. At 37°, the initial rate (i.e. in the first 6 hr) of accumulation of Cd^{2+} was larger than at later stages (from 6

to 24 hr). Cd^{2+} uptake by LLC-PK₁ cells led to concentration gradients across cell plasma membrane of more than 2000 after 24 hr of incubation. In contrast, uptake was virtually suppressed when incubation was carried out at $4^{\circ}C$ (Fig. 1).

2. Effect of Zn^{2+} on Cd^{2+} uptake: as shown in Fig. 2, addition of Zn^{2+} in the apical medium at either 12.5 or 25 Zn/Cd molar ratios decreased Cd^{2+} uptake. This inhibition was most notable after 4 hr of incubation, and was directly related to the concentration of Zn^{2+}.

3. Cd^{2+} uptake from the apical or basolateral cell sides: in LLC-PK₁ cells grown on permeable supports, uptake of Cd^{2+} from the apical side into the cytosolic fraction was, at similar duration of exposure and Cd^{2+} concentrations in the incubation medium (1μM), nearly identical to that measured in cells grown on plastic dishes (70.2±14.8 pg Cd/mg protein) after 6 hr of incubation; (compare with Fig. 1). The cell uptake of Cd^{2+} added to the basolateral side was somewhat lower (45.1 ± 6.6), but the difference was not statistically significant, and Cd^{2+} uptake from the apical or basolateral sides were similar for incubations at 5μM Cd.

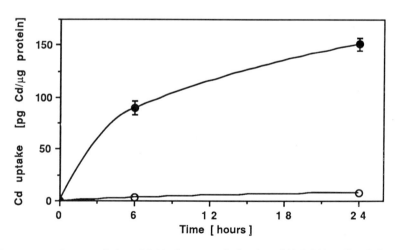

Figure 1.   Time-course of accumulation of Cd in the cytosolic fraction of LLC-PK1 cells. Cells at confluence were incubated with BM medium containing 1μ CdCl₂ during 6 or 24 hr at either 37° (closed symbols) or $4^{\circ}C$ (open symbols). Mean ± SE of 6 experiments.

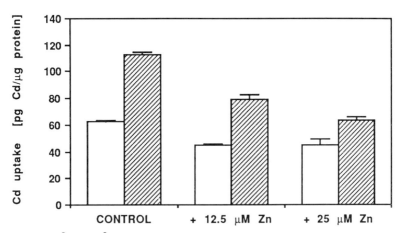

Figure 2.   Effect of Zn^{2+} on Cd^{2+} uptake into the cytosolic fraction of LLC-PK1 cells. Cells at confluence were incubated at 37° C with 1µM $CdCl_2$ during 2 (white columns) or 4 hr (filled columns) in the presence of O (Control), 12.5 or 25µM $ZnSO_4$. Mean ± SE of 4 dishes.

4. Transepithelial transfer of Cd^{2+}: after 6 hr of incubation at 37°C, negligible quantities of Cd^{2+}, corresponding to % of the total amount of the metal ion initially present in the incubation medium, were recovered in the compartment (apical or basolateral) opposite to that where Cd^{2+} was added. This transfer was markedly lower than that found to occur by simple diffusion through the filter alone, in the absence of the cell layer. After 6 hr of incubation, transepithelial gradients of Cd^{2+} ranged between approximately 50 and 100 (1µM added initially to either the apical or basolateral side).

5. Uptake of Cd by BBMV: for both Cd^{2+} (10 to 500µM) and Cd-Mt (10 to 200µM), uptake of the metal by BBMV was extremely rapid, and was nearly complete (80% of the maximal value) within 1 min at lower concentrations (10µM) of Cd^{+2} or Cd-Mt. At higher concentrations (200 and 500µM), the percent of Cd uptake during the first minute was smaller (approximately 50%), and a slower component of uptake appeared at these concentrations.

DISCUSSION

The use of in vitro cell culture systems, where epithelial cells can be grown on permeable supports, allows a direct investigation on the kinetics of uptake and possible transepithelial transfer of Cd. The results reported here, obtained in an established epithelial cell line with proximal tubule properties (12), confirm and extend observations previously published on the handling of Cd^{2+} and/or Cd-Mt by the kidney and the mucosal cells of the small intestine. Thus, the inhibition of apical Cd^{2+} uptake by Zn^{2+} in LLC-PK1 cells is reminiscent of the interaction between the two metals which has been observed in the intestine (13). It is noteworthy that, for identical Zn^{2+}/Cd^{2+} molar ratios (12.5 or 25), the level of inhibition of Cd^{2+} uptake by Zn^{2+} in LLC-PK1 cells was very similar to that observed in the jejunum (13).

Occurrence of Cd^{2+} uptake from the basolateral side of the renal tubular cells has been inferred from the fact that suppression of glomerular ultrafiltration did not prevent accumulation of Cd in the renal tissue (6,14). The present experiments provide a direct evidence that uptake of Cd^{2+} can occur at either side of the epithelial cell layer, and that the rate of uptake is approximately of similar magnitude at either side. In addition, it appears that no sizable transepithelial transfer of Cd^{2+} ions can be measured across a cell layer with proximal tubule characteristics and that, under these experimental conditions, nearly all the Cd^{2+} removed from either the basolateral or the apical side is accumulated in the cells. Whether prolonged exposure of the epithelial cells to Cd, resulting in higher intracellular concentrations, may result in a transepithelial transfer of Cd remains to be investigated.

The finding of a very rapid binding of Cd^{2+} and of Cd-Mt to renal brush border vesicles is in line with previous, similar observations in renal and intestinal apical membrane vesicles (8,2), and points again to the fact that this initial binding presumably represents the first step of intracellular incorporation of Cd when exposure occurs on the luminal side of the epithelium.

ACKNOWLEDGEMENTS

This study was supported by Swiss National Science Foundation.

REFERENCES

1.   Foulkes EC, McMullen DM: Kinetics of transepithelial movement of heavy metals in rat jejunum. Am J Physiol 253: G134-G138, 1987.

2.   Bevan C, Foulkes EC: Interaction of cadmium with brush-border membrane vesicles from the rat small intestine. Toxicology 54: 297-309, 1989.

3.   Foulkes EC: Renal tubular transport of cadmium- metallothionein. Toxicol Appl Pharmacol 45: 505-512, 1978.

4.   Felley-Bosco E, Diezi J: Fate of cadmium in rat renal tubules: a microinjection study. Toxicol Appl Pharmacol 91: 204-211, 1987.

5.   Felley-Bosco E, Diezi J: Fate of cadmium in rat renal tubules: a micropuncture study. Toxicol Appl Pharmacol 98: 243-251, 1989.

6.   Diamond G, Cohen JJ, Weinstein SL: Renal handling of cadmium in perfused rat kidney and effects on renal function and tissue composition. Am J Physiol 251: F784-F794, 1986.

7.   Cherian MG: The synthesis of metallothionein and cellular adaptation to metal toxicity in primary rat kidney epithelial cell cultures. Toxicology 17; 225-231, 1980.

8.   Selenke W, Foulkes EC: The binding of cadmium metallothionein to isolated renal brush border membranes. Proc Soc Exp Biol Med 167: 40-44, 1981.

9.   Fauth C, Rossier BC, Roch-Ramel F: Transport of tetraethylammonium by kidney epithelial cell line (LLC-PK$_1$). Am J Physiol 254: F351-F357, 1988.

10. Booth AG, Kenny AJ: A rapid method for the preparation of microvilli from rabbit kidney. Biochem J 142: 575-581, 1974.

11. Hopfer U, Nelson K, Perrotto J, Isselbacher KJ: Glucose transport in isolated brush border membrane from rat small intestine. J Biol Chem 248: 25-32, 1973.

12.   Gstraunthaler GJA: Epithelial cells in tissue culture. Renal Physiol Biochem 11: 1-41, 1988.

13. Foulkes EC: Interactions between metals in rat jejunum: implications on the nature of cadmium uptake. Toxicology 37: 117-125, 1985.

14. Foulkes EC: Excretion and retention of cadmium, zinc and mercury by rabbit kidney. Am J Physiol 227: 1356-1360, 1974.

56

RAT KIDNEY METALLOTHIONEIN AFTER CADMIUM EXPOSURE

M.P. Iniesta, M.I. Sanchez Reus and B. Ribas

Institute of Biochemistry, CSIC-Complutense Unversity, Faculty of Pharmacy, 28040 Madrid, Spain

INTRODUCTION

The relatively low molecular mass of metallo-thionein (MT) and its high affinity to metals, are important characteristics to exploit as an early molecular marker for nephrotoxicity, because of its easy renal filtration and ease of analysis. Cadmium is incorporated and retained by liver and kidney cells more than any other organ. Its absorption is increased in rats lacking iron or suffering ferropenic anaemia (1).

In kidney cortex from human autopsies, there is an age-dependent increase of Cd, Zn and Cd/Zn quotient reported (2) with a peak at mid-age and a subsequent unexplained decline. Cadmium is transferred to the kidney bound to low molecular weight complexes that can be freely filtered through the glomeruli, and it is also bound to the metallothionein, which is re-absorbed in the proximal tubules (3). The chronic administration of cadmium induces its accumulation in kidney and necrotic damage to the renal tubular epithelia, similar to that caused by a single injection of cadmium-bound metal-lothionein (4). The injection of isolated and labeled MT causes severe necrotic damage to the kidney, contradicting the theory that MT assumes a biological protective role by binding toxic heavy metals (5).

MT carries out its physiological and biochemi-cal functions intracellularly, but the toxic action of this protein should be explained as a function of the toxic heavy metal bound to MT (6). The inter-relationships between metals that bind proteins, is heightened by the multiple molecu-lar isoforms of MT found in blood and urine. This raises the possibility of testing these iso-forms as biochemical markers of nephrotoxicity in epidemiology and diagnosis of nephropa-thies.

It is suggested that the metallic composition of metallothionein in mammals is partly deter-mined by the nature and extension of the exposure of the body to different metals. Zinc, cadmium, copper and mercury have been de-tected in tissues in connection with MT (7), nevertheless, the metal composition depends also on the organ origin, metal content of the environment and diet (8). The renal accumula-tion of Cd^{2+} was similar in both sexes and was recovered in the MT fraction and associated with an increased zinc concentration in liver and kidney. The results on Cu^{2+} incorporation are unequivocal but the cadmium increase is corre-lated with higher levels of MT in the liver and kidney of rats (9). In humans and horses in-tense research has been performed with similar results by several authors (10,11), except for Cu^{++}, which are contradictory. This work is a preliminary report trying to consider MT as an early molecular marker to ameliorate and to prevent renal toxicity, induced by cadmium (4,12-15).

METHODS

Male Wistar rats weighing 200±10g were used. Cadmium chloride was given to one group at the dose of 0.1mg Cd/kg/day ip for 6 consecutive days. Controls received saline of the same ionic strength. Blood was withdrawn by cardiac puncture under light ether anaesthesia and the animals killed, kidneys dissected, frozen or MT extracted by the classical purification technique (16). Kidneys were homogenized with an Ultra Turrax in Tris-HCl buffer 2.5×10^{-2}M pH 7.5 (1:2; w:v) and the extracts ultracentrifuged at 1000,000 x g for 60 min and supernatants filtered through Millipore 0.4 μm membranes. An aliquot, of standard protein concentration for each experiment was applied to a Sephadex G-50 column (2.5 x 70 cm) previously calibrated with authentic proteins: beta-lactoglobulin, lysozyme, ribonuclease and cytochrome c. The elution profile was monitored at 253nm (MT does not absorb at 280nm because of the lack of aromatic aminoacids) and metal content of Zn^{2+} and Cd^{2+} determined by atomic absorption spectrophotometry. Total proteins were determined by the method of Lowry et al. (17). The peak of low MW proteins and MT content, was collected between the fraction 25-30 and submitted to high performance liquid chromatography (HPLC) as described (18,19). An aliquot of 1 μg Cd^{2+} of the MT extract is, if necessary, diluted with buffer A: Tris-HCl 2.5×10^{-2}M pH 7.5, used in the gradient, being buffer B: buffer A with 60% Acetonitrile, and separated on hyperchrome column Lichrosorb RP-18, 10 μM particle size and MN-300-7C4 (18-20).

RESULTS

Figure 1 shows the elution profile from the Sephadex G-50 column of two protein peaks, the high and low Mw proteins of the kidney extract from Cd^{2+} treated rats. The second peak, fraction 27, shows the contents of Cd^{2+} bound to MT, determined by atomic absorption spectrophotometry. Control animals did not show Cd^{2+} content. The molecular weight of the protein fraction of the second peak, compared to the elution profile of authentic molecules was in the region of 7000 daltons, and absorbed optically at 253nm with a maximum corresponding to MT, having a high Cd^{2+} content. Zn is also detected in fraction 27 using the same method.

The separations with the kidney extracts from the rat groups shows, that the control group has 4 peaks coinciding with 4 MT peaks from rabbit liver extracts, used here to establish the standard conditions for kidney extract (Sigma Chemical Co. Catalog Nr: 5392). The rat peaks appear in Figure 2A with retention times of: 25.4; 30.9; 31.4 and 42.5 min. MT-1 is absent in control animals, but it is highly induced after Cd^{2+} treatment. In contrast to the other 4 multiple molecular isoforms, as it is shown in figure 2B, the peak of highly induced MT-1 has a retention time of 20.4 min.

DISCUSSION

Several physiologic functions have been described for MT (16), one of which is the protection of the organism from toxic effects of harmful heavy metals, especially from cadmium (4,12-15). MT is interesting from the metabolic and from the toxicologic point of view, dealing with its high accumulation, sequestering and releasing metallic ions, for the catalytic molecules, the enzymes, and also for metallic proteins and peptides. During exposure or intoxication with heavy metals, MT is induced and its multiple molecular isoforms could serve as early molecular marker of nephrotoxicity. Cadmium has become a serious and wide-spread environmental contaminant during the last decades, and consecutive recommendations of the WHO stress the necessity to study this heavy metal which is now considered a toxic element.

In this work it is shown by HPLC of kidney extracts from rats treated with cadmium, that the peak of MT-1, the first in the profile of Figure 2B, is higher than of the other MT-isoforms, which it is not seen in the chromatograms of the control extracts. This first peak of MT-1 by HPLC, could be used in future experiments as a more selective molecular marker of nephrotoxicity. There is a need to establish its significance under low doses of cadmium. This result could emphasize the application of the isometallothionein separation by HPLC in order to establish its usefulness in the control of the effect of nephrotoxic agents.

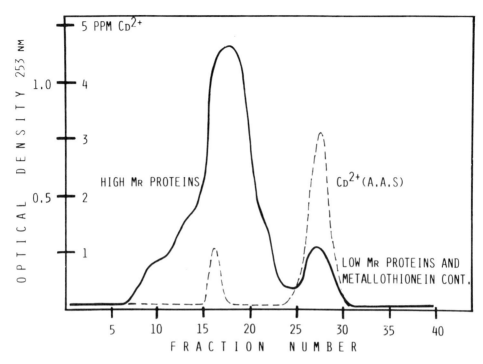

Figure 1. Elution profile from Sephadex G-50 of high and low Mw proteins of kidney of rats treated with cadmium.

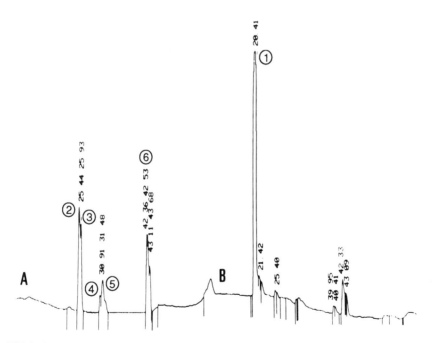

Figure 2. HPLC elution profile of isometallothioneins from rat kidney. A: in control rats MT-1 is absent; B: in treated rats, MT-1 is highly induced under Cadmium exposure.

The topographic origin of MT, during a Cd^{2+} nephrotoxic disease was proposed recently (21), using the MT-antigenicity, detected in the cytoplasm of proximal tubular cells. If the pathological process is exacerbated, the MT-immunofluorescence is increased within the distal tubule and the collecting duct. No specific staining was observed in the glomerulus, vascular endothelial cells and connective tissues (21). The renal damage by Cd^{2+} could be explained not only by the capacity of the kidney to synthesise MT and by the limited rate of excretion of both cadmium and Cd-MT, but also on the reabsorptive function of the renal system. MT in urine or blood, as an early marker of nephrotoxicity, does not originate from renal damage, but comes from a MT-induction after low cadmium exposure.

The separations by HPLC of the rat kidney extracts shows that the control group has 4 peaks coinciding with 4 MT peaks from standard rabbit liver extracts. The high resolution of isometallothioneins in independent peaks, as shown here, favours the application of this technique to the analysis of iso-metallothioneins excretion in urine, or its concentration in blood, as a molecular marker of cadmium exposure. The different isoforms separated in this work show that it is possible to compare the specificity of each isoform with different metals, the relationship between metals in each isoform, and as markers of nephrotoxicity occurring as a result of environmental pollution.

REFERENCES

1. Hamilton DL, Valberg LS: Relationship between cadmium and iron absorption. Am J Physiol 227: 1033-1037, 1974.

2. Chung J, Nartey NO, Cherian MG: Metallothionein levels in liver and kidney of Canadians - A potential indicator of environmental exposure to cadmium. Arch Environ Health 41: 319-323, 1986.

3. Foulkes EC: Role of metallothionein in transport of heavy metals. In: Foulkes EC (ed); Biological roles of metallothionein. North Holland-New York, Elsevier, 1982, pp. 131-140.

4. Suzuki KT: Studies of cadmium uptake and metabolism by the kidney. Environ Health Perspect 54: 21-30, 1984.

5. Cherian MG: Studies on toxicity of metallothionein in rat kidney epithelial cell culture. In: Foulkes EC (ed); Biological roles of metallothionein. North Holland-New York, Elsevier, 1982, pp. 193-202.

6. Cherian MG, Goyer RA, Delaguerrire-Richardson L: Cadmium metallothionein induced nephropathy. Toxicol Appl Pharmacol 38: 399-408, 1976.

7. Nordberg M, Kojima Y: Kgi JHR, Nordberg GF (eds); Metallothionein. Basel, Birkhauser Verlag, 1979, pp. 41-124.

8. Webb M: The Chemistry, Biochemistry and Biology of Cadmium. Amsterdam, Elsevier, 1979, pp. 195-266.

9. Stonard MD, Webb M: Influence of dietary cadmium on the distribution of the essential metals copper, zinc and iron in tissues of the rats. Chem Biol Interact 15: 349-363, 1976.

10. Piscator M: On cadmium in normal human kidneys together with a report on the isolation of metallothionein from livers of cadmium exposed rabbits. Nord Hyg Tidskr 45: 76-82, 1964.

11. Nordberg M, Elinder CG, Rahnster B: Cadmium, zinc and copper in horse kidney metallothionein. Environ Res 20: 341-350, 1979.

12. Lauwerys RR, Buchet JP, Roels HA: The relationship between cadmium exposure or body burden and the concentration of cadmium in blood and urine in man. Arch Occup Environ Health 36: 275-282, 1976.

13. Shaikh ZA, Smith LM: Biological indicators of cadmium exposure and toxicity. Experientia 40: 36-41, 1984.

14. Friberg L, Piscator M, Nordberg GF, Kjellstrom T: Cadmium in the environment. 2nd ed. CRC-Press, Cleveland 1974.

15. Piotrowski JK, Bolanowska W, Sapata A: Evaluation of metallothionein content in animal tissues. Acta Biochim Pol 20: 207-215, 1973.

16. Kägi JHR, Nordberg M eds. Metallothionein: Ist Inter Meeting. Birkhauser Verlag, Basel, 1979.

17. Lowry OH, Rosebrough NJ, Farr AL, Randall RJ: Protein measurement with Folin phenol reagent. J Biol Chem 193: 265-275, 1951.

18. Klauser S, Kägi JHR, Wilson KJ: Characterization of isoprotein patterns in tissue extracts and isolated samples of metallothioneins by reverse-phase high pressure liquid chromatography. Biochem J 209: 71-80, 1983.

19. Hunziker PE, Kägi JHR: Human hepatic metallothioneins: Resolution of six isoforms. In: Kägi JHR, Kojima Y (eds); Metallothionein II, Experientia Supplementum Vol 52, Basel-Boston, Birkhauser Verlag, 1987, pp. 257-264.

20. Ribas B, Iniesta MP: Induction of metallothionein 1 with cadmium, by high presure liquid chromatography. Anal Real Acad Farm 55:533-540, 1989.

21. Tohyama C, Nishimura H, Nishimura N: Immunohistochemical localization of metallothionein in the liver and kidney of cadmium or zinc treated rats. Acta Histochem Cytochem 21: 91-102, 1988.

57

EFFECTS OF Ni AND Cd ON PROTEOGLYCAN SYNTHESIS BY THE ISOLATED GLOMERULUS AND GLOMERULAR CELLS IN CULTURE

D. M. Templeton and J. Sheepers

University of Toronto, Department of Clinical Biochemistry, 100 College St., Toronto, Canada M5G 1L5

INTRODUCTION

The renal glomerulus is a dynamic anatomical structure involved in the formation of the plasma ultrafiltrate, and consequently in the filtration of numerous toxic substances, including many metal cations. Little is known about the susceptibility of the glomerulus to direct toxic insult. Numerous instances of glomerular involvement in human and experimental metal poisoning have been noted (1). In most situations, the question remains whether primary glomerular insult precedes functional or histopathological changes that occur secondary to systemic or tubulointerstitial effects. For example, immune complex-mediated glomerulonephritis can result from the release of cellular antigens from damaged tissues (2), while disturbances in glomerulotubular feedback secondary to proximal tubular damage, can impair glomerular function (3). However, the glomerulus is a specialized structure with a well-defined architecture, and is potentially susceptible to toxic insult at both cellular and extracellular levels.

The glomerulus contains at least five distinct cell types (4), including the fenestrated capillary endothelium, visceral epithelium forming foot processes along the glomerular basement membrane (GBM), and the parietal epithelium of Bowman's capsule. Both macrophage-like and smooth muscle-derived cells reside in the mesangium, the latter retaining contractile properties that aid in regulating capillary flows.

In addition, two distinct extracellular matrices are present. The GBM serves as the basal lamina of both endothelium and visceral epithelium, and is the primary determinant of glomerular permselectivity (5). Its structure depends on specific interactions of type IV collagen and several adhesive glycoproteins (laminin, fibronectin, nidogen, entactin, etc.), as well as the heparan sulphate proteoglycan (HSPG) (6). The more amorphous mesangial matrix contains additional types of collagen, as well as dermatan (DSPG) and perhaps chondroitin (CSPG) sulphate proteoglycans (7), and constitutes the bulk of the glomerular interstitium. Most glomerular pathology develops as a progression from mesangial inflammation and hypercellularity, to GBM thickening and mesangial expansion, to sclerosis and eventual replacement of the glomerulus with fibrotic tissue. The general nature of these changes (8) further hampers attempts to deduce the exact etiology of toxic glomerulopathies.

In order to investigate potential mechanisms of toxicity operating in the glomerulus, we have developed in vitro procedures for studying isolated rat glomeruli, glomerular cells in culture, and preparations of glomerular extracellular matrix. Here we consider the role of the epithelial and mesangial cells in synthesizing PGs, and report the effects of Ni^{2+} and Cd^{2+} on the cell-specific synthesis of these matrix components in vitro.

METHODS

Isolated glomeruli and cell culture: Glomeruli were prepared from kidneys of male Wistar rats (150-250 g) by graded sieving, suspended in RPMI 1640 medium containing penicillin G and streptomycin, and incubated at 37°C in a humidified atmosphere of 5% CO_2, as described elsewhere (9). Viability was assessed by Trypan blue exclusion following extensive disruption of the extracellular matrix with collagenase, necessary because adsorption of the dye to the matrices of intact glomeruli prevents visualization of individual cells (10). Routinely, 40,000 glomeruli are obtained from a pair of rat kidneys, with less than 3% contamination with tubular fragments and 90±5% cell viability. To establish primary cultures of glomerular cells, amphotericin B (0.25 ug/ml) and 20% (v/v) calf serum were included in the initial incubation mixture. Initial outgrowths were observed at 24-48 hr and by 5 days appeared as islands of typical polygonal epithelial cells surrounding attached glomeruli (9). They were used in primary culture at 5-9 days. The identity of these early cells as epithelial is well established (4,11), although their origin from parietal or visceral epithelium remains controversial (12). Mesangial cells appear later in primary culture after most other cells have regressed. When plated at high split ratio after 30 days, clones of contractile mesangial cells are easily identified by their characteristic spindle shape (Fig. 1a).

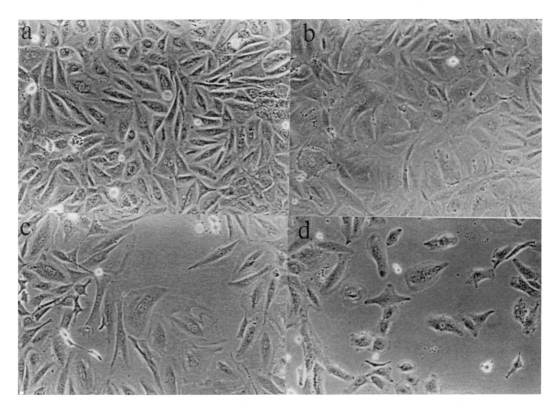

Figure 1. Phase contrast photomicrographs of confluent cultures of rat mesangial cells. Control (a) and after 16 hr exposure to 1 x 10^{-6} M Cd acetate (b), 5 x 10^{-5} M $NiCl_2$ (c) or 5 x 10^{-4} M $NiCl_2$.

The experiments reported here were carried out with a mesangial cell line obtained from Dr. Karl Skorecki, Department of Medicine, University of Toronto.

Other methods: PGs were labelled by the addition of carrier-free [35S]sulphuric acid at 0.2 mCi/ml to stationary incubations of freshly isolated glomeruli after a 2 hr recovery period. After 16 hr, medium was harvested and lyophilized and the glomeruli were resuspended twice in Hank's balanced salt solution, then extracted for 24 hr at 4°C with 4 M guanidine-HCl/50 mM sodium acetate/1% Triton X-100, pH 5.8, containing protease inhibitors, as described elsewhere (13). Cultured cells were labelled under the same conditions as intact glomeruli. Lyophilized media and extracts from both glomeruli and cell cultures were transferred to 7 M urea/50 mM sodium acetate/0.15 M NaCl, pH 6.0, by chromatography on Sephadex G-50. Pooled void volume fractions were applied to DEAE-Sephacel and eluted with a salt gradient of 0.15 - 1.15 M NaCl in urea-acetate buffer. Pooled PG peaks were further characterized by chemical and enzymatic degradation using HNO_2 (specific for the heparan sulphate side chains of HSPG), chondroitinase AC (CSPG-specific) and chondroitinase ABC (degrading both CSPG and DSPG). Full details are given elsewhere (13). Protein synthesis was measured as the incorporation of [3H]-leucine into protein over 16 hr. Concentrated stock solutions of Nickel chloride ($NiCl_2$) and Cadmium Acetate (($CH_3COO)_2Cd$) were prepared in equilibrated culture medium and sterilized by filtration. Aliquots were set aside prior to use, in order to check the concentrations by Zeeman-corrected electrothermal atomic absorption spectrophotometry. Solubility of the metals in the medium was confirmed at the highest concentrations reported. Test solutions were equilibrated in centrifuge tubes in the incubator overnight. The tubes were then centrifuged and the top and bottom halves were collected for separate analysis.

RESULTS

Incubation of glomeruli with $^{35}SO_4$ produces two populations of labelled PGs which are sep-

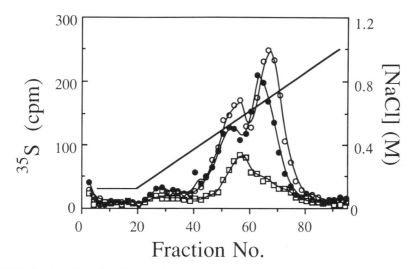

Figure 2. DEAE-Sephacel fractionation of PGs labelled by glomeruli in vitro. Control (open circles), 2×10^{-4} M $NiCl_2$ (closed circles), 2×10^{-5} M Cd acetate (squares).

arable based on their charge densities (Fig. 2). The first peak, eluting at lower salt concentration, is predominatly HSPG, with smaller amounts of DSPG, whereas the second peak is mainly DSPG. The pooled peaks generally contain less than 5% CSPG. Full details of the characterizations are presented elsewhere (13). It is important to note that, while the ratio of the two sulphated populations (and hence of HSPG to DSPG) is variable, dependent on the age of the donor rat and the ambient concentration of sulphate, all experiments reported here were performed under conditions that reproduce the profile of Fig. 2 for control glomeruli. When PGs were labelled in primary cultures of epithelial cells, a single peak was eluted from the DEAE-Sephacel column (Fig.3a), which corresponded in position to the material of lower charge density produced by intact glomeruli. This peak was resistant to degradation by chondroitinase enzymes, but was almost completely degraded by HNO_2 treatment, confirming its nature as HSPG (Table 1). Similar experiments with cultured mesangial cells resulted in broader elution of more highly charged material (Fig. 3b), containing significant quantities of HSPG and CSPG in addition to its major component, DSPG (Table 1). We conclude that the low charge density HSPG labelled by the intact glomerulus is a product of the epithelial cell, whereas the DSPG is contributed by the mesangial cell.

Protein synthesis in the isolated glomerulus was much more sensitive to Cd^{2+} than to Ni^{2+}. When measured over 16 hr in culture, at least 2×10^{-3} M $NiCl_2$ was required to depress protein

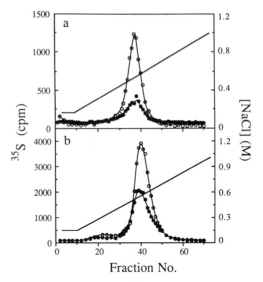

Figure 3. DEAE-Sephacel fractionation of PGs labelled by cultured glomerular cells, in the presence (closed circles) or absence (Control; open circles) of 1×10^{-4} M $NiCl_2$. (a) epithelial cells, (b) mesangial cells.

synthesis by 50%. The same effect is observed with $(CH_3COO)_2Cd$ at a 100-fold lower concentration. At 2×10^{-5} M Cd^{2+}, PG synthesis is decreased to a greater extent than total protein synthesis, however, and there is a preferential obliteration of higher charge density material, with a relative sparing of HSPG (Fig. 2). In contrast, 2×10^{-4} M Ni^{2+} decreases PG sulphation and total protein synthesis to a comparable extent (not shown), with no indication of a preferential reduction in either PG peak (Fig. 2).

The tolerance of relatively high levels of Ni by isolated glomeruli is also a property of cultured glomerular cells. As previously reported (1), concentrations in excess of 1×10^{-4} M $NiCl_2$ are necessary to inhibit the outgrowth of epithelial cells from glomeruli over 5 days. However, morphological signs of toxicity are quite apparent after exposure of cultured mesangial cells to 5×10^{-5} M $NiCl_2$ for only 16 hr, and are marked at 5×10^{-4} M (Fig. 1). The effects of Ni on the synthesis of PGs by cultured epithelial and mesangial cells were studied, in order to determine if the lack of specific effects in the

Table 1: Proteoglycans sulphated by cultured glomerular cells (% distribution of ^{35}S in cell layer).

PG	Mesangial cells	Epithelial cells
HSPG	21	97
DSPG	63	3
CSPG	16	-

intact glomerulus extended to the putative cells of origin, or was a property of the tissue as a whole. When epithelial cells were exposed to 1×10^{-4} M $NiCl_2$ for 16 hr, the total amount of sulphate incorporated into PGs was decreased by 63% (Fig. 3a). Exposure of confluent cultures of mesangial cells to the same concentration of Ni showed a smaller effect, causing a decrease in PG sulphation of only 41% (Fig. 3b).

These results provide some evidence that glomerular epithelial cells are more susceptible to damage by Ni than are mesangial cells, although these differences are modest and not obvious in the pattern of PG synthesis by the intact glomerulus. Both cell types were resistant to relatively high concentrations of Ni. The mesangial cells showed morphological signs of 16 hr toxicity only at 5×10^{-5} M Ni, with 5×10^{-4} M Ni causing marked damage (Fig. 1). In contrast, Cd^{2+} was toxic to glomeruli at 10^{-5} M, and resulted in death and detachment of all mesangial cells when used at this concentration for 16 hr. Changes in growth pattern and cellular morphology were apparent when mesangial cells were exposed to 10^{-6} M Cd for 16 hr (Fig. 1), and protein and PG synthesis were markedly reduced.

DISCUSSION

Striker et al. (14) reported that HSPG was a product of the glomerular epithelial cells, while the mesangial cells made primarily CSPG-like species. This early cell culture study has not until now been confirmed by ion exchange purification and quantitative analysis of the PGs. The synthetic profile of the endothelium remains unclear. However, the assignment of HSPG synthesis to the visceral epithelial cell, and of mainly DSPG synthesis to the mesangial cells, is consistent with the anatomical distribution of the PGs. HSPG is the major, if not exclusive, PG of the GBM. On the other hand, chondroitin sulphates are found throughout the mesangial matrix (7). We conclude that changes in HSPG production by the glomerulus mainly reflect changes in epithelial cell activity,

while depression of DSPG and CSPG is indicative of mesangial cell suppression.

Disturbed mesangial cell function could play an important role in Cd nephropathy. Lauwerys et al. (15) have found evidence of glomerular involvement in individuals occupationally exposed to Cd. A subgroup of those developing proteinuria exhibited mainly the high molecular weight type, with elevated ratios of urinary albumin to $beta_2$-microglobulin. The marked decreases in DSPG production upon treatment of the isolated glomerulus with Cd could arise from specific toxicity to the mesangial cells. In contrast, there is no evidence of specificity in the cellular effects of Ni, and relatively high levels of Ni are tolerated by the glomerulus and its cells. This conclusion is consistent with the known effects of Ni on the kidney. Acute exposures are generally well tolerated, and nephrotoxicity is not a prominent feature of chronic exposure to Ni (1,16).

The sensitivity of mesangial cells to Cd is further highlighted by comparison with the work of Cherian (17). No morphological changes were seen in rat kidney epithelial cells after 24 hr in the presence of Cd^{2+}, below 10^{-4} M, whereas 10^{-6} M Cd^{2+} has a clear effect on cultured mesangial cells over 16 hr (Fig. 1b). However, epithelial cells of similar origin were found to be relatively resistant to Ni^{2+}, exhibiting toxicity only after 16 hr exposure to 1×10^{-4} M metal (18), in excellent agreement with our results (Fig. 1c,d).

We conclude that the in vitro methods described here are helpful in studies of the nephrotoxic effects of metals. The synthesis of unique proteoglycans by different populations of glomerular cells serves as a useful indicator of cellular targets of toxicity. The mesangial cell is a preferential target of Cd, but not Ni. This may account for a glomerular component in the nephropathy occurring with chronic Cd exposure.

REFERENCES

1. Templeton DM. Nickel at the renal glomerulus: Molecular and cellular interactions. In:

Nieboer E, Aitio A (eds.); Nickel and Human Health: Current Perspectives. New York, John Wiley, In Press.

2. Druet P, Bernard A, Hirsch F, Weening JJ, Gengoux P, Mahieu P, Birkeland S: Immunologically mediated glomerulonephritis induced by heavy metals. Arch Toxicol 50: 187-194, 1982.

3. Oken DE: Acute renal failure caused by nephrotoxins. Environ Hlth Perspect 15: 101-109, 1976.

4. Striker GE, Striker LJ: Glomerular cell culture. Lab Invest 53: 122-131, 1985.

5. Kanwar YS: Biophysiology of glomerular filtration and proteinuria. Lab Invest 51: 7-21, 1984.

6. Timpl R: Recent advances in the biochemistry of glomerular basement membrane. Kidney Int 30: 293-298, 1986.

7. Kanwar YS, Rosenzweig LJ , Jakubowski ML: Distribution of de novo synthesized sulfated glycosaminoglycans in the glomerular basement membrane and mesangial matrix. Lab Invest 49: 216-225, 1983.

8. Klahr S, Schreiner G, Ichikawa I: The progression of renal disease. New Engl J Med 318: 1657-1666, 1988.

9. Templeton DM, Khatchatourian M: Synthesis of heparan sulfate proteoglycans by the isolated glomerulus. Biochem Cell Biol 66: 1078-1085, 1988.

10. Templeton DM, Chaitu N: Effects of divalent metals on the isolated rat glomerulus. Toxicology 61:119-133, 1990.

11. Harper PA, Robinson PM, Hoover RL, Wright TC , Karnovsky MJ: Improved methods for culturing rat glomerular cells. Kidney Int 26: 875-880, 1984.

12. Nörgaard JOR: Rat glomerular epithelial cells in culture: Parietal or visceral epithelial origin? Lab Invest 57:277-290, 1987.

13. Templeton DM, Castillo G: Variability of proteoglycan expression in the isolated rat glomerulus. Biochim Biophys Acta 1033:235-242, 1990.

14. Striker GE, Killen PD, Farin FM: Human glomerular cells in vitro: Isolation and characterization. Transplantation Proc 12(Suppl 1):88-99, 1980.

15. Lauwerys R, Buchet J-P, Roels H, Brouwers J, Stanescu D: Epidemiological survey of workers exposed to cadmium: Effect on lung, kidney and several biological indices. Arch Environ Health 28:145-148, 1974.

16. Sunderman FW Jr: Nickel. In: Seiler HG, Sigel H (eds); Handbook on Toxicity of Inorganic Compounds. New York, Marcel Dekker, 1988, pp.453-468.

17. Cherian MG: Rat kidney epithelial cell culture for metal toxicity studies. In Vitro Cell Develop Biol 21:505-508, 1985.

18. Helmut M, Libert C, Sunderman FW Jr: Nickel toxicity in primary epithelial cell cultures of rat kidney. Ann Clin Lab Sci 15:346-347, 1985.

58
ACUTE EFFECTS OF Ni^{2+} ON THE RAT KIDNEY

D. Palmer and M. Dobrota

Toxicology Unit, Robens Institute of Health and Safety, University of Surrey, Guildford, Surrey, GU2 5XH, UK

INTRODUCTION

Administration of high doses of NiCl$_2$ (2-5mg Ni^{2+}/kg) to rats by parenteral routes causes proteinuria and aminoaciduria (1). From minor structural changes observed in the glomerular basement membrane (GBM) it appears that nickel-induced proteinuria is attributable to glomerular injury (1). The reports of aminoaciduria suggest that nickel may also cause tubular effects (2). It is, however, not clear from the urinalysis data whether the proteinuria is of the high or low molecular weight type. If the major component of the proteinuria is albumin, this may be due to such effects as neutralisation of the GBM anionic barrier by Ni^{2+} or to increased filtration of albumin due to alteration in the albumin charge by bound nickel (3).

In this study we have examined the effects of acute doses of Ni^{2+} in order to characterise morphological changes in the glomeruli and tubules and compare these with proteinuria and enzymuria profiles of the rat kidney.

METHODS

Nickel chloride was administered intraperitoneally (i.p.) in male Wistar albino rats (230g body weight) at doses of 1.5, 3 and 6 mg Ni^{2+}/kg. Chronically dosed animals received 5 daily i.p. injections of 10 μg Ni^{2+}/kg. Kidney morphology and urinary parameters were examined at 12, 24 and 48hr after the single acute dose and at 48hr after the last injection of the chronically exposed animals. For ultrastructural observations the kidneys were perfused with Karnovsky's fixative (4) by a retrograde arterial perfusion based on the method of Maunsbach (5). After fixation in 10% neutral buffered formalin sections of the kidney were stained by standard Haematoxylin and Eosin (H+E), periodic acid Schiff (PAS) and Niagara blue 4B (6) for examination by light microscopy. Small pieces of kidney cortex were fixed in 2% glutaraldehyde, counterfixed in 2% osmic acid and after dehydration, embedding and sectioning, were examined by electron microscopy.

The animals were placed in metabolism cages overnight (12-15hr) just before sacrifice in order to collect urine samples for various measurements. The urines were analysed for total protein, creatinine, alkaline phosphatase (alk.phos), lactate dehydrogenase (LDH), N-acetyl-β-D-glucosaminidase (NAG) and also for protein profiles by SDS polyacrylamide gel electrophoresis.

RESULTS

Histopathology of the kidneys at even the highest doses revealed no significant or gross structural changes. Whilst no glomerular lesions were observed by light microscopy, some fusion of podocyte foot processes was observed by electron microscopy with 6 mg Ni/kg at 48hr (Figure 1). Some damage in the tubular brush border could be identified by light microscopy in the PAS stained sections (not illustrated) although this type of lesion was not apparent when examined by electron microscopy.

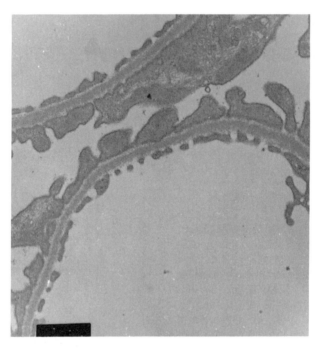

Figure 1. High resolution electron micrograph of glomerulus from a male rat 48hr after receiving 6mg Ni^{2+}/kg. Note the slightly flattened and fusing podocyte foot processes. The GBM appears normal.

In view of the very minor ultrastructural changes observed in the kidney after acute doses of nickel it was surprising to find significantly increased proteinuria and increases in the urinary levels of alkaline phosphatase, LDH and NAG. These increases in urinary protein and enzymes are summarised in Figure 2 as percentages of control values. LDH increases significantly with dose of Ni^{2+} at each time point and suggests that some intracellular contents (cytosolic) are released into the filtrate, most probably due to cellular turnover induced by the nickel treatment. It is considered unlikely that a significant component of LDH activity in urine attributable to serum isoenzymes of LDH could account for the 8-fold increase in urinary activity found at 48hr with 6mg Ni^{2+}/kg. The enzyme of lysosomal origin, NAG, is also significantly increased with time and at higher concentrations of Ni^{2+}. It is, however, not clear why NAG is also elevated at the chronic dose of Ni^{2+}. The urinary alk.phos. which is of brush border origin, shows a slightly different response in being elevated at all three doses only at the later timepoint of 48hr.

The increase in total proteinuria, also illustrated in Figure 2, shows that with 1.5 and 3 mg Ni^{2+}/kg there is a steady increase over the three time points but with 6·mg Ni^{2+}/kg the increase is already maximal at the earliest time point of 12hr. Examination of protein profiles in the urine samples by SDS polyacrylamide gel electrophoresis (Figure 3) indicates that much of the proteinuria is attributable to increase in the urinary albumin (66kd) and some high mol.wt. proteins, which probably represent transferrin (76kd), haptoglobin (86kd) and ceruloplasmin (132kd) at all three time points of the higher doses of Ni^{2+} treatment. As the intensity of the major low mol.wt protein, α-2-microglobulin (18kd) is very high in the control and treated samples it is not clear from these profiles if there is a significant increase in the low mol.wt proteins attributable to Ni-induced tubular damage.

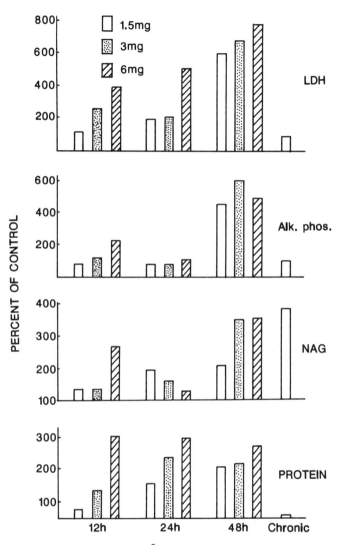

Figure 2. Effect of acute and chronic doses of Ni^{2+} on urinary enzyme and total protein. For simplicity and ease of comparison, all enzyme activities and protein values are expressed as percent of the control. Each value is a mean of 3 observations.

DISCUSSION

Minimal ultrastructural changes observed in the glomeruli are consistent with previously reported transient and reversible glomerular damage caused by acute doses of Ni^{2+} (1). Increased total proteinuria, which appears to be attributed mainly to high mol.wt proteins (especially albumin) is also consistent with glomerular damage. From the observations

that at least three major proteins of higher mol.wt than albumin are also increased by acute Ni^{2+} treatment it would appear that factors other than neutralisation of the charge on albumin by Ni^{2+} are also responsible for increased permeability of the GBM.

From the protein profiles obtained by electrophoresis (Figure 3) it is not clear if nickel significantly affects the tubular reabsorption of

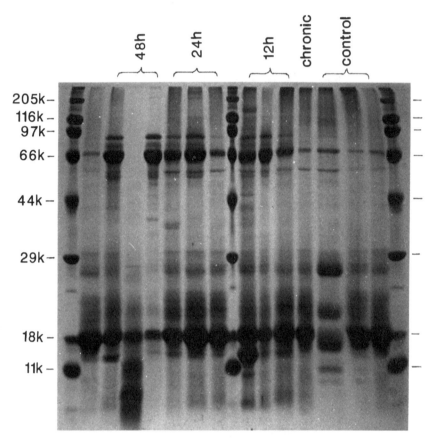

Figure 3. Proteinuria profiles obtained by SDS-polyacrylamide gel electrophoresis. Tracks 1, 9, 17 (right to left) contain mol wt. markers. Tracks 2, 3 and 16 are urines from control male rats. Track 4 is urine from a control female rat. Urines from Ni^{2+} treated rats are arranged in three sets which correspond to time points of 12, 24 and 48hr. Each set of these three tracks contains, from right to left, urines from animal dosed with 1.5, 3 and 6 mg/kg.

low mol.wt proteins. However the dramatic increases in urinary LDH, NAG and alkaline phosphatase, which are all of tubular origin, strongly suggest that a transient tubular dysfunction has been induced by the acute dose of Ni^{2+}. Interestingly the three enzymes chosen as markers of various cellular compartments differ in their response to the dose of Ni^{2+} and the time after treatment. It thus appears that acute doses of nickel produce complex and multifactorial effects in the tubules with cell leakage, indicated by permeability changes in the tubular cell membrane (LDH), occurring before any changes in the lysosomal compart-

ment (NAG) or the actual loss of the brush border (alk.phos).

This significant enzymuria is highly indicative of marked tubular dysfunction and is consistent with increased urinary concentration of β-2-microglobulin in nickel workers and with increased NAG activity in the urine of rats dosed with 6mg NiCl$_2$/kg (7). It is, however, not possible to unequivocally attribute the tubular changes to a direct effect of nickel since it is possible that any form of high mol.wt proteinuria may impair tubular function by overloading the tubular protein reabsorption.

REFERENCES

1. Gitlitz PH, Sunderman FW Jr, Goldblatt PJ: Aminoaciduria and proteinuria in rats after a single intraperitoneal injection of Ni(II). Toxicol Appl Pharmacol 34:430-440, 1975.

2. Foulkes EC, Blanks S: The selective action of nickel on tubule function in rabbit kidneys. Toxicology 33:245-249, 1984.

3. Templeton DM: Interaction of toxic cations with the glomerulus: binding of Ni to purified glomerular basement membrane. Toxicology 43:1-15, 1987.

4. Karnovsky MJ: A formaldehyde-glutaraldehyde fixative of high osmolality for use with electron microscopy (Abs). J Cell Biol 27:137A, 1965.

5. Maunsbach AB: The influence of different fixation methods on the ultrastructure of the rat kidney proximal tubule cells. J Ultrastruct Res 15:242-282, 1966.

6. Puchtler H, Meloan SN, Waldrop FS: Are picrodye reactions for collagens quantitative? Chemical and histochemical considerations. Histochemistry 88:243-256, 1988.

7. Sunderman FW Jr, Horak E: Biochemical indices of nephrotoxicity, exemplified by studies of nickel nephropathy. In: Brown SS, Davies DS (eds): Chemical indices and mechanisms of organ-directed toxicity. Pergamon Press, Oxford, pp. 55-67, 1981.

59
SEX DIFFERENCE OF NEPHROTOXICITY BY METHYLMERCURY IN MICE

A. Yasutake (1), K. Hirayama (2) and M. Inouye (3)

Biochemistry Section, National Institute for Minamata Disease, Minamata City, Kumamoto 867 (1), Kumamoto University College of Medical Science (2) and Research Institute of Environmental Medicine, Nagoya University (3)

INTRODUCTION

A series of experiments on sex-related differences in the response to methylmercury (MeHg) in mice has shown that after a non-toxic dose of MeHg chloride (MMC) (20 µmol/kg), male mice showed markedly higher renal uptake and urinary excretion rates of MeHg compared to females in various mouse strains. This might account, in part, for lower Hg levels in various tissues except for the kidney in males (1). The sex-related difference in the renal handling of MeHg is closely related to the difference of glutathione turnover rate in the kidney, a feature which is thought to be under hormonal control (2). In the case of successive administration, rapid renal uptake of MeHg in male mice sometimes caused an adverse effect; the kidney was quickly saturated with Hg leading to inhibition of urinary Hg excretion at an earlier time than in females (3). Accordingly, the kidney might be one of the critical organs by which susceptibility to MeHg toxicity was determined.

The present study was undertaken to obtain further information about the susceptibility of the kidney to MeHg toxicity, renal Hg levels, biotransfomation, and extent of renal failure were examined after administration of various doses of MMC in C57BL mice.

MATERIALS AND METHODS

Animals. Male and female C57BL/6N Jcl mice (aged 8 weeks) were orally dosed with MMC at dose levels of 20, 40, 80, 120, 160 and 200 µmol/kg.

Survival rates. For 7 days following MMC administration, changes of body weight and survival rates of the mice (6 for each dosing group) were examined.

PSP excretion test. 24 hr after MMC administration, distilled water (22.5 ml/kg) was given to mice (4 for each group) 30 min prior to PSP injection. An aqueous solution of PSP sodium salt was intravenously injected to mice (4 µmol/mouse) under pentobarbital anesthesia. Urine excreted during the following 30 min was collected and the ratio of PSP excreted in the urine was determined by the absorption at 560 nm after alkalification.

Hg analysis. Hg contents in plasma and kidney were determined by the method of oxygen combustion-gold amalgamation method (4). MeHg levels in the kidney were determined as described previously (2). To determine renal inorganic Hg, an aliquot (0.5 ml) of the homogenate in a micro-centrifuge tube (1.5 ml) was acidified with 0.2 ml of 6 N HCl. The acidified sample was vigorously shaken with 0.65 ml of benzene for 3 min, centrifuged at 12,000 x g for 3 min, and then the organic phase was sucked off to leave an insoluble material at the interface. Benzene extraction was repeated 6 times to remove MeHg completely. Then, the aqueous portion was neutralized with an equal volume of 1.71

N NaOH. Hg levels in the mixture thus obtained were determined as described above.

Plasma creatinine. An aliquot of plasma deproteinized with the aid of acetonitrile was chromatographed using a Waters SCX cation exchange column with 25 mM Na phosphate buffer (pH 3.65, 2.5 % acetonitrile) as an eluent, and the absorption at 215 nm was detected.

Induction of nephrotoxicity by HgCl₂. Four groups of mice (5 in each group) were intravenously injected with $HgCl_2$ (2, 4, 10 and 20 µmol/kg). 24 hr after administration, mice were subjected to the PSP excretion test, and Hg levels in plasma and kidney were determined.

Effects of selenite on nephrotoxicity. Five individual mice in each of the 5 groups were treated with one of the following: MMC (120 µmol/kg, po), MMC (120 µmol/kg, po) + Na_2SeO_3 (20 µmol/kg, iv), $HgCl_2$ (20 µmol/kg, iv), $HgCl_2$ (20 µmol/kg, iv) + Na_2SeO_3 (20 µmol/kg, iv) or Na_2SeO_3 (20 µmol/kg, iv). 24 hr after administration, PSP excretion rate and Hg levels in plasma and kidney were determined.

Statistical analysis. Statistical analysis of the data obtained was performed according to Student's t-test.

RESULTS

In the previous studies, male C57BL mice survived much longer than females after successive administration of 20 µmol MMC/kg/day (3). Following single administration of a higher dose, however, females showed markedly higher survival rates than males as shown in Table 1. All the females survived for more than 7 days after MMC administration at dose levels up to 160 µmol/kg, and 1/3 of the mice receiving the highest dose (200 µmol/kg) died on day 7. On the other hand, 1/3 of males died on day 6 at a dose level as low as 80 µmol/kg, and no mouse survived more than 4 days after a dosage of 200 µmol/kg.

Table 1. Survival rates (%) of MMC-treated mice during 7 days after administration was completed

Dose (µmol/kg)	Sex	Day 1	Day 2	Day 3	Day 4	Day 5	Day 6	Day 7
40	M	100 --						100
	F	100 --						100
80	M	100 -----------------------------			100	67	33	33
	F	100 --						100
120	M	100 -----------------------------			100	33	33	33
	F	100 --						100
160	M	100 -----------------------------			100	67	33	33
	F	100 --						100
200	M	100	100	17	0			
	F	100 ---					100	33

With the increase in the dose level up to 200 μmol/kg, the changes of the renal Hg levels 24 hr after the administration showed biphasic features in both sexes (Fig. 1). Although the Hg concentration linearly increased in the first phase up to the level of around 85 μg/g with the increasing dose, further increase of the dose resulted in a reduced rate of increase in the Hg levels. The doses by which the renal Hg level reached the plateau were 80 and 120 μmol/kg for males and females, respectively.

Normal C57BL mice excreted about 30% of injected PSP in urine for 30 min after injection in both sexes. PSP excretion at 24 hr after MMC administration was markedly inhibited (96%) in males at a dose level of 80 μmol/kg, at which the renal Hg reached the plateau level, and was inhibited completely by higher doses (Fig. 1). In females, however, no such inhibition was observed even when the renal Hg level was saturated after treatment with 120 μmol/kg MMC. The plasma creatinine values drastically increased concomitantly with the inhibition of urinary PSP excretion in male mice, whereas its increase was rather small even when PSP excretion in females was inhibited (Fig. 1).

Since mercuric mercury, such as $HgCl_2$ is well known to cause damage to the renal tubules (5), the possibility of participation of this mercurial species, which was biotransformed from MeHg (6,7), in the renal failure observed here was examined. The ratio of inorganic Hg (Hg-i) in the kidney of MMC-treated mice was 2-4% of total Hg at 24 hr after administration, except in the groups of males given 120 and 160 μmol/kg, which showed a 2 to 3 times higher ratio of Hg-i than the others (data not shown). The renal Hg-i levels and PSP excretion rates of MMC and $HgCl_2$-treated mice are summarized in Table 2. Male and female mice treated wih MMC showed renal failure with Hg-i levels as low as 2.45 and 2.74 μg/g, respectively, whereas renal accumulation of Hg-i after $HgCl_2$ administration did not disturb the renal function, even with levels as high as 12.2 and 6.9

μg/g, respectively. This indicates that the renal dysfunction caused by MMC administration would not be due to Hg-i, which was biotransformed from MeHg. Furthermore, although co-administration of Na_2SeO_3 resulted in increased plasma Hg, decreased renal Hg and recovered PSP excretion in $HgCl_2$-treated mice, these events in MMC-treated group were not affected by Na_2SeO_3 (Table 3).

The pathological changes in the kidney were evident in the proximal tubules of $HgCl_2$-treated mice; the epithelial cells were swollen and exfoliated into the tubular lumen (data not shown). On the other hand, the changes were slight in MMC-treated animals.

DISCUSSION

The present study demonstrated that toxic doses of MMC caused severe renal dysfunction, indicated by the reduced PSP excretion and increased plasma creatinine level, within 24 hr after administration in C57BL mice. Although the renal function of male mice was readily inhibited after MMC dosing by which the kidney was saturated with Hg, that of females was not inhibited when the renal Hg reached saturation. Preliminary experiments revealed that the Hg distribution and susceptibility of the kidney of castrated male mice after MMC administration aproached that of females, whereas that of castrated females remained unchanged. These results indicate that susceptibility of the kidney to MeHg toxicity might, at least partly, be under androgen control. Previously, we found that the efflux rate of renal glutathione, which has a high affinity for MeHg, was 2 times higher in males than in females (2), and that most of renal MeHg would be secreted in the lumenal space as its glutathione-conjugate (8). Thus, the renal tubules of male mice would be damaged more easily by a higher concentration of MeHg metabolite(s) in the lumen because of the higher efflux of glutathione-MeHg conjugate from the renal cells, even if renal MeHg levels were comparable to that of females.

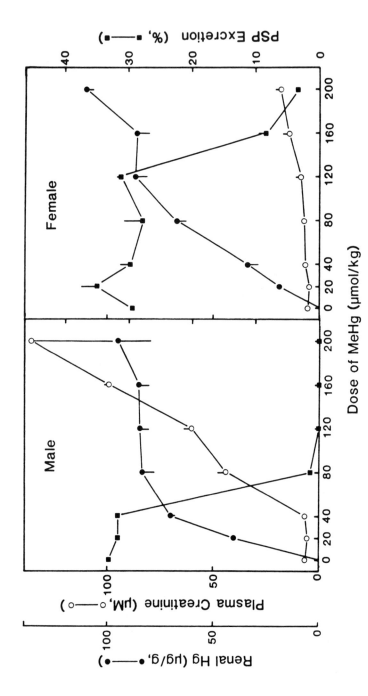

Figure 1. Dose-dependent changes of renal Hg, PSP excretion and plasma creatinine levels in MMC-treated mice. 24 hr after MMC administration, mice were subjected to PSP excretion test, then plasma and kidney were excised. Values represent mean ± SE obtained from 4 mice.

Table 2. Inorganic Hg levels in the kidney and PSP excretion rates of MMC and HgCl₂-treated mice[a]

Treatment	Sex	Inorganic Hg (μg/g)	PSP excretion (%)
MMC (μmol/kg, po)			
80	M	2.45 ± 0.82	1.3 ± 1.0
	F	1.90 ± 0.57	27.8 ± 9.2
120	M	9.09 ± 1.11	0.1
	F	3.02 ± 0.13	31.2 ± 2.4
160	M	7.36 ± 2.55	0.0
	F	2.74 ± 0.89	8.3 ± 3.7
HgCl₂ (μmol/kg, iv)			
2	M	8.22 ± 0.45	42.7 ± 4.2
	F	3.97 ± 0.37	35.7 ± 3.2
4	M	12.22 ± 0.27	42.2 ± 1.6
	F	6.89 ± 1.35	37.5 ± 5.1
10	M	19.35 ± 1.55	26.3 ± 18.0
	F	18.11 ± 1.50	1.9 ± 0.6
20	M	28.56 ± 0.87	0.3 ± 0.1
	F	32.22 ± 4.37	0.4 ± 0.2

[a] Values represent mean ± SD obtained from 5 mice.

Table 3. Effect of selenite co-administration on Hg levels in plasma and kidney and on PSP excretion 24 h after treatment in male mice[a]

Treatment	Plasma Hg (μg/ml)	Renal Hg (μg/g)	PSP excretion (%)
MMC	5.76 ± 1.25	93.8 ± 9.0	0.6 ± 0.3
MMC + Na₂SeO₃	5.54 ± 0.52	104.2 ± 9.8	0.6 ± 0.4
HgCl₂	1.04 ± 0.28*	28.7 ± 3.0*	0.2 ± 0.1*
HgCl₂ + Na₂SeO₃	5.40 ± 0.54	17.7 ± 1.4	20.1 ± 3.9
Na₂SeO₃	-	-	36.0 ± 2.3

[a] MMC (120 μmol/kg) was administered orally, and HgCl₂ and Na₂SeO₃ (20 μmol/kg for each) were administered intravenously. *Significantly different ($p<0.01$) from selenite co-administered group. Values represent mean ± SD obtained from 5 mice.

Although the neurotoxic action of MeHg is well documented in various animal species (3,9-11), its nephrotoxic action is still not well defined. A few investigators have reported renal injury by MeHg in rats 8 days after successive administration of MeHg for 7 days (11) or after feeding of a MeHg containing diet for 130 weeks (12). Since the ratio of Hg-i in the kidney increased to more than 40% of the total Hg as early as 10 days after MeHg single administration in rats (6), and Hg-i was a potent nephrotoxin (5), some contribution of Hg-i in the above-mentioned renal failure could well have been expected.

In the present study, the renal function was already disturbed as early as 24 hr after MMC treatment with dose levels of 80 and 160 μmol/kg for males and females, respectively. Although a similar disturbance was observed after treatment with $HgCl_2$ with dose levels exceeding 10 μmol/kg in both sexes, the renal Hg-i levels after toxic doses of MMC treatment were much lower than the levels after $HgCl_2$ administration of toxic doses (see Table 2). Thus, the involvement of Hg-i in the renal failure caused by MMC administration would be negligible; MeHg itself possibly caused the renal disturbance observed here. That co-administration of selenite, which decreases the acute nephrotoxicity of mercuric mercury (13,14), did not depress the nephrotoxic action of MeHg, is consistent with the notion described above.

The present results suggest that the kidney is one of the critical tissues by which susceptibility to MeHg acute toxicity is determined, and that the kidney of male mice has markedly higher susceptibility to MeHg toxicity than that of females.

ACKNOWLEDGEMENTS

We thank Mrs. Naoko Uemura and Mrs. Tamiko Terada for technical assistance.

REFERENCES

1. Hirayama K, Yasutake A: Sex and age differences in mercury distribution and excretion in methylmercury-administered mice. J Toxicol Environ Health 18: 49-60, 1986.

2. Hirayama K, Yasutake A, Inoue M: Effect of sex hormones on the fate of methylmercury and on glutathione metabolism in mice. Biochem Pharmacol 36: 1919-1924, 1987.

3. Yasutake A, Hirayama K: Sex and strain differences of susceptibility to methylmercury toxicity in mice. Toxicology 51: 47-55, 1988.

4. Jacobs MB, Yamaguchi S, Goldwater LJ, Gilbert H: Determination of mercury in blood. Am Ind Hyg Assoc J 21: 475-480, 1960.

5. Ganote CE, Reimer KA, Jennings RB: Acute mercuric chloride nephrotoxicity. An electron microscopic and metabolic study. Lab Invest 31: 633-647, 1974.

6. Norseth T, Clarkson TW: Studies on the biotransformation of [203]Hg-labeled methyl mercury chloride in rats. Arch Environ Health 21: 717-727, 1970.

7. Mehra M, Choi BH: Distribution and biotransformation of methylmercuric chloride in different tissues of mice. Acta Pharmacol Toxicol 49: 28-37, 1981.

8. Yasutake A, Hirayama K, Inoue M: Mechanism of urinary excretion of methylmercury in mice. Arch Toxicol 63:479-483, 1989.

9. Iverson F, Downie RH, Paul C, Trenholm HL: Methylmercury. Acute toxicity, tissue distribution and decay profiles in the guinea pig. Toxicol Appl Pharmacol 24: 545-554, 1973.

10. Takeuchi T, Eto K: Pathogenesis of chronic Minamata Disease (Chronic methylmercury poisoning). Adv Neurol Sci 18: 845-860, 1974.

11. Klein R, Herman SP, Brubaker PE, Lucier GW: A model of acute methyl mercury intoxication in rats. Arch Path 93: 408-418, 1972.

12.   Mitsumori   K, Maita   K, Shirasu   Y: Chronic toxicity of methylmercury chloride in rats: Pathological study. Jpn J Vet Sci 46: 549-557, 1984.

13.   Chmielnicka   J, Komsta-Szumska   E, Jedrychowski R: Organ and subcellular distribution of mercury in rats as dependent on

the time of exposure to sodium selenite. Environ Res 20: 80-86, 1979.

14.   Naganuma A, Ishii Y, Imura N: Effect of administration sequence of mercuric chloride and sodium selenite on their fates and toxicities in mice. Ecotoxicol Environ Safety 8: 572-580, 1984.

60

INCREASE OF Ia EXPRESSION ON B CELLS DURING THE COURSE OF MERCURY-INDUCED AUTOIMMUNE DISEASE IN BROWN NORWAY RATS

C. Dubey, B. Bellon, J. Kuhn, M. Goldman* and P. Druet

Pathologie rénale et vasculaire, INSERM U28, Hôpital Broussais, 96 rue Didot, 75674 Paris Cedex, FRANCE. *Laboratoire Pluridisciplinaire de Recherche Experimentale Biomédicale, Université Libre de Bruxelles, route de Lennik 808, B-1070 Bruxelles, BELGIQUE

INTRODUCTION

Brown Norway (BN) rats injected with $HgCl_2$ develop an autoimmune disease (1) characterized by T cell dependent-B cell activation (2) leading to lymphocytic proliferation (3) and hyper-immunoglobulinaemia affecting mainly IgE (4). Numerous autoantibodies of various specificities (5) are also produced, particularly anti-glomerular basement membrane (GBM) antibodies which are responsible for an autoimmune glomerulonephritis (GN) characterized by linear and then granular IgG deposits along the glomerular capillary walls (1). All these autoimmune phenomena occur transiently and are no longer observed during the third month of $HgCl_2$ injections.

It has been shown in mice (6,7) as well as in humans (8-10) that IgE hyper production is Interleukin(IL)-4 dependent. As this cytokine, not yet characterized in the rat, is also known to specifically enhance Ia antigen expression on B cells (11,12) we studied in vivo MHC class II expression on B cells during the course of mercury autoimmune disease (MAID) to investigate further the role of IL-4 involvement in this drug-induced disease.

METHODS

Animals originated from CSEAL (Orleans, La Source, France) BN rats were bred in our own animal facilities. 8 to 12 week old male and female rats were used.

Induction of mercury autoimmune disease (MAID)

BN rats were injected subcutaneously thrice weekly with 100µg $HgCl_2$ per 100g body weight. On days 3, 6, 15 and 30 after the first $HgCl_2$ injection, rats were bled to death and spleens and lymph nodes (LN) (para-aortic and mesenteric LN) were removed. Control rats were injected with acidic (pH 3.8) H_2O instead of $HgCl_2$.

IgE

Circulating IgE concentration was measured in an ELISA as already described (13).

Cell staining and fluorescence activated cell sorting (facs) analysis

OX6 (anti-rat Ia antigen) monoclonal antibody (Mab) was purified from ascitic liquid by affinity chromatography using protein A sepharose (Pharmacia Uppsala, Sweden) and then fluoresceinated using FITC as described (1). MARK-I Mab (anti-rat K chain) was kindly provided by Dr H Bazin and biotinylated by incubation with biotin succinimide ester (Calbiochem Behring, La Jolla, USA).

Spleens and lymph nodes were teased apart in Hanks' buffer and the resultant cells suspended in the same buffer.

Double immuno-staining experiments were carried out as follows: 5×10^5 cells were suspended in 100µl phosphate buffered-saline

(PBS) containing 1% of normal rat serum (NRS) and 0.1% NaN_3 were incubated together with optimal dilutions of FITC-OX6 Mab and biotinylated MARK-I for 30 min on ice, then washed twice with cold PBS-NRS-NaN_3 before a further incubation with 10µl phycoerythrin conjugated streptavidin (Amersham, UK). The last wash was done with cold PBS-NaN_3, and cells were finally suspended in 1ml of PBS containing 1% paraformaldehyde. Cellular Ia expression was measured on a logarithmic scale by the mean fluorescence intensity (MFI) of Ia staining determined with a fluorescence activated cell sorter (FACScan, Becton Dickinson). In order to compare MFI between samples analyzed on different days MFI values of cells from $HgCl_2$ injected rats were expressed as percentages of the mean MFI value of cells from H_2O injected rats stained the same day.

Statistical analysis

Comparisons between groups were done using Student's t-test.

RESULTS

IgE

Circulating IgE level of $HgCl_2$ injected rats peaked to 6000±200µg/ml at day 15 and went down to 1100±300µg/ml at day 30 (Figure 1). Circulating IgE level of H_2O injected rats stayed around 10µg/ml during all the experiment (Figure 1).

Ia antigen expression on B cells

Splenic B cells. The MFI for Ia antigens was higher in splenic B cells from $HgCl_2$ injected rats than in splenic B cells from control rats on days 6, 15 and 30 and reached 50%, 62% and 25% respectively of control values. Increase of Ia antigen expression (Figure 2) was highly significant on days 6 (p = 0.01) and 15 (p = 0.0004).

Lymph nodes B cells. The MFI for Ia antigen was higher on LN B cells from $HgCl_2$ injected rats than on LN B cells from control rats on days 3, 6 and 15 of injections and respectively reached 35%, 76% and 18% of control values. Increase of Ia expression was always highly significant (p = 0.003, p = 0.004, p = 0.004 on

days 3, 6 and 15 respectively). No increase of Ia antigen expression was observed on day 30 (Figure 2).

DISCUSSION

These data show that during the course of MAID Ia expression increases in B cells from both spleen and LN. In LN, this increase occurred as early as 3 days after the first $HgCl_2$ injection but had decreased to control values by 30 days. In the spleen, a significant increase of Ia antigen expression was observed on day 6 and persisted on day 30 but to a lesser extent. This transient enhancement of Ia antigen expression in B cells during the course of MAID is reminiscent of the transitory auto-immune hallmarks of the mercury disease (1) and interestingly parallels the kinetics of total serum IgE level (13).

In humans and mice, IL-4 has been described to be involved in IgE synthesis (6-10) and more specifically to enhance Ia expression on B cells (11,12). It is likely that in our model an early effect of $HgCl_2$ leads to increased IL-4 production and consequently to enhanced Ia antigen expression in LN B cells as early as the third day of injections. And so far it is the earliest marker of the immunotoxic effects of $HgCl_2$.

Since B cells expressing increased levels of Ia antigens could stimulate anti-self helper T cells to proliferate and to release lymphokines and in turn could be strongly activated to secrete immunoglobulins, the increased expression of Ia antigens in B cells could be a pivotal pathological event (14,15). In that respect it is of interest that anti-Ia autoreactive T cells are present in MAID (16).

Rat IL-4 has not yet been cloned and it is difficult to definitely relate the increase of Ia expression in B cells and IgE hyperproduction to IL-4, as it is the case in mice. Work is in progress in our laboratory to clone rat IL-4 and produce anti-rat IL-4 antibodies. It is postulated that the increased production of IL-4 could be the earliest marker of MAID and possibly of other drug-induced autoimmune disorders.

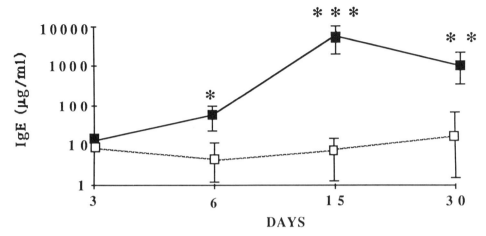

Figure 1. Kinetics of circulating IgE level in HgCl2 (black squares) and H2O (open squares) injected rats.
IgE concentrations are expressed on a logarithmic scale (mean ± SD)
* p < 0.05; ** p < 0.01 and *** p < 0.001

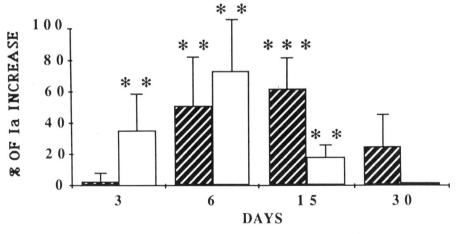

Figure 2. Spleen (hatched bars) and LN (open bars) cells were double stained with FITC anti Ia (OX6) and
biotinylated antiK chain (MARK I). Results are expressed as percentages (mean ± SD) of MFI values observed in control rats. ** p < 0.01; *** p < 0.001

ACKNOWLEDGEMENTS

We wish to thank Maryse Blin for typing the manuscript and Michel Paing for photographic assistance. Caroline Dubey is a recipient of a grant from Ministère de la Recherche et de la Technologie.

REFERENCES

1. Sapin C, Druet E, Druet P. Induction of anti-glomerular basement antibodies in the Brown-Norway rat by mercuric chloride. Clinical Exp Immunol 28:173-179, 1977.

2. Hirsch F, Couderc J, Sapin C, Fournié G, Druet P. Polyclonal effects of $HgCl_2$ in the rat, its possible role in an experimental autoimmune disease. Eur J Immunol 12:620-625, 1982.

3. Pelletier L, Pasquier R, Guettier C, Vial MC, Mandet C, Nochy D, Druet P. $HgCl_2$ induces T and B cells to proliferate and differentiate in Brown Norways rats. Clin Exp Immunol 71:336-342, 1988.

4. Prouvost-Danon A, Abadie A, Sapin C, Bazin H, Druet P. Induction of IgE synthesis and potentiation of anti-ovalbumin IgE antibody response by $HgCl_2$ in the rat. J Immunol 126:699-702, 1981.

5. Bellon B, Capron M, Druet E, Verroust P, Vial MC, Sapin C, Girard JF, Foidart JM, Mahieu P, Druet P. Mercuric chloride induced autoimmune disease in Brown-Norway rats: sequential search for anti-basement membrane antibodies and circulating immune complexes. Eur J Clin Invest 12:127-133, 1982.

6. Finkelman FD, Katona IM, Urban JF, Snapper CM, Ohara J, Paul WE. Suppression of in vivo polyclonal IgE responses by monoclonal antibody to the lymphokine B-cell stimulatory factor 1. PNAS USA 83:9675-9680, 1986.

7. Finkelman FD, Katona IM, Urban JF,; Holmes J, Ohara J, Tung AS, Sample JG, Paul WE. IL-4 is required to generate and sustain in vivo IgE responses. J Immunol 141:2335-2341, 1988.

8. Hofman FM, Brock M, Taylor CR, Lyons B. IL-4 regulates differentiation and proliferation of human precursor B cells. J Immunol 141:1185-1190, 1988.

9. Saryan JA, Leung DYM, Geha RS. Induction of human IgE synthesis by a factor derived from T cells of patients with hyper-IgE states. J Immunol 130:242-247, 1983.

10. Romagnani S, Maggi E, Del Prete GF, Ricci M. IgE synthesis in vitro induced per T cell factors from patients with elevated serum IgE levels. Clin Exp Immunol 52:85-94, 1983.

11. Monroe JG, Cambier JC, Mody EA, Pisetsky S. Hyper-Ia antigen expression on B cells from B6-lpr/lpr mice correlates with manifestations of the autoimmune state. Clin Immunol Immunopathol 34:124-135, 1985.

12. Polla BS, Poljak A, Ohara J, Paul WE, Glimcher H. Regulation of class II gene expression: analysis in B cell stimulatory factor-1 inducible murine pre-B cell lines. J Immunol 137:3332-3337, 1986.

13. Sapin C, Hirsch F, Delaporte JP, Bazin H, Druet P. Polyclonal IgE increase after $HgCl_2$ injections in BN and LEW rats: a genetic analysis. Immunogenetics 20:227-236, 1984.

14. Rosenberg YJ, Steinberg AD, Santoro TJ. The basis of autoimmunity in MRL lpr/lpr mice: a role for self Ia-reactive T cells. Immunol Today 5:64-67, 1984.

15. Janeway CA, Bottohly K, Babich J. Quantitative variation in Ia antigen expression plays a central role in immune regulation. Immunol Today 5:99-105, 1984.

16. Pelletier L, Pasquier R, Hirsch F, Sapin C, Druet P. Autoreactive T cells in mercury-induced autoimmune disease: in vitro demonstration. J Immunol 137:2548-2554, 1986.

17. Adelman NE, Watling DL, McDewitt HO. Treatment of (NZB/NZW)F_1 disease with anti-Ia monoclonal antibodies. J Exp Med 158:1350-1361, 1983.

61

LEAD-INDUCED CHANGES IN AVIAN RENAL HAEMODYNAMICS

A. Hawkins, D.N. Prashad (1) and R.O. Blackburn (2)

School of Biological Sciences and Environmental Health, Thames Polytechnic, London, SE18 6PF (1) and Department of Life Sciences, University of London, Goldsmiths' College, Deptford, London SE8 3BU

INTRODUCTION

The manifestations of lead poisoning include a wide range of physiological and structural effects on numerous organ systems. It has been reported from work on humans (1) and laboratory animals (2) that the cardiovascular, hepatic and renal systems act as depositories for lead. Morgan et al (3) have shown that some 50% of experimentally administered lead is located in these organ systems and that up to 20% of the absorbed lead is found in the kidneys.

Absorbed renal lead has been shown (1) to have a cortico-medullary distribution ratio of 50:1 and indeed primary changes appear to take place mainly in the proximal tubular cells of affected individuals, leading to structural and functional abnormalities. Animal studies have revealed that patho-morphological alterations include formation of intra-nuclear inclusions (4), and in rats and mice these inclusions were seen within 6 hr of intra-cardiac injection of 30µg/g lead (5). Such alterations may affect the activity of normal functions of the proximal tubules and so lead to a massive disruption in water and electrolyte homeostasis. Further, physiological changes in response to toxic insults with lead result in pronounced aminoaciduria, glycosuria and phosphaturia (2). In addition, lead is known to have various metabolic effects, such as inhibition of certain enzymes (6), binding to and therefore altering the physico-chemical status of membranes (2) and inhibiting sodium and potassium dependent ATPase activity (7).

Since much of the lead in the glomerular filtrate is reabsorbed (8) and a fall in GFR has been noted (9), it is likely that changes in normal glomerular activity may indirectly contribute to a significant retention of the cation. There is very little evidence to suggest that glomerular morphology is influenced by the presence of lead over the short term and it may be that a reduction in GFR results from lead-induced changes in renal haemodynamics.

The current study is designed to investigate glomerulo-tubular activity in hens treated with lead acetate in the presence or absence of heavy metal chelating agents, the ferric and magnesium salts of ethylene diamine tetraacetic acid (FeEDTA and MgEDTA respectively).

METHODS

Seventeen RIRxLS hens of approximately the same age (14 weeks) and weight (1.3 ± 0.2kg) were starved of food for 12 hr prior to experimentation but provided with water ad libitum.

The left brachial vein of each hen was cannulated for the continuous infusion of physiological saline (0.93% NaCl) containing an admixture of inulin (0.25%), para-aminohippuric acid (PAH) (0.025%) and mannitol (8%). This infusion mixture was delivered at a constant rate (0.5ml/min) for the duration of the experiment. After establishing adequate urine flows, the ureters of each hen were cannulated for collection of uncontaminated urine samples. The external iliac vein of each hen was then cannulated for the slow (0.10ml/min) infusion of either saline (group A, n=5), 1% FeEDTA (group B, n=6) or 1% MgEDTA (group C, n=6). After allowing for a blood-urine equilibrium period of 1 hr urine samples were taken from each group of hens at 10 min intervals for 60 min. Following this, a single, intravenous injection of lead acetate (270µg Pb) was administered to each hen in all 3 groups, and urine samples were taken at 10-min intervals. Blood samples were taken at the mid-point of each urine collection period in all hens. Inulin and PAH levels in blood and urine samples were determined by standard spectrophotometric methods and renal clearances of inulin (GFR) and PAH (ERPF) were calculated, using the equation UV/B, where UV is the rate of excretion of inulin or of PAH, and B that of the corresponding blood constituent.

RESULTS

Intravenous injection of 270µg of lead to group A (saline infused) hens resulted in a significant ($p < 0.02$) reduction in urine flow (UF) over the 30 minute experimental period. This amounted to an overall 65% decline in UF (Fig. 1, A). Lead-injected group B (FeEDTA infused) hens showed a 40% reduction ($p < 0.05$) in UF over the same period (Fig. 1, B). In group C (MgEDTA infused) hens, no significant changes were observed when control values were compared with those seen at 10, 20 and 30 min after lead treatment ($p > 0.1$; Fig. 1, C). The reduction in UF seen in group A birds may be attributable to the sharp ($p < 0.002$) decline of about 80% in GFR observed over the experimental period (Fig. 2, A).

In group B hens, the decrement in GFR was 49%, considerably less than that seen in group A hens (Fig. 2, B), suggesting that the ferric chelate reduces the effects of lead in terms of UF and GFR, and thereby offers some degree of protection from the toxic effects of the metal.

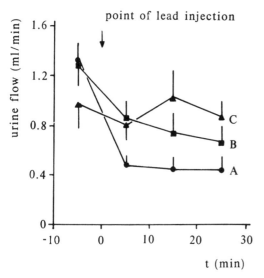

Figure 1. Urine flow rates (mean ± se) in hens treated with lead and infused with saline (A), FeEDTA (B) or MgEDTA (C).

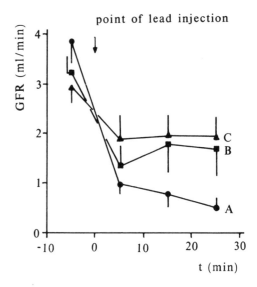

Figure 2. GFR (mean ± se) in hens treated with lead and infused with either saline (A), FeEDTA (B) or MgEDTA (C).

Group C hens showed an insignificant decline in GFR during the experiment (Fig. 2, C).

In group A birds consequent to lead treatment, there was a significant fall in ERPF (p<0.02) and this pattern of decline paralleled that observed in group B hens (p<0.02). However, in hens infused with MgEDTA (group C), there was a 60% increase (p<0.05) in ERPF over the 30 minutes after lead treatment (Fig. 3, C).

The changes observed following lead intoxication in each group of birds was not attributable to the infusion of either isotonic saline solution, FeEDTA or MgEDTA, since in separate experiments, where these constituents were infused continuously over a three hour period, no marked differences were noted in UF, GFR or ERPF.

DISCUSSION

The present study has shown that short-tern intravenous injection of lead causes a sponta neous reduction in the rate of urine flow. This lead-induced oliguria may have arisen from either increased reabsorbtion of water by renal tubules and/or from changes in glomerular haemodynamics. The first possibility seems unlikely, since all hens used in these experiments were in a state of osmotic diuresis. The observed decline in UF paralleled that of GFR when values from single kidneys were compared (n=30, r=0.7, p<0.001), suggesting that lead exerted an inhibitory effect on normal glomerular activity.

A decline in GFR could result from a combination of factors, including a fall in the hydrostatic pressure within the glomerular capillaries, and increases in oncotic and/or Bowman's capsular pressures. It is unlikely that the oncotic pressure would have increased in this study, as the birds were exposed to a continuous infusion of saline. There is no evidence currently available to suggest that changes in Bowman's capsular pressure occur in lead intoxication.

Although no work seems to have been done to determine arterial pressure in lead-poisoned hens, long-term studies in guinea-pigs (10)

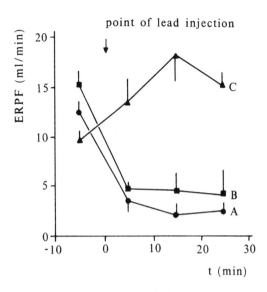

point of lead injection

Figure 3. ERPF (mean + se) in hens treated with lead and infused with either saline (A), FeEDTA (B) or MgEDTA (C).

have shown a reduction in renal blood flow and GFR. This latter study also suggested that renal hypoxia was associated with experimental lead poisoning. In addition, vasoconstriction of renal blood vessels has been noted (11); this forms part of the generalised vasoconstriction associated with lead poisoning.

In the context of the present experiments, a significant decline in ERPF was noted after lead treatment; it is likely that this resulted from the vasoconstriction of either renal arterioles or a redistribution of blood away from the kidneys.

The lead-induced changes in UF, GFR, and ERPF in group A hens were largely similar to those observed in birds infused with FeEDTA (group B), except that in the latter group the declines in these parameters were lower.

In contrast, group C hens (infused with MgED-TA) showed non-significant fluctuations in UF, and a slight decline in GFR over the experimental period. There was, however, a significant increase in ERPF, this rise in ERPF may result from a rapid shunting of blood to the kidneys, and may act to facilitate the renal excretion of the toxic cation. However, the mechanisms whereby MgEDTA influences changes in glomerular haemodynamics in lead-poisoned birds remain largely unresolved.

REFERENCES

1. Barry PSI: A comparison of concentrations of lead in human tissues. Brit J Ind Med 32: 119-139, 1975.

2. Choie DD, Richter GW: Effects of lead on the kidney. In: Singhal RL, Thomas JA (eds); Lead Toxicity. Baltimore-Munich, Urban and Schwarzenberg, 1980, pp. 187-212.

3. Morgan A, Holmes A, Evans JC: Retention, distribution and excretion of lead by the rat after intravenous injection, B J Ind Med 34: 37-42, 1977.

4. Goyer RA, Rhyne BC: Pathological effects of lead. In: Richter GW, Epstein MA (eds); International Review of Experimental Pathology 12, New York, Academic Press, 1973, pp. 1-77.

5. Choie DD, Richter GW, Young LB: Biogenesis of intranuclear lead-protein inclusions in mouse kidney. Beitr Path 155; 197-203, 1975.

6. Nordberg GF: Effects and dose-response relationships of toxic metals. New York, Elsevier Scientific Publishing Co., 1976.

7. Nechay BR, Saunders JP: Inhibitory characteristics of lead chloride in sodium- and potassium-dependent adenosinetriphosphatase preparations derived from kidney, brain and heart of several species. J Toxicol Environ Health 4: 147-159, 1978.

8. Vander AJ, Taylor DL, Kalitis K, Mouw DR, Victery W: Renal handling of lead in dogs: clearance studies. Am J Physiol 233: F532-F538, 1977.

9. Cramer K, Goyer RA, Jagenberg R, Wilson MH: Renal ultrastructure, renal function and parameters of lead toxicity in workers with different periods of lead exposure, B J Ind Med 31: 123-127, 1974.

10. Secchi GC, Alessio L, Cirla AM, Schweizer M: Effects of experimental lead poisoning on some enzymatic activities of the kidney. Clin Chim Acta 27: 467-474, 1970.

11. Cirla AM, Vercello G, Chiappino G: Azione vasospastica del piombo plasmatico. Med Lav 62: 14-21, 1971.

62

IMMUNOSUPPRESSIVE AND IMMUNOENHANCING EFFECTS OF GOLD

S. Ueda, R. Azemoto, Y. Wakashin, M. Ogawa, H. Yoshida, Y. Mori, M. Wakashin and M. Ohto

First Department of Internal Medicine, School of Medicine, Chiba University, Chiba, Japan

INTRODUCTION

Sodium aurothiomalate (gold) is known as an immunosuppressant and is used in the treatment of rheumatoid arthritis, but it sometimes causes renal injuries, a serious clinical complication (1-4). Using Hartley guinea pigs, we have demonstrated that injection of gold produces tubulointerstitial nephritis with anti-tubular basement membrane (TBM) auto-antibody and immune complex nephropathy with anti-renal tubular epithelial (RTE) antibody (5). It is of interest that autoantibodies are induced by gold treatment. Furthermore, we have reported that appropriate low doses of gold induce interstitial nephritis in genetically resistant C57BL/6 mice, suggesting that gold could depress the activity of TBM specific suppressor T cells (6). In this paper, we attempted to prove clearly that gold has not only suppressive effect but also phenotypically enhancing effect on the immune system according to the condition of the immune system of the host.

MATERIALS AND METHODS

Animals Six-week-old BALB/c mice were purchased from Shizuoka Animal Center (Shizuoka, Japan). Random-bred ddY mice were also obtained from the same source.

Preparation of Murine TBM Antigen TBM antigen was prepared from TBM of normal kidneys from BALB/c (BALB TBM antigen) and ddY mice (ddY TBM antigen). The purification procedures have been described (7).

Experiment I: Effect of Gold on Development of Interstitial Nephritis (IN).

Forty BALB/c mice were divided into 4 groups (n = 10 each). The animals of groups 1, 2 and 3 were immunized twice 0.05 mg of BALB TBM antigen with 0.05 ml of complete Freund's adjuvant (CFA) with a 2-week interval. In groups 2 and 3, in addition to TBM antigen immunization, the animals were injected with 0.01 mg (group 2) or 0.1 mg (group 3) of sodium aurothiomalate (gold) once a week for 4 weeks, starting 1 week before the first TBM antigen injection. In group 4, the animals were injected with saline and 0.05 ml CFA without the antigen or gold.

Experiment II: Effect of Gold on the Activity of TBM-Specific Suppressor T Cells Thymocytes from BALB/c mice that had been immunized with TBM antigen without CFA have suppressive activity on development of IN in the mice that had been immunized with TBM antigen with CFA. In this experiment, we studied whether gold can depress the suppressor activity of the TBM antigen primed thymocytes, or not. Forty BALB/c mice were divided into 4 groups (n = 10 each). All of these mice received intra-peritoneal injections of 0.1 mg of TBM antigen twice at a two-week interval. In three groups, animals were injected with 0.1 mg, 0.05 mg, or 0.01 mg of gold once a week for 4 weeks, starting 1 week before the first TBM antigen injection. TBM antigen-primed thymocytes (TBM-Thy) were obtained from these mice two weeks after the second injection of antigen. In vivo suppressor activity of TBM-Thy from four groups were assayed by a transfer study. TBM-Thy were suspended in RPMI 1640 medium at a concentration of 2×10^8 Viable cells/ml. These thymocytes were then transferred to (0.25 ml/mouse) BALB/c mice that had been immunised with 0.05 mg of ddY TBM antigen with 0.05 ml of CFA twice, after which the decrement of severity of IN and the titer of anti-TBM antibody were examined.

Histological Examination   Ten animals from each experimental group were sacrificed 8 weeks after the final immunization. Renal tissues were obtained; and the specimens were fixed in 10% buffered formalin for routine histological examination by light microscopy. The severity of interstitial changes was graded by the degree of mononuclear cell infiltration per cross section of cortex as follows: 0; no or rare small foci of interstitial cell accumulation; 1+: distinct small area of infiltration and tubular damage involving 5 to 10% of the cortex; 2+: focal areas of involvment up to approximately 25% of the cortical area; 3+: focal areas of involvement up to 50% of the cortical area as well as other changes seen in a typical interstitial nephritis; 4+, focal areas of involvement of more than 50% of the cortical area.

Direct Immunofluorescent Study of Diseased Kidneys   Small blocks of kidney obtained at sacrifice were quickly frozen in acetone dry ice, and 4 µm cryostat sections cut and stained with FITC-labeled goat IgG antibody fraction against mouse IgG (Cappel Lab. Inc., PA). Intensity of staining was graded 0 to 4 by the standard methods of this laboratory.

Titration of Anti-TBM Antibody   Titration of anti-TBM antibody was carried out by enzyme-linked immuno-sorbent assay (ELISA). In brief, flat-bottom microplates (NUUC, Denmark) were coated with TBM antigen, and 0.2 ml of sample serum diluted 1:500 with phosphate-buffered 0.15 M-NaCl, pH 7.2; containing 0.05% Tween 20 (PBST), was added to each well. After 5 hr of incubation at room temparature, the plates were washed with PBST. Goat anti-mouse gamma-globulin IgG-peroxidase (EY Lab. Inc., San Mateo, CA) was diluted 1:1000 with PBST and added to the plates.

After 16 hr the plates were washed and the amount of peroxidase that bound to the well was determined using 5-aminosalicylic acid (Sigma Ltd) as substrate. Reaction in the individual well was stopped by the addition of 0.05 ml of 1 N-NaOH after a suitable incubation period at room temperature. The absorbence was measured at 450 nm using a 580 Microelisa Auto Reader (Dynatech Inst., Inc., Torrence, CA). All samples were measured in triplicate. The titer of anti- TBM antibody was expressed in values of OD.

RESULTS

Induction of Interstitial Nephritis (IN) and Titer of Anti-TBM Antibody in Mice Treated with Gold (Experiment 1).   Two immunizations with syngeneic TBM antigen and CFA induced typical IN in all BALB/c mice, and the mean histological score was 3.4. The more notable interstitial changes were seen to be mononuclear cell infiltration into the interstitium: interstitial fibrosis, destruction of the TBM and tubules, and periglomerular fibrosis (Figure 1). Four injections with 0.01 mg of gold definitely depressed the frequency and grade of IN in the mice. The mean histological score of them was 1.4. Furthermore, the frequency decreased to 50% in the group with 0.4 mg of gold, and mean histological score of this group was 0.9 (Table 1).

Sera were obtained 14 days after the final immunization. The mean titer of the mice without gold was 0.594. Treatment with 0.04 mg of gold decreased the mean titer of sera to 0.264. The titers in the group with 0.4 mg of gold were lower, and the mean titer of them was 0.228. Anti-TBM antibody was not detected at all in the animals injected with saline and CFA (Table 1).

Assessment of In Vivo Suppressive Activity of TBM Antigen-Sensitised Thymocytes from the Mice with and without Gold Treatment (Experiment 2).   Thymocytes from BALB/c mice that had been immunized with TBM antigen without adjuvant were transferred to BALB/c mice that had been immunized with TBM antigen with adjuvant. TBM antigen-sensitized thymocytes were also prepared from the mice without treatment with gold (TBM-Thy), the mice with treatment with 0.4 mg of gold (Gold-0.4mg-TBM-Thy), the mice with 0.2 mg of gold (Gold-0.2mg-TBM-Thy), and from the mice with 0.04 mg of gold (Gold-0.04mg-TBM-Thy).

Induction of IN in the mice was remarkably suppressed by the transfer of TBM-Thy. Transfer of TBM-Thy decreased the mean histological score from 3.4 to 0.2 (Figure 2). Deposition of IgG along the TBM (Figure 3) and antibody formation (Figure 4) was also clearly suppressed by the transfer of TBM-Thy. This suppressive activity of gold-0.4mg, 0.2 mg, and 0.04 mg-TBM-Thy on development of IN and antibody response decreased in a dose dependent manner (Figure 2, 3 and 4).

DISCUSSION

Gold is used as an immunosuppressant chiefly in the treatment of rheumatoid arthritis, but it sometimes causes renal injuries (1-4). We have reported that injection of gold produces interstitial nephritis (IN) with anti-TBM antibody in guinea pigs (5). Autoimmune IN is also induced experimentally by immunization with TBM antigen in many animal species, such as guinea pigs (8,9), rats (10,11) and mice (12,13). IN is characterized by unique renal interstitial lesions accompanied by anti-TBM autoantibody. There are strain differences in susceptibility to IN even among the same species, and genetic control of this suceptibility in mice has been studied (12,13). SJL/J and BALB/c strain mice were genetically highly susceptible to IN and showed high immune response to TBM antigen. However, C57BL/6 mice were resistant to development of interstitial lesions when they are immunized with TBM antigen. We induced typical IN with high titers of anti-TBM antibody in C57BL/6 by treating them with gold and immunizing them with TBM antigen in CFA, suggesting that gold depressed the activity of TBM-specific suppressor T cells (6). A pilot study (unpublished data) showed that TBM antigen sensitized thymocytes from BALB/c mice that had been immunized with syngeneic or allogeneic TBM antigen without adjuvant have a strong suppressive activity on induction of IN and antibody response to the antigen. Using this system, we designed two experiments to clarify the effects of gold on immune system.

Table 1. Induction of interstitial nephritis and titration of anti-TBM antibody in gold treated BALB/c mice.

	Treated by	Occurrence of IN (positive/tested)	Histological score (mean)	Titer of antibody (Mean)
Group I	TBM Ag + CFA	10/10	3.4	0.594
Group II	TBM Ag + CFA Gold (0.04 mg)	7/10	1.4	0.264
Group III	TBM Ag 4 CFA Gold (0.4 mg)	5/10	0.9	0.228
Group IV	Saline + CFA	0/10	0	not detected

Histological examination was carried out in the 8th week after the second immunization. Severity of interstitial nephritis (IN) was graded according to the degree of interstitial changes as described in the text. The titer of antibody was measured on 14 days after the second immunization, and was expressed in values of OD 450.

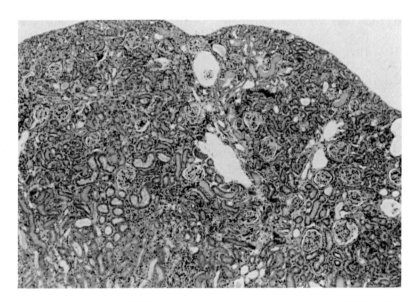

Figure 1. Typical IN induced in a BALB/c mouse that had been immunized with TBM antigen with CFA
(H&E, x100).

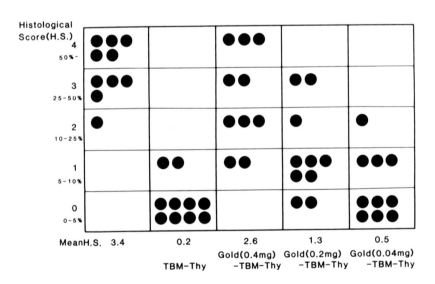

Figure 2. Induction of IN in donor mice transferred with TBM-primed thymocytes.

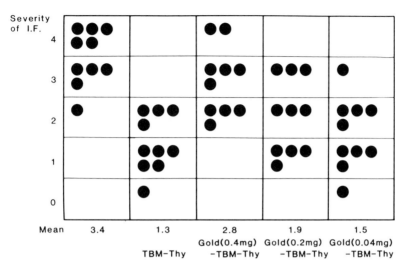

Figure 3. Deposition of IgG along the TBM in the donor mice transferred with TBM-primed thymocytes. Direct immunofluorescent study of the kidney was carried out in the 8th week after the second immunization. Intensity of staining was graded from 0 to 4.

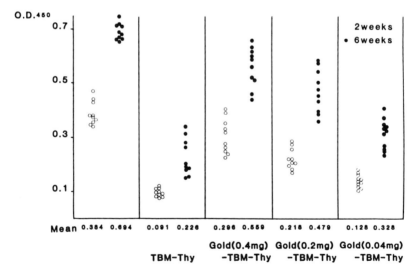

Figure 4. Titer of anti-TBM antibody in donor mice anti-TBM antibody was measured by ELISA 2 and 4 weeks after the second immunization.

Gold definitely depressed the frequency and grade of IN in BALB/c mice that had been immunized with TBM antigen in CFA. Antibody response to TBM antigen was also depressed by gold. These phenomena were dose dependent, indicating that gold acted as an immunosuppressant in this experiment. However, we cannot determine which region of immune system (macrophages, helper T cells, effector T cells, or B cells ?) was suppressed by gold. On the other hand, in the experiment using TBM-sensitized thymocytes, gold clearly decreased the activity of TBM antigen specific suppressor T cells in a dose dependent manner.

Based on the present study, we are able to suggest that gold always suppresses activity of all immune cells, and gold has phenotypically both immunosuppressive and immunoenhancing effects according to the condition of the immune system of the host.

REFERENCES

1. Derot M, Kahn A, Mazalten A: Nephrite anurique aique mortelle apres tritment aunique chrysocyanose associee. Bull Soc Med Hop Paris 70: 234-239, 1954.

2. Lee JC, Dushkin M, Eyring EJ: Renal lesions associated with gold therapy. Light and electron microscopic studies. Arch Rheum 8: 1-13, 1965.

3. Silverberg DS: Kidd EG, Shnitka TK, Ulan RA: Gold nephropathy. A clinical and pathologic study. Arch Rheum 13: 812-825, 1970.

4. Watanabe I, Whittier FC, Moore J: Gold nephropathy. Ultrastructural, fluorescence, and electron microscopic studies of two patients. Arch Pathol Lab Med 100: 632-635, 1976.

5. Ueda S, Wakashin M, Wakashin Y, Yoshida H, Iesato K, Mori T, Mori Y, Akikusa B, Okuda K: Experimental gold nephropathy in guinea pigs: Detection of autoantibodieas to renal tubular antigens. Kidney Int 29: 539-548, 1986.

6. Ueda S, Wakashin M, Wakashin Y, Mori T, Yoshida H, Mori Y, Iesato K, Ogawa M, Azemoto R, Kato I, Okuda K: Suppressor system in murine interstitial nephritis. Analysis of tubular basement membrane (TBM)- specific suppressor T cells and their soluble factor in C57BL/6 mice using syngeneic system. Clin Immunol Immunopathol 45: 78-91, 1987.

7. Wakashin Y, Takei I, Ueda S, Mori Y, Iesato K, Wakashin M, Okuda K: Autoimmune interstitial disease of the kidney and associated antigen. Purification and characterization of a soluble tubular basement membrane antigen. Clin Immunol Immunopathol 19: 360-371, 1981.

8. Steblay RW, Rudofsky U: Renal tubular disease and autoantibodies against tubular basement membrane induced in guinea pigs. J Immunol 107: 589-594, 1971.

9. Hyman LR, Steinberg AD, Colvin RB, Bernard EF: Immunopathogenesis of autoimmune tubulointerstitial nephritis. I. Demonstration of differential susceptibility in strain II and strain XIII guinea pigs. J Immunol 16: 327-335, 1976.

10. Lehman DH, Wilson CB, Dixon FJ: Interstitial nephritis in rats immunized with heterologous tubular basement membrane. Kidney Int 5: 187-195, 1974.

11. Krieger A, Thones GH, Gnther E: Genetic control of autoimmune tubulointerstitial nephritis in rats. Clin Immunol Immunopathol 21: 301-308, 1981.

12. Rudofsky UH, Dilwith RL, Tung KSK: Susceptibility differences of inbred mice to induction of autoimmune renal tubulointerstitial lesions. Lab Invest 43: 463-470, 1980.

13. Ueda S, Wakashin M, Wakashin Y, Yoshida H, Azemoto R, Iesato K, Mori T, Mori Y, Ogawa M, Okuda K: Autoimmune interstitial nephritis induced in inbred mice. Analysis of mouse tubular basement membrane antigen and genetic control of immune response to it. Am J Pathol 132: 304-318, 1988.

PART XII
IN VITRO

63

EFFECT OF VALPROATE ON AMMONIAGENESIS IN ISOLATED HUMAN KIDNEY-CORTEX TUBULES

G. Baverel, G. Martin, D. Durozard and J. Besson

INSERM U 80 and CNRS UA 1177, Laboratoire de Physiologie Rénale et Métabolique, Faculté de Médecine Alexis Carrel, rue Guillaume Paradin, 69008 Lyon, France

INTRODUCTION

Valproate (dipropylacetate), a branched-chain fatty acid, administered as the sodium salt or as valproic acid, is a widely used and effective anticonvulsant (1); drug administration may result in an increase in the blood concentration of ammonia rarely associated with clinical manifestations (2,3). This adverse effect of valproate has been attributed to a reduced hepatic conversion of ammonia into urea secondary to a fall of the hepatic content of acetyl-glutamate which is an activator of carbamyl-phosphate synthetase, a key-enzyme in ureagenesis (4).

Another possible explanation for this hyper-ammonemia is an increased release of ammonia by extra-hepatic tissues; on the basis of arterio-venous difference measurements across the human and rat kidney (5-7), recently it has been proposed that valproate accelerates glutamine metabolism in this organ resulting in an increased renal venous release of ammonia.

The purpose of the present study was to examine the possible mechanisms by which valproate stimulates the renal production of ammonia in the human kidney. For this, human kidney-cortex tubules were isolated and incubated with glutamine or glutamate as substrate in the absence and presence of valproate. In addition to providing the first information available on the in vitro metabolism of glutamine and glutamate in adult human kidney tubules, our data indicate that, in this experimental model,

valproate stimulates renal ammoniagenesis by increasing primarily flux through glutaminase.

MATERIALS AND METHODS

Fresh normal kidney cortex was obtained from the uninvolved pole of kidneys removed for neoplasm from adult patients fasted for 18 hr. Specimens of cortex were immediately dissected and placed in ice-cold Krebs-Henseleit (pH 7.40) buffer gassed with a mixture of O_2/CO_2 (19:1) until the beginning of the tubule isolation period (usually within 10 min). Kidney tubules were prepared by collagenase treatment of renal cortical slices as described previously (8,9).

Incubations were performed at 37^oC in a shaking water bath in 25 ml stoppered Erlenmeyer flasks, each with a center well, in an atmosphere of O_2/CO_2 (19:1). The tubules obtained were incubated for 60 min in 4 ml of Krebs-Henseleit medium (10) with 1 mM $L[1^{14}C]$-glutamine or 1 mM $L[1^{14}C]$-glutamate as substrate in the absence or presence of valproate (sodium salt). The flasks were prepared in duplicate for all experimental conditions. Incubations were terminated by adding perchloric acid (2% final concentration). In all experiments, zero-time flasks were prepared with and without substrate by adding perchloric acid before the tubules. Collection and measurement of the $^{14}CO_2$ formed from radioactive glutamine and glutamate were carried out as previously described (11). After removal of the denatured protein by centrifugation (4000 x g for 10 min), the supernatant was neutralized with 20% KOH for metabolite determination. Glutamine, glutamate, ammonia, alanine, aspartate, pyruvate, lactate, alpha-ketoglutarate, fumarate, malate, citrate, glucose, glycogen and also the dry weight of the amount of tubules added to the flasks were determined as described (8,11).

Net substrate utilization and product formation were calculated as the difference between the total contents of the flask (tissue + medium) at the start (zero-time flasks) and after 60 min of incubation. The $^{14}CO_2$ production from radioactive glutamine or glutamate was calculated by dividing the radioactivity in $^{14}CO_2$ by the specific radioactivity of the labeled glutamine or glutamate determined in the zero-time samples for each experiment. Flux through glutamate dehydrogenase was taken as the difference between the $^{14}CO_2$ released and the alanine found. The metabolic rates are expressed in micromoles of substance removed or produced per hour per g dry wt of tubule fragments. They are given as means ± S.E.M.. The results were analyzed by Student's t-test for paired data, comparing values obtained in the presence and absence of valproate.

L-Glutamine, L-glutamate, glutaminase (grade V), amino-oxyacetate and rotenone were supplied by Sigma Chemical Co. (St Louis, MO., USA), other enzymes and coenzymes came from Boehringer (Meylan, France) and sodium valproate was supplied by Sanofi Recherche (Montpellier, France). L-[1^{14}C]-glutamate (50 mCi/mmol) was obtained from the Radiochemical Centre (Amersham, Bucks, U.K.) and L-[1^{14}C] glutamine was synthesized by the method of Baverel and Lund (11). The other chemicals used were of analytical grade.

RESULTS

As shown in Table 1, valproate stimulated glutamine utilization by human kidney tubules in a dose-dependent manner, and also increased the formation of ammonia, $^{14}CO_2$, lactate and alanine, as well as the accumulation of pyruvate. Calculations from the data of

Table 1 show that, under certain conditions, the increase in ammonia synthesis caused by valproate was greater than the increase in the glutamine removed. This means that valproate stimulated not only flux through glutaminase, which releases as ammonia the amide nitrogen of glutamine, but also flux through glutamate dehydrogenase, which releases as ammonia the amino nitrogen of the glutamate formed from glutamine via glutaminase. As shown in Table 1, the flux through glutamate dehydrogenase was slightly stimulated by 0.1 and 1 mM valproate. No significant accumulation of intermediates of the tricarboxylic acid cycle, aspartate or glycogen was observed.

In contrast with the finding with glutamine as substrate, no significant change in glutamate removal or in ammonia and $^{14}CO_2$ production was observed in the presence of valproate (Table 2). The addition of valproate did, however, cause a concentration-dependent increase in pyruvate accumulation and in lactate and alanine synthesis; but this increase was less than that observed with glutamine as substrate. As shown in Table 2, valproate did not alter flux through glutamate dehydrogenase when glutamate was the substrate used. Similarly, no accumulation of glycogen, aspartate or of intermediates of the tricarboxylic acid cycle was observed in the absence or the presence of valproate.

DISCUSSION

The present study establishes that valproate stimulates the removal of glutamine and the production of ammonia by human kidney tubules. Increased glutamine removal may have resulted from a stimulatory effect of valproate on glutaminase and/or from an augmented removal of glutamate (synthesized from glutamine via glutaminase), a potent end-product inhibitor of renal glutaminase (12). The fact that the increase in alanine synthesis was less than the increase in glutamine removal (see Table 1) strongly suggests that this compound stimulated glutamine utilization not only by increasing glutamate metabolism (mainly by alanine aminotransferase), but also by stimulating glutaminase. Additional evidence that the

Table 1. Effect of valproate on the metabolism of 1mM L-[1-^{14}C]glutamine in human kidney tubules.

Experimental Condition	GLN 1mM	GLN 1mM +VP 0.001mM	GLN 1mM +VP 0.01mM	GLN 1mM +VP 0.1mM	GLN 1mM +VP 1mM	GLN1mM +VP 10mM
Metabolite Removal or Production						
Glutamine	-142.1 ±25.7	-175.0 ±16.0	-217.8. ±30.9	-262.3. ±42.4	-275.9. ±35.4	-267.5. ±50.9
Glutamate	+37.6 ±8.5	+38.6 ±8.6	+34.4 ±6.4	+30.6 ±5.1	+41.0 ±4.7	+33.6 ±3.7
Ammonia	+350.4 ±61.1	+383.0 ±8.7	+457.1... ±86.3	+498.8.. ±87.0	+527.7. ±85.8	+483.3. ±69.1
Alanine	+17.5 ±2.2	+37.3 ±9.8	+66.9... ±13.4	+86.3. ±8.9	+81.4.. ±13.2	+107.5... ±24.0
Glucose	+52.9 ±5.6	+53.8 ±5.6	+50.1 ±6.5	+38.2... ±2.8	+19.2... ±4.3	+9.1. ±2.3
Pyruvate	+3.2 ±0.6	+4.9 ±1.4	+12.5 ±4.1	+16.9.. ±2.5	+21.7.. ±3.8	+30.5... ±6.9
Lactate	+6.4 ±5.7	+9.0 ±7.6	+23.8 ±12.4	+47.4.. ±4.3	+68.1.. ±4.9	+56.6. ±3.2
^{14}CO$_2$	+118.2 ±16.2	+135.3 ±17.2	+176.3. ±24.2	+201.7. ±27.7	+198.7. ±28.4	+207.9. ±28.9
Flux through Glutamate dehydrogenase	100.7 ±16.7	98.0 ±16.3	109.4 ±16.3	115.4... ±19.8	117.3.. ±16.2	100.4 ±13.1

Kidney tubules (7.8±1.5 mg dry wt per flask) were incubated for 60 min as described in the Methods section. Results (μmol/g dry wt.) for metabolite removal (-) or production (+) are reported as means ± SEM for 4 experiments. GLN = Glutamine; VP = Valproate. * = P<0.05; ** = P<0.02; *** = P<0.01

stimulatory effect of valproate was exerted primarily on glutaminase was obtained by the addition of valproate plus amino-oxyacetate, an inhibitor of transaminases (13), which did not abolish the large increase in both glutamine removal and ammonia formation caused by valproate despite the suppression of the increase in alanine synthesis (results not shown, n=4). The fact that stimulation of flux through glutamate dehydrogenase was observed only with glutamine and not with glutamate as substrate indicates that, with glutamine as substrate, this stimulation was not a primary event in the effect of valproate but was secondary to the stimulation of flux through glutaminase which appears to be the primary target of valproate in its stimulatory effect of renal ammoniagenesis. However, valproate failed to alter assayed glutaminase activity in isolated human kidney tubules incubated in the presence of 5 mM glutamine and rotenone (results not shown, n=2). This suggests that valproate affected flux through glutaminase in human kidney tubules in vitro (and probably in vivo) by some indirect mechanism which remains to be elucidated.

REFERENCES

1. Simon D, Penry JK: Sodium di-n-propylacetate(DPA) in the treatment of epilepsy: a review. Epilepsia 16: 549-573, 1975.

2. Coulter DL, Allen RJ: Hyperammonemia with valproic acid therapy. J Pediatr 99: 317-319, 1981.

3. Marescaux C, Warter JM, Rumbach L, Micheletti G, Chabrier G, Imler M: Valproate-induced hyperammonemia: Role of diet. Wld rev. nutr. Diet 43: 174-178, 1984.

Table 2. Effect of valproate on the metabolism of 1mM L-[1-14C]glutamate in human kidney tubules.

Experimental condition	GLU 1mM	GLU 1mM +VP 0.001mM	GLU 1mM +VP 0.01mM	GLU 1mM +VP 0.1mM	GLU 1mM +VP 1mM	GLU 1mM +VP 10mM
Metabolite Removal or Production						
Glutamate	-133.7 ±17.1	-130.7 ±17.5	-152.7 ±22.8	-164.8 ±27.6	-149.2 ±17.3	-145.4 ±18.4
Ammonia	+137.8 ±4.3	+128.2 ±8.9	+140.3 ±11.6	+143.9 ±11.6	+135.0 ±10.3	+133.1 ±5.4
Alanine	+31.7 ±9.4	+35.1 ±10.7	+51.2... ±13.9	+55.6. ±8.9	+47.4... ±9.4	+65.9. ±8.0
Glucose	+48.9 ±6.1	+46.1 ±4.8	+44.1. ±6.4	+25.1. ±5.8	+10.3. ±2.9	+2.7. ±2.1
Pyruvate	+3.4 ±1.1	+3.9 ±1.5	+5.2 ±1.6	+11.8... ±2.1	+13.3... ±3.4	+10.3.. ±0.8
Lactate	+7.6 ±0.9	+8.5 ±0.6	+13.8 ±3.6	+38.1. ±5.0	+41.2.. ±6.8	+36.1.. ±6.0
$^{14}CO_2$	+148.5 ±31.4	+148.3 ±33.2	+161.5 ±35.2	+161.9 ±35.5	+145.1 ±25.8	+151.3 ±26.4
Flux through Glutamate dehydrogenase	116.8 ±24.7	113.2 ±25.9	110.3 ±26.8	106.3 ±25.0	97.7 ±17.4	85.4 ±22.3

Kidney tubules (7.6±3.5 mg dry wt per flask) were incubated for 60 min as described in the Methods section. Results (µmol/g dry wt.) for metabolite removal (-) or production (+) are reported as means ± SEM for 4 experiments. GLU = Glutamate; VP = Valproate. * = P<0.05; ** = P<0.02; *** = P<0.01

4. Coudé FX, Grimber G, Parvy P, Rabier D, Petit F: Inhibition of ureagenesis by valproate in rat hepatocytes. Role of N-acetylglutamate and acetyl-CoA. Biochem J 216: 233-236, 1983.

5. Warter JM, Imler M, Marescaux C, Chabrier G, Rumbach L, Micheletti, Krieger J: Sodium valproate-induced hyperammonemia in the rat: role of the kidney. Eur J Pharmacol 87: 177-182, 1983.

6. Warter JM, Marescaux C, Chabrier G, Rumbach L, Micheletti B, Imler M: Métabolisme rénal de la glutamine chez l'homme au cours des traitements par le valproate de sodium. Rev Neurol (Paris) 140: 370-371, 1984.

7. Ferrier B, Martin M, Baverel G: Valproate-induced stimulation of renal ammonia production and excretion in the rat. J Clin Chem Clin Biochem 26: 65-67, 1988.

8. Baverel G, Bonnard M, d'Armagnac de Castanet E, Pellet M: Lactate and pyruvate metabolism in isolated renal tubules of normal dogs. Kidney Int 14: 567-575, 1978.

9. Baverel G, Bonnard M, Pellet M: Lactate and pyruvate metabolism in isolated human kidney tubules. FEBS Lett 101: 282-286, 1979.

10. Krebs HA, Henseleit K: Untersuchungen über die Harnstoffbildung im Tierkörper. Hoppe-Seylers Z Physiol Chem 210: 33-66, 1932.

11. Baverel G, Lund P: A role for bicarbonate in the regulation of mammalian glutamine metabolism. Biochem J 184: 599-606, 1979.

12. Goldstein L: Relation of glutamate to ammonia production in the rat kidney. Am J Physiol 210: 661-666, 1966.

13. Braunstein AE: Binding and reactions of the vitamin B6 coenzyme in the catalytic center of aspartate transaminase. Vitam Horm (N.Y.) 22: 451-484, 1964.

64

MAINTENANCE OF GLUCOSE UPTAKE IN PRIMARY CULTURE OF HUMAN PROXIMAL TUBULAR CELLS

J. Mclaren[1,2,3], *P. H. Whiting*[2], *J. Simpson*[4] *and G. M. Hawksworth*[1,3]

Departments of Medicine & Therapeutics[1], *Clinical Biochemistry*[2], *Pharmacology*[3] *and Pathology*[4], *University of Aberdeen, UK*

INTRODUCTION

The proximal tubule (PT) is an important site for drug and xenobiotic induced damage (1). Due to the morphological and functional complexity of the kidney, development of a well defined in vitro system is essential for the elucidation of the mechanisms responsible for nephrotoxicity. In this context the study of a homogeneous cell population in suspension and particularly the growth of cells in primary culture provide useful investigative tools. In addition, culture of human tissue eliminates the problems associated with extrapolation from animal data.

If human PT cells are to be used as an in vitro model for toxicity studies then they must retain certain renal functions such as the Na^+-dependent uptake of glucose, which is used as a marker of PT cell function (2). Using a modification of the method previously developed for rat PT cells (3) we have isolated and purified human PT cells and characterised these cells in terms of their ability to transport glucose in suspension and primary culture.

METHODS

Collagenase (0.22u/mg) was obtained from Boehringer Mannheim GmbH, Germany. Dulbecco's Modified Eagles Medium and the Penicillin/Streptomycin solution (500Iu/ml,500µg/ml) were obtained from Gibco, UK, and Hams F12 Medium from Flow Laboratories, UK. The cell culture supplements, insulin, hydrocortisone, human transferrin and the Percoll density solution were obtained from Sigma, UK.

Isolation and purification of human PT cells

Human proximal tubular cells were prepared from 10-14g samples of renal cortex, obtained from surgical nephrectomies. All samples used were considered histologically normal and the enzymatic digestion was initiated within 20 minutes of removal of the kidney. The isolation method used was essentially that described by Gordon et al (3) for the rat and involved collagenase digestion followed by Percoll density centrifugation (starting density 1.044g/ml). The isolation of human PT cells required a higher concentration of collagenase (0.2% w/v), a longer incubation (100 min) and mechanical dissocation.

Cell culture conditions.

Isolated cells were inoculated onto 100mm diameter collagen coated plates, at a plating density of 3×10^6 cells/plate. The cell culture medium used, SFFD, was a 50:50 mixture of Dulbecco's:Ham's F12 supplemented with 10mM Hepes buffer, sodium bicarbonate (3.8mg/ml), penicillin (500Iu/ml), streptomycin (500µg/ml), human transferrin (5µg/ml), insulin (5µg/ml), hydrocortisone (5×10^{-8}M) and 10% foetal calf serum (FCS). Cell attachment was determined after 24 hr, with the cultures being maintained in a humidified incubator at 37°C. Thereafter the medium was changed every 2 days. At confluence the cells were passed using a trypsin (0.1%) versene (0.05%) solution. Trypsinisation did not exceed 3 min, with gentle shaking of the plates increasing cell detachment. Detached cells were washed in serum-supplemented medium and then subcultured in a 1:3 ratio.

Glucose uptake.

Glucose uptake was assessed using a non-metabolizable analogue, alpha-methylglucoside (AMG). The method employed was modified from that used for rabbit PT cells (4) and required the incubation of PT cell suspensions and primary cell monolayers in a Krebs-Hepes buffer containing 2mM glutamine, 0.25mM AMG and 0.05µCi/ml of ^{14}C-AMG, for 30 min at 25°C. The cell suspensions were incubated in a 1ml volume while primary cell monolayers were exposed to 2ml. The uptake reaction was terminated by the addition of excess ice cold Hanks buffer, after which the cells were washed 3 times in the same buffer before being solubilised in 1ml of a 50:50 mixture of Soluene:propan-2-ol. Primary culture monolayers were solubilised in 2ml of 0.5M NaOH and subsequently scraped from the plates and homogenised. Inhibition studies with phlorizin (0.5mM) were performed on both suspensions and primary cultures. Both preparations were assayed for protein by the method of Lowry et al (5) and the radioactivity measured using scintillation counting.

Cryopreservation.

Freshly isolated cells were cryopreserved with 10% dimethlysulphoxide in 10% serum-supplemented SFFD. 5x10^6 cells were suspended in 1ml of the cryoprotectant and left on ice for 10 min, after which time they were frozen at 1°C/min to -80°C. When required the cryopreserved cells were thawed rapidly to 37°C and washed with Krebs-Hepes buffer before assessment of viability by Trypan blue exclusion.

RESULTS AND DISCUSSION

Collagenase digestion of human cortex, followed by Percoll density centifugation resulted in the formation of two distinct bands (Table 1). Band A appeared at density 1.040g/ml and consisted of mainly single PT cells with high viability (93%), cell recovery and on microscopic examination an intact brush border, but some distal contamination. Band B at density 1.060g/ml, was made up of PT fragments, single PT cells and some distal contamination. The cells in band B were used throughout the study and these were successfully cryopreserved for 1 week with a viability of between 30-40% and a recovery of between 40-50% upon thawing.

Following isolation, PT cells were inoculated onto 100 mm diameter collagen coated plates with a plating efficiency of 40%. Following the rapid growth of the cells confluence was reached with 6 days (Figure 1). One of the major problems associated with the culture of PT cells in serum-supplemented medium is fibroblast contamination (6). The inclusion of 10% FCS in the growth medium used in this study, resulted in only minimal fibroblast contamination over the 7 days in primary culture. This was confirmed following immunohistochemical analysis using monoclonal antibodies. Cultured cells stained negative for Thy 1.1, fibronectin, collagen IV and actin, which are typical markers for mesangial cells. They were also negative for the endothelial markers factor VIII, MHC class II and the monocyte/leucocyte antigens. The positive staining by the epithelial markers; Common All, epithelial and cytokeratin confirmed that the cells in primary culture were mostly epithelial in origin (7).

Table 1. Viability and recovery of human proximal tubular cells.

	Viability %	Proximal tubular cells/ g of cortex x10^6
Before Percoll gradient	85 ± 3	15 ± 5
After Percoll		
A	93 ± 3	5 ± 2
B	91 ± 4	9 ± 4

All results are expressed as mean ± SD. (n=4)

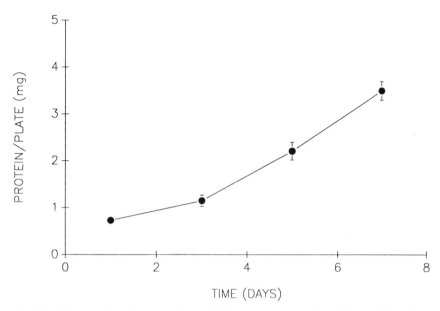

Figure 1. Growth of proximal tubular cells over 7 days in primary culture. Mean ± SD of 5 experiments.

In our study human PT cells in suspension demonstrated an AMG uptake of 1.87±0.23 nmol/mg of protein which was maintained at 1.46±0.22 nmol/mg over the 7 days in primary culture (Table 2). The uptake in both suspension and primary culture was sensitive to inhibition by 0.5mM phlorizin (a known compe-titive inhibitor of the Na^+-dependent glucose uptake), inhibition being greater in suspension (96%) than primary culture (67%). This and other work (8) supports the hypothesis that glucose uptake is mediated by a Na^+-glucose cotransport system, situated on the apical membrane of the cell, and which is maintained over 7 days in primary culture.

AMG uptake was maintained over the 7 days in primary culture, prior to the attainment of confluence and indicates that this is not a pre-requisite for optimal transport. This contrasts with studies in the LLC-PK1 cell line in which confluence is required for optimal transport (9). Glucose transport also appears to be inde-pendent of the rate of cell growth.

The possibility that AMG transport is affected by trypsinisation was investigated. The results demonstrated that AMG uptake, in particular its sensitivity to 0.5mM phlorizin, was maintained for at least two passages after which time the uptake and sensitivity fell (Table 3). This is consistent with some susceptibility of the cells following trypsinisation.

Table 2. The effects of Phlorizin (0.5mM) on AMG uptake in human proximal tubular cells .

	AMG uptake	Phlorizin (0.5)mM	% inhibition
	(nmol/mg of protein)		
Suspension Primary culture	1.87 ± 0.23	0.10 ± 0.08	95
Day 1	1.40 ± 0.15	0.39 ± 0.10	72
Day 3	1.58 ± 0.20	0.42 ± 0.13	73
Day 5	1.45 ± 0.15	0.42 ± 0.16	68
Day 7	1.40 ± 0.25	0.41 ± 0.09	70

All values are expressed as mean ± SD. (n=4)

Table 3. The effect of trypsinisation on AMG uptake.

	AMG uptake	Phlorizin (0.5mM)
	(nmol/mg of protein)	
1st Passage	1.50 ± 0.28	0.40 ± 0.09
2nd Passage	1.45 ± 0.32	0.49 ± 0.12
3rd Passage	0.64 ± 0.08	0.54 ± 0.10
4th Passage	0.35 ± 0.10	0.40 ± 0.07

All values are expressed as mean ± SD.

In conclusion we have shown that human PT cells can be isolated and purified to a high degree using a process of collagenase digestion followed by Percoll density centrifugation. Furthermore these cells can be successfully cultured in a serum-supplemented medium with only minimal fibroblast contamination. We have also shown that glucose is taken up by the cells in suspension and that this functional characteristic of PT cell function is maintained over 7 days in primary culture.

Future work will involve further characterisation of proximal tubular cells, with particular attention being paid to the use, in culture, of porous membranes. This offers several advantages for growing and studying epithelial cells, (10) in particular the measurement of organic anion and cation transport where access to the baso-lateral membrane is essential.

ACKNOWLEDGEMENTS

This work was supported by a grant from the University Advisory Committee on Research. The authors appreciate the help given by the Consultant Urologists, Mr J H Steyn, Mr W H H Garvie and Mr L E F Moffat, and the assistance provided by Keith N Stewart.

REFERENCES

1. Kuo C, Hook JB. Depletion of renal glutathione content and nephrotoxicity of Cephaloridine in rabbits, rats and mice. Toxic Appl Pharmacol 63:292, 1982.

2. Tune BM, Burg MB. Glucose transport by proximal renal tubules. Am J Physiol 221:580-585, 1971.

3. Gordon EM, Whiting PH, Simpson JG, Hawksworth GM. Isolation and characterisation of rat renal proximal tubular cells. Biochem Soc Trans 15:457, 1987.

4. Sakhrani LM, Badie-Dezfooly B, Trizna W, Mikhail N, Lowe AG, Taub M, Fine LG. Transport and metabolism of glucose by renal proximal tubular cells in primary culture. Am J Physiol 246:F757-F764, 1984.

5. Lowry OH, Rosebrough NJ, Farr AL, Randall RJ. Protein measurement with folin phenol reagent. J Biol Chem 193:265, 1951.

6. Chuman L, Fine LG, Cohen A, Saier MH jr. Continuous growth of proximal tubular kidney epithelial cells in hormone-supplemented serum-free medium. J Cell Biol 94:506-510, 1982.

7. Abbott F, Jones S, Lockwood CM, Rees AJ. Autoantibodies to glomerular antigens in patients with Wegner's granulomatosis. Nephrol Dial Transplant 4:1-8, 1989.

8. Kleinzeller A, Kolinska J, Benes I. Transport of monosaccharides in kidney cortex cells. Biochem J 104:852-860, 1967.

9. Moran A, Turner RJ, Handler JS. Regulation of sodium-coupled glucose transport by glucose in a cultured epithelium. J Biol Chem 258:15087, 1983.

10. Steele ME, Preston AS, Johnson JP, Handler JS. Porous bottom dishes for culture of polarized cells. Am J Physiol 251:136-139, 1986..

65

EFFECT OF MEDIUM COMPONENT DEPRIVATION ON A PRIMARY CULTURE OF RABBIT PROXIMAL TUBULE CELLS: THE EFFECT OF PHOSPHATE AND GLUCOSE

J.P. Morin, H. Toutain, N. Vauclin-Jacques and J.P. Fillastre

I.N.S.E.R.M. U-295, U.E.R. Médecine-Pharmacie de Rouen, BP 97, Saint Etienne du Rouvray, FRANCE

INTRODUCTION

An important aspect of renal cell culture is the continuing search for cells of renal origin that exhibit specific renal characteristics and function at a level that is quantitatively and qualitatively similar to a given nephron segment in vivo. Closely related to this, is the problem of altered phenotype in culture-adapted cells, a problem present in most, if not all, cultures derived from the kidney (1). The kidney is a heterogeneous structural system where compartmentation of metabolic pathways in different parts of the nephron is particularly marked. In that respect, enzymes of the glycolytic pathway were found to be abundant throughout the distal tubule and were low in the proximal convoluted and straight tubule (2), while enzymes of the gluconeogenic pathway and the capacity to form glucose seem to be restricted to the proximal tubule (3). Metabolic studies with isolated nephron segments confirm that the proximal tubule does not produce significant amounts of $^{14}CO_2$ from ^{14}C-glucose while distal tubule oxidizes ^{14}C-glucose to a considerable extent (4,5).

These observations led to the conclusion that glucose is not one of the preferred substrates for proximal tubule cells in vivo, since they are capable of fatty acid oxidation, glutamine metabolism and utilization of gluconeogenic substrates (6).

The aim of the present study was to assess the role of glucose and phosphate on the alter-ation of the phenotype of rabbit proximal tubule cells in primary culture.

MATERIALS AND METHODS

Primary culture of rabbit proximal tubule cells:

New Zealand white rabbits weighing 1.5 to 2.0 kg were used in these experiments. We used a modification (7) of the isolation method for proximal tubules described by Brendel (8). The suspension of pure proximal tubule was concentrated over a 40µm nylon sieve and incubated for 5 min at 37°C in 50 ml RK1 medium plus collagenase (0.125 mg/ml plus trypsin inhibitor 0.0025 %), poured onto a 40µm nylon sieve, gently washed with a spray of culture medium, and gently forced through this sieve. The material passed through the sieve, was collected and poured onto a 20µm nylon sieve. Proximal tubule fragments were then collected. The protein concentration of the inoculum was measured using the Bradford protein assay on a sonicated aliquot. Proximal tubule fragments were plated generally at 0.6 mg protein per 60 mm diameter petri dish or 25 cm^2 flask or 0.25 mg protein per 35 mm diameter petri dish and grown in RK2 medium consisting of medium RK1, insulin (5µg/ml), transferrin (5µg/ml), sodium selenite (5ng/ml), penicillin (25IU/ml), streptomycin (25µg/ml) and hydrocortisone (10^{-7}M).

At day 1 of first medium change was done and cells were grown in the appropriate medium: RK2 medium, glucose free RK2 medium or phosphate-free RK2 medium. Biochemical pattern analysis and morphologic examination were performed at days 3, 7 and 11.

Biochemical assays

Enzyme activities were measured in homogenates of both the starting inoculum of proximal tubule fragments and cultured cells scrapped from two 60mm diameter petri dishes. Each determination was done in duplicate in two homogenates for each point. Data were collected from 6 independent primary cultures.

Gamma-glutamyl transpeptidase, ouabain-sensitive Na-K-ATPase, N-acetyl-beta-D-glucosaminidase, cathepsin B, alkaline phosphatase, glucose-6-phosphatase and alanine aminopeptidase were assayed by established methods (9). Lactate dehydrogenase, hexokinase were determined according to Bergmeyer (10) and Bergmeyer and Bernt (11) glutathione-S-transferase was assayed according to Habig (12), succinate dehydrogenase was assayed according to Pennington (13). Protein concentrations were determined either by the technique of Bradford (14) or according to the method of Lowry et al. (15).

Morphologic study

Morphologic examination of the cultured cells was done using optical phase contrast microscopy, transmission and scanning electron microscopy, the monolayers being fixed, dehydrated and embedded in situ in the tissue culture dishes for transmission electron microscopy and fixed, dehydrated and 'sputter' coated in situ in the culture dishes for scanning electron microscopy.

RESULTS

Glucose-free medium

Results concerning the time-course evolution of the biochemical pattern of primary cultures of rabbit proximal tubule cells grown in control and glucose free media are reported in Table 1.

Glucose deprivation in the medium induced significant decrease in GGT, Na-K-ATPase,

LDH, and HK activities at days 7 and 11. SDH, CAT B, NAG, Alk.P and GSH-S-T were not, or only slightly affected by medium glucose deprivation. AAP activity levels were sustained at a slighly higher level in glucose-free than in control medium. The drop in glucose-6-phosphatase activity which occurred very early in control primary cultures was delayed by medium glucose deprivation. Cell growth was moderately inhibited by medium glucose deprivation as reflected by tissue culture dishes protein content.

Morphologic examination of the cultures by means of phase contrast microscopy revealed a more homogeneous and apparent cobblestone aspect of the monolayers grown in glucose-free medium when compared to control conditions. Furthermore, in cells grown in glucose-free medium, numerous refringent cytoplasmic vesicles were clearly seen 24 to 48 hr after the first medium change. Both conditions led to numerous domes formation at monolayer confluency.

Morphologic examination of the cultures by means of transmission electron microscopy revealed that epithelium height was higher and brushborder microvilli were more developed at the apical side of the cells grown in glucose-free medium than in control medium. Furthermore, more numerous lysosomes were seen in cells grown in glucose-free medium.

Morphologic examination of the monolayer surface by means of scanning electron microscopy confirmed the marked difference in brushborder development between both culture conditions as clearly shown in the micro graphies.

Phosphate free medium

Growth in phosphate-free medium led to higher residual activities of AAP, GGT, Alk.P, G-6-Pase, CAT B, and NAG. SDH and GSH-S-T activity levels were unaffected by medium phosphate deprivation while Na-K-ATPase, LDH and HK activities were decreased by medium phosphate deprivation. Cell growth was markedly reduced by medium phosphate depri-

Table 1: Comparative study of 11 marker enzyme activities measured in primary cultures of rabbit proximal tubules cells grown in control conditions or in glucose-free medium.

	DAY 3	DAY 7	DAY 11
Control AAP	44.10± 21.4	13.50± 3.5	10.90± 3.5
Glucose⁻	45.60± 20.3	19.40± 5.0	16.60± 6.5
Control GGT	117.00± 42.5	80.80± 22.1	43.20± 11.6
Glucose⁻	114.00± 42.3	49.20± 10.5	25.60± 5.4
Control Alk.P	197.00± 105	16.70± 6.6	6.70± 5.1
Glucose⁻	154.00± 66.6	21.70± 5.6	8.50± 2.1
Control Na-K-ATPase	134.00± 71.5	221.00± 101	269.00± 116
Glucose⁻	146.00± 56.4	172.00± 48.2	151.00± 39.4
Control NAG	43.40± 9.3	37.80± 4.5	43.70± 5.9
Glucose⁻	43.80± 9.1	36.90± 8.8	25.80± 3.8
Control CAT B	4.16± 0.50	5.44± 0.58	5.32± 0.60
Glucose⁻	4.30± 0.69	5.36± 0.77	5.36± 0.64
Control SDH	0.74± 0.05	0.60± 0.09	0.69± 0.14
Glucose⁻	0.62± 0.17	0.65± 0.16	0.46± 0.25
Control LDH	330.00± 30	812.00± 201	1960.00± 220
Glucose⁻	340.00± 60	460.00± 40	480.00± 210
Control HK	13.90± 4.8	33.00± 4.9	39.50± 6.4
Glucose⁻	10.70± 4.0	15.50± 1.7	19.80± 3.0
Control G-6-Pase	32.20± 15.0	8.35± 8.3	3.72± 3.2
Glucose⁻	77.30± 52.7	13.50± 10.6	7.48± 5.1
Control GSH-S-T	1174.00± 267	1029.00± 99.6	1034.00± 104
Glucose⁻	1074.00± 204	1113.00± 95.5	1239.00± 36.5
Control Proteins	477.00± 114	1062.00± 159	1388.00± 217
Glucose⁻	475.00± 135	747.00± 182	827.00± 185

Results are expressed as µmoles/min/g protein for all enzymes except for succinate dehydrogenase which are expressed as O.D. units/min/g protein. Each value is the mean ± S.D. of 6 independent primary cultures. AAP = Alanine aminopeptidase, GGT = gamma-glutamyl transpeptidase, Alk. P = Alkaline phosphatase, NAG = N-acetyl-beta-D-glucosaminidase, CAT B = Cathepsin B, SDH = Succinate dehydrogenase, LDH = Lactate dehydrogenase, HK = Hexokinase, G-6-Pase = Glucose-6-phosphatase, GSH-S-T = Glutathione-S-transferase.

vation as shown by protein content of culture dishes.

Examination of the culture by means of optical phase contrast microscopy showed cells with low contrast and refregence and confirmed the inhibition of cell growth. Cells grown in phosphate-free medium did not reach monolayer confluency.

DISCUSSION

Glucose metabolism in the kidney differs in several respects from that of other tissues.

Table 2: Comparative study of 11 marker enzyme activities measured in primary cultures of rabbit proximal tubules cells grown in control conditions or in phosphate-free medium.

	DAY 3	DAY 7	DAY 11
Control AAP	44.10±21.4	13.50±3.5	10.90±3.5
Phosphate⁻	51.40±25.1	29.80±11.8	24.40±4.5
Control GGT	117.00±42.5	80.80±22.2	43.20±11.7
Phosphate⁻	135.00±60.4	104.00±19.9	97.30±13.2
Control Alk. P	196.00±105	16.70±6.7	6.72±5.1
Phosphate⁻	140.00±76.6	45.70±26.5	22.60±6.6
Control Na-K-ATPase	134.00±71.5	221.00±101	269.00±116
Phosphate⁻	134.00±67.7	142.00±39.1	189.00±101
Control G-6-Pase	32.20±15.0	8.35±8.3	3.72±3.24
Phosphate⁻	51.90±27.7	11.90±9.8	6.70±6.12
Control CAT B	4.16±0.50	5.44±0.59	5.32±0.60
Phosphate⁻	5.14±1.20	10.40±1.37	8.64±1.41
Control NAG	43.40±9.3	37.80±4.55	43.60±5.86
Phosphate⁻	47.50±12.6	63.90±10.3	59.10±4.33
Control SDH	0.74±0.06	0.60±0.09	0.69±0.10
Phosphate⁻	0.61±0.13	0.69±0.10	0.64±0.25
Control LDH	0.33±0.03	0.81±0.20	1.96±0.22
Phosphate⁻	0.32±0.05	0.52±0.07	0.47±0.21
Control HK	13.90±4.81	33.10±4.99	39.50±6.43
Phosphate⁻	13.70±3.75	24.10±3.78	23.90±3.23
Control GSH-S-T	1174.00±267	1029.00±99.6	1034.00±104
Phosphate⁻	1191.00±292	1233.00±111	1201.00±36.5
Control Proteins	477.00±114	1062.00±159	1388.00±217
Phosphate⁻	402.00±100	494.00±126	516.00±102

Results are expressed as μmoles/min/g protein for all enzymes except for succinate dehydrogenase which are expressed as O.D units/min/ protein Protein ar expresse a μg protein/6cm petri dish. Each value is the mean ± S.D. of 6 independent primary cultures.

Whereas many cell types in the body appear to require glucose as a carbon source, the proximal tubule cells consume this carbohydrate only sparingly and appear to function mainly as a glucose forming (gluconeogenic) structure, its energy production depending mainly on glutamine utilisation or fatty acid oxidation (6). This pattern of glucose utilisation by the freshly isolated proximal tubules contrasts sharply with that exhibited by cells maintained in culture which display a highly active glycolysis. These cells, grown in control medium, have undergone a major alteration in metabolic strategy in the process of adapting to culture, a change that may be in part responsible for the phenotypic alterations that occur in primary cultures of proximal tubule cells. It should be noticed that similar alterations concerning glucose metabolism have been reported in rat hepatocytes in primary cultures (16).

The use of glucose-free medium, although diminishing the cell culture growth rate, is of interest since it partially prevents the cellular shift in metabolism towards glycolysis and allows preservation of the polarized structure with well developed brushborder microvilli at the apical pole of the cells. These two points are of great interest in the search for culture conditions which lead to the least alteration of initial phenotype during cell adaptation to culture conditions.

Primary cultures in hormonally defined medium allow study of the role of medium components on the alteration of cellular phenotype. These studies may bring interesting information to design culture conditions leading to in vitro models capable of expression of cellular functions and structural organization which mimic the in vivo situation of cells from defined nephron segments.

ACKNOWLEDGEMENTS

This work was supported by grants from Rhône Poulenc Santé.

REFERENCES

1. Gstraunthaler G: Epithelial cells in tissue culture. Renal Physiol Biochem 11:1-42, 1988.

2. Guder WG, Ross BD: Enzyme distribution along the nephron. Kidney Int 26: 101-111, 1984.

3. Burch HB, Narins RG, Chu C, Fagioli S, Choi S, McCarthy W, Lowry O: Distribution along the rat nephron of three enzymes of gluconeogenesis in acidosis and starvation. Am J Physiol 235:F246-F253, 1978.

4. Klein KL, Wang MS, Torikai S, Davidson WD, Kurokawa K: Substrate oxidation by isolated single nephron segments of the rat. Kidney Int 20:29-35, 1981.

5. Le Bouffant F, Hus-Citharel A, Morel F: In vitro $^{14}CO_2$ production by single pieces of rat cortical ascending limbs and its coupling to active salt transport. In: Morel F (ed); Biochemistry of Kidney Functions, Amsterdam, Elsevier Biomedical Press, 1982, pp. 363-370.

6. Guder WG, Wagner S, Wirthensohn G: Metabolic fuels along the nephron: pathways and intracellular mechanisms of interaction. Kidney Int 29:41-45, 1986.

7. Toutain H, Fillastre JP, Morin JP: Preparative free flow electrophoresis for the isolation of two populations of proximal cells from the rabbit kidney. Eur J Cell Biol. 49:274-280, 1989.

8. Brendel K, Meezan E: Isolation and properties of a pure preparation of proximal kidney tubules obtained without collagenase treatment. Fed Proc 34:803, 1975.

9. Hjelle JT, Morin JP, Trouet A: Analytical cell fractionation of isolated rabbit renal proximal tubules. Kidney Int 20:71-77, 1981.

10. Bergmeyer HU: Hexokinase assay. In: Bergmeyer HU (ed); Methods of enzymatic analysis. New York, Academic Press, 1974, pp. 473-475.

11. Bergmeyer HU, Bernt E: Lactate deshydrogenase UV-assay with pyruvate and NADH. In: Bergmeyer HU (ed); Methods of enzymatic analysis. New York, Academic Press, 1974, pp. 574-579.

12. Habig WH, Pabst MJ, Jakobi WB: Gluthion-S-transferases: the first enzymatic step in mecapturic acid formation. J Biol Chem 249:7130-7139, 1974.

13. Pennington RJ: Biochemistry of dystrophic muscle: mitochondrial succinate tetrazolium reductase and adenosine triphosphatase. Biochem J 80: 649-654, 1961.

14. Bradford MM: A rapid and sensitive method for quantification of microgram quantities of protein utilizing the principle of protein dye binding. Anal Biochem 72:248-254, 1976.

15. Lowry OH, Rosebrough NJ, Farr AL, Randall RJ: Protein measurement with the folin

phenol reagent. J Biol Chem 193:265-275, 1951.

16. Bissell DM, Levine GA, Bissell MJ: Glucose metabolism by adult hepatocytes in primary cultures and cell lines from rat liver. Am J Physiol 234:C122-C130, 1978.

66

PURIFICATION OF RABBIT PROXIMAL TUBULE CELLS: A TOOL FOR IN VITRO NEPHROTOXICITY STUDIES

H. Toutain, N. Vauclin-Jacques, J.P. Fillastre and J.P. Morin

I.N.S.E.R.M. U-295, U.E.R. de Médecine-Pharmacie de ROUEN, BP 97, 76800 Saint Etienne du Rouvray, FRANCE

INTRODUCTION

The studies of renal metabolism and drug-induced nephrotoxicity in vivo are clearly hampered by the metabolic and morphologic heterogeneity of the nephron. In vitro techniques, such as tubule suspensions (1,2) and isolated microdissected tubules (3) have been designed to solve this problem. Microdissected structures offer the advantage of leading to well-identified segments that allowed biochemical and metabolic characterizations of each portion of the nephron. In contrast, this complex methodology presented the disadvantage of producing minute amounts of biological sample. In recent studies, isolated cells, obtained from renal cortex (4,5) and from papillary collecting duct (6) were established as useful tools for a better understanding of cell metabolic and transport properties. However, the cortical isolated cells presented a large contamination with glomerulus and distal cell types. The objective of the present study was to investigate a new methodology that would allow the preparation of a larger amount of pure proximal tubular cells without any glomerulus contamination.

MATERIALS AND METHODS

Isolated proximal tubule cell suspension. Adult female New Zealand white rabbits were used in all experiments. The method developed for the cell isolation which avoids any proteolytic treatment, was derived from Carlson (2) and Heidrich and Dew (7). Cells were isolated in 95% O_2, 5% CO_2 Earle's balanced salt solution, supplemented with 60 mM sucrose, 26 mM $NaHCO_3$, 4 mM glutamine, 5 mM glucose, 5 mg/l BSA, pH 7.4, 330 mOsm. The suspension of purified proximal tubules was poured in the isolation medium, supplemented with 2.8 mM citrate as Ca-binding agent, for 10 min. The proximal tubules were then washed with the oxygenated isolation medium (citrate-free) and pressed through a 40 µm pore size nylon sieve. The suspension obtained was then passed through a 20 µm pore size nylon sieve. After two centrifugations at 150 g for 5 min, the isolated cells were resuspended in the appropriate medium (depending on the type of the experiment). Protein concentration was determined (8).

Enzyme determinations. The activity of the marker enzymes was assayed on cortical homogenates, proximal tubule suspensions and on the isolated proximal tubular cells. Alanine aminopeptidase, N-acetyl-beta-D-glucosaminidase and cathepsin B were measured according to the procedure previously described by (9). Gamma-glutamyl transpeptidase, alkaline phosphatase, glucose-6-phosphatase and sodium potassium ATPase were measured (10). Hexokinase and lactate dehydrogenase were assayed by established methods (11,12). Catalase activity was assessed by the decomposition of hydrogen peroxide at 240 nm (13). The activity of hormone-sensitive adenylate cyclase was determined by a modification of methods previously described (14) in a final volume of 200µl for 30 min at 30°C. The production of cyclic

427

AMP was assayed by a radiocompetition assay (15) using purified human erythrocyte membranes as binding protein (16).

Oxygen consumption was measured at 37°C with a Clarke oxygen electrode (Gilson Medical Inc., Meddleton, USA) on 1.3 ml of isolated proximal cells suspended in an HEPES buffer containing (in mM) 0.87 $CaCl_2$, 2.68 KCl, 1.47 KH_2PO_4, 0.47 $MgCl_2$, 137 NaCl, 8 Na_2HPO_4, 20 HEPES, 5 glucose, 1 alanine, 4 lactate. Cell concentration was 2-4 mg protein/ml. The cells were continuously oxygenated for 15 min before O_2 consumption measurement.

Glucose production was measured (17) at 37°C on isolated cell suspensions resus-pended in a Krebs-Ca buffer pH 7.4, continuously bubbled with O_2 95%, CO_2 5% at 37°C for 1 hr before use in the presence of succinate or pyruvate at a final concentration of 10 mM.

Cell ATP content was determined by incubating 2 ml of the isolated cell suspension at 37°C in a saturated oxygen Krebs-Ca buffer, for various lengths of time with 10 mM succinate or pyruvate substrate. Just after the experiment, ATP levels were determined accordingly (18).

RESULTS

Marker enzyme studies. Ten marker enzyme activities were assessed on isolated proximal

Table 1. Enzymatic characterization on cortical homogenates, proximal tubules and isolated proximal cells.

	Cortical homogenates	Proximal tubules	Isolated cells
Gamma-glutamyl transpeptidase	94.80 ± 28.42 (6)	75.28 ± 30.02 (6)	103.13 ± 14.87 (6)
Alkaline phosphatase	248.73 ± 31.28 (6)	308.89 ± 31.81 (6) a**	313.96 ± 21.31 (6) a**
N-acetyl-beta-D glucosaminidase	42.73 ± 16.48 (6)	53.28 ± 17.46 (6)	44.20 ± 19.81 (6)
Alanine aminopeptidase	29.83 ± 3.03 (6)	41.63 ± 6.94 (6) a**	66.87 ± 10.67 (6) a***, b***
Glucose-6-phosphatase	56.51 ± 10.40 (5)	91.07 ± 29.58 (5) a*	123.66 ± 31.92 (6) a***
Na^+-K^+-ATPase	139.81 ± 34.98 (5)	218.89 ± 15.20 (4) a**	547.46 ± 65.32 (4) a***, b***
Cathepsin B	11.97 ± 3.30 (6)	16.81 ± 4.16 (6)	13.31 ± 3.76 (6)
Catalase	11.32 ± 1.80 (5)	10.26 ± 1.06 (6)	10.01 ± 1.34 (6)
Lactate dehydrogenase	185.09 ± 33.03 (6)	94.13 ± 21.97 (6) a**	49.23 ± 6.96 (6) a***, b***
Hexokinase	8.44 ± 1.31 (6)	3.46 ± 1.45 (6) a***	4.60 ± 0.94 (6) a***

All enzyme activities are given as $\mu mol.min^{-1}.g\ protein^{-1}$. Statistical analysis was made: (a) versus cortical homogenates, (b) versus proximal tubules. The statistical analysis was made using the paired Student's test: *P<0.05, **P<0.01, ***P<0.001. Values are means ± SD of (n) experiments.

cells (Table 1) compared with isolated proximal tubules and cortical homogenates.

Glucose-6-phosphatase activity, a gluconeogenesis marker enzyme, was significantly increased in the isolated proximal cells compared with proximal tubules or cortical homogenate activities (1.4-fold and 2.2-fold respectively). Activities of 2 brush border enzymes, alkaline phosphatase and alanine aminopeptidase were enhanced by 26% and 124% respectively, in the isolated proximal cells compared with the cortical homogenate activities. Na-K-ATPase, which is located in the basolateral membrane, and glucose-6-phosphatase activities presented a similar pattern. The activities of gamma-glutamyl transpeptidase, a brush border enzyme, N-acetyl-beta-D-glucosaminidase and cathepsin B, lysosomal marker enzymes and catalase, a peroxysomal enzyme, appeared to be stable along the cell isolation procedure. Lactate dehydrogenase and hexokinase activities (glycolysis enzymes) were significantly lower in the isolated proximal cells compared with cortical homogenate activities (-73% and -45% respectively).

ATP levels. The ability of the isolated proximal cells to maintain their ATP content (Table 2) was also evaluated. The cell ATP level remained constant over 60 min when incubated with either pyruvate or succinate substrate.

Oxygen consumption. The basic cell oxygen consumption was reduced by 58% by the addition of ouabain (100 µM) in the incubation medium (Table 3). In contrast, the endogenous respiration rate was enhanced by 155% after succinate substrate application.

Gluconeogenesis capacity. The rate of glucose production (Table 4) was linear up to 80 min from pyruvate substrate (10 mM) by isolated proximal cells. Glucose production appeared to be 2-fold higher from pyruvate compared with succinate substrate. Parathyroid hormone addition in the incubation medium induced a 18% increase in glucose production from pyruvate substrate.

Adenylate cyclase activity (AC). AC was measured in the absence or presence of stimulation on cortical homogenates and isolated proximal cells (Table 5). The concentrations of NaF and hormones were determined to give the maximal AC response and were consistent with published data (3). The highest stimulated to basal AC activity ratios (S/B ratios) in the renal cortex were obtained with PTH and NaF action (10.67, p; 8.57, p). Nevertheless, ISO, SCT and AVP induced a slight increase in S/B ratio with 1.79 ($p<0.01$), 1.76 ($p<0.01$), 2.44 ($p<0.001$) respectively. The basal AC specific activity was reduced in the isolated proximal cells compared with the renal cortex activity (a 5-fold decrease). Among the hormones and components used in our report to stimulate AC activity in isolated proximal cells, only PTH and NaF were able to induce a marked response in isolated cells. The ratio of NaF and PTH-stimulated AC activities were 62 and 52, respectively.

DISCUSSION

The present results describe the potential of a pure suspension of rabbit proximal tubular cells

Table 2. ATP content of isolated proximal cells.

	n	ATP levels (nmol/min/mg protein)		
Time (minutes)		0	30	60
+ Succinate 10 mM	4	6.00 ± 0.78	6.00 ± 0.90	6.03 ± 0.23
+ Pyruvate 10 mM	4	5.51 ± 0.71	6.71 ± 1.35	6.43 ± 1.02

Values are means $\pm$ SD of (n) experiments.

Table 3. Oxygen consumption of the isolated proximal cells

	n	cell oxygen consumption
Basal	4	9.21 ± 1.53
+ Ouabain 100 µM	4	3.87 ± 0.25
+ Succinate 10 mM	4	23.48 ± 2.02

Values are means $\pm$ SD of (n) experiments. Oxygen consumption are given as nmol O_2/min/mg protein

Table 4. Gluconeogenesis capacity of the isolated proximal cells

	n	Glucose formed
Pyruvate 10 mM	6	345.67 ± 23.69
Succinate 10 mM	4	155.33 ± 11.93
Pyruvate 10 mM + PTH 10 µg/ml	3	419.67 ± 38.28
Pyruvate 10 mM + cAMP 0.1 mM	3	382.00 ± 9.89

Values are means $\pm$ SD of (n) independant experiments. Glucose production are expressed as nmol glucose/min/g protein.

isolated by a new simple methodology combining mechanical treatment, short exposure to Ca-binding agent and several sieving steps on a pure suspension of proximal tubules. The first step of the isolation procedure led to isolated proximal tubules without any glomerular contamination (2). The second step prepared a single cell suspension with a complete removal of cellular debris, subcellular organelles, tubule fragments and cell aggregates by the combination of three washes and filtration on nylon sieves and glass wool layer.

Divalent chelating media containing EDTA, were shown to induce cell morphological and respiratory damage (19). A short time incubation of isolated proximal tubules in sodium citrate media, followed by Ca-concentration increase led to morphologically intact isolated proximal cells. The cell respiratory rate in basal- and succinate-stimulated conditions was consistent with previously reported data from isolated chick renal cells (4) and from rabbit

isolated renal cortical cells (5). In this study, ouabain inhibition of the cell oxygen consumption (-58%) was similar to that measured on isolated proximal tubules (20) and 2-fold higher compared with data reported by Poujeol and Vandewalle (5) from isolated renal cortical cells obtained by mechanical dissociation alone. While these authors correlated the decrease in ouabain responsiveness to the reduction in Na/K-ATPase activity along the cell isolation procedure, our results showed that this enzyme activity was increased in the isolated proximal cells. This high activity of the Na^+ pump combined with the cellular ATP content should allow the cell to maintain high potassium and low sodium content.

It is now well established that the renal gluconeogenesis pathway is located in the convoluted proximal portion of the nephron (21,22). The proximal characteristics of these isolated cells, shown by transmission electron microscopy, were emphasized by their capacity to convert noncarbohydrate substrates to glucose through the gluconeogenesis process. Increase of the glucose production by PTH action was consistent with data previously reported (22) and demonstrated the membrane receptor integrity and the cell ability to modulate the metabolic response through the cellular cyclic AMP level.

The key enzymes involved in glycolysis are located in the distal part of the nephron (23). The loss of distal glycolytic enzyme activity (hexokinase and lactate dehydrogenase), along the cell isolation procedure, clearly demonstrated the decrease of distal cellular contamination in the isolated proximal cells. On the basis of our data, it is feasible to postulate that the isolated cell suspension mainly consists of cells from the convoluted portion of the proximal tubule. These findings were recently ascertained by the separation of this cell suspension in two populations of proximal cells by free flow electrophoresis, one from the convoluted part and the other from the straight part of the proximal tubule (24).

In another part of the experiments adenylate cyclase responsiveness to various polypeptidic

Table 5. Adenylate cyclase activity in isolated proximal cells.

	Renal cortex	Isolated cells
Basal act.	150.27 ± 13.5 (1.00)	29.42 ± 2.69 (1.00)
NaF 5 mM	1258.60 ± 80.29 (8.57)	1488.53 ± 104.10 (52.1)
PTH 10 μg/ml	1557.55 ± 73.09 (10.6)	1916.05 ± 138.77 (61.7)
ISO 10^{-6} M	267.97 ± 19.61 (1.79)	53.35 ± 4.66 (1.85)
AVP 10^{-6} M	357.29 ± 12.83 (2.43)	47.16 ± 4.12 (1.62)
SCT 500 ng/ml	265.48 ± 25.89 (1.77)	53.68 ± 4.66 (1.84)

Values are means ± SEM of 6 independent experiments and are expressed as pmole cAMP formed/30 minutes/mg of proteins. Values between brackets give the S/B ratio (stimulated activity/basal activity). (PTH, parathyroid hormone; NaF, sodium fluoride; ISO, isoproterenol; AVP, arginin vasopressin; SCT, synthetic salmon calcitonin).

hormones and beta-adrenergic agonist was evaluated in order to assess the purity of the cell preparation. Indeed, several studies (25, 3) clearly established that among PTH, ISO, SCT and AVP, only PTH was able to stimulate adenylate cyclase in the proximal tubules. In contrast, adenylate cyclase present in the distal portion of the nephron was responsive to PTH, ISO, SCT and AVP. Adenylate cyclase response to the different stimulations in renal cortex rendered an account of cell diversity present in this preparation and was consistent with data previously reported (5). Adenylate cyclase activity in the isolated proximal cells was only markedly increased by the PTH stimulation and gave a PTH Stimulation/Basal ratio similar to that obtained by Morel (25) from microdissected convoluted proximal tubules. This last point clearly shows the removal of nonproximal cell types by the isolation method.

In conclusion, the present report describes a simple technique for isolating pure proximal tubular cells, without any glomerular contamination, and with a large decrease in distal elements. These isolated proximal cells were shown to possess morphological integrity and a high metabolic capacity. This isolation method was shown to be suitable in order to go ahead in the preparative isolation of structures from the proximal tubule of the rabbit kidney. Indeed, Toutain et al. (this proceedings) described the preparative separation of cells from the pars convoluta and the pars recta by means

of high voltage free flow electrophoresis from this pure suspension of rabbit proximal tubular cells. This method also gives suitable material for the development of primary culture of proximal tubular cells. All these methodologies should provide useful tools to enhance the knowledge of proximal cell physiology and its interactions with drug-induced nephrotoxicity.

ACKNOWLEGMENTS

This work was supported by grants from Rhône-Poulenc Santé.

REFERENCES

1. Vinay P, Gougoux A, Lemieux G: Isolation of a pure suspension of rat proximal tubules. Am J Physiol 241:F403-F411, 1981.

2. Carlson EC, Brendel K, Hjelle JT, Meezan E: Ultrastructural and biochemical analysis of isolated basement membranes from kidney glomeruli and tubules and brain and retinal microvessels. J Ultrastruct Res 62:26-53, 1978.

3. Morel F: Sites of hormone action in the mammalian nephron. Am J Physiol 240:F159-F164, 1981.

4. Liang CT, Barnes J, Cheng L, Balakir R, Sacktor B: Effects of 1,25(OH)2D3 administrated in vivo on phosphate uptake by isolated chick renal cells. Am J Physiol 242:C312-C318, 1982.

5. Poujeol P, Vandewalle A: Phosphate uptake by proximal cells isolated from rabbit kidney: role of dexamethasone. Am J Physiol 249:F74-F83, 1985.

6. Stokes JB, Grupp C, Kinne RKH: Purification of rat papillary collecting duct cells: functional and metabolic assessement. Am J Physiol 253:F251- F262, 1987.

7. Heidrich HG, Dew ME: Homogeneous cell populations from rabbit kidney cortex: proximal, distal tubule and renin active cell isolated by free flow electrophoresis. J Cell Biol 74:780-788, 1977.

8. Bradford MM: A rapid and sensitive method for quantification of microgram quantities of protein utilizing the principle of protein dye binding. Anal Biochem 72:248-254, 1976.

9. Toutain H, Olier B, Fillastre JP, Morin JP: Influence of Muzolimine, a new diuretic, on experimental gentamicin nephrotoxicity. Nephrol Dial Transplant 2:520-525, 1987.

10. Hjelle JT, Morin JP, Trouet A: Analytical cell fractionation of isolated rabbit renal proximal tubules. Kidney Int 20:71-77, 1981.

11. Bergmeyer HU: Hexokinase assay. In: Bergmeyer HU (ed); Methods of enzymatic analysis. New York, Academic Press, 1974, pp. 473-475.

12. Bergmeyer HU, Bernt E: Lactate dehydrogenase UV-assay with pyruvate and NADH. In: Bergmeyer HU (ed); Methods of enzymatic analysis. New York, Academic Press, 1974, pp. 574-579.

13. Aebi H: Catalase UV-assay. In: Bergmeyer HU (ed); Methods of enzymatic analysis. New York, Academic Press, 1974, pp. 674-678.

14. Torikai S, Wand MS, Klein KL, Kurokawa K: Adenylate cyclase and cell cyclic AMP of rat cortical thick ascending limb of Henle. Kidney Int 20:649-654, 1981.

15. Gilman A: A protein binding assay for adenosine-3',5'-cyclic monophosphate. Proc Natl Acad Sci USA, 67:305-312, 1970.

16. Levine MA, Downs RW, Singer M, Marx SJ, Aurback GD, Spiegel AM: Deficient activity of guanine nucleotide regulatory protein in erythrocytes from patients with pseudohypo. parathyroidism. Biochem Biophys Res Comm 94:1318-1324, 1980.

17. Bergmeyer HU, Bernt E, Schmidt F, Stork H: D-glucose determination with hexokinase and glucose-6-phosphate dehydrogenase. In: Bergmeyer HU (ed); Methods of enzymatic analysis. New York, Academic Press, 1974, pp. 1196-1201.

18. Lamprecht W, Trautschold I: Determination of adenosine triphosphate with hexokinase and glucose-6-phosphate dehydrogenase. In: Bergmeyer HU (ed); Methods of enzymatic analysis. New York, Academic Press, 1974, pp. 2101-2110.

19. Baur H, Kasperek S, Pfaff E: Criteria of viability of isolated liver cells. Hoppe-Seyler's Z Physiol Chem 356:827-838, 1975.

20. Mandel LJ: Primary active sodium transport, oxygen consumption, and ATP: coupling and regulation. Kidney Int 29:3-9, 1986.

21. Burch HB, Narins RG, Chu C, Fagioli S, Choi S, McCarthy W, Lowry O: Distribution along the rat nephron of three enzymes of gluconeogenesis in acidosis and starvation. Am J Physiol 235:F246-F253, 1978.

22. Wang MS, Kurokawa K: Renal gluconeogenesis: axial and internephron heterogeneity and the effect of parathyroid hormone. Am J Physiol 246: F59-F66, 1984.

23. Guder W, Ross BD: Enzyme distribution along the nephron. Kidney Int 26: 101-111, 1984.

24. Toutain H, Fillastre JP, Morin JP: Preparative free flow electrophoresis for the isolation of two populations of proximal cells from the rabbit kidney. Eur J Cell Biol 49:274-280, 1989.

25. Morel F, Chabardes D, Imbert-Teboul M: Methodology for enzymatic studies of isolated tubular segments: Adenylate Cyclase. In Martinez- Maldonado M (ed); Methods in Pharmacology. New York, Plenum Press, 1978, Ch 11, 4B, pp. 297-323.

67

BIOCHEMICAL AND FUNCTIONAL CHARACTERIZATION OF A PRIMARY CULTURE OF RABBIT PROXIMAL TUBULE CELLS: A TIME-COURSE STUDY

J.P. Morin, H. Toutain, N. Vauclin-Jacques and J.P. Fillastre

I.N.S.E.R.M. U-295, U.E.R.de Médecine-Pharmacie de Rouen, BP 97, 76800 Saint Etienne du Rouvray, FRANCE

INTRODUCTION

In the last 15 years, many investigators have found kidney tubular epithelial cells in culture to be a very useful system for studies of kidney functions, differentiation, morphogenesis, pathophysiology and carcinogenesis (1). Renal epithelial cell cultures may serve as an alternative model system to study those renal cell functions in vitro which, as a consequence of the heterogeneity of the kidney, cannot be assessed in vivo. Because the various cell populations may react differently to injurious stimuli, a well defined and characterized in vitro system would be valuable for studies of pathogenetic mechanisms involved in nephrotoxicity and malignant transformations.

MATERIALS AND METHODS

Isolation of proximal tubule fragments

New Zealand white rabbits weighing 1.5 to 2.0 kg were used in these experiments. We used a modification of the isolation method for proximal tubules described by Brendel and Meezan (2) which is reported in Toutain et al. (3). The suspension of pure proximal tubule was concentrated over a 40μm nylon sieve and incubated for 5 min at 37°C in 50 ml RK1 medium plus collagenase (0.125 mg/ml plus trypsin inhibitor 0.0025%), poured onto a 40μm nylon sieve, gently washed with a spray of culture medium, and gently forced through this sieve. The material passed through the sieve was collected and poured onto a 20μm nylon sieve. Proximal tubule fragments were then collected. The protein concentration of the inoculum was measured using the Bradford protein assay on a sonicated aliquot. Proximal tubule fragments were plated generally at 0.6 mg protein per 60 mm diameter petri dish or 25 cm^2 flask or 0.25 mg protein per 35 mm diameter petri dish and grown in RK2 medium consisting of medium RK1, insulin (5μg/ml), transferrin (5μg/ml), sodium selenite (5ng/ml), penicillin (25UI/ml), streptomycin (25μg/ml) and hydrocortisone (10^{-7}M).

Biochemical assays

Enzyme activities were measured in homogenates of both the starting inoculum of proximal tubule fragments and cultured cells scrapped from two 60mm diameter petri dishes. Each determination was done in duplicate in two homogenates for each point. Data was collected from at least 6 independent primary cultures.

Gamma-glutamyl transpeptidase, ouabain-sensitive Na-K-ATPase, N-acetyl-glucosaminidase, cathepsin B, alkaline phosphatase, glucose-6-phosphatase, alanine aminopeptidase were assayed by established methods (4). Lactate dehydrogenase and hexokinase were determined according to Bergmeyer (5) and Bergmeyer and Bernt (6), catalase was assayed according to Aebi (7), glutathione-S-transferase was assayed according to Habig (8), succinate dehydrogenase was assayed according to Pennington (9).

433

Membrane transport studies

Methyl glucoside transport was measured every two days using 3-11 day old primary cultures of rabbit kidney epithelial cells. Before the uptake period, the monolayers grown in 35 mm dishes were washed with a glucose free RK2 medium at $37^{o}C$. 1,5 ml glucose free RK2 medium containing ^{14}C-methyl glucoside ($10^{-3}M$) with a specific ^{14}C activity of 0.2 µCi/ml warmed to $37^{o}C$ was added to each dish. The cultures were then incubated in a humidified incubator (90%) in a 5% CO_2 95% air environment. After two washes, the cells were solubilized with 1 ml NaOH(1N) for 2 hours at $37^{o}C$ and a 500µl aliquot was used for label determination in a Rack beta (LKB) scintillation counter in Ready Safe (Beckman) scintillation fluid. The remainder of each sample was used for protein determination according to Lowry (10). The radioactive counts in each sample were then normalized with respect to proteins and were corrected for zero time uptake (label not removed by the washing procedure).

^{3}H thymidine and ^{3}H leucine incorporations

Precursor incorporation into DNA and proteins was measured every two days using 0-14 day old primary cultures of rabbit proximal tubules. ^{3}H thymidine (TRK 418 Amersham) 0.3 µCi/ml or ^{3}H leucine (TRK 510 Amersham) 0.25 µCi/ml are added to RK2 medium and 1.5 ml was added per 35 mm dish. Cultures were incubated at $37^{o}C$ in a humidified (90%) atmosphere in a 5% CO_2 95% air environment for 24 hr. After the final wash, 1 ml 10% trichloroacetic acid was added in each dish. Samples were centrifuged (3000 g for 20 min). Supernatants were discarded and pellets digested for one hour as described above and aliquots used for label and protein determination. The radioactive counts in each sample were then normalized to protein and corrected for zero time uptake.

Protein assays

Protein concentrations were determined either by the technique of Bradford (11) or according to the method of Lowry (10).

RESULTS

Cultured Cells

Within a few hours, tubular fragments were observed to attach to the plastic of tissue culture flasks and dishes. Those which did not attach were subsequently removed with the first medium change 72 hr after plating. 24 to 48 hr after seeding, discrete islands of cells migrated out from each attached tubule fragment. Day zero of the culture was generally considered 48 hr after seeding. With each successive day in culture the island increased in size as the cells divided. At day 4 of the culture, the islands were all alkaline phosphatase positive. By day 6-7 the islands became continuous, forming a confluent sheet, with cobblestone appearance and multiple dome formation. Dome formation was reversed by the addition of ouabain (10^{-5} M) to the culture medium and restored after ouabain withdrawal from the culture medium. By day 12-14, the domes disappeared from the monolayer and focal cell necrosis was seen to develop after day 14.

Time-course study of enzymatic pattern

Time-course patterns of 12 enzyme activities were followed every 2 days from seeding till day 16 of the culture. These enzyme activities were chosen for their distributions along the nephron and involvement in key pathways of cellular metabolism.

Brushborder enzymes. The activity of brushborder enzymes i.e. alanine aminopeptidase, gamma-glutamyl transpeptidase and alkaline phosphatase decreased from day 0 to day 6 to reach a plateau value between day 6 and day 16. Plateau levels were about 2%, 12% and 34% of proximal tubule specific activities for alkaline phosphatase, alanine aminopeptidase and gamma-glutamyl transpeptidase respectively.

Na-K-ATPase activity, a basolateral membrane marker, was depressed during the cell growth phase and recovered partially at confluency. Specific activity was then approximately 75% of that of isolated proximal tubules.

Lysosomal enzyme activities were slightly depressed at the onset of the culture and were thereafter sustained at a plateau level of 68% and 59% of that of isolated proximal tubules for NAG and cathepsin B respectively.

Succinate dehydrogenase, a mitochondrial marker activity, was depressed early in the culture and was thereafter sustained at a plateau level between days 2 and 16 at approximately 45% of that of isolated proximal tubules.

Catalase, a peroxisomal marker activity, decreased from day 0 to day 4 to reach a plateau level from day 4 to day 16 at about 25% of the isolated proximal tubule value.

Glutathione-S-transferase activity, a cytosolic enzyme, remained constant and similar to that observed in isolated proximal tubules throughout the study.

Glucose-6-phosphatase decreased rapidly at the beginning of the culture to reach very low activity (3% of isolated proximal tubule value) from day 6.

Glycolytic marker enzymes underwent a dramatic and regular increase from day 0 to days 8-10 to reach 17 and 48-fold the activities observed in isolated proximal tubules for hexokinase and lactate dehydrogenase respectively.

Thymidine and leucine incorporations

Thymidine incorporation into the TCA precipitable fraction of cells was followed every two days from day 3 to day 15. Thymidine incorporation rate decreased from day 3 (0.55 ng/mg protein/24 hr) to day 9 (0.08 ng/mg protein/24 hr), was sustained from day 9 to day 13 and was practically 0 at day 15.

Leucine incorporation rates into the TCA precipitable fraction of cells remained almost constant over the duration of the study (15 to 20 ng/mg protein/24 hr).

Alpha-methyl-D-glucoside (AMG) transport

Kinetic of AMG uptake was studied at day 3 during exponential growth and at day 7 at monolayer confluency. At both time-points AMG incorporation was linear as a function of time over a 240 min period at 37°C. Incorporation rates were 0.722 nMole/min/mg protein (r=0.992) and 0.503 nMole/min/mg protein (r=0.989) at days 3 and 7 respectively.

AMG incorporation was followed between days 3 and 11. Incorporations were performed at 37°C over a 120 min incubation period. A slight decrease in incorporation rate was seen between day 3 and day 5 and a plateau level was seen between day 5 and 11 at a rate of about 0.5 nMole/min/mg protein.

Inhibition studies were performed between days 3 and 11. The uptake of AMG was strongly inhibited (95% inhibition) by phloridzin (5×10^{-4}M). The amplitude of inhibition was similar at all the experimental delays. Phloretin (10^{-4}M) produced a 50% inhibition of AMG uptake. Again, the amplitude of inhibition was similar at all the experimental time-points.

DISCUSSION

This paper has investigated the time course pattern of 12 enzyme activities, the profile of thymidine and leucine uptakes and the AMG transport in primary cultures of rabbit kidney proximal tubule cells grown in hormonally defined medium. The primary cultures derived from highly purified proximal tubules and retained many distinctive properties typical of rabbit proximal tubule cells, the levels of which may differ from those observed in freshly isolated proximal tubules.

In an attempt to further characterize our primary isolates and their behaviour in culture we have measured the activities of marker enzymes such as gamma-glutamyl transpeptidase, alkaline phosphatase and alanine aminopeptidase, which were chosen because of their association primarily with the microvilli of proximal tubule cells (12, 13). Na-K-ATPase was chosen because of its association with the basolateral membrane of the epithelial cells of kidney tubules (14), N-acetyl glucosaminidase and cathepsin B were chosen as lysosomal markers, catalase as peroxysomal marker, succinate dehydrogenase as a mitochondrial marker, glutathione-S-transferase as a cytosolic marker of proximal tubule cells, Glucose-6-phosphatase as a marker for gluconeogenesis, and hexokinase and lactate dehydrogenase as marker for glycolytic activity based on the data of Guder and Ross (15).

Brushborder enzyme specific activities decreased with the age of the culture between days 0 and 6 and reached a plateau level between days 6 and 16. As reported in other studies (16, 17), alkaline phosphatase was more depressed than other brushborder marker enzymes. It should be stressed, however, that alkaline phosphatase activities reported in our study are similar to those reported by Bell (18) in mouse, and Smith and Acosta (1986) in rat kidney primary cultures, and superior to that reported for human (17) and rabbit (16) kidney primary cultures. The decrease in brushborder enzyme activity during the first 7 days in culture may be related to the ultrastructural observations of shorter microvilli in cells of monolayers as opposed to primary isolates. Variation in the amplitude of the decrease in brushborder enzyme specific activity could be in part due to specific regulation by substrate concentrations in the culture medium.

Ouabain Na-K-ATPase activity, a basolateral membrane marker enzyme is depressed during exponential growth and restored at monolayer confluency concomitantly with dome formation. The sensitivity of domes to the addition of ouabain in the culture medium confirms the capacity of active transepithelial transport by these cells.

Catalase specific activity followed a similar time-course pattern to that of gamma-glutamyl transpeptidase. It should be kept in mind that the distribution of peroxisomes along the rabbit nephron closely parallels that of gamma-glutamyl transpeptidase (15).

Glutathione-S-transferase, a soluble enzyme involved in drug detoxication exclusively distributes in proximal tubule without any concentration gradient along this structure. No variation in specific activity was seen for this enzyme with the age of the culture. This point is of particular importance to confirm the proximal nature of our cultured cells.

Enzymes of glucose metabolism undergo dramatic changes in activity with culture aging. Glucose-6-phosphatase, which is reported to be an exclusive proximal tubule enzyme in the kidney essentially in the pars convoluta (19), is rapidly depressed in the culture to become barely detectable after day 6. This dramatic decrease in glucose-6-phosphatase activity, which is consistent with that reported by Trifillis et al. (17) in human primary cultures, may be explained by the presence of high amounts of insulin used as a growth factor in the medium, and the presence of high amounts of glucose (3.15 g/l) in the culture medium. These components are expected to depress the gluconeogenic pathway (19) and to orient the cellular metabolism towards other pathways.

Hexokinase and lactate dehydrogenase, two enzymes involved in the glycolytic pathway were increased at day 10 by a factor 16 and 47 respectively, suggesting a cellular orientation towards glucose utilization through the glycolytic pathway. The levels of Hexokinase and lactate dehydrogenase reached in our primary cultures at day 10-12 are similar to those observed in either MDCK or LLC-PK1 cell lines (20). These authors concluded that the adaptation to culture of the kidney cell lines caused a strict dependence on glycolysis resulting in high activities of glycolytic enzymes. Similar findings concerning glucose metabolism and utilization were reported for rat hepatocytes in primary cultures compared to permanent cell lines, with a progressive adaptation as hepatocytes aged in primary culture shifting toward the pattern exhibited by the permanent cell line (21). The shift in glucose metabolism and utilization observed in our model seems to be due to functional adaptation to cell culture conditions i.e. high insulin high glucose levels more than to the overgrowth of other kidney epithelial cell types.

An important function of the proximal tubule is the reabsorption of sugars from the lumen of the tubule back to the blood. To determine whether the proximal tubule cells in culture possess this hexose-transport system located on the apical membrane for its sodium-dependent component and on the basolateral surface for the sodium-independent component (22, 23), the incorporation of AMG, a non-metabolisable sugar, was studied. AMG uptake study was performed at 37°C in glucose-free culture medium containing labelled and unlabelled AMG in a CO_2 5%-air 95% environment in order to more closely mimic culture conditions. These conditions differ from the usual incorporation media consisting of buffered salt solutions (18) or modified Krebs Ringer solution (16). These uptake conditions led to a linear incorporation of AMG as a function of time for at least 4 hours at 37°C at a rate of 0.5 to 0.7 nM/min/mg protein as a function of the age of the culture. Salt solutions led to lower incorporation rates of about 0.13 nM/min/mg protein at 23°C with a linear period of 120 min (16) and 0.3 nM/min/mg protein with a linear period of 60 minutes at 23°C (18). The AMG carrier is mainly located on apical membranes. The slight decrease of rate seen between day 3 and day 5 appears to be consistent with the decrease in either gamma-glutamyl transpeptidase or alanine aminopeptidase which occur during the same period suggesting a decrease in the relative amount of apical membrane in the culture. The inhibition ratios of AMG uptake by phloretin and phloridzin remained constant throughout the study, suggesting that transporter characteristics are not altered by culture aging.

It is generally agreed that the proximal tubule is an important site of toxic and carcinogenic effects, and may play a key role in most hypotheses concerning the pathogenesis of acute renal failure (24). For these reasons, the isolation of purified rabbit proximal tubule structures, their primary culture and their extensive characterization may provide a well defined in vitro system for the host of future studies concerning nephrotoxicity and transport phenomena.

ACKNOWLEDGEMENTS

This work was supported by grants from Rhône-Poulenc Santé.

REFERENCES

1. Gstraunthaler G: Epithelial cells in tissue culture. Renal Physiol Biochem 11:1-42, 1988.

2. Brendel K, Meezan E: Isolation and properties of a pure preparation of proximal kidney tubules obtained without collagenase treatment. Fed Proc 34:803, 1975.

3. Toutain H, Fillastre JP, Morin JP: Preparative free flow electrophoresis for the isolation of two populations of proximal cells from the rabbit kidney. Eur J Cell Biol 49:274-280, 1989.

4. Hjelle JT, Morin JP, Trouet A: Analytical cell fractionation of isolated proximal tubules. Kidney Int 20:71-77, 1981.

5. Bergmeyer HU: Hexokinase assay. In: Bergmeyer HU (ed); Methods of enzymatic analysis. New York, Academic Press, 1974, pp. 473-475.

6. Bergmeyer HU, Bernt E: Lactate deshydrogenase UV-assay with pyruvate and NADH. In: Bergmeyer HU (ed); Methods of enzymatic analysis. New York, Academic Press, 1974, pp. 574-579.

7. Aebi H: Catalase UV assay. In: Bergmeyer HU (ed); Methods of enzymatic analysis. New York, Academic Press, 1974, pp. 674-678.

8. Habig WH, Pabst MJ, Jakobi WB: Glutathione-S-transferases : the first enzymatic step in mecapturic acid formation. J Biol Chem 249:7130-7139, 1974.

9. Pennington RJ: Biochemistry of dystrophic muscle: mitochondrial succinate tetrazolium reductase and adenosine triphosphatase. Biochem J 80:649-654, 1961.

10. Lowry OH, Rosebrough NJ, Farr AL, Randall RJ: Protein measurement with the folin phenol reagent. J Biol Chem 193:265-275, 1951.

11. Bradford MM: A rapid and sensitive method for quantification of microgram quantities of protein utilizing the principle of protein dye binding. Anal Biochem 72:248-254, 1976.

12. Spater HW, Poruchynsky MS, Quintana N, Inoue M, Novikoff KM: Immuno cytochemical localization of gamma-glutamyl transferase in rat kidney with protein A-horseradish peroxydase. Proc Natl Acad Sci, USA 79:3547-3552, 1982.

13. Mondorf AW, Kinne R, Scherberich JE, Falkenberg F: Isolierung, enzymatische und immunologische Charakterisierung einer Plasma-membranfraktion vom Proximal en Tubulus der menschlichen Niere. Clin Chim Acta 37:25-32, 1972.

14. Katz AL, Doucet A, Morel F: Na^+,K^+-ATPase activity along the rabbit, rat and mouse nephron. Am J Physiol 237:F114-F120, 1979.

15. Guder WG, Ross BD: Enzyme distribution along the nephron. Kidney Int 26:101-111, 1984.

16. Chung SD, Alavi N, Livingston D, Hiller S, Taub M: Characterization of primary rabbit kidney cultures that express proximal tubule functions in a hormonally defined medium. J Cell Biol 95:118-126, 1982.

17. Trifillis AL, Regec AL, Trump BF: Isolation, culture and characterization of human renal tubular cells. J Urol 133:324-329, 1985.

18. Bell CL, Tenenhouse HS, Scriver CR: Initiation and characterization of primary mouse kidney epithelial cultures. In Vitro Cell Develop Biol 24: 683-695, 1988.

19. Burch HB, Narins RG, Chu C, Fagioli S, Choi S, McCarthy W, Lowry O: Distribution along the rat nephron of three enzymes of gluconeogenesis in acidosis and starvation. Am J Physiol 235:F246-F253, 1978.

20. Gstraunthaler G, Pfaller W, Kotanko P: Biochemical characterization of renal epithelial cell cultures (LLC-PK1 and MDCK). Am J Physiol 248:F536-F544, 1985.

21. Bissell DM, Levine GA, Bissell MJ: Glucose metabolism by adult hepatocytes in primary cultures and cell lines from rat liver. Am J Physiol 234:C122-C130, 1978.

22. Kinne RH, Murer H, Kinne-Safran E, Thees M, Sachs G: Sugar transport by renal plasma membrane vesicles. J Membr Biol 21:375-395, 1975.

Smith MA, Acosta D: Development of a primary culture system of rat kidney cortical cells to evaluate the nephrotoxicity of xenobiotics. Fd Chem Toxic 24:551-556, 1986.

23. Beck JC, Saktor B: The sodium electrochemical potential-mediated uphill transport of D-glucose in renal brushborder membrane vesicles. J Biol Chem 253:5531-5535, 1978.

24. Zalem RC, McDowell EM, Nagle RB, McNeil JS, Flamenbaum W, Trump BF: Studies on the pathophysiology of acute renal failure. II. A histochemical study of the proximal tubule of the rat following administration of mercuric chloride. Virchows Arch B Cell Pathol 22:197, 1976.

68

DEVELOPMENT OF A PRIMARY RAT CELL CULTURE MODEL FOR INVESTIGATIONS OF RENAL PROXIMAL TUBULAR DAMAGE

E.T. Barron, I. Pratt and M.P. Ryan

Department of Pharmacology, University College Dublin, Dublin 4, Ireland

INTRODUCTION

There has been an increasing ethical, commercial and scientific need for reliable, well-characterised and appropriate in vitro models for the study of renal toxicology. The nephron is structurally and functionally complex with many specialised functions occurring in morphologically discrete segments. It is therefore relevant to adapt a molecular and mechanistic approach to investigations of site-specific processes and the site-specific perturbations produced by chemicals and drugs. In these investigations in vitro systems offer many advantages over more conventional in vivo systems, in that specific nephron segments may be studied individually.

A number of such systems are currently under study, ranging from the isolated perfused kidney to brush border membrane vesicles. Renal cell lines have been much used and have yielded much valuable information; however, they may be limited in that dedifferentiation may occur with loss of specific characteristics of the original cell of origin. Primary cultures of specific segments of the nephron should overcome these limitations. The present study was undertaken to develop a method for the isolation of rat renal proximal tubule fragments for the purpose of preparing primary cell cultures of the proximal epithelium.

METHODS

Tissue Preparation.

Kidneys from 3-4 Wistar rats were used per preparation. The kidneys were perfused in situ with ice-cold Krebs-Henseleit Salts (KHS) buffer previously saturated with 95% O_2/5% CO_2. They were excised, the cortices removed and minced with scalpel blades. The minced cortices were suspended in KHS containing 0.15% collagenase (BDH) and then digested for 20 min at 37°C in an atmosphere of 95% O_2/5% CO_2. Following the digestion period, the tubules were separated from the undigested portion by washing through a tea-strainer. The resulting tubule mixture was resuspended in 45% iso-osmotic Percoll and subjected to centrifugation for 20 minutes at 20,000 rpm at 6°C (1). The fraction containing primarily proximal tubules was removed, washed and resuspended in DMEM tissue culture medium containing 10% fetal calf serum and 0.1mM gentamicin. Samples were taken at this point for measurement of brush border marker enzymes (2-3) and protein content (4). The tubules were plated at a density of approximately 0.5 mg protein per well.

Isotope Studies

Prior to incubation with isotope, cells were washed twice with incubation medium (unmodified DMEM). To study thymidine incorporation into DNA and leucine incorporation into protein, cells were incubated in 1 ml of DMEM containing 0.25µCi/ml [³H]thymidine and [¹⁴C]leucine, respectively, for the appropriate time interval. Similarily, cells were incubated with 0.25µCi/ml. alpha-Methyl D-[^{14}C]pyranoside, a D-glucose analogue, to study the cellular hexose transport system. Following incubation, cells were washed twice with ice-cold KHS, solubilised with 2% SDS and radioactivity counted.

RESULTS

Enrichment of the proximal fraction with proximal tubules was demonstrated by increase in the brush border marker enzymes alkaline phosphatase and gamma-glutamyltranspeptidase (90% and 52%, respectively) and a reduction in the distal marker enzyme hexokinase (62%). Viability of the tubules was demonstrated by a double fluorescent viability technique using ethidium bromide and acridine orange.

48 hr following inoculation outgrowth of cells of typical epithelial morphology was apparent. The cells exhibited mitotic activity as demonstrated by daily linear [^{3}H]thymidine incorporation for a further two days, after which cell division decreased significantly. Electron microscopic examination of the cells at day 4 of growth provided evidence for the epithelial nature of the cells, including the presence of microvilli.

The cells in culture were further characterised by the presence of Na^{+}-dependent phloridzin-inhibitable hexose transport system, a characteristic of the proximal epithelial cell. Alpha-Methyl D-[^{14}C]pyranoside, a D-glucose analogue, was transported into the cells in a time-dependent manner. This transport was significantly inhibited in a Na^{+}-free medium and was inhibited by phloridzin in a dose-dependent manner. The presence of oubain-sensitive rubidium (^{86}Rb) uptake also indicated that these cells retain biochemical integrity.

Cisplatin (CP), a nephrotoxic anti-cancer drug was selected as a model nephrotoxin, to conduct preliminary toxicity studies using these primary cultures. ^{195}Pt-CP was transported

Table 1. Alpha-Methyl D-[^{14}C]pyranoside uptake into primary cultures of rat renal proximal tubules.

Alpha-Methyl D-[^{14}C]pyranoside uptake (nmoles/mg protein)		
Na^{+} containing	Na^{+} free	Phloridzin(1uM)
36±8.0	4.0±0.5	14.0±2.0

Uptake was measured in the presence and absence of 142mM Na^{+} and in the presence of 1.0µM Phloridzin. Equimolar choline chloride and choline bicarbonate was substituted.
Values represent the mean and standard errors of three experiments carried out in triplicate. Incubation period = 60 min.

Table 2. The effect of increasing concentrations of cisplatin on [^{3}H]thymidine and [^{14}C]Leucine incorporation into rat proximal tubule cells.

Cisplatin µg/ml	Precursor incorporation (% of control)	
	[^{3}H] Thymidine	[^{14}C] Leucine
0	100	100
1	75±10	91±9
2.5	37±6	54±5
5.0	22±4	32±8
7.5	19±2	25±5
10.0	16±5	18±6

Values represent the mean and standard errors of three experiments carried out in triplicate. Incubation period = 24 hr.

slowly into the cells, this transport was partially inhibited by the metabolic inhibitors potassium cyanide and iodoacetate (30µM) suggesting an element of active transport of CP. CP caused a dose-dependent inhibition of [^{3}H]thymidine and [^{14}C]leucine incorporation, significant inhibition occurring at 24 hours with a dose of 1.0µg/ml CP. Inhibition of [^{3}H]thymidine incorporation by 5.0µg/ml (16µM) CP occurs as early as 8 hr following drug treatment.

DISCUSSION

In this study, it was demonstrated that proximal tubules of good purity and viability could be obtained. Cultures developing from these tubular fragments displayed typical epithelial morphology and were shown to maintain transport properties characteristic of the renal proximal epithelium, such as Na^+-dependent hexose transport. In preliminary toxicity studies, Cisplatin, a known nephrotoxin, was shown to rapidly inhibit thymidine incorporation at low doses. It may be concluded that such primary cell cultures, which appear to retain many properties of the cells of origin, offer potiential for mechanistic studies of target cell toxicity.

ACKNOWLEDGEMENTS

This work was supported by a Strategic Research Programme Grant from Eolas, the Irish Science and Technology Agency.

REFERENCES

1. Gesek FA, Wolff DW and Standhoy JW. Improved separation method for rat proximal and distal renal tubules. Am J Physiol 253:F358-365, 1987.

2. Lansing AI, Belkhode ML, Lynch WE and Lieberman I. Enzymes of plasma membranes of liver. J Biol Chem 94:721-734, 1965.

3. Tate SS, and Meister A. Interaction of gamma-glutamyltranspeptidase with amino acids, peptides, and derivatives and analogues of glutathione. J Biol Chem 249:7593-7602, 1974.

4. Lowry OH, Rosenbrough NJ, Farr AL and Randall RJ. Protein measurement with the Folin phenol reagent. J Biol Chem 193:265-275, 1951.

69

OXIDATIVE INJURY IN ISOLATED RAT RENAL PROXIMAL AND DISTAL TUBULAR CELLS

L.H. Lash and J.J. Tokarz

Department of Pharmacology, Wayne State University School of Medicine, 540 East Canfield Avenue, Detroit, MI 48201, U.S.A.

INTRODUCTION

Each cell type of the nephron differs structurally, biochemically, and hence functionally from one another. As a consequence of this heterogeneity, mechanisms of chemical toxicity or pathological injury in the kidney cannot be adequately described at the level of the whole organ, but must be evaluated at the level of a particular region or cell type. Several examples are known in which exposure of kidneys, either in vivo or in vitro, to nephrotoxic chemicals or to pathological conditions produces specific patterns of injury.

Isolated renal cells in suspension have been a useful in vitro model system in which to study drug metabolism, transport and chemical toxicity (1-7). To study nephron heterogeneity with respect to susceptibility to chemical and pathological injury on a biochemical level, we developed an in vitro system using isolated cell preparations from rat renal cortex. These are highly enriched populations of cells derived from specific regions of the nephron which could be obtained in large numbers and extended viability (8). In a previous study with this cell preparation (8), we exposed isolated rat renal proximal tubular (PT) and distal tubular (DT) cells to the nephrotoxic cephalosporin antibiotic cephaloridine and found selective cytotoxicity in PT cells.

Many diseases and chemical toxicities are associated with the production of active oxygen species or other reactive metabolites that alter the redox balance of the cell, producing an "oxidative stress" (9-12). This is particularly important in the kidney because of its high basal rate of aerobic metabolism. In the present work, we exposed PT and DT cells to three cytotoxic agents, menadione (MD), tert-butyl hydroperoxide (tBH) and hydrogen peroxide (H_2O_2), each of which produces an oxidative stress. This enabled us to study and to compare the susceptibility of renal PT and DT cells to this form of chemical injury.

METHODS

Isolation of rat renal PT and DT cells. Isolated renal cortical cells were prepared from male Fischer 344 rats (200-300 g) by collagenase perfusion (1). To obtain enriched populations of PT and DT cells, cortical cells were subjected to density-gradient centrifugation in Percoll (8). Briefly, cortical cells (5 ml, 5-8 x 10^6 cells/ml) were layered on 35 ml of 45% (v/v) isosmotic Percoll solution in 50-ml polycarbonate centrifuge tubes and were centrifuged at 4°C for 30 min at 20,000 g in a Sorvall RC2B centrifuge using a SS34 rotor. The density-gradient produced (1.016 g/ml to 1.120 g/ml) was continuous and concave with an inflection point at 1.057 g/ml. PT cells were identified by measurement of gamma-glutamyltransferase and alkaline phosphatase activities as marker enzymes (13) and DT cells were identified by measurement of hexokinase activity as a marker enzyme (13).

Before incubations, cells were diluted 5-fold with Krebs-Henseleit buffer containing 25 mM Hepes, 2% (w/v) bovine serum albumin, and substrates (5 mM glucose, 5 mM glutamine; omitted when substrate specificity of respiration was measured), were washed to remove Percoll, and were resuspended in fresh buffer at concentrations of 1-4 x 10^6 cells/ml. Cell concentrations were determined in the presence of 0.2% (w/v) Trypan blue in a hemacytometer, and cell viability was estimated by measuring the fraction of cells that exclude Trypan blue or by measuring the leakage of lactate dehydrogenase (LDH) (14). All buffers were equilibrated with and incubations were performed at 37°C under an atmosphere of 95% O_2/5% CO_2 in a shaking water bath.

Statistical analyses were performed by paired t-tests and differences with two-tail probabilities less than 0.05 were considered significant.

RESULTS

Selected biochemical properties of the isolated renal PT and DT cell preparation are summarized in Table 1. The two commonly employed measures of cell viability, Trypan blue exclusion and LDH leakage, show that the PT and DT cells are greater than 90% viable at the time of isolation. Rates and characteristics of cellular oxygen consumption, cellular concentrations of ATP and glutathione, and distribution of marker enzymes indicate that the two cell populations are metabolically competent and exhibit properties characteristic of the PT and DT regions of the nephron.

Succinate stimulated respiration in PT cells, but not in DT cells, indicative of the selective presence of a brush-border membrane trans-

TABLE 1. Characteristics of Renal Proximal and Distal Tubular Cell Preparation.

Parameter	Proximal Tubules	Distal Tubules	n
Yield per preparation using kidneys from 1 rat (x 10^6 cells)	30.1 $\pm$ 11.6	12.8 $\pm$ 5.1	29
Viability measurement			
Trypan blue exclusion (%)	94.5 $\pm$ 2.8	93.7 $\pm$ 2.9	20
LDH leakage (%)	9.94 $\pm$ 5.94	8.62 $\pm$ 5.57	11
Oxygen consumption (nmol/min per 10^6 cells)			
Basal	12.4 $\pm$ 1.9	35.3 $\pm$ 2.2	7
+ 5 mM Succinate	16.7 $\pm$ 1.8	31.6 $\pm$ 1.7	7
+ 0.25 mg Nystatin/ml	17.7 $\pm$ 3.2	45.3 $\pm$ 3 3[a]	3
+ 0.1 mM Ouabain	7.8 $\pm$ 2.7	17.3 $\pm$ 4.0[a]	3
+ 1 mM Amiloride	10.1 $\pm$ 3.2	8.4 $\pm$ 3.5[a]	3
ATP (nmol/10^6 cells)	2.87 $\pm$ 0.33	6.58 $\pm$ 1.48	3
Glutathione (nmol/10^6 cells)	15.1 $\pm$ 1.2	12.1 $\pm$ 0.1	3
Marker enzymes (nmol/min)			7
Alkaline phosphatase	403.0 $\pm$ 113	117.0 $\pm$ 34	
Gamma-glutamyltransferase	1481.0 $\pm$ 282	186.0 $\pm$ 25	
Hexokinase	111.0 $\pm$ 48	785.0 $\pm$ 235	

Data are means $\pm$ S.E. [a]Significantly different (p< 0.05) from basal.

port system for succinate localized in the PT region (15,16). In contrast, amiloride selectively inhibited respiration in DT cells. The rate of oxygen consumption was also responsive to changes in the activity of the $(Na^+ + K^+)$-stimulated ATPase; in agreement with previous results by Mandel and colleagues (17-19) in isolated proximal tubules, stimulation of the $(Na^+ + K^+)$-stimulated ATPase activity in both PT and DT cells with the monocation ionophore nystatin increased the rate of respiration and inhibition of the $(Na^+ + K^+)$-stimulated ATPase with ouabain decreased the rate of respiration. This finding indicated that both cell types devote a significant portion of their energy supply to active transport. Glutathione concentration, as previously reported (20), was slightly (25%) higher in PT cells than in DT cells.

Having established the identity and enrichment of the two cell populations, we could now employ this in vitro preparation to study susceptibility to oxidative injury. The concentration dependence of tBH-, MD-, and H_2O_2-induced cytotoxicity was examined by incubating PT and DT cells for 1 hr with various concentrations of the three agents and measuring LDH leakage (Fig. 1). Marked differences occurred in the susceptibility of the two cell types to injury; tBH, at the highest concentration used (2 mM), reduced PT cell viability from 85% to 63%, but reduced DT cell viability from 85% to 18%. Similarly, MD (1 mM) reduced PT cell viability to 51%, but reduced DT cell viability to 14% and H_2O_2 (1 mM) reduced PT cell viability to 53%, but reduced DT cell viability to 22%.

Differences in the pattern of the time courses of tBH-, MD-, and H_2O_2- induced cytotoxicity in PT and DT cells also occurred (Fig. 2). For all three agents, cytotoxicity developed more slowly in PT cells than in DT cells, indicative of the greater sensitivity of the latter cells to these chemicals. Significant agent-induced decreases in PT cell viability occurred after 60 or 120 min of incubation. In contrast, significant decreases in DT cell viability occurred after 30 or 60 min of incubation, depending on the agent used. As with the concentration dependence of cytotoxicity, the decreases observed in DT

cells were much larger than those observed in PT cells.

DISCUSSION

We have developed a separation procedure for obtaining two populations of isolated cells from rat kidney cortex, one enriched in cells from the proximal tubular region and one enriched in cells from the distal tubular region. The procedure differs from other separation methods for these two nephron regions (21-23) in that isolated, single cells in suspension, rather than isolated tubules, are obtained. Analysis of yield, viability (Trypan blue exclusion, LDH leakage), respiratory properties, ATP and glutathione concentrations, and marker enzyme activities in the two cell populations (Table 1) demonstrates that they are suitable for study of renal function and metabolism on a cellular and molecular level because the cells have adequate concentrations of key metabolites (e.g. ATP, glutathione) and respond to external stimuli by altering some reaction or process in an integrated manner (e.g. respiratory response to modulation of $(Na^+ + K^+)$-ATPase activity).

Isolated rat kidney cortical cells, which are predominantly of proximal tubular origin (1,3), have been used in the study of drug metabolism (1,2), transport (4,7), and mechanisms of cytotoxicity (5,6). The goal of this research was to study all of the above, but with a focus on how the various regions of the nephron compared with each other and what factors determined their differences. In the present work, susceptibility to oxidative stress was examined by comparing effects of three cytotoxic agents, tBH, MD, and H_2O_2, each known to act via generation of reactive oxygen metabolites (24,25).

DT cells exhibited a much greater sensitivity to injury (5- to 10-fold, depending on the agent used) than did PT cells. The relative resistance of PT cells may allow the kidney to deal more efficiently with this form of injury because the proximal tubule is the region of the nephron that is most dependent on oxidative metabolism for its energy-dependent functions (17-19) and is

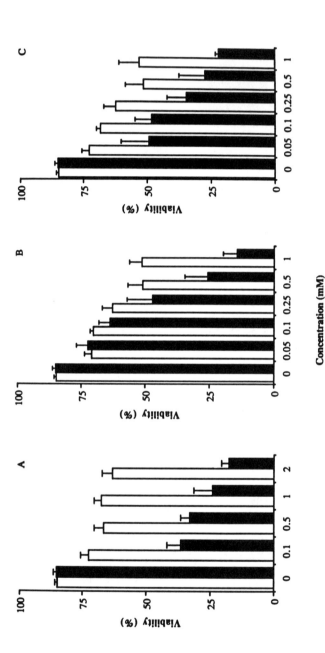

Fig. 1. Concentration dependence of oxidative injury. Isolated renal PT (open bars) and DT (filled bars) cells were incubated for 1 hr at 37°C with the indicated concentration of tBH (A), MD (B), or H_2O_2 (C). Viability was measured as the fraction of cells that did not leak LDH. Results are means ± S.E. of three cell preparations. For PT cells, all additions except 1 mM H_2O_2 produced significantly lower ($p < 0.05$) cell viability compared to control (0 addition). For DT cells, all additions except 0.05 and 0.25 mM MD and 0.05 mM H_2O_2 produced significantly lower ($p < 0.05$) cell viability compared to control (0 addition).

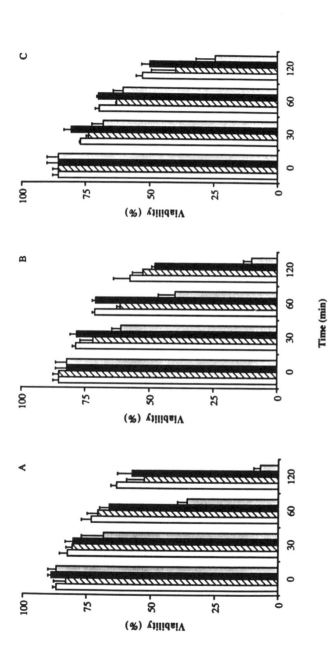

Fig. 2. Time course of oxidative injury. Isolated renal PT and DT cells were incubated for the indicated times at 37°C with either 1 mM tBH (A), 0.25 mM MD (B), or 0.25 mM H₂O₂ (C). Viability was measured as the fraction of cells that did not leak LDH. Results are the means ± S.E. of three cell preparations. PT cells + buffer (open bars); PT cells + agent (striped bars); DT cells + buffer (dark filled bars); DT cells + agent (light filled bars). For PT cells, addition of tBH at 60 min, MD at 60 min, and H₂O₂ at 60 min produced significantly lower (p< 0.05) cell viability compared to control. For DT cells, addition of tBH at 120 min, MD at 30, 60, and 120 min, and H₂O₂ at 120 min produced significantly lower (p<0.05) cell viability compared to control.

the region that would be exposed to the greatest extent to toxicants and other xenobiotics that might produce oxidative injury. Additionally, there were differences in the sensitivity of the two cell types to the three agents tested: Based on the concentration dependence (Fig. 1) and time course (Fig. 2) of cytotoxicity, MD was the most cytotoxic of the three compounds; H_2O_2 was slightly more cytotoxic than tBH, which may reflect differences in intracellular metabolism of the two peroxides.

Activities of detoxication enzymes in PT and DT cells, such as catalase, glutathione peroxidase, and superoxide dismutase, may be important in determining these responses. Glutathione status is of particular importance for redox homeostasis in renal cells (26); differences in content of glutathione and in activities of glutathione-dependent enyzmes may therefore contribute to susceptibility to oxidative damage. In addition to the slightly higher concentration of glutathione in PT cells as compared to DT cells (Table 1 and ref. 20), we have found that activities of glutathione peroxidase and glutathione reductase are significantly higher in PT cells than in DT cells (Lash and Tokarz, unpublished data). This indicates that DT cells have a reduced ability to counteract challenges to normal redox status, which may be partially responsible for the higher susceptibility of those cells to oxidative stress.

In conclusion, we have employed a preparation of highly enriched, isolated PT and DT cells in suspension to study nephron heterogeneity with regards to susceptibility to oxidative injury. Employing three different pro-oxidant chemicals, we have shown clearly that the DT region of the nephron is much more sensitive to oxidative stress than is the PT region.

ACKNOWLEDGEMENT

This work was supported in part by a Pharmaceutical Manufacturer's Association Foundation Starter Grant and by National Institutes of Health Grant DK40725.

REFERENCES

1. Jones DP, Sundby G-B, Ormstad K, Orrenius S: Use of isolated kidney cells for study of drug metabolism. Biochem Pharmacol 28: 929-935, 1979.

2. Ormstad K, Jones DP, Orrenius S: Characteristics of glutathione biosynthesis by freshly isolated rat kidney cells. J Biol Chem 255: 175-181, 1980.

3. Ormstad K, Orrenius S, Jones DP: Preparation and characteristics of isolated kidney cells. Methods Enzymol 77: 137-146, 1981.

4. Lash LH, Jones DP: Uptake of the glutathione conjugate S-(1,2-dichlorovinyl)-glutathione by renal basal-lateral membrane vesicles and isolated kidney cells. Mol Pharmacol 28: 278-282, 1985.

5. Lash LH, Anders MW: Cytotoxicity of S-(1,2-dichlorovinyl)glutathione and S-(1,2-dichlorovinyl)-L-cysteine in isolated rat kidney cells. J Biol Chem 261: 13076-13081, 1986.

6. Lash LH, Elfarra AA, Anders MW: S-(1,2-Dichlorovinyl)-L-homocysteine-induced cytotoxicity in isolated rat kidney cells. Arch Biochem Biophys 251: 432-439, 1986.

7. Lash LH, Anders MW: Uptake of nephrotoxic S-conjugates by isolated rat renal proximal tubular cells. J Pharmacol Exp Ther 248: 531-537, 1989.

8. Lash LH, Tokarz JJ: Isolation of two distinct populations of cells from rat kidney cortex and their use in the study of chemical-induced toxicity. Anal Biochem 182:271-279, 1989.

9. Cadenas E, Sies H: Oxidative stress: Excited oxygen species and enzyme activity. Adv Enz Regul 23: 217-237, 1985.

10. Fridovich I: Biological effects of the superoxide radical. Arch Biochem Biophys 247: 1-11, 1986.

11. Halliwell B: Oxidants and human disease: Some new concepts. FASEB J 1: 358-364, 1987.

12. Kehrer JP, Mossman BT, Sevenian A, Trush MA, Smith MT: Free radical mechanisms in chemical pathogenesis. Toxicol Appl Pharmacol 95: 349-362, 1988.

13. Guder WG, Ross BD: Enzyme distribution along the nephron. Kidney Int 26: 101-111, 1984.

14. Moldéus P, Högberg J, Orrenius S: Isolation and use of liver cells. Methods Enzymol 52:60-71, 1978.

15. Wright SH, Kippen I, Wright EM: Stoichiometry of Na^+-succinate cotransport in renal brush-border membranes. J Biol Chem 257: 1773-1778, 1982.

16. Fukuhara Y, Turner RJ: Sodium-dependent succinate transport in renal outer cortical brush-border membrane vesicles. Am J Physiol 245: F374-F381, 1983.

17. Balaban RS, Mandel LJ, Soltoff SP, Storey JM: Coupling of active ion transport and aerobic respiratory rate in isolated renal tubules. Proc Natl Acad Sci USA 77: 447-451, 1980.

18. Harris SI, Balaban RS, Barrett L, Mandel LJ: Mitochondrial respiratory capacity and Na^+- and K^+-dependent adenosine triphosphatase-mediated ion transport in the intact renal cell. J Biol Chem 256: 10319-10328, 1981.

19. Harris SI, Patton L, Barrett L, Mandel LJ: (Na^+,K^+)-ATPase kinetics within the intact renal cell: The role of oxidative metabolism. J Biol Chem 257: 6996-7002, 1982.

20. Brehe JE, Chan AWK, Alvey TR, Burch HB: Effect of methionine sulfoximine on glutathione and amino acid levels in the nephron. Am J Physiol 231: 1536-1540, 1976.

21. Scholer DW, Edelman IS: Isolation of rat kidney cortical tubules enriched in proximal and distal segments. Am J Physiol 237: F350-F359, 1979.

22. Vinay P, Gougoux A, Lemieux G: Isolation of a pure suspension of rat proximal tubules. Am J Physiol 241: F403-F4111, 1981.

23. Gesek FA, Wolff DW, Strandhoy JW: Improved separation method for rat proximal and distal renal tubules. Am J Physiol 253: F358-F365, 1987.

24. Smith MT, Evans CG, Thor H, Orrenius S: Quinone-induced oxidative injury to cells and tissues. In: Sies H (ed); Oxidative Stress. London, Academic Press, 1985, pp.91-113.

25. Sies H: Hydroperoxides and thiol oxidants in the study of oxidative stress in intact cells and organs. In: Sies H (ed); Oxidative Stress. London, Academic press, 1985, pp.73-90.

26. Lash LH, Jones DP, Anders MW: Glutathione homeostasis and glutathione S-conjugate toxicity in the kidney. Rev Biochem Toxicol 9: 29-67, 1988.

70

SEPARATION OF CELLS FROM THE CONVOLUTED AND STRAIGHT PORTIONS OF THE PROXIMAL TUBULE FROM THE RABBIT KIDNEY BY FREE-FLOW ELECTROPHORESIS

H. Toutain and J.P. Morin

I.N.S.E.R.M. U-295, U.E.R. de Médecine-Pharmacie de ROUEN, BP 97, 76800 Saint Etienne du Rouvray, FRANCE

INTRODUCTION

Free flow electrophoresis is a carrier free method used for cell and subcellular particle separations with different electrophoretic mobilities (1,2). The electrophoretic mobility is related to the electrokinetic potential (zeta potential) dependant on the cell vector medium and the cell surface properties under the effect of an applied electrical field. This method has been successfully used for the preparative separation of different cell populations from the rabbit kidney cortex: one from the proximal tubule and one from the distal part of the nephron (2-4). The procedure, leading to cell suspensions prepared for free flow electrophoresis separation, must avoid any proteolytic treatment (2).

In the present study, we report the preparative isolation of two cell populations from the proximal tubule of the rabbit kidney by coupling high voltage free flow electrophoresis and the use of an originally designed buffer system. The quality of the separation of different isolated cell populations was evaluated by using enzymatic markers with specific localizations along the proximal tubule. After the electrophoretic run, the cell integrity and the metabolic properties were determined.

MATERIALS AND METHODS

Preparation of the cell suspension. The method developed for cell preparation was derived from a combination of the techniques of Brendel and Meezan (5), Carlson et al. (6) and Heidrich and Dew (2). Cell preparation procedure was undertaken in 95% O_2 / 5% CO_2 Earle's balanced salt solution supplemented with (in mM) 60 sucrose, 26 $NaHCO_3$, 4 glutamine, 5 glucose, 5mg/l BSA, pH 7.4, final osmolality 330 mOsm (isolation medium). The pure proximal tubules were poured in isolation medium supplemented with sodium citrate (2.8 mM) as Ca-binding agent, for 10 min. This medium was oxygenated for 20 min before use. After this time period, the proximal tubules were washed with the isolation medium (free of citrate) and pressed on a 40 µm mesh nylon sieve. The suspension obtained (containing isolated cells and tubule pieces) was then passed through a 20 µm mesh nylon sieve. Protein content of the isolated cell suspension was measured according to Bradford (7).

Enzyme characterization. Enzyme activities were measured both on the cortical homogenates, the proximal tubule suspensions and on the proximal isolated cells. Some of them were also measured in each of the different fractions from the free flow electrophoretic run. Gamma-glutamyl transpeptidase, Na-K-ATPase, N-acetyl-beta-D-glucosaminidase and alkaline phosphatase activities were assayed as previously described (8-10). Lactate dehydrogenase and hexokinase activities were measured as described by Bergmeyer (11,12). True glucose-6-phosphatase (8) was assessed in cortical homogenates, proximal tubules, isolated cells (600 µl), and in each of the electrophoretic fractions (by trapping on a 0.45 μm filter, in duplicate) and washed free of the electrophoresis phosphate buffer.

Free flow electrophoresis chamber buffer. Homogeneity of the electric field with two different chamber buffers. Media to be used for preparative free-flow cell electrophoresis must be adjusted to fixed variables for three physical parameters, pH 7.2-7.4, conductivity 600-800 μS, and osmolality 290-330 mOsm. pH and electrical conductivity were measured in each fraction collected from the electrophoretic run, using two different chamber buffers i) a triethanolamine buffer (1) which contains (in mM) 270 sucrose, 11 triethanolamine, 11 acetic acid, 5 D-glucose, 5μM $CaCl_2$, 2.5 μM $MgCl_2$, 5 mg/l BSA; ii) a novel phosphate buffer containing (in mM) 210 sucrose, 100 glycine, 1 NaH_2PO_4, 4 Na_2HPO_4, 5 glucose and 5μM $CaCl_2$, 2.5 uM $MgCl_2$, 5mg/l BSA. Physical properties were the same for both media: pH 7.4, conductivity 650 μS, osmolality 330 mOsm. Operating conditions were 150 V/cm, 100 mA, 4°C buffer flow rate 2ml/fraction/hr.

Cell oxygen consumption with the two chamber buffers. Cell oxygen consumption mesurements were performed at 37°C by an oxypolarographic technique. After 10, 30 and 60 min in one of the two electrophoretic chamber buffers, described above, the cells were centrifuged and resuspended in 1.3 ml of an Hepes buffer containing (in mM) 0.87 $CaCl_2$, 2.68 KCl, 1.47 KH_2PO_4, 0.47 $MgCl_2$, 137 NaCl, 8 Na_2HPO_4, 20 HEPES, 5 glucose, 1 alanine and 4 lactate, prior to the respiration rate determination in the presence of 10 mM succinate as substrate. The cells were continuously oxygenated for 15 min before O_2 consumption measurement.

Free flow electrophoresis separation. After the cell preparation procedure, the cells were rinsed twice in electrophoresis phosphate chamber buffer, before the filtration on a thin glass wool layer and resuspended in oxygenated chamber buffer at a concentration of 0.5 mg protein/ml. The suspension was then injected into the free flow electrophoresis apparatus. The electrophoresis was carried out in a VAP 21 apparatus (Bender & Hobein - München, Germany). The run was performed at 4°C, 114 mA, 170 V/cm, buffer flow rate 2 ml/fraction/hr, sample injection 3.5 ml/hr. The fractions were used immediately for glucose-6-phosphatase determination and the excess was frozen at - 20°C.

Transmission electron microscopy. After the electrophoretic run, all the cell-containing fractions were pooled in order to determine the morphological state of the cells. This examination was also performed on the cell sample prior to the electrophoresis separation. Isolated cells were fixed in 2% glutaraldehyde in 120 mM cacodylate buffer. After a 1 hr fixation, cells were rinsed in cacodylate-sucrose buffer, postfixed with osmium tetroxide and embedded in epon. Sections were viewed with a CM 10 Philips microscope.

Cell oxygen consumption. All the cell-containing fractions were pooled after the electrophoresis run and centrifuged at 150 g for 5 min and then resuspended in the Hepes medium described below, prior to oxygen consumption measurement with 10 mM succinate substrate. Oxygen consumption was measured as described in the above section.

RESULTS

Enzyme characteristics. This first set of experiments investigated the nature of the cell-content of the preparation by measuring reliable marker enzymes. Enzymatic marker activities were assessed in each proximal cell preparation and compared with isolated proximal tubules and cortical homogenates. These data are presented by Toutain et al. in this volume. The conclusion of the enzymatic study is that isolated cells were highly purified proximal tubule cells.

Buffer Stability. The triethanolamine buffer presented an instability zone between the fractions 1 and 25. The pH appeared to be out of the physiological values between the fractions 9 and 18. This point can probably explain the difficulties encountered in the region of the injection port of the sample which is located at the vertical of fraction 15, when this buffer was used for the separation. In contrast, the phosphate chamber buffer presented a satisfactory stability in the migration zone between fractions 15 and 72 (Figure 1).

Effect of the incubation in the two chamber buffers on isolated cell oxygen consumption. Compared to the control levels, made in Hepes buffer, the triethanolamine buffer induced a decrease in cell respiration rate (Table 1) by 49% after 1 hr. In contrast, the phosphate chamber buffer only slightly reduced the oxygen consumption (ca. 7%) after a one hour incubation period. Indeed, all the electrophoresis separations were performed with the new designed phosphate chamber buffer.

Separation of isolated cells by free flow electrophoresis. The cell protein content was measured in each fraction after the electrophoretic run and enzyme marker activities were used to characterize the different cell populations separated by free flow electrophoresis. The cell sample was injected in the apparatus above the fraction 15 at the top of the electrophoretic chamber and the cells were migrated to the chamber anodic side.

The mean cell protein pattern of five separate experiments, is illustrated by Figure 2. The examination of this profile indicated that the main cell peak was found between the fraction 53 and 66 and represented 74% of the cells collected after the free flow electrophoresis separation (on the protein basis). A second

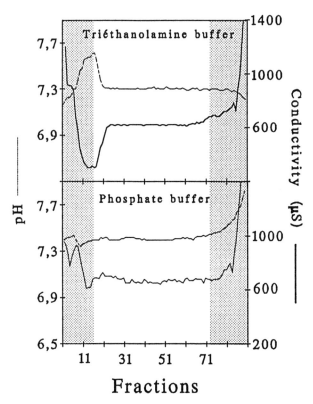

Figure 1. Electrical conductivity and pH stability in the migration chamber with two different electrophoresis chamber buffer systems: a triethanolamine buffer and a phosphate buffer. The light part between fractions 15 and 72 represents the migration zone.

shoulder peak came into view between the fraction 45 and 53 and represents 18% of the collected cells.

Glucose-6-phosphatase (G6Pase) is an enzyme of the gluconeogenesis metabolic pathway which is a marker of the cells from the convoluted part of the proximal tubule (13). The G6Pase profile is presented in the Figure 2. The highest G6Pase specific activities were located in the cell fractions with high electrophoretic mobilities corresponding to the main peak of cell proteins (53-64). Compared to the cell sample, the G6Pase specific activity was markedly enriched in the fractions 54-64 (1.9-fold increase in fraction 58) and decreased in the fractions 38-52. The amount of G6Pase activity of the fractions 45-53 only represents 12% of total cell activity.

Gamma-glutamyl transpeptidase (GGT) is a brush border marker enzyme which is mainly located in the cells from the straight proximal tubule (14). The examination of this enzyme pattern, illustrated in Figure 2, had shown that the highest specific activity of this enzyme was not found in the region of the main protein peak (53-66) but rather located in the cathodic protein peak (45-53). The GGT specific activity significantly rose in the fractions 43-52 compared with the cell sample activity and the fraction 49 presented a 2.9-fold increase. On the other hand, the GGT specific activity was reduced in the fractions 54-67.

Evaluation of morphological integrity and metabolic properties of cells after free flow electrophoresis. After the free flow electrophoresis separation all the cell-containing fractions were pooled in order to evaluate the cell integrity. Cells appeared to possess long microvilli on their surfaces (Figure 3). All the subcellular structures are well preserved. The cell integrity was not modified by the application of high field strength during the separation procedure. By another way, cell oxygen consumption appeared to be reduced by about 22% after the electrophoretic run.

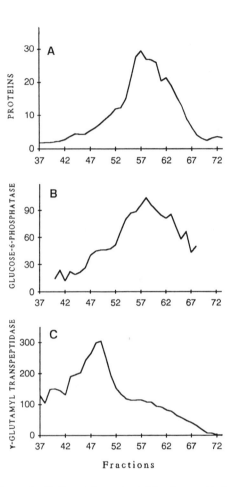

Figure 2. Cell protein content (A), glucose-6-phosphatase activity (B) and gamma glutamyl transpeptidase activity (C) in each fraction separated by free flow electrophoresis. Enzyme activities are given in UI/g prot. and proteins as µg/ml. Values are means of 5 independent experiments.

DISCUSSION

The most frequently used techniques to obtain isolated cell suspensions require enzyme treatment of tissues with collagenase alone or with a combination of proteolytic enzymes (15-17). This methodology allowed the preparation of a large amount of intact isolated cells from the kidney cortex of the rabbit. Such cell preparations were used for the isolation of cortical cell sub-populations by free flow electrophoresis. The results had shown that the

Table 1. Electrophoresis chamber media and oxygen consumption capacity.

	Oxygen consumption $(nmol\ O_2 \cdot min^{-1} \cdot mg\ protein^{-1})$		
Time (min)	10	30	60
Hepes buffer	28.86 ± 2.56	28.95 ± 5.19	30.50 ± 8.71
Phosphate buffer	25.34 ± 6.07	26.05 ± 8.44	28.46 ± 9.96
Triethanolamine buffer	17.10 ± 5.22	16.63 ± 6.03	15.60 ± 3.91

Incubation periods were carried out at 4°C in the different media and oxygen consumption was determined in Hepes buffer at 37°C with succinate 10 mM as substrate. Values are means ± standard deviation of 4 independent experiments.

proteolytic action induced alterations of the cell surface charge and prevented good separation experiments (2). Several authors had described cell isolation procedures that avoided any enzymatic treatment by using Ca-binding agents combinated with gentle mechanical forces (2,18). Vandewalle (4) presented a successful separation of two different cell populations (proximal and distal) from a cortical cell suspension, obtained after a Ca-binder action, by using free flow electrophoresis. In the present study, an original preparation of proximal tubular cells was obtained by associating the action of a Ca-binding ion on a pure suspension of proximal tubules (free of glomeruli), gentle mechanical dissociation and sifting on nylon meshes. This method originates from a combination of two modified techniques previously reported (2,6). The entire isolation procedure was carried out without any proteolytic treatment and led to a single-cell suspension that can be suitable for cell separation by free flow electrophoresis. It is now well established that Ca-free media, containing EDTA, can induce morphological injury and depressed cell respiration (19). It should be pointed out that a 10 min incubation in sodium citrate did not modify the cell morphological integrity.

After the isolated cell characterization (Toutain et al., this volume) we examined whether the separation of this proximal cell suspension

in different sub-populations could be obtained by means of high voltage free flow electrophoresis. Several studies performed on isolated cortical cells did not lead to the separation of different cell populations from the proximal tubule by means of free flow electrophoresis but only reported the isolation of proximal and distal cells (2-4). In order to solve this problem three main parameters were modified in our study: i) the cell sample consisted of pure proximal tubular cells with few other contaminating cell types ii) a new electrophoretic chamber medium was developed which had a better pH and conductivity stability under the applied electrical field (2,4) iii) this novel chamber medium which provides a constant electric field over the separation area allowed the use of a higher electric field strength that improved the separation of cells with only small difference in surface charge. The new phosphate chamber buffer also offers the advantage of preventing alterations in cell respiration.

This new experimental approach led to the isolation of two proximal cell populations that were characterized by biochemical markers. The cells in the slow-moving electrophoresic fractions (43-52) expressed both a higher GGT activity and a lower G6Pase activity compared to the injected cell sample. According to previously reported data, GGT activity is mainly located in the straight (S3) portion of the proximal tubule (14,20). In contrast, the cells of the

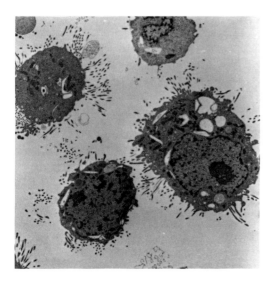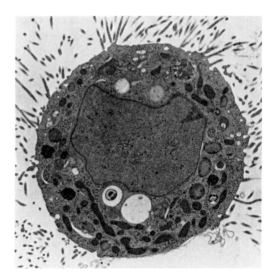

Figure 3. Electron micrographs of isolated proximal cell suspension before the electrophoresis (A, x 3900) and a typical isolated cell after the electrophoretic run (B, x 6610).

main peak (fractions 54-64) had a high G6Pase activity and a low GGT activity. Burch et al. (13) clearly established that the glucose-6-phosphatase activity is markedly higher in the early convoluted part of the proximal portion of the nephron (S1 segment). Our results show that, on the protein basis, the first cell population represents 18.5% of the total collected cells while the convoluted proximal cells comes to 73.8%. This finding supports the hypothesis previously expressed (Toutain et al., this volume) that the isolated cell preparation mainly consisted of proximal convoluted cells. The results of our study are consistent with those reported by Heidrich and Dew (2) and show that the cell integrity was well preserved after a short exposure to high field strength during the free flow electrophoresis run.

In conclusion, the present study describes a new simple method to isolate a pure suspension of proximal cells without enzymatic treatment. These metabolically active and morphologically intact cells retained their own cell surface charge properties and can be separated in two different sub-populations by means of high voltage free-flow electrophoresis. Such

study, which to our knowledge is the first to present a preparative method to separate intact and viable isolated cells from straight and convoluted part of the rabbit proximal tubule, allows physiological and biochemical experiments requiring cells of well-defined origin along the nephron. This methodology should allow the development of primary culture models from convoluted and straight portion of the proximal tubule of the rabbit kidney.

ACKNOWLEGMENTS

This work was supported by grants from Rhône-Poulenc Santé.

REFERENCES

1. Hannig K: Continuous free flow electrophoresis as an analytical and preparative method in biology. J Chromatogr 159:183-191, 1978.

2. Heidrich HG, Dew ME: Homogeneous cell populations from rabbit kidney cortex: Proximal, distal tubule and renin active cell isolated

by free flow electrophoresis. J Cell Biol 74:780-788, 1977.

3. Heidrich HG: Cell population from the renal proximal and distal tubule isolated by free flow electrophoresis: Cell function and differentiation. New York, AR Liss, 1982, pp 115-126.

4. Vandewalle A, Kopfer-Hobelsberger B, Heidrich HG: Cortical cell populations from rabbit kidney isolated by free flow electrophoresis: Characterisation by measurement of hormone-sensitive adenylate cyclase. J Cell Biol 92:505-513, 1982.

5. Brendel K, Meezan E: Isolation and properties of a pure preparation of proximal kidney tubules obtained without collagenase treatment. Fed Proc 34:803, 1975.

6. Carlson EC, Brendel K, Hjelle JT, Meezan E: Ultrastructural and biochemical analysis of isolated basement membranes from kidney glomeruli and tubules and brain and retinal microvessels. J Ultrastruct Res 62:26-53, 1978.

7. Bradford MM: A rapid and sensitive method for quantitation of microgram qualities of protein utilizing the principle of protein dye binding. Anal Biochem 72:248-254, 1976.

8. Hjelle JT, Morin JP, Trouet A: Analytical cell fractionation of isolated rabbit renal proximal tubules. Kidney Int 20:71-77, 1981.

9. Morin JP, Viotte G, Vandewalle A, Van Hoff F, Tulkens P, Fillastre JP: Gentamicin induced nephrotoxicity: a cell biology approach. Kidney Int 18: 583-590, 1980.

10. Toutain H, Olier B, Fillastre JP, Morin JP: Influence of muzolimine, a new diuretic on experimental gentamicin nephrotoxicity. Nephrol Dial Transplant 2:520-525, 1987.

11. Bergmeyer HU: Hexokinase assay. In: H.U. Bergmeyer (ed): Methods of enzymatic analysis. Verlag Chemie Academic Press 1974, pp 473-475.

12. Bergmeyer HU, Bernt E: Lactate dehydrogenase UV-assay with pyruvate and NADH. In: HU Bergmeyer (ed); Methods of enzymatic analysis. Verlag Chemie Academic Press, 1974, pp 574-579.

13. Burch HB, Narins RG, Chu C, Fagioli S, Choi S, McCarthy W, Lowry O: Distribution along the rat nephron of three enzymes of gluconeogenesis in acidosis and starvation. Am J Physiol 235:F246-F253, 1978.

14. Shimada H, Endou H, Sakai F: Distribution of gamma-glutamyl transpeptidase isoenzymes in the rabbit single nephron. Jpn J Pharmacol 32:121-129, 1982.

15. Rosenberg MR, Michalopoulos G: Kidney proximal tubular cells isolated by collagenase perfusion grow in defined media in the absence of growth factors. J Cell Physiol 131:107-114, 1987.

16. Taub M, Sato G: Growth of functional primary cultures of kidney epithelial cells in defined medium. J Cell Physiol 105:369-378, 1980.

17. Thimmappayya B, Reddy RR, Bhargava PM: Preparation of kidney cell suspension and respiration of kidney and liver cell suspensions. Exp Cell Res 63:333-340, 1970.

18. Poujeol P, Vandewalle A: Phosphate uptake by proximal cells isolated from rabbit kidney: Role of dexamethasone. Am J Physiol 249:F74-F83, 1985.

19. Baur H, Kasperek S, Pfaff E: Criteria of viability of isolated liver cells. Hoppe-Seyler's Z Physiol Chem 356:827-838, 1975.

20. Guder WG, Ross BD: Enzyme distribution along the nephron. Kidney Int 26:101-111, 1984.

71

BULK ISOLATION OF STRAIGHT AND CONVOLUTED PROXIMAL TUBULES FROM RABBIT KIDNEYS: DIFFERENTIAL GLUCOSE-DEPENDENT PROTECTION DURING ANOXIA

C.E. Ruegg and L.J. Mandel

Division of Physiology, Department of Cell Biology, Duke University Medical Center, Box 3709, Durham, North Carolina 27710, U.S.A.

INTRODUCTION

Earlier studies by Ruegg et al (1) and Wolfgang et al (2) have demonstrated that straight (PST) and convoluted (PCT) regions of the renal proximal tubule within positional renal slices could be selectively injured following in vitro exposure to a variety of chemicalagents or anoxia. These in vitro studies demonstrated that regioselective nephrotoxicity induced by several agents could result from innate cellular mechanisms within these nephron segments independent of blood flow delivery patterns or tubuloglomerular feedback mechanisms proposed from several in vivo studies. However, the investigation of innate cellular mechanisms responsible for selective PCT or PST injury were difficult to study in slices since all biochemical and physiological measurements represent the average response of the entire slice, while selective injury occurs only in specific nephron segments. Hence, in the present study we describe and characterize a method to independently isolate PCT and PST, in milligram quantities, such that the mechanisms underlying selective injury within each segment could be studied.

In vitro exposure of PCT and PST to anoxia will be investigated in this paper since it was previously shown in slices that anoxia induces selective injury to the PCT (1). The underlying mechanisms responsible for selective PCT injury and PST protection during anoxia however

remains unclear. Since Ross and Guder (3) have shown that the activities of most glycolytic enzymes associated with the metabolism of glucose to pyruvate are higher in PST relative to PCT, we will also investigate glucose-dependent metabolic differences during anoxia as a possible mechanism of PST protection.

METHODS

PCT and PST Isolation: Suspensions of PCT and PST were prepared from female New Zealand White rabbit kidneys following in situ retrograde perfusion with ice cold Dulbecco's Modified Eagle's/ Ham's Nutrient Mix F-12 (DME/F12) medium containing 15 mM HEPES, 15 mM NaHCO$_3$ and 2 mM heptanoate. Following decapsulation, the outer cortical cortices from both kidneys, used to isolate PCT, were removed with a Stadie-Riggs microtome. The remaining kidney tissue was sliced perpendicular to its polar axis into 2 mm slabs. Each slab was trans-illuminated on a light table and the outer stripe of the medulla, used to isolate PST, was dissected from the surrounding tissue. Each fraction was then minced and separately digested for 50 min at 37°C in 15 ml of DME/F12 medium supplemented with: collagenase (125 U/ml), hyaluronidase (300 U/ml), bovine serum albumin (1 mg/ml) and deoxyribonuclease (0.1 mg/ml). Tubules were collected from the supernatant fraction every 15 min during digestion to maximize tissue viability and yield. Following digestion, the PCT and PST were isolated from other nephron segments on separate discontinuous (40-90%) isotonic Percoll gradients. Proximal tubular bands were then collected from each gradient (at or below the 55% Percoll step) and washed 3 times before resuspending in DME/F12 medium. Following isolation, each tissue band collected from the discontinuous Percoll gradient was characterized by measuring the proximal tubular enzyme marker leucine aminopeptidase, the distal tubular marker hexokinase, and protein recoveries by standard methods (4,5).

Differential Effects of Anoxia: PCT and PST suspensions (1 mg/ml) in DME/F12 medium were preincubated for 1 hr at $37^\circ C$ under an Air/CO_2 atmosphere. Following preincubation, each suspension was divided in half and exposed for an additional 40 min to either anoxic (95% N_2/5% CO_2) or control (Air/CO_2) conditions. All fractions were then allowed to recover in Air/CO_2 for 1 hr. Samples for analysis were collected from all groups at the end of each experimental phase.

Glucose-Dependent Protection during Anoxia: To investigate if the PCT and PST differences observed following anoxia (see results) were dependent on anaerobic utilization of glucose, proximal tubular fractions were preincubated as described above before each flask was split, centrifuged (144 x g), washed twice and resuspended in an equal volume of nutrient buffer with or without glucose. The buffer composition was (in mM): NaCl, 103; NaHCO$_3$, 20; HEPES, 10; NaH$_2$PO$_4$, 2; KCl, 5; MgSO$_4$, 1; CaCl$_2$, 1; malate, 5; glutamate, 5; lactate, 4; valerate, 1; alanine, 1; glucose, 0 or 5; and dextran (0.6%). Each flask was then made anoxic by gassing with 95% N_2/5% CO_2 for 30 min. Following anoxia, each fraction was washed back into DME/F12 medium for a 60 min recovery period. Samples for analysis were taken at the end of each experimental phase.

Analytical Procedures: Oxygen consumption (QO_2) was measured polarographically in a 0.3 ml custom-made glass chamber maintained at $37^\circ C$ and fitted with a Clark-style electrode calibrated with dithionite and 21% oxygen (room air). ATP was measured by HPLC from perchloric acid extracts according to the method of Hull-Ryde et al (6). Intracellular potassium content was measured by atomic absorption after tubules were spun through a mixture (1:2) of dioctylphthalate:n-butylphthalate and extracted into 8% perchloric acid. Lactate dehydrogenase (LDH) activity was measured according to the method of Bergmeyer (7) and reported as a "percent release". Protein was used to normalize all the data and was measured according to Bradford (4). Statistical differences ($p<0.05$) were analyzed by analysis of variance (ANOVA) followed by Fisher's least significant difference test to determine which groups were statistically different.

RESULTS

Characterization of Proximal Tubular Isolation Methods The hexokinase, leucine aminopeptidase and protein distributions along the bands of the discontinuous Percoll gradient are shown in Table 1. Since hexokinase activities are very low in proximal tubules relative to other nephron segments (3,8), it appears that the tubular segments banding at and below the 55% Percoll gradient step (i.e. below a density of 1.066) are enriched in proximal tubules. The hexokinase activity measured in these proximal tubular bands is quantitatively very close to the activities measured in microdissected proximal tubules (4-6 Units/gm protein; (8)) demonstrating the enzymatic purity of these proximal tubular bands.

The enrichment of leucine aminopeptidase, an enzyme found only in the proximal tubular brush border membrane (3), also demonstrates that the proximal tubules band at and below the 55% Percoll gradient step. A 23% enzymatic enrichment factor (90/FT) can be calculated for the proximal tubular bands isolated from the cortical cortices which closely approximates that expected for this kidney region which contains 80 to 90% PCT. Likewise, an enzymatic enrichment factor of 62% can be calculated for the outer stripe preparation which approximates to the expected value for this region which contains about 40% PST (9). The presence of leucine aminopeptidase activity in the 40, 45 and 50% Percoll bands demonstrates that although these bands contain mainly distal tubular fragments (high hexokinase activity) they are also contaminated by more buoyant proximal tubular fragments damaged during digestion. The enzymatic purity of these proximal tubular bands was again demonstrated since leucine aminopeptidase activities were similar to those measured in microdissected tubules (3).

The tissue yield of PCT (pooled 55 and 90% Percoll bands) isolated from the cortical cortices represents 72% of the total protein layered on top of the gradient (fraction total (FT)). Since in vivo the cortical cortices contain 80 to 90% PCT before isolation, this 72% value represents an isolation efficiency between 80 and 90%. The remaining PCT are distributed among the upper Percoll gradient bands (see leucine aminopeptidase data) or lost during collagenase digestion. Similarly, the protein yield of PST isolated from the outer stripe represents 27% of the total protein for an isolation efficiency of only

Table 1: Percoll Density Gradient Distribution of Proximal and Distal Tubular Marker Enzymes and Protein Recoveries.

	Tubular Density limits	Hexokinase* (distal)	LAP# (Proximal)	Recovery mg protein
Cortex Cortices (for PCT isolation)				
FT		13.1 ± 0.9	251 ± 12	53.1 ± 6.0
40%	- 1.053	$22.0 \pm 2.8E$	$111 \pm 8D$	---
45%	1.054 - 1.059	$21.2 \pm 2.5E$	$209 \pm 22D$	---
50%	1.060 - 1.065	13.5 ± 1.4	270 ± 10	---
55%	1.066 - 1.070	$4.2 \pm 0.6D$	$289 \pm 10E$	6.3 ± 1.0
90%	1.071 - 1.123	$2.8 \pm 0.4D$	$308 \pm 19E$	30.9 ± 4.1
Outer Stripe (for PST isolation)				
FT		19.3 ± 2.6	184 ± 5	57.7 ± 5.5
40%	- 1.053	24.8 ± 2.3	$124 \pm 9D$	---
45%	1.054 - 1.059	23.2 ± 2.5	160 ± 11	---
50%	1.060 - 1.065	$12.5 \pm 1.1D$	$213 \pm 11E$	---
55%	1.066 - 1.070	$5.1 \pm 0.8D$	$287 \pm 24E$	6.0 ± 0.5
90%	1.071 - 1.123	$4.1 \pm 0.5D$	$298 \pm 6E$	8.5 ± 0.8

Each value represents the mean $\pm$ SE from at least 6 experiments.
* units/gm prot. where 1 unit phosphorylates 1 umol glucose/min (25°C).
# Leucine aminopeptidase (LAP) reported as nmol beta-Napthylamine released from L-Leucyl-beta-Napthylamide/min/mg protein at 37°C.
FT = Total fraction before Percoll separation.
E or D = Activity is enriched (E) or de-enriched (D) from FT (p<0.05)

68%, since this region of the kidney contains approximately 40% PST before isolation. Light microscopic examination confirmed these enzymatic data showing that the proximal tubular bands of both groups were 98% pure.

Differential Effects of Anoxia in PCT and PST (Table 2). Following 40 min of anoxia and 60 min of recovery, the basal QO_2 (nmol O_2/min/mg protein) of PCT dropped 70% from 39.5±3.7 to 11.9±1.3. In contrast, the QO_2 of PST declined by only 50% from 49.2±4.6 to 24.8±2.8, indicating that the PCT was more susceptible to anoxic injury than PST. Similarly, after 40 min of anoxia, the ATP content (nmol/mg protein) of PCT decreased 90% from 10.03±1.7 to 1.06±0.10 while the ATP content of PST decreased only 78% from 11.5±1.3 to 2.53±0.46. Although these ATP contents were significantly reduced from controls, the PST maintained an ATP content 2.4 times higher than PCT (p<0.05) following 40 min of anoxia. After 60 min of recovery from anoxia, the PST

recovered 53% of their original ATP content, while the ATP content of PCT did not change significantly during recovery. The cytosolic enzyme lactate dehydrogenase (LDH), released from PCT and PST following anoxic exposure, was used as an indicator of irreversible plasma membrane damage. During anoxia, a 60±7% LDH release was observed from the PCT group, while only a 40±7% LDH release came from the PST group exposed to the same conditions. During recovery from anoxia, no additional LDH release was observed from either group. These results correlate with the changes in QO_2 and ATP described above and demonstrate that the cellular injury occurs during the anoxic phase of these experiments rather than during reoxygenation. In contrast to the changes observed in QO_2, ATP and LDH, the intracellular potassium content of both PCT and PST decreased by more than 70% following anoxia with no differential responses being observed during anoxia or following recovery. This apparent lack of differential response may

Table 2: Differential Effects of Anoxia on PCT and PST.

		Oxygen consumption (nmol O_2/min/mg)	ATP (nmol/mg)	LDH (% release)	Potassium (nmol/mg)
Control	PCT	39.5±3.7	10.30±1.70	12.6±1.6	334±37
	PST	49.2±4.6	11.50±1.30	8.9±1.1	314±33
40' Anoxia	PCT	---	1.06±0.10[ab]	60.3±7.5[ab]	79±22[a]
	PST	---	2.53±0.46[a]	40.4±7.0[a]	114±32[a]
40' Anoxia &	PCT	11.9±1.3[ab]	2.26±0.45[ab]	66.0±5.9[ab]	197±51[ac]
60' Recovery	PST	24.8±2.8[a]	5.60±0.83[ac]	46.7±7.5[a]	217±40[ac]

Each value represents the mean ± SE from at least 5 experiments.
[a] = Different from paired control (p<0.05).
[b] = PCT different from PST under same condition (p<0.05).
[c] = Changed significantly during recovery when to anoxia (p<0.05).

be a function of the phthalate step (used to separate tubules from the medium) which selects for intact (more viable) tubules, thereby blunting the measurement of differential responses.

PCT and PST Dependence on Anaerobic Glucose Utilization. Since most of the measurements made above showed that PST were more resistant to anoxic exposure than PCT, the anaerobic mechanisms associated with this relative protection were investigated by examining changes in oxygen consumption and LDH release (Table 3). Following 30 min of anoxia in glucose-containing buffer, and recovery in DME/F12 medium, the basal oxygen consumption (QO_2) (nmol O_2/min/mg protein) of PCT decreased 70% from 31.0 ± 2.8 to 9.2 ± 1.5 while the QO_2 of PST remained unchanged from controls. This differential response between PCT and PST was dependent on the presence of exogenously added glucose during anoxia since removing this substrate from the buffers during anoxia abolished the enhanced respiration of PST bringing it to the PCT level of respiration. In contrast to these changes in QO_2, significant release of lactate dehydrogenase (LDH) was observed mainly in the PCT groups ($\pm$ glucose). Although the QO_2 of PST incubated in glucose-free buffer was significantly reduced compared to PST incubated in glucose-containing buffer, the release of LDH from these groups were not significantly different. Since LDH release only occurs when the plasma membrane is ruptured, these results indicate that PST exposed to 30 min of anoxia in glucose-free buffer exibited minimal plasma membrane damage despite the significant inhibition in QO_2. In contrast, when PST were exposed to 30 min of anoxia in glucose-containing buffer, they were able to totally recover their QO_2 functions and showed no plasma membrane damage as measured by LDH release.

Table 3: Glucose-Dependent Effects on Oxygen Consumption and LDH Release.

Glucose		Oxygen Consumption (nmol O_2/min/mg protein)		Lactate dehydrogenase (% Release)	
		+	-	+	-
Control	PCT	31.0 ± 2.8	28.4 ± 2.0	12.1 ± 3.6	12.0 ± 4.3
	PST	31.4 ± 4.3	33.2 ± 3.2	10.6 ± 1.9	8.8 ± 1.3
30' Anoxia*					
	PCT	9.2 ± 1.5^a	11.8 ± 1.9^a	41.2 ± 5.5^a	53.5 ± 4.0^{ac}
	PST	27.0 ± 3.6^{bc}	15.0 ± 2.8^a	18.0 ± 3.9^b	22.0 ± 2.6^{ab}

Each value represents the mean $\pm$ SE from 5 experiments.

* = Anoxia QO_2 values were measured after 60 min Air/CO_2 recovery in DME/F12 medium. Lactate dehydrogenase values were measured after 30 were measured after 30 min of anoxia and were unchanged during recovery.

a = Different from paired control (p<0.05).

b = PST different from PCT under same condition (p<0.05).

c = $\pm$ glucose pairs are different (p<0.05).

DISCUSSION

The bulk isolation procedure described here provides a means of separately isolating PCT from the cortical cortices (a region devoid of PST) and PST from the outer stripe of the medulla (a region devoid of PCT) (9) in milligram quantities. These segments were highly enriched (98%) following discontinuous Percoll separation as shown by the proportional enrichment of leucine aminopeptidase and de-enrichment of hexokinase activities (Table 1) which were quantitatively very close to the activities measured in microdissected proximal tubules (3,8). Since the PCT and PST represent the two major anatomical divisions of the proximal nephron which can be selectively injured following exposure to a wide variety of chemical agents and anoxia (1,2,10), we investigated the differential responses between PCT and PST following in vitro anoxia.

The higher ATP content and lower LDH release from PST during anoxia (and recovery) as well as the higher rate of QO$_2$ in PST following recovery from anoxia, all demonstrate that PCT are more susceptible to anoxia than PST (Table 2). Furthermore, during anoxia the ATP content of PST was maintained 2.4 times higher than PCT, suggesting that the mechanism of PST protection may be related to the higher glycolytic capacity of PST relative to PCT (3). Since the differential PST protection observed during anoxia could be blocked by removing glucose from the suspension buffer during anoxia (Table 3), we conclude that the glucose-dependent protection of PST during anoxia is due to its increased glycolytic capacity relative to PCT.

Although PST injury is most often observed following ischemia in vivo, this site of injury is probably a function of the no-reflow phenomenon described by Glaumann and Trump (11) as opposed to an innate cellular susceptibility of PST segments which are protected following "ischemia" in vitro (1). Since anoxia acts by inhibiting mitochondrial oxidative phosphorylation, other nephrotoxic agents that inhibit electron transport should also express a glucose-dependent PST protection relative to PCT

segments, given equal access of the toxicant within PCT and PST segments.

Using this bulk preparation, mechanistic differences between nephrotoxicant transport and biotransformation can now be investigated directly in the target cell types to delineate the events responsible for regioselective nephrotoxicity within proximal tubular segments.

Complete description and discussion of these results are presented in two articles in the American Journal of Physiology 259:F164-F175 and F176-F185, 1990.

REFERENCES

1. Ruegg CE, Gandolfi AJ, Nagle RB, Brendel K: Differential patterns of injury to the proximal tubule of renal cortical slices following in vitro exposure to mercuric chloride, potassium dichromate, or hypoxic conditions. Toxicol Appl Pharmacol 90: 261-273, 1987.

2. Wolfgang GHI, Gandolfi AJ, Krumdieck CL, Brendel K: Evaluation of organic nephrotoxins using rabbit renal cortical slices. Toxicol In Vitro 3:341-350, 1989.

3. Ross BD, Guder WG: Heterogeneity and compartmentation in the kidney. In: Sies H (ed); Metabolic Compartmentation. New York, Academic, 1982, p. 363-409.

4. Bradford MM; A rapid and sensitive method for the quantification of microgram quantities of protein utilizing the principle of protein-dye binding. Anal Biochem 72: 248-254, 1976.

5. Brannan TS, Corder CN, Rizk M: Histochemical measurement of rat kidney hexokinase (38616). Proc Soc Expt Biol Med 148: 714-719, 1975.

6. Hull-Ryde EA, Cummings RG, Lowe JE: Improved method for high energy nucleotide analysis of canine cardiac muscle using reverse phase high performance liquid chromatography. J Chromatogr 275: 411-417, 1983.

7. Bergmeyer HU, Bernt E, Hess B: Lactic dehydrogenase. In: Bergmeyer HU (ed); Meth-

ods of Enzymatic Analysis. New York, Academic, 1963, p. 736-740.

8. Vandewalle A, Wirthensohn G, Heidrich HG, Guder WG: Distribution of hexokinase and phosphoenolpyruvate carboxykinase along the rabbit nephron. Am J Physiol 240: F492-F500, 1981.

9. Kaissling B, Kriz W: Structural analysis of the rabbit kidney. Adv Anat Embryol Cell Biol 56: 1-123, 1979.

10. Weinberg JM: Issues in the pathophysiology of nephrotoxic renal tubular cell injury pertinent to understanding cyclosporine nephrotoxicity. Transplant Proc 17 Suppl 1:81-90, 1985.

11. Glaumann B, Trump BF: Studies on the pathogenesis of ischemic cell injury: III. Morphological changes in the proximal pars recta tubules (P3) of the rat kidney made ischemic in vivo. Virchows Arch B 19: 303-323, 1975.

72

METABOLIC STUDIES ON ISOLATED RAT GLOMERULI: A VALUABLE TOOL TO INVESTIGATE GLOMERULAR DAMAGE

S. Kastner (1), M.F. Wilks (2), M. Soose (1), P.H. Bach (2), H. Stolte (1)

Division of Nephrology, Hannover Medical School, Konstanty-Gutschow Str. 8, 3000 Hannover 61, Germany (1) and Nephrotoxicity Research Group, Robens Institute, University of Surrey, Guildford GU2 5XH, UK (2)

INTRODUCTION

Metabolic changes in glomeruli have been suggested to contribute to the decline of kidney function in renal disease (1). Thus, the assessment of glomerular metabolism may help to further elucidate the causes and pathogenesis of renal lesions. There is, however, little information on metabolic differences in superficial (cortical) versus juxtamedullary glomeruli. Such differences might be crucial to the development of target-specific nephrotoxicity, since it has recently been suggested that the nephrotic syndrome caused by administration of the anti-cancer drug adriamycin (ADR) to experimental animals is due to selective damage of the juxtamedullary glomerular population by ADR-semiquinone radicals (2).

Highly purified glomeruli can be isolated by the sieving method (3) to give intact cellular structures able to carry out metabolic processes, involving the incorporation of tritiated amino acids in macromolecules and the oxidation of radiolabeled substrates such as carbohydrates and fatty acids to CO_2 (1,4).

The aim of the present study was firstly to compare the metabolic properties of freshly isolated cortical and juxtamedullary glomeruli and secondly to study if an ADR-pretreatment of rats (causing a model nephrotic syndrome) is related to metabolic changes in the two glomerular populations. Macromolecular synthesis and glucose oxidation were chosen as parameters of glomerular metabolic activity.

Animals

Female W/A rats (University of Surrey strain), 75-119 days, 182 ± 13 g, were housed in groups of 5 in plastic cages in a controlled environment ($20\text{-}22^{o}C$, 40-60% humidity) with a 12 hour light/dark cycle and received food and tap water ad libitum. For the adriamycin experiments, the rats were injected via the tail vein with a single dose of 5 mg/kg of ADR (Farmitalia, Carlo Erba Ltd, UK).

Preparation of glomeruli

Control and ADR-treated rats were sacrificed by cervical dislocation on day 7 after treatment. At this time-point micropuncture studies had shown no changes in proteinuria of superficial glomeruli, but overall protein excretion was significantly elevated compared to controls (2). The kidneys were removed and decapsulated. After bisectioning, the outer cortex (with cortical glomeruli) and the cortico-medullary junction (with juxtamedullary glomeruli) were separated from the rest of the kidney.

The procedure for glomerular isolation was essentially the same as described by Misra (3). The tissue was minced in small fragments and suspended in HEPES-buffered Earle's balanced salt solution (EBSS). The glomeruli were isolated by forcing the chopped tissue through a number of stainless steel sieves (Endecotts LTD, London, UK): from a 250 μm sieve which disrupted the tissue, through a 150 μm sieve which trapped tubular fragments, down to a 75 μm sieve which retained glomeruli. After washing twice, the final preparation was approximately 95% pure as assessed by phase contrast microscopy.

Assessment of glomerular metabolism

The isolated glomeruli were suspended in EBSS, and 1 ml aliquots of the glomerular suspensions were incubated with 2.5 µCi L-5-^{3}H proline (30 Ci/mmol; Amersham International, UK) or 0.5 µCi D-U-^{14}C glucose (56 mCi/mmol; Amersham International, UK) at 37°C in a shaking water bath. At appropriate time points the incubations were terminated.

^{3}H proline incorporation was quantified by precipitation of the total protein with ice-cold 6% (w/v) TCA and subsequent washing and filtration onto glass fibre discs followed by drying with absolute alcohol. After removal of residual TCA with diethyl ether, the precipitate was dissolved in 0.5 M NaOH and after addition of 4 ml scintillant (OptiPhase Safe, LKB) counted in a LKB 1219 beta scintillation counter.

Oxidative metabolism was measured by trapping $^{14}CO_2$ with NaOH-soaked filter strips in capped Erlenmeyer flasks. The incubation periods were stopped at appropriate time points with 1 ml 0.2 M HCl, the filter strips were transferred into scintillation vials and were quantified as described above (for details of the method see (5)).

Glomerular protein concentrations were determined by the Coomassie Blue Dye Binding Method (6) using bovine serum albumin as a standard.

Statistics

The results are expressed as picomoles substrate incorporated or oxidized per mg glomerular protein. All data are given as mean and standard deviation. Statistical significance was calculated using the two sided Student's t-test for independent measurements with a level of significance $p < 0.05$.

RESULTS

Both proline incorporation and glucose oxidation in isolated glomeruli were constant at glomerular protein concentrations ranging from 23-268 µg/ml (Fig. 2). The glomerular protein concentration in the final suspension was 257 ± 62 µg/ml for cortical glomeruli and 103 ± 36 µg/ml for juxtamedullary glomeruli.

As shown in figure 3, the glomeruli maintained their metabolical activity for an incubation period of 4 to 5 hours for both groups (control glomeruli and those isolated from the kidneys of ADR-pretreated rats). Cortical and juxtamedullary glomeruli showed distinctly different metabolic activities. In control experiments proline incorporation in cortical glomeruli was twice that of juxtamedullary glomeruli ($p < 0.001$). However, the glucose oxidation rate of cortical glomeruli was about 25% less than that of the juxtamedullary population (not significant at 4 hour time-point).

Glomerular metabolism was markedly influenced by in vivo administration of ADR. Proline incorporation was significantly increased in both glomerular populations, but more pronounced in juxtamedullary glomeruli. Glucose oxidation was significantly elevated in juxtamedullary glomeruli, whereas in cortical glomeruli no changes could be observed after ADR-treatment (Fig. 3).

DISCUSSION

The cellular material in isolated glomerular preparations varies according to the number of animals and the dilution of the final suspension. Since there is no guarantee for uniformity of preparations, it was important to establish a possible dependence of the rate of glomerular metabolism on the glomerular protein concentration. In our system, both proline incorporation and glucose oxidation were independent of the amount of glomerular material in the final suspension at protein concentrations ranging from 23-260 µg/ml.

The anatomical heterogeneity of cortical and juxtamedullary glomeruli was reflected in a heterogeneity of glomerular metabolism. While proline incorporation was higher in cortical compared to juxtamedullary glomeruli, glucose oxidation was lower. The reason for these dif-

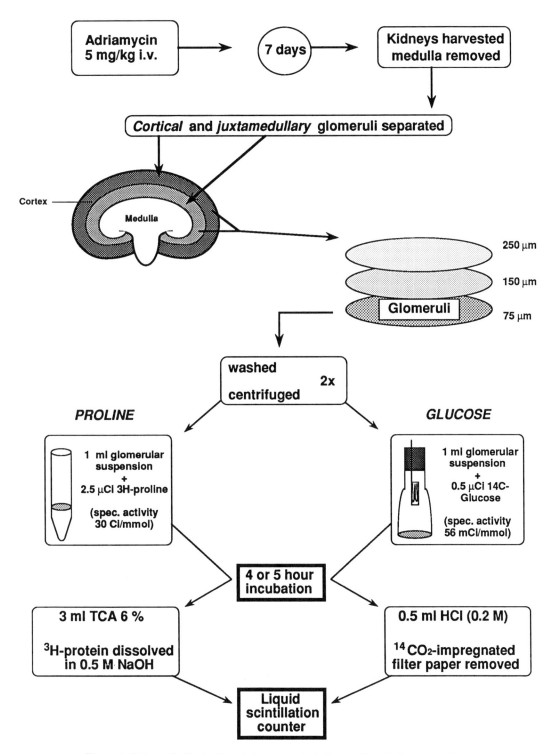

Figure 1. Schematic illustration of glomerular isolation and incubation procedure.

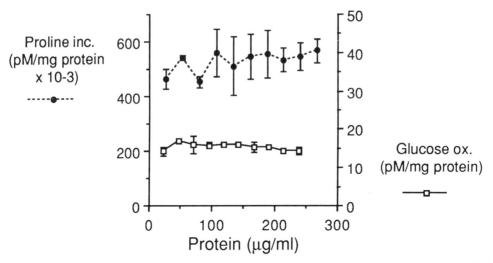

Figure 2. Proline incorporation and glucose oxidation at different glomerular protein concentrations in the final suspension (incubation time 4 hr).

ferences is not readily apparent, but may have implications on the susceptibility of the two glomerular preparations to toxins. It should be noted that there are strain differences in the metabolic heterogeneity, since glomeruli isolated from MWF-rats, a strain with a high number of superficial glomeruli, showed no difference in the rate of proline incorporation between cortical and juxtamedullary glomeruli (7).

Following ADR-treatment, proline incorporation and glucose oxidation were stimulated; the implications of such a different response of cortical and juxtamedullary glomeruli to ADR are discussed elsewhere (7). The increased proline incorporation could be due to an enhanced activity of macromolecular synthesis of glomerular cells. This would be in accordance with morphologi cal changes, described by Bertani et al (8). An important morphological alteration induced by ADR is the thickening of the glomerular basement membrane, occurring from the epithelial side (9). This could be caused by the enhanced macromolecular syn-

thesis of epithelial cells. A possible explanation for the enhanced glucose oxidation rate is an elevated   activity of glucose-6-phosphatase and the tricarboxylic acid cycle enzymes (10).

It is proposed that the pathophysiological changes described here are one step in the cascade of ADR-nephrotoxicity, eventually leading to an altered protein permeability of the (juxtamedullary) glomerular filtration barrier (Fig. 4). As far as the applied model is concerned, it could be shown that isolated glomeruli from control animals as well as from ADR-treated animals retain their viability over an incubation period of up to 5 hours by maintaining their metabolic activities in vitro and also reflect drug-induced metabolic alterations in the glomerulus. The data shows that metabolic studies with isolated glomeruli are a valuable tool for studying and quantifying the effects of nephrotoxins on the kidney glomerulus and help identify the mechanistic basis for such effects.

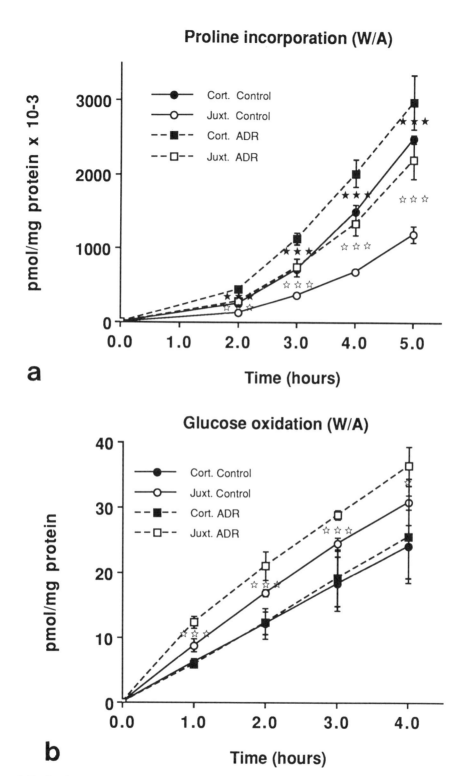

Figure 3. Proline incorporation (a) and glucose oxidation (b) [pmol/mg protein] as a function of incubation time. Cortical control vs. cortical ADR (closed symbols, *** p<0.001), juxtamedullary control vs. juxtamedullary ADR (open symbols, * p<0.05, *** p<0.001).

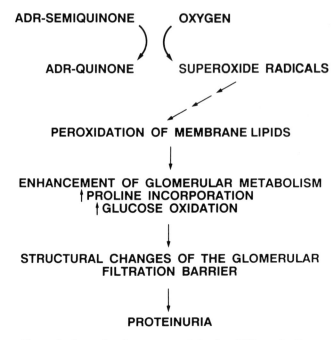

Figure 4. Cascade of processes following ADR-application.

ACKNOWLEDGEMENTS

The authors wish to thank Drs Neill J Gregg and Enoch N Kwizera for their valuable help throughout the experiments. This research was supported by the European Commission's Biotechnology Action Programme, and, in part, by the Dr Hadwen Trust for Humane Research and the Humane Research Trust. MFW was a recipient of a postdoctoral fellowship by Deutsche Forschungsgemeinschaft.

REFERENCES

1. Brendel K, Meezan E: Properties of a pure metabolically active glomerular preparation from rat kidney. II. Metabolism. J Pharmacol Exp Ther 187: 342-351, 1973

2. Soose M, Haberstroh U, Rovira-Halbach G, Stolte H: Heterogeneity of glomerular barrier function in early adriamycin nephrosis of MWF rats. Clin Physiol Biochem 6: 310-315, 1988

3. Misra RP: Isolation of glomeruli from mamalian kidneys by graded sieving. AJCP 58: 135-139, 1972

4. Hjelle JT, Carlson EC, Brendel K, Meezan E: Biosynthesis of basement membrane matrix by isolated renal rat glomeruli. Kidney Int 15: 20-32, 1979

5. Wilks MF, Kwizera EN, Bach PH: Assessment of heavy metal nephrotoxicity in vitro using isolated glomeruli and proximal tubular fragments. Renal Physiol Biochem 13:275-284, 1990

6. Bradford MM: A rapid and sensitive method for the quantitation of microgramm quantities of protein, utilizing the principle of protein-dye binding. Anal Biochem 72: 248-254, 1976

7. Kastner S, Wilks MF, Gwinner W, Soose M, Bach PH, Stolte H: Metabolic heterogeneity of isolated cortical and juxtamedullary glomeruli in adriamycin nephrotoxicity. Renal Physiol Biochem, in press.

8. Bertani T, Poggi A, Pozzoni R, Delaini F, Sacchi G, Thoua Y, Mecca G, Remuzzi G, Donati MB: Adriamycin induced nephrotic syndrome in rats. Sequence of pathological events. Lab Invest 46: 16-23, 1982

9. Kurtz SM, Feldman JD: Experimental studies on the formation of the glomerular basement membrane. J Ultrastruc Res 6: 19-27, 1962

10. Dubach UC, Recant I: Enzymatic activity of the isolated glomerulus in normal and nephrotic rats. J Clin Invest 39: 1364-1371, 1960.

73

PROBLEMS WITH THE USE OF FURA IN FRESHLY ISOLATED RAT PROXIMAL TUBULES

C.E.M. Jones

Department of Pharmaceutical Sciences, Aston University, Birmingham, UK.

INTRODUCTION

It is widely acknowledged that ionized calcium plays a key role in various physiological processes (1,2) and different methods have been used to study cytosolic Ca^{2+} in renal tissues (3,4). In recent years, however, perhaps the most prevalent method has involved the use of the fluorescent calcium indicators e.g. Quin and Fura. These indicators seem to have been used mainly in cultured renal cell systems (5) rather than in freshly isolated whole tubule systems.

Previous work in this laboratory has examined and characterised variously isolated rat proximal tubule (PT) samples. The evidence suggested that PT samples isolated mechanically were superior in both structural and functional integrity to PTs isolated by collagenase perfusion techniques.

As a result of this work, it was decided to attempt to utilise whole PTs (isolated by both mechanical and enzymatic means) in cytosolic calcium studies. The aim was to see whether it was possible to develop a successful system, involving Fura, for measuring cytosolic Ca^{2+} in whole PTs and whether results obtained with this system differed from those obtained with cultured renal cells.

METHODS

Tubule Isolation

PTs were prepared by either a) Mechanical Separation or b) Perfused Enzyme Separation.

In both cases two 250-300g Fischer rats were anaesthetised, dissected for renal perfusion and renal blood was washed out by a heparinised normal saline flush. The renal cortex was then subjected to one of the two methods;

a. Mechanical Separation.

Renal perfusion with a 0.5% Fe_3O_4 suspension was followed by removal and mincing of the cortex region for homogenisation with 2-3 strokes of a loose, round pestle.

b. Perfused Enzyme Separation.

A 0.05% solution of collagenase was perfused at 37°C for ~3 mins and then removed by a normal saline flush. This was followed by a perfusion of 0.05% Fe_3O_4 with subsequent removal and mincing of the blackened cortex.

After either treatment, the PTs were released from their respective cortex sample by disrupting the tissue with graded mesh. The Fe_3O_4 loaded glomeruli were removed with a magnet and the PTs were separated out from the tubule "soup" by sieving on a 64µm nylon mesh.

Fura Measurements

PT samples from each of the two isolation methods were suspended in an incubation media containing KHS, 5mM HEPES (pH 7.4), 3% dextran and 10mM pyruvate. Aliquots of each suspension (containing approximately 2mg protein per incubation) were incubated with 500nM Fura in DMSO for 15 mins at 25°c. The PTs were washed free of the Fura and resuspended in 2 ml of fresh incubation medium. The PT samples were monitored at 25°c in a Perkin Elmer fluorimeter at 510nm emission with continuous excitation at 340nm. Calibration was performed by the standard method of Triton and EGTA (5).

RESULTS

Heavy Metal Quenching

Potential quenching of the Fura signal by the iron oxide used in the isolation procedure was examined with the use of the lipid soluble chelator N,N,N'N-tetrabis(2-pyridylmethyl)ethylenediamine (TPEN) (7). On addition of 20μm (final concentration) TPEN to Fura loaded, mechanically isolated PT samples, no alteration in the Fura signal was seen. Even when the concentration of TPEN was increased to 60μm no rise in the Fura signal was seen. This would appear to indicate that the iron oxide had virtually no residual quenching effect on the Fura signal.

Basal Calcium Levels and Fura Leakage

The calculation of basal calcium levels and Fura leakage were made according to the methodology of Smith et al (5). The results are summarised in Table 1.

Effect of Ionomycin on Basal Calcium.

The ionophore Ionomycin was added to Fura loaded PTs isolated by both the mechanical and perfused enzyme techniques to see whether they could elicit a rise in basal calcium levels. The traces obtained are shown in Figures 1 and 2. Ionomycin elicited a significant rise in collagenase isolated PTs only.

DISCUSSION

Maintenance of cellular polarity and intercellular connections are believed by many researchers to be vital to cellular regulation. One of the drawbacks of studying cytosolic Ca^{2+} in cultured renal cell suspensions is the loss of intercellular connections - even monolayer measurements may seldom be adequate (6). It was hoped that using Fura in freshly isolated PT fragments might ameliorate this potential defect and give an indication of

Table 1. Basal Ca^{2+} levels and leakage rates for Mechanical and Collagenase isolated PTs.

	Basal Ca^{2+}	Leakage (over 10 mins)
MECHANICAL ISOLATES	523±55nM (n = 6)	8%
COLLAGENASE ISOLATES	182±14nM (n = 6)	13%

whether intercellular connections influenced Ca^{2+} levels. Perhaps predictably, however, progress in this area was not without problems.

After ensuring that Fura-2AM was being converted to Fura in both PT preparations, the next technical concern was with the possible chelating effect of the iron oxide used during the tubule isolation procedure. Chelation of Fura by heavy metals, with subsequent quenching, is known to be a problem (7). Addition of the lipid soluble chelator TPEN showed, however, that the iron oxide had virtually no residual quenching effect on the Fura signal.

Nevertheless, despite this, basal Ca^{2+} levels in the PT fragments were significantly higher than that of around 100nm usually obtained in their cultured counterparts. Although the Ca^{2+} levels obtained in the collagenase isolated PTs were comparable to levels obtained by other workers using similar preparations (8), the basal Ca^{2+} levels in the mechanically isolated PTs were particularly high and variable (Table 1). Leakage was also higher in PT fragments compared with cultured cells (5), though the rate of leakage was higher with the collagenase rather than the mechanically isolated PTs. Both PT samples were loaded and monitored at $25^{o}C$ rather than at higher temperatures in order to reduce the level of leakage. Probenecid was not employed to attenuate leakage as it was felt that its additional effects on transport etc. might create more problems than it solved. However, the recent use of sulfinpy-

Fluorescence

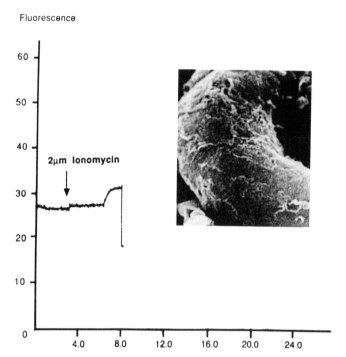

Figure 1. Effect of Ionomycin on the cytosolic Ca^{2+} concentration of mechanically isolated PTs. Trace showed that Ionomycin produced only a slight rise in Ca^{2+} levels. **Inset.** SEM of a mechanically isolated PT showing a well preserved basal surface structure and copious amounts of connective tissue.

Fluorescence

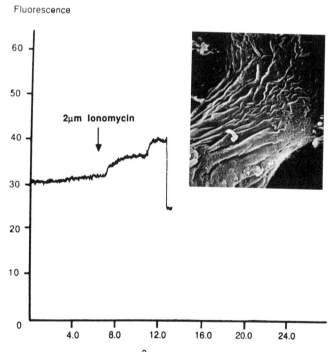

Figure 2. Effect of Ionomycin on the cytosolic Ca^{2+} concentration of collagenase isolated PTs Trace showed significant rise in Ca^{2+} levels with Ionomycin. **Inset.** SEM of a collagenase isolated PT showing no obvious connective tissue residues, but significant basolateral deterioration.

razone in attenuating leakage may in future prove a useful alternative to probenecid.

Finally, addition of the ionophore Ionomycin appeared to produce a rise in cytosolic Ca^{2+} with the collagenase isolated PTs only - although it was possible that any rise induced in the mechanically isolated PTs might well have been masked by their high basal Ca^{2+}.

It was difficult to know exactly why the responses of Fura in the two PT preparations differed from each other and from those of cultured proximal cells. Damage during preparation, cellular heterogeneity and dye sequestration are all possibilities. However, another less obvious factor may be involved - which might also explain some of the anomalous responses between the collagenase and mechanically isolated PTs.

Initial characterisation work on both PT preparations indicated that the mechanically isolated PTs had superior structural preservation and greater longevity than their collagenase isolated counterparts, with the most obvious structural disparities seen at the basolateral surfaces of the two PT preparations. As shown in the SEM photographs (Figure 1 and 2 insets), the mechanically isolated PTs showed an essentially intact basement membrane whilst the collagenase isolated PTs showed gross membrane distortion. This difference might account for the higher level of Fura leakage from the collagenase isolated PTs. However, a potentially more significant feature in this case were the connective tissue residues left on the PT surface by the mechanical, but not the collagenase, isolation technique.

Preliminary experiments in this laboratory have shown that 54% of the FURA signal from mechanically isolated PTs was located on the surface of the cells, whereas collagenase isolates exhibited an external signal of only 11%. Indeed other workers have also recently observed external binding whilst using QUIN in whole PTs (10). This finding then begs the question of to what exactly is the FURA bound?

The most obvious answer might seem the copious connective tissue residues present on the surface of the mechanically isolated PTs. The FURA might bind to the connective tissue itself or perhaps to the Ca^{2+} ions contained in this region which form the "3rd compartment" involved in renal Ca^{2+} kinetics (9). Equally the FURA might possibly bind to the calcium contained in proteins within the basement membrane. These external sources of Ca^{2+} would not be distinguished by FURA from cytosolic pools and hence would yield spuriously high basal Ca^{2+} levels.

In addition the external FURA coating might cause physical antagonism of agonists and could account for the lack of response to Ionomycin, though this is highly speculative. The above would not be problems in cultured renal cells as the basement membrane region is usually lost or significantly attenuated during proliferation.

It is probably also worth observing that higher basal Ca^{2+} levels found in whole PTs might reflect genuine differences with cultured cell systems, i.e. cultured renal cells undergo significant de-differentiation and can lose not only basement membranes but can have attenuated organelle levels, e.g. mitochondria. This could result in a "down regulation" in cellular chemistry which might manifest in part as a lower cytosolic Ca^{2+} level.

In conclusion, this preliminary evidence would seem to suggest that the use of FURA in whole PT systems is not without difficulty and currently appears to offer no immediate advantages over cultured systems in FURA measurements of cytosolic renal calcium.

ACKNOWLEDGEMENTS

Thanks are extended to SERC for the research studentship and to Ms L Tompkins (Birmingham University) for her histology expertise. Dr E.S Harpur is also acknowledged in this work.

REFERENCES

1. Goligorsky MS, Hruska KA: Hormonal modulation of cytoplasmic calcium concentration in renal tubular epithelium. Mineral Electrolyte Metab 14:58-70, 1988.

2. Frindt G, Lee CO, Yang JM, Winhager EE: Potential role of cytoplasmic calcium ions in the regulation of sodium transport in renal tubules. Mineral Electrolyte Metab 14:40-47, 1988.

3. Mandel LJ, Murphy E: Regulation of cytosolic free calcium in rabbit proximal renal tubules. J Biol Chem 259:11188-11196, 1984.

4. Snowdowne KW, Freudenrich CC, Borle AB: The effects of anoxia on cytosolic free calcium, calcium fluxes and cellular ATP levels in culture kidney cells. J Biol Chem 260:11619-11626, 1985.

5. Smith MW, Ambudkar IS, Phelps PC, Regec AL, Trump BF: $HgCl_2$-induced changes in cytosolic Ca^{2+} of cultured rabbit renal tubular cells. Biochimica et Biophysica Acta 931:130-142, 1987.

6. Rink TJ: Measurement of cytosolic calcium: Fluorescent calcium indica tors. Mineral Electrolyte Metab 14:7-14, 1988.

7. Arslan P, DiVirgilio F, Beltrame M, Tsien RY, Pozzan T: Cytosolic Ca^{2+} homeostasis in Ehrlich and Yoshida carcinomas. J Biol Chem 260:2719-2727, 1985.

8. Llibre J, LaPointe MS, Batlle DC: Free cytosolic calcium in renal proximal tubules from the spontaneously hypertensive rat. Hypertension 12:399-404, 1988.

9. Uchikawa T, Borle AB: Studies of calcium-45 desaturation from kidney slices in flow through chambers. Am J Physiol 234:R34-R38, 1978.

10. Filburn CR, Harrison S: Parathyroid hormone regulation of cytosolic Ca^{2+} in rat proximal tubules. Am J Physiol 258:F545-552, 1990.

PART XIII
MARKERS OF NEPHROTOXICITY

74

ABNORMALITIES ALONG THE NEPHRON AS ASSESSED BY EARLY MARKERS OF RENAL DAMAGE IN PATIENTS ON LONG-TERM LITHIUM TREATMENT

A. Rasi, MC. Bocchi, A. Mutti, R. Alinovi, E. Bergamaschi, L. Marinelli, M. Spaggiari
and I. Franchini

Laboratory of Industrial Toxicology, Institute of Clinical Medicine and Nephrology, University of
Parma, Via Gramsci 14, I-43100 Parma, Italy

INTRODUCTION

Lithium salts, mainly lithium carbonate, have been used for 40 years to prevent relapses of manic-depressive illness. Impaired renal ability to acidify and concentrate urine is a common finding among patients on lithium (1). It is usually regarded as a minor side-effect of the drug, i.e. a pharmacologically-induced physiologic impairment of distal tubules and collecting ducts, such a target-selective effect being usually reversible after discontinuation of the therapy.

Although, by the end of 1970s, several case reports of lithium-induced chronic renal insufficiency had been published (2,3), the overall evidence suggesting progressive renal damage in patients taking lithium would be rather limited, because of some methodological weaknesses in human studies (4). However, that long-term treatment with lithium salts may lead to tubulo-interstitial nephropathies, is also indicated by animal data. Experimentally-induced focal fibrosis, tubular atrophy, and cystic dilatation of distal tubuli were obtained by exposing animals to toxic doses (5,6).

In addition to tubular effects, the occurrence of nephrotic syndrome in psychiatric patients has been attributed to long-term treatment with lithium salts (7,8). Thus, although case-reports do not constitute evidence, there is some indication that lithium may adversely affect the kidney function both at the glomerular level and in other segments along the nephron.

The present study was aimed at evaluating whether early markers of kidney damage and dysfunction could detect other abnormalities among patients on lithium, in addition to distal tubular dysfunction.

METHODS

Subjects

This study was designed as a cross-sectional investigation involving 30 patients on lithium carbonate. Their age was 50.9 (SD 14.7). The duration of treatment ranged from 1 to 18 years (9.4 years on average, SD 5.1). The dose was adjusted to maintain serum lithium within the range of 0.6 to 1.0 mEq/l.

Two control groups of healthy subjects and psychiatric patients, respectively, were simultaneously examined. Since sex and age were used as matching criteria for both control groups, the distribution of these variables was the same in all groups.

The first control group was recruited among blood donors living in the same area, and psychiatric patients (taking drugs other than lithium carbonate) were from the same clinic as the patients on lithium.

All subjects examined, including those under study, fulfilled the following admission criteria:

(i) no signs or history of previous renal disease; (ii) no intake of other potentially nephrotoxic drugs, namely antibiotics, analgesics, etc.; (iii) no occupational exposure to heavy metals and/or organic solvents; (iv) no signs or symptoms of infectious disease.

Analytical methods

The urinary excretion of plasma and tissue proteins was measured by sensitive immuno-chemical methods. Albumin (9) and beta2-microglobulin (10) were chosen as markers of increased glomerular permeability and impaired tubular reabsorption, respectively. Brush border antigens (BB-50) revealed by monoclonal antibodies were also measured by specific ELISA procedures (11,12).

The urinary excretion of plasma proteins was expressed as a function of creatinine, which was measured by a picrate reaction with a Technicon Auto-Analyzer. Since BB-50 is not filtered, it was related to the renal mass, as expressed by the GFR (13).

Statistical analysis

All urinary parameters from patients on lithium showed a markedly skewed distribution. Statistical analysis was thus based on log-transformed values, which were consistent with a normal distribution (Kolmogorov-Smirnov non-parametric test). ANOVA and Duncan's multiple range test were used to assess any difference between groups, whereas any eventual correlation between variables was assessed by evaluating the Pearson's correlation coefficient.

RESULTS

The urinary excretion of plasma and brush-border proteins was markedly increased in patients on lithium as compared to both control groups (table 1).

The cumulative frequency distribution of albuminuria from patients on lithium was shifted markedly towards higher figures as compared to both control groups (Fig. 1).

Table 1: Results of investigation of albumin, beta2-microglobulin and brush borders antigens excretion in psychiatric and control group.

Variable	Patients on Lithium		Psychiatric Patients		Control Group	
	GM	GDS	GM	GSD	GM	GSD
Albuminuria						
mg/gr.creat.	20.60	5.10**	6.70	1.60	4.70	1.70
B2-microglobulin						
µg/gr. creat.	275.50	2.30**	46.50	3.60	73.80	2.00
BB-50						
U/ml GFR	0.34	2.80*	0.20	2.20	0.17	1.80

Significantly increased as compared to both control groups: *p<0.05;
**p<0.01 (ANOVA and Duncan's multiple range test).

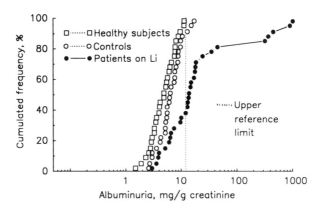

Figure 1. Cumulative frequency distribution of albuminuria in patients on lithium, healthy and psychiatric controls.

Whereas only 3 psychiatric controls and no healthy subjects showed increased albuminuria, 18/30 patients on lithium exceeded the upper reference limit. Five of them and none of the controls showed macroalbuminuria or clinically significant high molecular weight proteinuria, i.e values exceeding 200 mg/g of creatinine.

Although less evident, consistent increases in the urinary excretion of beta2-microglobulin (Fig. 2A) and brush-border antigens (Fig. 2B) were recorded among patients on lithium as compared to both control groups. About one third of patients on lithium showed abnormally high values of such markers, which on average were more than double those of both healthy subjects and psychiatric controls, thus suggesting that increased glomerular permeability was associated with both damage and dysfunction to proximal tubules.

All such markers showed slight but statistically significant correlations with the duration of lithium therapy (Table 2).

The relationship between duration of treatment and albuminuria would also be indicated by the fact that all patients with macroalbuminuria were treated with lithium carbonate for more than six years. Albuminuria was also correlated with serum lithium levels.

DISCUSSION

Early markers of kidney damage showed that lithium-induced renal dysfunction and/or lesion is not confined to distal tubules. At variance from what was reported by Hansen et al. (14), our findings point to significant injury to proximal tubuli and glomeruli, in addition to the well known reduced ability to concentrate urine. It ought to be noted that the dose administered to the patients we studied was rather low, i.e. adjusted to maintain lithium below 1 mEq/l, thus far from the toxic range.

Whereas the mixed type of proteinuria observed in some patients raises interpretative problems with several possible explanations, the increased excretion of brush-border antigens can only be interpreted as a consequence of cell necrosis or increased turnover along the proximal tubules (15-16). Furthermore, such an approach combines the analytical advantages of immunochemical methods with the presumed target selectivity of enzymuria (11). If injury to proximal tubule is clearly shown by both low molecular weight proteinuria and brush-border antigens, it seems also unlikely that such damage may account for the 5 cases with macroalbuminuria. As a result, early markers indicate the coexistence of glomerular and tubular lesions in the kidneys of patients on lithium.

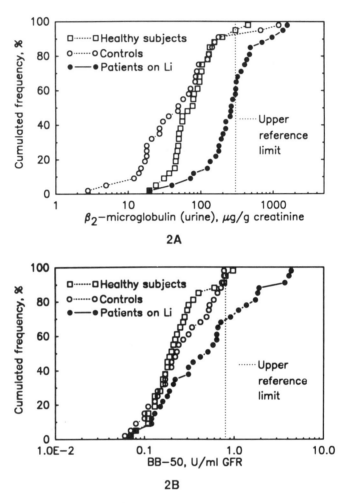

Figure 2. Cumulative frequency distribution of beta2-microglobulin (A) and brush-border antigens (B) in patients on lithium, healthy subjects and psychiatric controls.

Although we cannot extrapolate any long-term consequences from a cross- sectional investigation, the present study supports the view that patients on lithium represent an additional group at risk as far as chronic renal disease is concerned.

Chronic renal damage following long-term treatment with lithium salts has been reported by several workers. Cohen et al. (2) showed that - according to various authors (17-27) - a proportion of cases ranging from 0 to 50% (median 8%) of patients on lithium may eventually develop chronic renal insufficiency evolving towards end-stage renal disease. The relative risk for chronic renal disease associated with lithium therapy cannot be assessed easily, because of major methodological problems, but some considerations are possible on the basis of indirect evidence.

Lithium-induced nephropathy was mentioned for three patients in the EDTA-ERA registry as the cause of end-stage renal failure requiring renal replacement therapy in 1985 and 1986 (28). This would suggest that lithium-induced

Table 2: Correlation matrix between independent variables and renal markers.

Variable	Albumin	B2m	BB-50	Osm
Dose	.12	-.08	.01	.01
S-Li	.37*	.23	.24	-.08
Duration	.28*	.27	.32*	-.29*

* p<0.05

nephropathy is a minor problem. On the other hand, the relative risk for end-stage renal disease might be very high, owing to the limited number of patients belonging to this highly selected group. In fact, the incidence of end-stage renal disease among patients on lithium seems to be much higher than that of 50-60 new patients per million recorded for the general population.

Such an increased risk may still be regarded as acceptable, especially as compared to the benefits of such a therapeutic approach to serious psychiatric problems. Thus, fear of renal disease may not require the therapy to be stopped. However, a close monitoring of renal function is strongly recommended. Since increased serum creatinine reflects only late, nonspecific degenerative changes, it may not be sufficient to adequately protect subjects at risk from developing chronic renal disease (29).

ACKNOWLEDGEMENTS

Supported in part by the Commission of the European Communities (contr. EV4V-0190-I-A) and by Regione Emilia Romagna (Ricerca Sanitaria Finalizzata).

REFERENCES

1. Batelle D, Gaviria M, Grupp M, Arruda JA, Wynn J, Kurtzman NA: Distal nephron function in patients receiving lithium therapy. Kidney Int 21: 477-486, 1982.

2. Cohen JJ, Harrington JT, Kassirev JP: Lithium and the kidney. Kidney Int 19: 374-387, 1981.

3. Walker RG, Davies BM, Holwill BJ, Dowling JP, Kincaid-Smith P: A clinico-pathological study of lithium nephrotoxicity. J Chron Dis 35: 685-695, 1982.

4. Lippmann S: Lithium's effects on the kidney. Postgrad Med 71: 99-108, 1982.

5. Ottosen PD, Sigh B, Kristensen J, Olsen S, Christensen S: Lithium induced interstitial nephropathy associated with chronic renal failure. Acta Path Microbiol Immunol Scand Sect 92: 447-454, 1984.

6. Walker RG, Escott M, Birchall I, Dowling JP, Kincaid-Smith P: Chronic progressive renal lesions induced by lithium. Kidney Int 29: 875-881, 1986.

7. Depner TA: Nephrotic syndrome secondary to lithium therapy. Nephron 30: 286-289, 1982.

8. Richman AV, Masco HL, Rifkin SI, Acharya MK: Minimal-change disease and the nephrotic syndrome associated with lithium therapy. Ann Intern Med 92: 70-72, 1980.

9. Alinovi R, Mutti A, Bergamaschi E, Franchini I: Competitive enzyme-linked immunosorbent assay (celisa) of urinary albumin. Clin Chem 34: 993, 1988.

10. Vincent C, Revillard JP: Beta2-microglobulin. In: Bergmeyer HU (ed); Methods of Enzymatic Analysis:Proteins and Peptides. Weinheim, VCH, 1986, pp.248-265.

11. Mutti A, Lucertini S, Valcavi P: Urinary excretion of brush-border antigen revealed by monoclonal antibody: early indicator of toxic nephropathy. Lancet 2: 914-917, 1985.

12. Mutti A: The study of urinary excretion of kidney antigens to reveal early effects of exposure to exogenous chemicals. In: Foa' V, Emmett EA, Maroni M, Colombi A (eds); Occupational and Environmental Chemical

Hazards. Chichester, Ellis Horwood Limited, 1987, pp. 315-322.

13. Thornley C, Dawnay A, Cattel WR: Human Tamm-Horsfall glycoprotein: urinary and plasma levels in normal subjects and patients with renal disease determined by a fully validated radioimmunoassay. Clin Sci 68:529-535, 1985.

14. Hansen HE, Mogensen CE, Sorensen JL, Norgaard K, Heilskov J, Andersen A: Albumin and beta$_2$-microglobulin excretion in patients on long-term lithium treatment. Nephron 29: 229-232, 1981.

15. Mutti A, Alinovi R, Bergamaschi E, Fornari M, Franchini I: Monoclonal antibodies to brush border antigens for the early diagnosis of nephrotoxicity. Arch Toxicol Suppl 12: 162-165, 1988.

16. Mutti A: Detection of renal diseases in humans: developing markers and methods. Toxicol Letters 46: 177-191, 1989.

17. Hestbech J, Hansen HE, Andisen A, Olsen S: Chronic renal lesions following long-term treatment with lithium. Kidney Int 12: 205-213, 1977.

18. Hansen HE, Hestbech J, Sorensen JL, Norgaard K, Heilskov J, Amdisen A: Chronic interstitial nephritis in patients on long-term lithium treatment. Q J Med 48: 577-591, 1979.

19. Burrows GD, Davies B, Kinkaid-Smith P: Unique tubular lesion after lithium. Lancet i: 1310, 1978.

20. Kinkaid-Smith P, Burrows GD, Davies BM, Holwill B, Walter M, Walker RG: Renal biopsy findings in lithium and pre-lithium patients. Lancet 2. 700-701, 1979.

21. Rafaelson OJ, Bolwing TG, Ladefoged J, Brun C: Kidney function and morfology in long-term lithium treatment. In:Cooper TB, Gershon S, Kline NS, Schou M (eds); Lithium: Controversies and Unresolved Issues. Excerpta Medica, Amsterdam, 1979, p. 578.

22. Vestergaard P, Amdisen A, Hansen HE, Schou M: Lithium treatment and kidney function. A survey of 237 patients in long-term treatment. Acta Psychiatr Scand 60: 504-520, 1979.

23. Hallgren R, Alm PO, Hellsing K: Renal function in patients on lithium treatment. Br J Psychiatr 135: 22-27, 1979.

24. Hullin RP, Coley VP, Birch NJ, Thomas TH, Morgan DB: Renal function after long-term treatment with lithium. Brit Med J 1: 1475-1495, 1979.

25. Donker AMJ, Prins E, Meijer E, Sluiter WJ, van Berkestijn JWBM, Dols LCW: A renal function study in 30 patients on long-term lithium therapy. Clin Nephrol 12: 254-262, 1979.

26. Muller-Oerlinghausen B, Drescher K: Time course of clinical-chemical parameters under long-term lithium therapy. Int J Clin Pharmacol Biopharm 17: 228-235, 1979.

27. Colt EWD, Igel G, Fieve RR, Dunner DL: Lithium associated nephropathy. Am J Phsychiatr 136: 1098-1099, 1979.

28. Wing AJ, Brunner FP, Geerlings W, Broyer M, Brynger H, Fassbinder W, Rissoni G, Selwood NH, Tufeson G: Contribution of toxic nephropathies to end-stage renal failure in Europe: a report from the EDTA-ERA registry. Toxicol Lett 46:281-292, 1989.

29. CEC-IPCS Consensus Statement on the Health Significance of Nephrotoxicity. Toxicol Lett 46: 1-12, 1989.

75

KIDNEY AND URINE N-ACETYL-BETA-D-GLUCOSAMINIDASE LEVELS FOLLOWING CYCLOSPORIN A TREATMENT IN THE RAT

A.J. Burnett and P.H. Whiting

Department of Clinical Biochemistry, Aberdeen University, Foresterhill, Aberdeen AB9 2ZD, UK

INTRODUCTION

The structural, functional and biochemical heterogeneity demonstrated by the kidney predisposes it to the site-specific toxicity which results from exposure to many chemicals and environmental agents. Although all segments of the nephron are susceptible to site-specific damage depending on the toxicant, the proximal renal tubule is a favoured site in this regard. The reasons for this may be related to the large surface area of brush border essential for its reabsorptive function. This segment of the nephron consequently has a high requirement for effective energy generation, reflected in the large numbers of mitochondria found in proximal tubular cells, the presence of cytochrome P-450-dependent drug metabolism, large numbers of lysosomes and marked gluconeogenesis with respect to carbohydrate metabolism (1).

The acute toxicity associated with Cyclosporin A (CsA) is characterised functionally by a reduction in glomerular filtration rate and structurally by a tubulopathy involving the proximal renal tubule both in experimental animals and in transplant recipients treated with the drug (2,3). Other biochemical alterations associated with CsA nephrotoxicity include glycosuria, Tamm Horsfall proteinuria and enzymuria (4,5). In this context, increased urinary excretion of the lysosomal hydrolase N-acetyl-beta-D- glucosaminidase (NAG), brush border enzyme gamma-glutamyl transferase and glutathione-S-transferase, found in the cytosol, have all been demonstrated (7,8).

All these enzymes are found in high concentration in the proximal renal tubule (1).

The lysosomal hydrolase NAG in particular has been used as an important adjunct to the diagnosis of drug-induced nephrotoxicity which may predate alterations in GFR (9). This assumes that increased cell content of NAG, reflecting lysosomal induction following cell injury, is parallelled by its excretion into the urine. This study investigates the relationship between NAG activity in both the urine and kidney following exposure to a known toxic dose of CsA.

METHODS

Animals: Adult, male Sprague-Dawley rats (mean weight 280g) were used and allowed free access to both food and water throughout the experimental period.

Cyclosporin A: CsA (Sandoz Ltd., Basle, Switzerland) was dissolved initially in absolute ethanol at room temperature and a 10% (v/v) solution in olive oil (Boots Co. Ltd., Nottingham, UK) prepared. CsA or its vehicle (10% ethanol in olive oil) was administered to conscious animals by gastric incubation using a No 4 FG cannula (Portex Ltd., Hythe, Kent, UK).

Experimental protocol: Groups of 5 rats received CsA (50 mg/kg body weight) or its vehicle daily for 4, 7, 10 or 14 days. After the last drug or vehicle treatment animals were placed in individual metabolic cages overnight (16 hr) and urine, free of faecal contamination, was collected. (Prior to the experiment each animal was placed in a metabolic cage for 16h periods on 3 consecutive days which allowed adaptation to the new environment to which they were exposed during subsequent urine collection periods.) Blood was obtained from the tail tip under light ether anaesthesia and serum separated by centrifugation. Both urine and serum samples were stored at -20°C until assayed. Renal function and urine activity of NAG were assessed on days 5, 8, 11 and 15 before the animals were sacrificed and kidney NAG activity measured. In addition, a group of untreated age matched controls were used to obtain pretreatment values.

Biochemical measurements: Creatinine clearance rates (CCR), glucose determinations and NAG activity measurements in both the kidney and urine were performed as described previously (10, 11). Kidney NAG activities are expressed as units per hour while urine activities are expressed as units/mmol urinary creatinine.

Statistics: Results (mean $\pm$ 1SD) were analysed using ANOVA followed by the appropriate Student's 't' test.

RESULTS

Compared to pretreatment values CsA-treated animals demonstrated a significant 3 fold increase and 50% decrease in urine flow rate (UFR) and C_{CR} respectively, by day 4 (Table 1), which was maintained until day 10. By day 14, however, mean C_{CR} values had slightly increased whilst the increased UFR was maintained. Total NAG enzymuria was elevated by 2-3 fold on days 4 and 7, peaked on day 10 demonstrating a 7 fold increase and although mean values were still elevated on day 14, results were variable ranging from 54 to 340 units/mmol. A similar pattern was also observed with respect to glycosuria and in addition a positive significant correlation was noted between this parameter and NAG enzymuria (r=0.7863, p<0.001). Plasma glucose levels, measured in all animals immediately prior to sacrifice, were only significantly increased in CsA-treated animals on day 7,

compared to both pretreatment and vehicle-treated results (15.8±2.7 versus 9.0±1.0 or 10.0±1.8 mmol/1; p<0.001). There was no apparent correlation between plasma and urine glucose concentrations over the experimental course in either treatment group.

Renal NAG levels: There was no significant effect on total renal NAG activity over the duration of the experiment with vehicle administration alone (Figure 1). CsA treatment caused a slight but significant 30% reduction in total NAG levels between days 4-7 when compared to pretreatment values (p< 0.05). However, on day 10, a 10-fold increase in renal levels was observed (p<0.001) which by day 14 had returned to pretreatment values. Over the 14 day experimental period a positive significant correlation between kidney and urine total NAG activity was observed (r=0.6400, p<0.01). Similar results were obtained when renal NAG activities were expressed as either units/g wet weight or units/mg protein. Over the course of the experiment, treatment with either CsA or its vehicle showed no significant effect on kidney protein content.

NAG isoenzyme studies: Vehicle treatment produced a reduction in both urine and kidney NAG-B isoenzyme activity, expressed as a proportion of total activity, from pretreatment values of around 20% to 8% by day 14. Compared to results from vehicle treated animals, CsA treatment resulted in a 2-fold increase in both kidney and urine NAG-B isoenzyme activity on day 7 (34.8±8.5 versus 16.9±4.8 and 41.8±6.4 versus 19.4±7.3 respectively, both p<0.001; expressed as a % of total activity) so predating the increase in total NAG activities observed on day 10.

DISCUSSION

The results of this study confirm and extend previous observations from this and other laboratories (2), on experimental CsA-nephrotoxicity in the Sprague-Dawley rat. CsA, administered at the known toxic dose of 50mg/kg/day for 14 days, produced a reduction in C_{CR} and increased UFR and glycosuria. Furthermore, coordinancy between urinary ex-

Table 1. The effect of CsA on renal function and NAG enzymuria.

Treatment duration (days)	UFR ml/h/kg	C_{CR} ml/h/kg	NAG U/mmol	Glycosuria mmol/l
Pretreatment	1.86±0.35	438±82	47±8	0.48±0.15
4	5.90±2.20[b]	229±47[c]	119±55[a]	1.01±0.44
7	3.73±1.90[a]	235±101[b]	148±29[c]	10.30±6.20[b]
10	3.97±1.11[b]	253±43[c]	279±47[c]	50.01±33.40[c]
14	4.00±1.90[a]	301±46[a]	120±123	20.20±30.90

Results are expressed as mean±1SD and there were 5 animals per group. CsA treatment values compared to pretreatment results as vehicle was without significant effect on any of the above parameters. a, $p<0.05$; b, $p<0.01$; c, $p<0.001$.

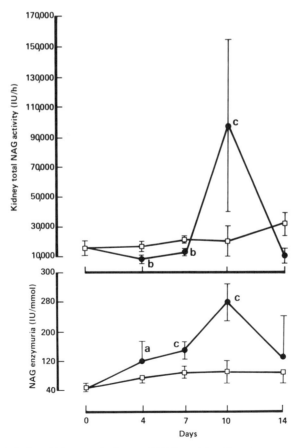

Figure 1. The effect of CsA on kidney and urine total NAG activity. Results (mean±1SD) compared to vehicle treated values at each time point. a, $p<0.05$; b, $p<0.01$; c, $p<0.001$.

cretion of NAG and kidney levels of NAG was observed. The observed correlations between urinary glucose and NAG levels, increased UFR and the absence of both frank hyperglycaemia and any relationship between plasma glucose levels and glycosuria, suggest that CsA treatment resulted in tubular damage and defective tubular reabsorption. Indeed, glycosuria has been suggested as being a sensitive indication of CsA-nephrotoxicity in renal transplant recipients (11), although abnormal glucose homeostasis has also been observed following treatment with the drug (12).

The increased urinary excretion and renal tissue activity of NAG is consistent with the autophagic response of the lysosomes to a sublethal cellular toxic insult. Previous observations from this laboratory (2) have demonstrated the presence of increased numbers of lysosomes and myeloid bodies throughout the proximal convoluted tubule when sublethal cellular damage was sustained following CsA treatment. In the present study increased lysosomes were also observed in the proximal tubules of CsA-treated rats on day 10 (results not shown), in addition to isometric vacuolisation and basal lipid droplet accumulation. The observed relationship between kidney and urinary total NAG activities also confirms the use of this enzymuria in mirroring a cellular response to a toxic insult.

The observation that both kidney and urinary NAG levels fell before the end of the treatment period may be due to simple cell depletion of the enzyme or reflect an acute response to injury. Similar patterns of tissue and urinary NAG activity have also been observed following treatment with gentamicin in the mouse (13) and low dose CsA nephrotoxicity in the rat (20mg/kg/day for 42 days) where fluctuations in C_{CR} and NAG enzymuria were associated with similar fluctuations in the circulating drug concentration (9). These in turn were related to hepatic cytochrome P-450-dependent monooxygenase activity. The similarity to gentamicin-induced fluctuations in renal function may be due to the association of both agents with lysosomes (14).

Increased activity of NAG-B isoenzyme has been suggested to be indicative of renal insult (15) and the results of this study demonstrate that NAG-B increased prior to the large increase observed in total activity. The prevalence of NAG-A and even more of NAG-B in the proximal tubule may be consistent with the view that modification of enzymuria, and urinary isoenzyme profile in particular, reflects an insult at this site.

REFERENCES

1. Guder WG, Ross BD: Enzyme Distribution along the Nephron. Kidney Int 26:101-111, 1984.

2. Thomson AW, Whiting PH, Simpson JG: Cyclosporin: Immunology, Toxicity and Pharmacology in experimental animals. Agents and Actions 15:306-327, 1984.

3. Mihatsch MJ, Thiel G, Basler V, Ryffel B, Landmann J, von Overbeck J, Zollinger HU: Morphological patterns in cyclosporin-treated renal transplant recipients. Transplant Proc 17 (suppl 1): 101-116.

4. Dawnay A, Lucey M, Thornley C, Beetham R, Neugerger JM, Cattell WR, Williams R: The effects of long-term low-dose cyclosporine A on renal tubular function. Transplant Proc 20 (suppl 3): 725-31, 1988.

5. McAuley FT, Simpson JG, Thomson AW, Whiting PH: The predictive value of enzymuria in Cyclosporin A-induced renal toxicity in the rat. Tox Let 32:165-171, 1986.

6. Backman L, Applekvist EL, Ringden O, Dallner G: Urinary Levels of Basic Glutathione Transferase as an indicator of Proximal Tubular Damage in Renal Transplant Recipients. Transplant Proc 21:1514-1516, 1989.

7. Price RG: Urinary N-acetyl-beta-D-glucosaminidase (NAG) as an indicator of renal diseases. In: Dubach UC, Schmidt U (eds); Diagnostic significance of Enzymes and Proteins in Urine. Bern, Huber, 1979, pp 150-165.

8. Duncan JI, Heys SD, Thomson AW, Simpson JG, Whiting PH: Influence of the hepatic

drug metabolising enzyme inducer phenobarbitone on Cyclosporine nephro- and hepatotoxicity in renal allografted rats. Transplantation 45:693-697, 1988.

9. Whiting PH, Simpson JG, Davidson RJL, Thomson AW: Pathological changes in rats receiving CsA at immunotherapeutic dosage for 7 weeks. Brit J Exp Path 64:437-443, 1983.

10. Ellis RB, Ikonne JU, Masson PK: DEAE-cellulose microcolumn chromatography coupled with automated assay: application to the resolution of N-acetyl-beta-D-hexosaminidase components. Analytical Biochem 63:5-11, 1975.

11. Chan P, Chapman JR, Morris PJ: Glycosuria: An Index of Cyclosporine Nephrotoxicity. Transplant Proc 19:1780, 1987.

12. Helmchen U, Schmidt WE, Siegel EG, Creutzfeldt W: Morphological and functional changes of pancreatic B-cells in cyclosporine A-treated rats. Diabetologia 27:416-418, 1984.

13. Whiting PH, Petersen J, Simpson JG: Gentamicin-induced nephrotoxicity in mice: protection by loop diuretics. Brit J Exp Path 62:200-206, 1981.

14. Dobrota M, Louis JR: In: Intracellular localization of cyclosporin A in the rat. Bach PH, Lock EA (eds); Nephrotoxicity: Extrapolation from in vitro to in vivo, and animals to man. London, Plenum Press, 1989, pp 325-330.

15. Bourbouze R, Baumann F-C, Bonnalet JP, Farman N: Distribution on N-Acetyl-beta-D-Glucosaminidase Isoenzymes along the Rabbit Nephron. Kidney Int 25:636-642, 1984.

76

CIRCADIAN RHYTHM OF PROTEINURIA IN RATS

E. Bergamaschi (1), A. Mutti (1), R. Alinovi (1), A. Rasi (1), C. Biagini (1), M. Giovanetti (1), I. Franchini (1) and A. Bernard (2)

(1) Laboratory of Industrial Toxicology, Institute of Clinical Medicine and Nephrology, University of Parma, Parma, Italy and (2) Unit of Industrial Toxicology and Occupational Medicine, Catholic University of Louvain, Brussels, Belgium

INTRODUCTION

Several factors accounting for the biological variability of proteinuria in man have been extensively investigated (1-4). Apart from the influence of sex and dietary factors (5) little is known about the variables affecting the renal handling of single plasma proteins in experimental animals. On the other hand, such a basic knowledge would be necessary both to correctly design experiments and to interpret data obtained from animals challenged with nephrotoxic chemicals. In fact, increased urinary excretion rates of single plasma proteins measured by immunochemical methods are regarded as sensitive markers of the selective dysfunctions of discrete segments along the nephron (6).

Two separate experiments were carried out to evaluate whether a circadian rhythm of the urinary protein excretion rate occurs in rats and whether such a rhythm is modified by exogenous factors, such as the inversion of the light/dark cycle.

METHODS

Animals

Twelve male and twelve female mature Sprague-Dawley rats were obtained from Charles River Italia (Calco, Como, Italy). Male rats weighing 240-270 g and aged about 10-12 weeks were used, whereas females had the same age but weighed 200-230 g.

After one week of acclimatisation, they were individually housed, under constant conditions of temperature and humidity, and an artificial light-dark cycle of 12:12 hr in plastic metabolic cages equipped with urine-faeces separators The 12-hr day-time was defined as from 6:00 to 18:00 hours and the correspondent night-time period as from 18:00 - 6:00 hr. Laboratory chow designed for maintenance in short- and medium-term studies, with a protein content of 19g% (Italiana Mangimi, Settimo Milanese, Milan, Italy) and filtered tap water were freely available throughout the study.

Study Design

First Experiment: The occurrence of a spontaneous circadian rythm for proteinuria was investigated in two groups of male and female rats, respectively. The animals from each group were randomly assigned to two subgroups starting urine collection during the night or during the day. The animals were followed for 5 days. The existence of a circadian rhythm was evaluated on data gathered from the last three days, the first 48 hr of the study being considered as conditioning period. Four collection periods were used during each experimental day: from 06:00 - 12:00, from 12:00 - 18:00, from 18:00 - 00:00, and from 00:00 - 06:00.

Second experiment: This experiment was designed to evaluate the relative effect of the light-dark cycle and of the time of day in male rats only. The animals were randomly divided into four subgroups. The first group started urine collection with artificial dark during the day

(DD), the second with artificial light during the night (NL), the third with artificial light during the day (DL), and the last with dark during the night (ND). The sequence of conditions was balanced between groups in accordance with a 4 x 4 Latin square design. Thus, each animal was subjected to four measurements on different experimental conditions during a 2-day study period.

Analytical methods

Urine samples were collected in cooling vials every six hours over NaN_3 as preservative. Urine volume was measured. Then, after centrifugation (1000 g X 10 min) samples were frozen ($-20^{o}C$) until analysis, with the exception of aliquots for IgG determination, which were kept at $4^{o}C$.

Albumin and alpha$_{2u}$-globulin were measured by competitive ELISA (7) using monospecific antisera and rat proteins. Rat albumin was purchased from Calbiochem (La Jolla, CA) and rabbit anti-rat albumin -IgG fraction- was from Bio Science Products (Emmenbrucke, Switzerland). Purified alpha$_{2u}$-globulin was a kind gift from Dr. E. Lock (ICI, Central Toxicology Laboratories, Alderley Park, UK). Beta$_2$-microglobulin and IgG by were determined by Latex immunoassay, as described previously (8).

SDS-PAGE electrophoresis of pooled and undiluted urine samples was performed on micro-gels (8-25% constant gradient) using a Phast-System apparatus (Pharmacia, Uppsala, SW) and double silver staining procedure.

Statistics

Experimental data is expressed as mean value and standard error of the mean (SEM). Analysis of variance (ANOVA) was used as the primary statistical technique, whereas Student's t test for paired data was used to assess differences between groups. The analysis of variance was adapted to a 4 X 4 Latin square design with repeated measurements, this model allowing simultaneous testing of sources of variation between (day sequence) and within (time of day) experimental conditions as well as some of the interactions between these. These tests were performed by using the statistical package SPSS/PC+ (Chigago, III) implemented on a Personal System/2 model 60 IBM computer (IBM UK Int. Products Ltd., Portsmouth, UK).

To determine the presence of a circadian rhythm, data from each 6 hr period was analysed by the Cosinor method (9). In this procedure the best cosine curve is fitted to the sequential data on the variable by means of the least-squares method. For statistically validated rhythms ($p<0.05$), the acrophase (i.e. the time at which the peak of the phenomenon is located) was assessed.

RESULTS

Table 1 summarizes the main findings of the first experiment. Urinary excretion rates of all proteins were much higher during night-time, with the exception of albumin in the male rats, which showed slightly higher values during daytime.

From the visual inspection of Fig. 1A, the existence of a circadian rhythm for both high (albumin) and low molecular weight plasma proteins (beta$_2$-microglobulin) in female rats can be envisaged. However, a somewhat different behaviour of IgG and alpha$_{2u}$-globulin was observed, although such proteins belong to the same groups of high and low molecular weight proteins, respectively (Fig. 1B).

An infradian rhythm could eventually be suggested for IgG, whereas a circadian rhythm, but with large day-to-day variations, was exhibited by alpha$_{2u}$-globulin.

ANOVA revealed that both the day of experiment and the period of sampling (night or day) influenced the excretion rate of plasma proteins. Significant differences were obtained both as a result of day sequence ($p<0.01$ for albumin and $p<0.01$ for IgG) and of varying times of days ($p<0.001$ for albumin; $p<0.01$ for alpha$_{2u}$-globulin; $p<0.001$ for beta$_2$-microglobulin; $p<0.01$ for IgG), a significant interactive effect emerging between day sequence and time of day for beta$_2$-microglobulin ($p< 0.001$).

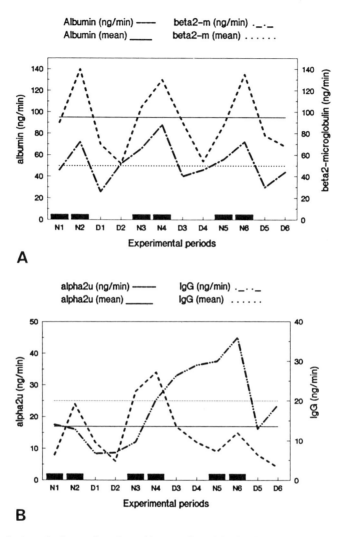

Figure 1. Circadian rhythm of urinary albumin and beta2-microglobulin (A) and variations of IgG and alpha2u-globulin in female rats (B) during the three days of experiment (D = day-time; N = night-time).

These findings are consistent with the existence of a circadian rhythm for urinary proteins. Data from every 6-hr period, analysed by the Cosinor method, revealed a circadian rhythm for albumin, alpha2u-globulin and beta2-microglobulin, but not for IgG.

Whereas the acrophase of albumin was located at 1:02 am (95% confidence limits: 19:32-5:09) in females, it occurred during day-time in male rats (9:00 am; 95% confidence limits: 4:35-16:12). Beta2-microglobulin, tested in females only, revealed the same trend with acrophase at 1:26 am (95% confidence limits: 18:54-5:01). Alpha2u-globulin also showed a circadian rhythm with acrophases around 2:00 am both in male and female rats, thus overlapping that of albumin in female, but not male rats. The urinary excretion of IgG showed a time-re-

Table 1: Urinary excretion of single plasmaproteins during day-time (from 06:00 - 18:00) and night-time (from 18:00 - 06:00).

| | Male rat | | | | Female rat | | | |
| | Day-time | | Night-time | | Day-time | | Night-time | |
	Mean	SEM	Mean	SEM	Mean	SEM	Mean	SEM
Albumin (ng/min)	250	44	218	30*	71.0	9.7	120.0	15.1***
Alpha$_{2u}$ (ng/min)	2630	123	4200	170**	15.5	3.9	24.3	4.7*
Beta$_2$-m (ng/min)	n.a.		n.a.		25.6	3.4	77.5	9.8***
IgG (ng/min)	n.a.		n.a.		18.2	2.0	21.7	2.6

*p<0.05; **p<0.01; ***p<0.05 as compared to day-time; n.a. = not available.

lated variability, as suggested by analysis of variance, but no hints of a circadian rhythm.

During the second experiment in male rats, our attention was focused on albumin and alpha$_{2u}$-globulin excretion rates (Fig. 2).

Under normal light-dark cycle (day-light/night-dark) day-to-night variations in albumin and alpha$_{2u}$-globulin excretion rates were consistent with the circadian rhythm of such proteins. Whereas albumin did not change significantly between day and night (255 ± 38 ng/min vs 232 ± 25 ng/min), alpha$_{2u}$-globulin showed much larger variations during the night-dark period (3870 ± 265 ng/min) than the one recorded during the day-light period (2430 ± 178 ng/min). Reversal of the light-dark cycle caused major changes in the excretion of these proteins. Albumin excretion was much more prominent under night-light conditions (372 ± 63.8 ng/min) as compared to both the day-dark (270 ± 42.1 ng/min) and night-dark conditions. The night-to-day variation of alpha$_{2u}$-globulin was flattened (night-light 3340 ± 230 ng/min vs 2264 ± 135 ng/min day-dark).

Accordingly, the alpha$_{2u}$-globulin/albumin ratio showed the highest value during the night dark period and the lowest during the night light condition. This trend was also suggested by the results of SDS-PAGE electrophoresis (not presented here).

DISCUSSION

The present investigation indicates the existence of a circadian rhythm of single urinary plasma proteins in rats. To our knowledge, it has not been reported before. Some authors have demonstrated that the urinary excretion of total protein among rats varies depending on either chronobiological parameters (10) and other related physiological factors, such as protein intake (5).

The influence of hemodynamic changes, like post-meal induced vasodilation and increases in plasma vasoactive hormones, leading to nocturnal changes of transglomerular pressure, has been suggested to explain such nycthemeral variations of proteinuria in rats (11). These findings are in agreement with recent reports showing the existence of circadian rhythms for urinary proteins in normal humans (2-4).

Since in man the urinary total protein and albumin achrophases are located in a time span common to that of glomerular filtration rate, the diurnal variation in the filtered load is probably the mechanism underlying both the circadian rhythm of the urinary excretion of high-molecular weight proteins and the renal response to other factors such as physical work load and protein intake. Competitive mechanisms between filtered proteins and peptides from

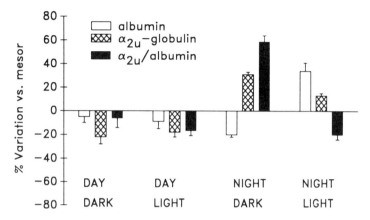

Figure 2. Percentage of variations vs. mesor (mean value) of urinary albumin and alpha2u-globulin in male rats following normal light-dark cycle (Day-Light; Night-Dark) and after reversal of cycle (Day-Dark; Night-Light).

ingested meat may also play a role by reducing the tubular uptake of low molecular weight proteins (12).

Since rats are nocturnal, proteinuria in female animals is consistent with chronobiological data obtained in volunteers, whereas the renal handling of plasma proteins in male rat is influenced by poorly understood mechanisms. Since in male rats $alpha_{2u}$-globulin (a sex specific low molecular weight protein) synthesis is under hormonal control, mainly androgens and corticosteroids (13), several factors may account for the sex-related differences found in the present study.

The much higher values of $alpha_{2u}$-globulin recorded in male rats were associated with the absence of a circadian rhythm for albumin, in spite of day-to-night variations (Table 1). A rhythm for albumin excretion rate was however suggested by findings obtained after the inversion of the light-dark cycle and subsequent reduction in $alpha_{2u}$-globulin excretion. By contrast, female rats showed a regular rhythmic pattern for the urinary excretion rates of all proteins, though the chronobiological parameters of single proteins were not the same.

In the first 48 hr of the experiment, surprisingly high values were recorded for all variables; moreover a circadian rhythm was not evident,

suggesting that handling procedures of animals might greatly influence the results from acute experiments. Adaptative responses to stressors could modify physiological and hemodynamic parameters, leading an additional source of variability when two or more groups or treatment are compared.

As a whole, these findings suggest that the biological variability may influence the results of experimental work. Thus, spontaneous changes in the pattern of proteinuria should be carefully considered when planning short-term exposures, where pronounced increases in proteinuria may occur independently of the treatment. During long-term studies standard collecting or sampling procedures should be adopted, in order to minimize the effect of physiological factors as sources of variability. Finally, preference should be given to female rats, since in this case extrapolation to man seems to be less affected by species-related problems.

ACKNOWLEDGEMENTS

Supported in part by the Commission of the European Communities (contr. EV4V-0190-I-A).

REFERENCES

1. Koopman MG, Krediet RT, Zuyderhaudt FJM, De Moor EAM, Arisz C: Circadian rhythm of proteinuria in patients with a nephrotic syndrome. Clin Sci 69: 395-401, 1985.

2. Montagna G, Buzio C, Calderini C: Relationship of proteinuria and albuminuria to posture and to urine collection period. Nephron 35: 143-144, 1983.

3. Buzio C, Arisi L, Capani F, Barani R, Quaretti P: Circadian rhythm of proteinuria in normal subjects but not in patients with glomerulonephritis. Ann Clin Res 19: 30-33, 1987.

4. Buzio C, Mutti A, Capani F, Andrulli S, Quaretti P, Alinovi R, Negro A, Rustichelli R: Circadian rhythm of proteinuria: Effects of an evening meat meal. Nephrol Dial Transpl 4: 266-270, 1989.

5. Neuhaus OW, Flory W, Biswas N, Holberman CE: Urinary excretion of alpha$_{2u}$-globulin and albumin by adult male rats following treatment with nephrotoxic agents. Nephron 28: 133-140, 1981.

6. CEC/IPCS (ILO-UNEP-WHO): Proceedings of the International Workshop on the Health Significance of Nephrotoxicity. Toxicol Lett 46: 1-12, 1989.

7. Alinovi R, Mutti A, Bergamaschi E, Franchini I: Competitive Enzyme-linked immunosorbent assay (CELISA) of urinary albumin. Clin Chem 34: 993, 1988.

8. Viau C, Bernard A, Lauwerys R: Determination of rat beta$_2$-microglobulin in urine and serum. I. Development of an immunoassay based on latex particles agglutinations. J Appl Toxicol 6: 185-189, 1986.

9. Halberg F, Tomg YL, Johnson EA: Circadian system phase, an aspect of temporal morphology: procedure and illustrative examples. In: Mayersbach H (ed); The Cellular Aspect of Biorhythms. Berlin, Springer-Verlag, 1967, pp. 20-48.

10. Cambar J, Toussaint C, Nguyen BC: Etude des rhythmes circadiennes de l'excretion des electrolytes et des proteines urinaires chez le rat. CR Soc Biol (Paris) 172: 103-109, 1978.

11. Cambar J, Lemaigne F, Toussaint C: Etude des variations nycthemerales de la filtration glomerulaire chez le rat. Experientia 35: 1607-1608, 1979.

12. Bernard C, Viau C, Ouled A, Lauwerys R: Competition between low- and high-molecular weight proteins for tubular uptake. Nephron 45: 115-118, 1987.

13. Vandoren G, Merteus B, Heyns W, Van Baclen H, Ramhaults W, Verhoeven G: Different forms of alpha-2u-globulin in male and female rat urine. Eur J Biochem 134: 175-181, 1983.

77

ELEVATED PLASMA FIBRONECTIN LEVELS IN IMMUNE AND TOXIC GLOMERULAR DISEASES

J. Quirós (1), J. González-Cabrero (2), G. Herrero-Beaumont (1) and J. Egido (2)

Departments of Rheumatology (1) and Nephrology (2). Fundación Jiménez Díaz, Universidad Autónoma, C.S.I.C., Madrid, Spain

INTRODUCTION

Fibronectin (FN) is a high molecular weight (440 Kd) dimeric glycoprotein, composed of two similar polypeptide chains, which are held together with disulphide bonds (1). Two major forms of FN have been characterized: cellular FN, present on the surface of many cells where it plays an important role in organizing the extracellular matrix, and plasma FN, that behaves as an opsonic protein promoting phagocytosis (2,3). Previous works have documented low plasma levels in various clinical situations, such as burn (4), disseminated intravascular coagulation (5), septic trauma and multiple organ failure (6). Normalization of plasma FN concentration correlated with a better clinical course (7). In connective tissue disease, FN was found increased at sites of inflammation, such as the dermis of involved skin by progressive systemic sclerosis (8) and rheumatoid synovial membrane and synovial fluid (9). Other authors (10) have reported a degradation of the fibronectin present in rheumatoid synovial fluid and a direct binding to immune complexes, suggesting the FN participation in tissue destruction and repair in inflammatory diseases. By contrast, moderately high plasma levels of FN have been reported in nephrotic syndrome patients (11). In the present work we studied the plasma fibronectin levels in the course of two nephropathies (toxic and immune) and its relation with the proteinuria and the glomerular lesions.

MATERIALS AND METHODS

Induction of the nephropathies Chronic nephritis was induced in female Wistar rats, according to the protocol of our group (12). Animals received an initial s.c. dose of 5 mg of ovalbumin in Freund's complete adjuvant, and 3 weeks later the same dose was repeated in incomplete adjuvant. A week later, daily i.p. administration of 10 mg of ovalbumin was started. Toxic nephropathy was induced by a single intravenous injection of 7.5 mg/Kg of adriamycin to female Wistar rats. Proteinuria was measured by the standard sulphosalicylic method. Serum creatinine, blood cholesterol and serum total proteins were measured by standard autoanalyzer.

Purification of fibronectin and preparation of anti-Rat fibronectin serum Rat plasma FN was purified by affinity chromatography on gelatin-Sepharose as described by Vuento and Vaheri (13). The purified FN showed a single line on Ouchterlony immunodiffusion vs anti-whole rat serum and a single major band at 440 Kd on sodium dodecyl sulfate polyacrylamide gel electrophoresis (SDS-PAGE) (14). Concentration of solutions (Tris 0.05M, NaCl 0.1M, pH 7.5) of purified fibronectin were determinated spectrophotometrically by assuming A (1% 1cm, 280)=12.8 (15).

Antiserum to rat fibronectin was raised in rabbit by subcutaneous injections of 500µg of purified fibronectin, conjugated with complete Freund's adjuvant, followed by several fortnightly boosters. Rabbits were bled and the serum was subjected to ammonium sulphate precipitation and dialysis against phosphate buffer saline (PBS) sodium azide.

Plasma fibronectin determinations Blood samples, collected by cardiac puncture, were anticoagulated with 10% ethylenediaminetetraacetic acid (EDTA), and supplemented with 5mM benzamidine to prevent degradation of fibronectin. The plasma were separated by centrifugation, frozen at -70°C and thawed just before assay.

Fibronectin concentration was determined by Rocket immunoelectrophoresis (Laurell's electroimmunoassay) (16) in 1% agarose (Mr = -13) containing monospecific antiserum a dilution (1/400) and 1% (w/v) polyethylene glycol. Electrophoresis was performed overnight at 1 Volt/cm at 15°C using Tris/barbital buffer (pH 8.6, I=0.02).

Tissue processing Renal tissue for light and electron microscopy was processed as previously described (17). Tissue for electron microscopy was fixed in glutaraldehyde in cacodylate buffer, post-fixed in osmiun tetroxide in veronal buffer, dehydrated in graded alcohols, embedded in Epon 812, stained with uranyl acetate and lead citrate and examined in a Zeiss M 109 electron microscopy.

Statistical methods The paired or unpaired Student's t-test was used to assess significance with the confidence level at 95%. Mean ± SD are presented.

RESULTS

Immune nephritic model Proteinuria prior to development of disease was 8.2 ± 2.2 mg/24 hr (n = 50 animals). As published before (12) proteinuria develops at the 3rd week after the first i.p. ovalbumin administration. At the 4th week around 70% of animals had proteinuria between 40-80 mg/24 hr. The group of rats with proteinuria within these values was studied during 15 days; then, animals were killed and kidney and blood samples taken. Total protein, cholesterol and creatinine serum levels are shown in Table 1.

In histological studies, the glomeruli were uniformly involved by mesangial hypercellularity with increase in mesangial matrix. Prominent and huge mesangial and subendothelial deposits, with thickening and irregularity of the glomerular capillary wall were also seen. Immunofluorescence studies showed initial mesangial deposits of IgG, appearing in the capillary wall when the animals presented proteinuria in nephrotic reach.

Fibronectin determinations in immune nephritis Fibronectin levels were significantly increased (863 ± 153 µg/ml, n=23) in nephritic rat with proteinuria 100 mg/24 hr compared to control rats (350 ± 46, p<0.0005). Nephritic rat with proteinuria <100 mg (53 ± 31 mg/24h) had also increased Fn levels (538 ± 69 µg/ml, p< 0.0005).   Immunised rats without proteinuria had higher FN levels (450 ± 90 µg/ml, p<0.01) than control rats, but less than rats with proteinuria (Figure 1).

Adriamycin nephropathy Proteinuria began on the 7th day after i.v. administration of adriamycin. All rats had heavy proteinuria from the 2nd week (Figure 2). Total protein, cholesterol and creatinine serum levels are shown in Table 1. At the 4th week animals showed striking abnormalities of glomerular epithelial cells with extensive fusion of foot processes and segmental detachment of epithelial cells from the underlying basement membrane.

Fibronectin determinations in adriamycin nephropathy Fibronectin increased significantly (580 ± 110 µg/ml, p<0.0005) from the first week, with greater levels in the 2nd and 3rd weeks (780 ± 133 and 923 ± 180 µg/ml respectively). As can be seen in Figure 2, a relationship was found in the increase of both proteinuria and fibronectin levels.

DISCUSSION

In the model of chronic serum sickness in rats, induced by repeated injections of OVA, we have previously described a functional deficit of Fc receptors (18) and an important role of inflammatory mediators, polymorphonuclear and

TABLE 1. Total protein, cholesterol and creatinine serum levels.

	Total Protein g/dl	Cholesterol mg/dl	Creatinine mg/dl
Control Rats	6.2 ± 0.54 n=7	50 ± 6 n=9	0.7 ± 0.07 n=9
Nephritic Rats Protein >100mg/24hr	4.2 ± 0.6 n=9 p<0.0005	215 ± 67 n=10 p<0.0005	1.2 ± 0.4 n=10 p<0.0025
Adriamycin	5 ± 1.15	202 ± 148	0.8 ± 0.8

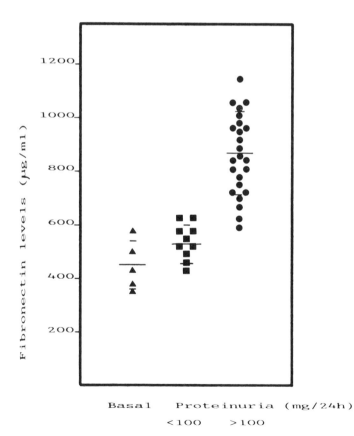

Figure 1. Plasma fibronectin levels in rats with serum sickness nephritis without (triangles) and with proteinuria less than 100mg/12h (squares); and more than 100mg/24h (circles).

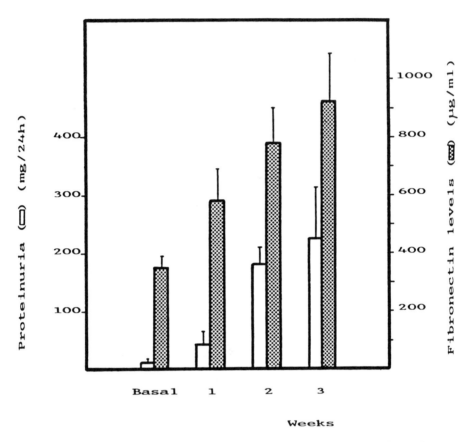

Figure 2. Follow up of proteinuria and FN levels in rats with adriamycin nephropathy.

macrophage cells, contributing to local conditions for immune complexes deposition (12). Adriamycin nephropathy has a clinico-histological picture similar to that observed in minimal change glomerulonephritis in humans, with podocyte alterations consisting of loss of foot processes. We have previously reported the importance of platelet activating factor in the induction of kidney damage in this last model (19). Our results show in both nephropathies that rats with proteinuria present elevated plasma FN levels. In both models, this rise of FN occurred in the early phases. In the immune nephritis moderately high FN levels were detected when proteinuria was not yet present and the glomerular lesions were localized only in the mesangial area. Moreover, these FN levels are progressively increased from the be-

ginning of proteinuria until they reach the nephrotic range (Figure 1). At this stage the glomeruli were uniformly involved with mesangial and subendothelial deposits and thickening of glomerular capillary wall. In the adriamycin nephropathy, FN increases from the 1st to 3rd week in parallel with the increase of proteinuria (Figure 2).

Elevated FN levels may be caused by increased hepatic synthesis, as is the case for other high molecular weight proteins in the nephrotic syndrome. Others have reported FN production by glomerular cells in vitro (20). Intraglomerular FN is localized only in the mesangial area in normal glomeruli. Pericapillary FN distribution occurs with advanced mesangial proliferation and correlated with IgG or C3 deposition in capillary walls (21). Patients with IgA nephropathy have FN-IgA complexes which are preferentially deposited in mesangial structures (22).

The significance of the increased FN is unknown, due to its extensive participation in sundry physiological processes. FN appears to be an opsonic probe for blood-borne and fluid phase tissue and cytoskeletal debris or products of intravascular coagulation and inflammation (6). FN induces an increase in the membrane expression of Fc, C3b (3,23) and C1q (24) receptors in monocytes, therefore enhancing adherence and ingestion of IgG-, C3b- and C1q-coated particles (3-24). Recently, there have been reports about the different actions that the fibronectin degradation products have in the activation of neutrophils and subsequent release of elastase (25) and in augmentation (26) or depression (27,28) of phagocytosis. These studies show the important role of FN in the maintenance of an adequate phagocytic state, in the formation and elimination of immune complexes and production and resolution of inflammatory lesions. Future studies must be carried out to evaluate the nature of the circulating form of the molecule in relation to its functional activity.

ACKNOWLEDGEMENTS

This work was supported by the Fondo de Investigaciones de la Seguridad Social (86/752) and by Fundación Iñigo Alvarez de Toledo.

REFERENCES

1. Mosesson MW, Amrani DL: The structure and biologic activities of plasma fibronectin. Blood 56: 145-158, 1980.

2. Saba TM, Jaffe E: Plasma fibronectin: Its synthesis by vascular endothelial cells and role in cardiopulmonary integrity after trauma as related to reticuloendothelial function. Am J Med 68: 577-593, 1980.

3. Pommier CG, Inada S, Fries LF, Takahashi T, Frank MM, Brown EJ: Plasma fibronectin

enhances phagotyctosis of opsonized particles by human peripheral blood monocytes. J Exp Med 157: 1844-1854, 1983.

4. Eriksen HO, Kalaja E, Jensen BA, Clemmensen I. Plasma fibronectin concentrations in patients with severe burn injury. Burns 10: 422-426, 1984.

5. Mosher DF, Williams EM. Fibronectin concentration is decreased in plasma of severely ill patients with disseminated intravascular coagulation. J Lab Clin Med 91: 729-735, 1978.

6. Saba TM: Plasma and tissue fibronectin: Its role in the pathophysiology of the critically ill septic injured patient. Critical care, state of the art. Edited by B Chernow and WC Shoemaker. Society of critical care medicine, California. Vol 7. 1986, pp 437-464.

7. Todd TR, Glynn MFX, Silver E, Redmond MD: A randomized trial of cryoprecipitate replacement of fibronectin deficiencies in the critically ill. Am Rev Resp Dis 129: A102, 1984.

8. Cooper SM, Keyser AJ, Bearliev AD, Ruoslahti E, Nimni ME, Quismorio FP. Increase in fibronectin in deep dermis of involved skin in progressive systemic sclerosis. Arthritis Rheum 22: 983-987, 1979.

9. Carsons S, Mosesson MW, Diamond HS. Detection and quantitation of Fibronectin in synovial fluid from patients with rheumatic disease. Arthritis Rheum 24: 1261-1267, 1981.

10. Herbert KE, Coppock JS, Griffiths AM, Williams A, Robinson MW, Scott DL. Fibronectin and immune complexes in rheumatic diseases. Annals of Rheum Dis 46: 734-740, 1987.

11. Cosio FG, Bakaletz AP: Abnormal plasma fibronectin levels in patients with proteinuria. J Lab Clin Med 104: 867-872, 1984.

12. Sánchez Crespo M, Alonso F, Barat A, Egido J: Rat serum sickness: possible role of inflammatory mediators allowing deposition of immune complexes in the glomerular basement membrane. Clin Exp Immunol 49: 631-638, 1982.

13. Vuento M, Vaheri A: Purification of Fibronectin from Human Plasma by Affinity Chromatography under Non-Denaturing Conditions. Biochem J 183: 331-337, 1979.

14. Weber K, Osborn M: The reliability of molecular weight determinations by dodecylsulphatepolyacrylamide gel electrophoresis. J Biol Chem 244: 4406-4412, 1969.

15. Mosesson MW, Chen AB, Huseby RM: The cold-insoluble globulin of human plasma studies of its essential structural features. Biochim Biophys Acta 386: 509-524, 1975.

16. Laurell CB: Electroimmunoassay. Scand J Lab Inves 29 Suppl. 124: 21-37, 1972.

17. Quirós J, González-Cabrero J, Herrero-Beaumont G, Egido J: Beneficial effect of fibronectin administration on chronical nephritis in rats. Arthritis Rheum 33:685-692, 1990.

18. Herrero-Beaumont G, Egido J, Sancho J, González E, Castañeda S, Escanero JF: Defective function of the mononuclear phagocytic system in rats with chronic nephritis. Evidence of a decreased degradation of IgG aggregates by Kupffer cells. Immunology 63: 87-92, 1988.

19. Egido J, Ramírez F, Robles A, Ortiz A, Arriba G, Rodríguez MJ, Mampaso F, Braquet P: PAF, adriamycin-induced nephropathy and ginkgolide B. Ginkgolides. Chemistry, Biology, Pharmacology and Clinical Perspectives. P. Braquet (Ed.), 1988, pp 631-640.

20. Oberley TD, Mosher DF, Mills MD. Localization of fibronectin within the renal glomerulus and its production by cultured glomerular cells. Ann J Path 96: 651-662, 1979.

21. Ikeya M, Nagase M, Honda N: Intraglomerular distribution of fibronectin in primary glomerular diseases. Clin Nephrol 24: 53-59, 1985.

22. Cederholm B, Wieslander J, Bygren P, Heinegard D: Circulating complexes containing IgA and fibronectin in patients with primary IgA nephropathy. Proc Natl Acad Sci USA 85: 4865-4868, 1988.

23. Bohnsack JF, O'Shea JJ, Takahashi T, Brown EJ: Fibronectin-enhanced phagocytosis of an alternative pathway activator by human culture-derived macrophages is mediated by the C4b/C3b complement receptor (CR1). J Immunol 135: 2680-2686, 1985.

24. Sorvillo JM, Gigli I, Pearlstein E: The effect of fibronectin on the processing of C1q- and C3b/bi-coated immune complexes by peripheral blood monocytes. J Immunol 136: 1023-1026, 1986.

25. Wachtfogel YT, Abrams W, Kucich U, Weinbaum G, Schapira M, Colman RW: Fibronectin degradation products containing the cytoadhesive tetrapeptide stimulate human neutrophil degranulation. J Clin Inves 81: 1310-1316, 1988.

26. Czop JK, Kadish JL, Austen KF: Augmentation of human monocyte opsonin-independent phagocytosis by fragments of human plasma fibronectin. Proc Natl Acad Sci USA 78: 3649-3653, 1981.

27. Ehrlich MI, Krushell JS, Blumenstock FA, Kaplan JE: Depression of phagocytosis by plasmin degradation products of plasma fibronectin. J Lab Clin Med 98: 263-271, 1981.

28. Rourke FJ, Blumenstock FA, Kaplan JE: Effect of fibronectin fragments on macrophage phagocytosis of gelatinized particles. J Immunol 132: 1931-1936 1984.

78

NEPHROTOXICITY SCREENING IN MARMOSETS: ESTABLISHMENT OF TEST CRITERIA AND VALIDATION USING AN AMINOGLYCOSIDE ANTIBIOTIC

R. Kuzel, T. Perry, G. Ainge and P. Trennery

Toxicology Department, Glaxo Group Research, Ware, Herts., UK

INTRODUCTION

The objectives of a good toxicity screen are to define the adverse effects of new chemical entities on a biological system using simple, rapid, repeatable and preferably non-invasive procedures. Zbinden et al (1) formulated a nephrotoxicity screening test based on the quantitative assessment of urinary components collected under standardised conditions in the Sprague-Dawley rat. Test criteria were based on the statistical distribution of a variety of measurements.

A non-human primate is often a necessary alternative to the dog as a non-rodent experimental animal in regulatory toxicology and because marmosets (Callithrix jacchus) readily breed in captivity and can be group housed they present an ethically more acceptable primate than many of the larger species. It was considered important, therefore, to establish a similar nephrotoxicity screening test for the marmoset.

Firstly, it was necessary to generate data in healthy animals to calculate test criteria for routine urine analyses. Secondly, to validate the procedure, the aminoglycoside antibiotic neomycin was used. Finally, we investigated whether the measurements selected were more sensitive and earlier indicators of neomycin-induced nephrotoxicity than blood urea or creatinine measurements or light and electron microscopy.

METHODS

1. <u>Establishment of Test Criteria</u> Marmosets of both sexes, approximately one year of age, were individually housed in stainless steel metabolism cages for periods of 16.5 hr. Urine was collected with animals having free access to drinking water, but not food. During routine safety evaluation studies, urine is collected into glass containers at room temperature; this procedure was also adopted in this exercise. Many enzymes are unstable in urine kept at room temperature and could, therefore, not be measured.

Water intake and total urinary volume were noted prior to the following measurements being performed on the fresh urine:

pH		)
Protein	g/l	)
Glucose	mmol/l	)
Ketones	mmol/l	)
Bilirubin	mg/dl	) Multistix 10-SG on
Blood	mg/dl free Hb	) Clinitek 200
Urobilinogen	mol/l	)
Nitrite	mol/l	)
Leucocytes	per l	)
Specific Gravity		)

N-Acetyl-a-D-glucosaminidase (NAG) (expressed as a ratio to urinary creatinine) mol/l:mmol/l

After centrifugation for 20 minutes at 400g, the sediment was stained with Modified Sternheimer - Malbin reagent and a sample examined under the microscope. The following were assessed:

Cumulative number seen in 5 objective fields (x40):

Epithelia - Squamous
Epithelia - Non-squamous
Spermatozoa (if more than 50, then 50 was recorded)
Erythrocytes
Leucocytes
Casts

Average percent cover of 5 objective fields (x40):

Bacteria
Crystals
Amorphous Debris

All data were stored in an RS1 (BBN Software Product Corp) statistical database on a VAX 8700 (128Mb) computer.

Test criteria were set at an error probability of 5%. Non-normally distributed data were ranked and non-parametric limits set by selecting the 2.5 and 97.5 percentiles.

2. Validation It was considered inappropriate to expose large numbers of marmosets to the effects of a known nephrotoxin. Therefore, four animals (2 male, 2 female) only were dosed on a daily basis with 35mg/kg/day neomycin (Neobiotic-Upjohn) intramuscularly. Whenever changes to blood urea and/or creatinine were noted, dosing was stopped and recovery monitored.

The above approach was designed to investigate which measures were useful as early indicators and their subsequent usefulness with continued treatment. A second experiment was employed to investigate whether urinary measurements proved to be earlier indicators of neomycin-induced nephrotoxicity than either blood parameters, light microscopy or electron microscopy. A further 4 marmosets were dosed for 3 days only with 35mg/kg/day neomycin. Urine was collected overnight on the third day and samples of blood taken for urea and creatinine measurements. One marmoset was then killed by barbiturate overdosage and the kidneys were fixed in formalin. Haematox-

ylin and eosin stained 5 μm paraffin sections and resin embedded Toluidine blue stained 1 μm sections were examined by light microscopy. For electron microscopy ultra-thin sections were examined in a Philips CM10 transmission electron microscope.

RESULTS

1. Test Criteria

The statistical data and subsequent test criteria established in both male and female marmosets are presented in Table 1.

2. Validation

Three measurements were identified in this study as being useful markers in the marmoset of nephrotoxicity caused by neomycin.

The presence of renal tubular cells was consistently seen as the first change but numbers returned to within established criteria if dosing was continued.

Although not as sensitive, urinary NAG:creatinine concentrations were elevated in all animals. Insufficient data were collected to establish test criteria with this measurement, but elevations were between 10- and 100-fold the mean value obtained from animals before treatment commenced and continued to increase until dosing was stopped.

The dip-stick test for glucose proved to be a good early indicator of damage. Inter-individual variation within our untreated marmosets was nil (dip-stick test) so this marker was also quite sensitive.

In the second experiment, we measured urinary glucose concentration using an automated technique and the results of these and other data are presented in Table 2.

The large numbers of renal tubular cells present in the urine was the most dramatic effect seen, with urinary NAG concentration also being significantly increased in all 4 animals. Plasma creatinine and BUN were not convincingly affected.

TABLE 1: Test criteria for urinary measurements in male and female marmosets.

Variable constituents	No.of samples M	F	Mean (sem) M	F	Median M	F	Skewness M	F	Kurtosis M	F	Distribution M	F	Test Criteria M	F
pH	114	122	6.13 (0.08)	5.88 (0.06)	6.0	6.0	0.16	0.21	-0.277	-0.54	D	D	5,7.5	5,7
PROT	126	122	0.15 (0.02)	0.17 (0.02)	0.05	0.05	3.14	2.95	10.09	9.09	D	D	0.05,1.0	0.05,1.0
GLU	113	122	1.4 (0.0)	1.4 (0.0)	1.4	1.4	-	-	-	-	D	D	1.4	1.4
KET	113	122	0.49 (0.06)	0.74 (0.06)	0.25	0.25	4.35	2.00	22.35	6.5	D	D	0.25,1.9	0.25,1.9
BILI	113	122	0.3 (0.02)	0.28 (0.01)	0.25	0.25	3.14	4.22	8.05	16.08	D	D	0.25,0.9	0.25,0.9
BLOOD	113	122	0.05 (0.007)	0.06 (0.007)	0.023	0.023	1.93	1.77	2.48	1.93	D	D	0.0075,0.3	0.0075,0.3
UROB	113	122	3.2 (0.0)	3.2 (0.0)	3.2	3.2	-	-	-	-	D	D	3.2	3.2
NIT	113	122	6.58 (0.31)	6.98 (0.29)	9.75	9.75	-0.05	-0.3	-2.03	-1.94	D	D	3.25,9.75	3.25,9.75
LEUC	113	128	0.13 (0.13)	1.02 (0.59)	0	0	10.63	9.09	113.0	91.42	D	D	0.0,0.0	0.0,15.0
SP.GR	113	122	1.02 (0.00)	1.02 (0.00)	1.015	1.02	0.31	-0.15	-0.76	-0.328	D	D	1.005,1.03	1.005,1.03
RBC	80	103	20.43 (6.27)	14.17 (1.16)	10.0	12.0	8.1	0.83	69.81	0.53	LN	N	1.0,164.75	1.0,48.025
WBC	81	103	3.77 (2.14)	10.05 (3.63)	0.00	0.0	7.12	6.58	54.91	49.85	NN	LN	1.0,159.0	1.0,300.7
CASTS	82	103	1.9 (0.96)	1.14 (0.33)	0.0	0.0	6.11	4.73	38.11	23.92	NN	NN	1,10.0	1,8.0
BACT	89	106	45.4 (3.44)	43.87 (2.75)	40.0	40.0	0.32	0.31	-1.41	-1.27	NN	NN	10,100	10,100
CRYS	81	103	4.3 (0.68)	3.3 (0.62)	0.0	0.0	1.44	2.21	2.7	5.39	NN	NN	0,10	0,10
SQ.EP	81	103	3.33 (0.43)	5.13 (0.81)	2.0	3.0	1.26	5.64	0.92	43.7	LN	LN	1,15.2	1,20.85
NON SQ.EP	80	103	0.28 (0.14)	0.64 (0.139)	0.00	0.00	5.65	2.43	34.14	5.54	NN	NN	0,6.0	0,3.0
SPERM	78	103	10.59 (4.63)	0.0 (0.00)	0.0	0.00	4.37	0.0	19.75	0.0	NN	NN	0,175.9	0.0,0.0
AMOR.DEB	81	104	0.37 (0.21)	0.19 (0.19)	0.00	0.00	4.99	10.20	23.54	104.0	NN	NN	0,10	0.0,0.0
URINE VOL	116	124	9.06 (0.8)	9.5 (0.68)	6.0	7.0	1.88	1.51	3.54	2.6	LN	LN	1,36.3	1,32.63
WATER IN	114	124	7.5 (0.8)	6.5 (0.95)	3.5	2.8	2.21	3.92	6.11	18.11	LN	LN	0.7,31.6	0.9,44.4
NAG:CREAT	18		20.4 (2.42)		18.85		0.95		0.21		NN	NN	8.84	31.34

N = Normal : NN = Non-normal : LN = Log Normal : D = Discreet

TABLE 2: The influence of 3 days dosing with 35mg/kg/day neomycin on selected blood and urinary measurements.

Animal Number	Predose	Day 3	
N147	10.87	15.30	Blood Urea Nitrogen
N175	10.02	7.88	(mmol/l)
N185	10.08	11.24	
N104	10.12	11.23	
N147	61	74	Plasma Creatinine
N175	56	47	(umol/l)
N185	50	58	
N104	57	70	
N147	9.6	31.5	(Urinary
N175	19.9	72.0	NAG:creatinine
N185	26.3	145.2	(umol/l:mmol/l)
N104	16.5	52.2	
N147	0	195	Urinary
N175	0	99	Renal Tubular Cells
N185	0	107	(No/ml)
N104	0	77	
N147	0.18	0.38	Urinary
N175	0.18	0.60	Glucose (mmol/l)
N185	0.15	0.51	
N104	0.27	0.27	

Examination of haematoxylin and eosin stained paraffin sections of the kidneys from marmoset N185 showed no abnormalities. However, 1 μm resin sections stained by Toluidine blue showed a dramatic increase in the number of secondary lysosomes present in proximal convoluted tubule cells. This finding was confirmed by electron microscopy which revealed that the lysosomes very often contained myeloid bodies. In addition, the shape of the mitochondria in such cells was more irregular than that seen in untreated marmosets of a similar age.

DISCUSSION

The test criteria for a number of routinely measured urinary parameters have been established. This study highlights the lack of specificity of a number of the routine measures undertaken. Variances were wide in normal urine (hence test criteria) and thus these measures were probably of limited use in routine screening procedures. They were, notably, red and white blood cells, water intake and the presence of bacteria in the urine. Conversely, a number of measurements exhibited only slight inter-individiual variation and thus, may have potential as markers of change.

Validation of the procedures using neomycin was performed following 2 dose regimes; the first to identify consistent markers with dosing over 9-15 days and the second to find the earliest markers after a much shorter exposure time to the nephrotoxin.

The first experiment showed the lack of changes in most of the measurements undertaken in the marmoset. There were three notable exceptions; urinary NAG, urinary glucose (when semi-quantitatively assessed by 'dip-stick test') and the presence of renal tubular cells in the urine.

Dosing for 3 days only was demonstrated to have caused ultrastructural changes which could be detected using the 3 markers above. Of the 3, presence of renal tubular cells in urine was the most dramatic effect with urinary NAG concentration also clearly elevated. Glucose concentration was not significantly altered in 1/4 marmosets, thus, perhaps indicating that this measurement is not as consistent a marker as the other two. The repeated dosing of neomycin for over a week revealed the ineffectiveness of renal tubular cells as detectors in a long term regime whereas both urinary glucose and NAG concentration were robust markers of nephrotoxic potential. These urinary criteria are not necessarily any earlier detectors of renal damage than electron microscopy, however, as increased secondary lysosomes were noted in the proximal tubule cells of rats as early as 48 hr after gentamycin treatment (2). The selected criteria do provide, however, a non-invasive method of detecting early renal damage by aminoglycoside antibiotics. Plasma urea and creatinine proved to be insensitive markers of this level of toxic insult.

Haematuria and the increased excretion of leucocytes, a frequent finding in rat studies following nephrotoxic insult (3), proved insensitive in the marmoset. Protein excretion, considered a sensitive marker in the clinical situation, was not particularly useful in the marmoset.

REFERENCES

1. Zbinden G, Kent K, Thouin MH. Nephrotoxicity screening in rats; general approach and establishment of test criteria. Arch Toxicol 61:344-348, 1988.

2. Kosek JC, Masse RI, Cousins MJ. Nephrotoxicity of Gentamycin. Lab Invest 30:48-57, 1974.

3. Fent K, Mayer E, Zbinden G. Nephrotoxicity screening in rats: a validation study. Arch Toxicol 61:349-358, 1988.

79

PROTON NUCLEAR MAGNETIC RESONANCE URINALYSIS AND CLINICAL CHEMICAL STUDIES ON THE PROGRESSION AND RECOVERY OF NEPHROTOXIC LESIONS INDUCED IN RATS BY BROMOETHANAMINE AND HgCl2

E. Holmes (1), F.W. Bonner (2), K.P.R. Gartland (1) and J.K. Nicholson (1)

Department of Chemistry, Birkbeck College, University of London, 29 Gordon Square, London WC1H 0PP UK (1) and Department of Toxicology, Sterling-Winthrop Research Centre, Northumberland UK (2)

INTRODUCTION

Proton nuclear magnetic resonance (PMR) spectroscopy is a powerful tool for determining novel biochemical markers of region-specific nephrotoxicity and monitoring the biochemical effects following nephrotoxic insult (1-5). In particular, PMR can be used to investigate the biochemical changes that occur at the onset and during the progression of the nephrotoxic lesion (1-5). However, little PMR work has been performed on the biochemical changes associated with recovery of renal function and renal tubular regeneration. In the present study we have investigated the biochemical changes associated with cellular regeneration following insult with HgCl2 (a proximal tubular toxin) and bromoethanamine hydrobromide (BEA, a toxin causing renal papillary necrosis). HgCl2 causes necrosis of the epithelial cells lining the pars recta of the proximal tubule and the primary mechanism of toxicity involves the combination with biological sulphydryl groups resulting in the inhibition of a number of key enzyme systems, especially those in Krebs cycle (1,6). BEA produces renal papillary necrosis (RPN) mimicking several of the clinical features associated with analgesic nephropathy. Following a single injection of BEA, the percentage of filtering juxtamedullary nephrons is markedly reduced (7). In the present study, conducted over 14 days, the changes in both endogenous and exogenous metabolites following single injections of BEA and HgCl2 were examined. PMR spectroscopy was used as the main analytical tool supported by renal histopathology and conventional clinical chemistry methods.

METHODS

Animals and treatments. Twenty-four male Fischer 344 rats were allocated to 3 groups (n=8) and given single i.p. injections of either 0.9% saline (control), 1 mg/kg HgCl2 or 150 mg/kg BEA in saline. Rats were housed individually in metabolism cages for a period of 2 days prior to dosing to permit acclimatisation, and urine was collected at the following time points: 0-8 hr (day 1), 8-24 hr (day 1), 0-8 hr (day 2), 8-24 hr (day 2), 8-24 hr (day 3), 8-24 hr (day 6), 8-24 hr (day 9), 8-24 hr (day 15). Rats were allowed free access to food and water throughout the experiment.

Clinical chemistry. Creatinine, lactate, alkaline phosphatase (ALP), gamma-glutamyl transpeptidase (GGT) and Lactic dehydrogenase (LDH) were measured in urine using Baker assay kits. Urinary volumes and osmolalities were also determined.

PMR Urinalysis. Urine was corrected for urinary flow rate by the method described previously (2), lyophilised and reconstituted in ^2H_2O. PMR spectra were recorded on Bruker WH400 and AM400 spectrometers at 400MHz at ambient probe temperatures (298 $\pm$ 1°K).

Water suppression was achieved using gated irradiation. For each urine sample 64 free induction decays (FIDs) were collected into 16,384 data points and zero-filled to 32,768 data points. The pulse width used was typically 45°, the acquisition time was 1.7 seconds and a 2-3 seconds delay between pulses was employed to ensure that the spectra were fully T_1 relaxed. An exponential line broadening function of 0.5 Hz was applied prior to Fourier transformation. Shifts were referenced to internal sodium 3-trimethylsilyl-[2,2,3,3,-^{2}H]-1-propionate

(TSP; d = 0 ppm). Resonance assignments were made by chemical shift, spin-spin coupling patterns, pH-dependencies of chemical shifts and ultimately standard addition employing the procedure adapted by Bales et al (8).

RESULTS AND DISCUSSION

Tables 1 and 2 demonstrate the overall patterns of change in urinary creatinine, lactate and selected enzymes following single i.p. injections of BEA or HgCl2. These are region-specific nephrotoxins affecting different

TABLE 1. Urinary creatinine, lactate, ALP, GGT and LDH from control and BEA-treated rats.

Time point	Creatinine (umol/hr)	Lactate (mmol/hr)	ALP (U/hr)	LDH (U/hr)	GGT (U/hr)
Control	3.3±0.47	0.34±0.05	179.0±37.6	20.8±2.7	719.4±142.0
Day 1	2.9±0.23	1.10±0.12	192.6±49.4	64.9±8.1	626.0±161.0
Day 2	3.6±0.31	0.61±0.09	208.4±80.7	34.8±7.3	823.5±247.7
Day 3	3.8±0.76	0.52±0.10	198.1±19.8	20.2±4.0	599.2±225.4
Day 6	3.9±0.38	0.44±0.04	178.1±41.0	17.9±2.7	646.5±135.5
Day 9	3.3±0.49	0.40±0.05	180.9±28.0	18.9±5.3	550.0±105.1

Values represent the mean ± the standard deviation of the 8-24 hr time points from the days listed. n = 8 rats for all groups.

TABLE 2. Urinary creatinine, lactate, ALP, GGT and LDH from control and HgCl2-treated rats.

Time	Creatinine (umol/hr)	Lactate (mmol/hr)	ALP (U/hr)	LDH (U/hr)	GGT (U/hr)
Control	2.9±0.07	0.33±0.04	174.7±44.6	19.5±3.3	595.2±84.7
Day1	3.4±0.27	1.78±1.2	1322.5±436.5	1013.6±488.7	9345.6±893.9
Day 2	3.3±0.30	8.9±1.8	530.1±254.7	800.9±246.5	2298.5±896.3
Day 3	4.0±0.46	5.7±1.9	118.0±20.1	58.1±14.0	359.2±80.6
Day 6	3.6±0.19	0.55±0.06	77.4±13.6	18.5±2.1	198.5±42.7
Day 9	3.0±0.19	0.42±0.03	78.8±20.1	13.0±5.8	236.9±44.7

Values represent the mean ± the standard deviation of the 8-24 hr time points from the days listed. n = 8 rats for all groups.

portions of the nephron and cause correspondingly different perturbations of urinary metabolites. Changes in PMR spectra of urine following nephrotoxic insult with BEA and HgCl$_2$ over a 15 day time course are shown in Figures 1 and 2 respectively.

Bromoethanamine: Conventional analysis indicates that BEA produces a marked reduction in urine osmolality and a considerable, sustained increase in volume from 0-8 hr on day 1 (data not shown). Modest enzymuria is also apparent (2,7). Metabolites of BEA appear in PMR spectra of urine within 8 hr after dosing (day 1) and are also present in minor quantities at 8-24 hr (day 1). Bach et al (9) observed as many as 10 urinary metabolites using high performance liquid chromatography but did not succeed in structurally identifying them. These metabolites remain unidentified. At day 3 urinary levels of succinate and 2-OG increase. Succinic aciduria is also a feature of urine from rats dosed with propylene imine (2), another papillary toxin. Elevations in urinary dimethylamine and trimethylamine-N-oxide are also a feature of BEA toxicity. Modest increases in lactate and glucose levels were seen by PMR urinalysis following BEA (Figure 1). PMR urinalysis indicates that a recovery of normal urinary metabolite levels following a single dose of BEA is achieved by day 6 and, further, that maximal metabolic perturbations occur throughout the 8-48 hr period after dosing.

Mercuric Chloride: Considerable elevations in glucose were seen at 8-24 hr (day 1) which were sustained until day 3 together with an elevation in taurine levels occurring as early as 0-8 hr post dosing. Other features include aminoaciduria (alanine, glutamine, lysine and valine) beginning at 0-8 hr (day 2) - alanine and lactate levels increasing during the earlier time point (Figure 2). HgCl$_2$ causes a progressive hypocitraturia, the lowest level of urinary citrate seen throughout the 8-24 hr period of day 2. 15. Succinate and 2-OG also decrease soon after dosing (Figure 2). Conventional analyses reveal a slight increase in urinary volume and a pulse in enzyme levels at 8h which return to control levels at day 3. The perturbed metabolite patterns discernible from PMR urinalysis results suggest that the maximal perturbations in renal biochemistry occur between 8 and 72 hr after HgCl$_2$ treatment. Urine spectra measured at day 6 are very similar to controls indicating that full tubular regeneration has occurred (Figure 2).

These results show that PMR urinalysis is clearly of value in following the time-course-related perturbations in renal biochemistry following nephrotoxic insult and that information relevant to cellular regeneration can also be obtained.

ACKNOWLEDGEMENTS

We thank Sterling-Winthrop and The National Kidney Research Fund, for financial support of this and related work. We thank the MRC for use of central NMR facilities. EH is grateful to the Science and Engineering Research Council for a studentship.

REFERENCES

1. Nicholson JK, Timbrell JA, Sadler PJ: Proton NMR spectra of urine as indicators of renal damage: Mercury-induced nephrotoxicity in rats. Mol Pharmacol 27: 644-651, 1985.

2. Gartland KPR, Bonner FW, Nicholson JK: Investigations into the biochemical effects of region specific nephrotoxins. Mol Pharmacol 35: 242-250, 1989.

3. Gartland KPR, Bonner FW, Nicholson JK: The biochemical characterisation of p-aminophenol-induced nephrotoxic lesions in the F344 rat. Arch Toxicol 63: 97-106, 1989.

4. Nicholson JK, Gartland KPR: A nuclear magnetic resonance approach to investigate the biochemical and molecular effects of nephrotoxins. In: Reed E, Cook GMW, Luzio JP (eds); Methodological Surveys in Biochemistry and Analysis. Vol. 17 (Cells, Membranes and Disease, Including Renal). London, Plenum Press, 1987, pp. 397-408.

5. Gartland KPR, Bonner FW and Nicholson JK. Application of proton NMR urinalysis to the

BROMOETHANAMINE

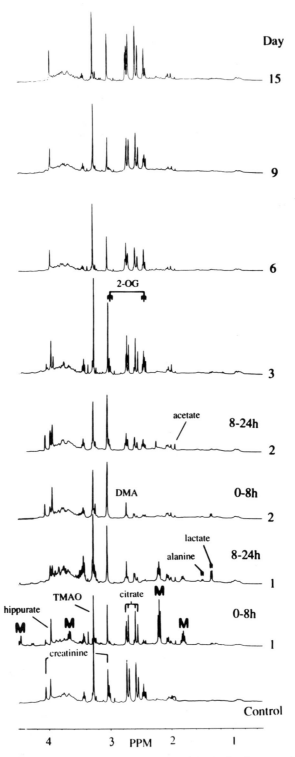

Figure 1. 400 MHz PMR spectra (region to low frequency of water) of urine from rats before (control) and at various times up to 15 days following 150 mg/kg BEA. See text for experimental conditions. DMA, dimethylamine; DMG, N,N-dimethylglycine; TMAO, trimethylamine N-oxide; M, metabolites of BEA.

MERCURIC CHLORIDE

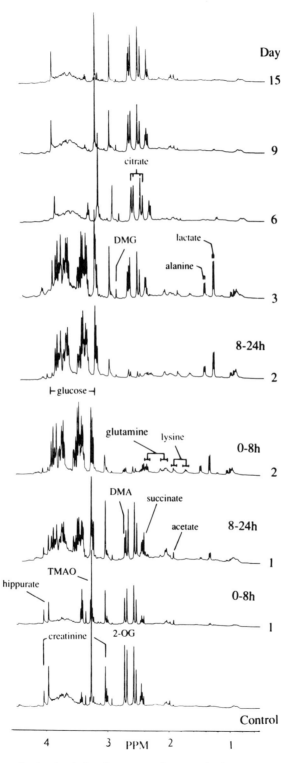

Figure 2. 400 MHz PMR spectra (region to low frequency of water) of urine from rats before (control) and at various times up to 15 days following 1 mg/kg HgCl₂. See text for experimental conditions. DMA, dimethy-lamine; DMG, N,N-dimethylglycine; TMAO, trimethylamine N-oxide

examination of nephrotoxic lesions induced in rats by HgCl2, hexachloro-1,3-butadiene, and propylene imine. In: Bach PH, Lock EA (eds); Nephrotoxicity: Extrapolation from in vitro to in vivo and from animals to man. London, Plenum Press, 1989, pp. 505-518.

6. Biber TUL, Mylle M, Baines AD, et al.: A study in micropuncture and microdissection of acute renal damage in rats. Am J Med 44: 664-705, 1968.

7. Sabatini, S. Pathophysiology of drug induced papillary necrosis. Fund Appl Toxicol 4: 909-921, 1984.

8. Bales JR, Higham DP, Howe I, et al.: The use of high resolution proton NMR spectroscopy for rapid multi-component analysis of urine. Clin Chem 30: 426-432, 1984.

9. Bach PH, Bridges JW, Grasso P et al.: Changes in medullary glycosaminoglycan histochemistry and microvascular filling during the developement of 2-bromoethanamine hydrobromide-induced renal papillary necrosis. Toxicol Appl Pharmacol 69: 333-344, 1983.

80

COMPUTER PATTERN RECOGNITION ANALYSIS OF PMR SPECTROSCOPIC DATA FROM URINE OBTAINED FROM RATS IN VARIOUS NEPHROTOXICITY STATES

K.P.R. Gartland (1), C.R. Beddell (2), J.C. Lindon (2) and J.K. Nicholson (1)

Department of Chemistry, Birkbeck College, University of London, Gordon House, 29 Gordon Square, London WC1H OPP U.K. (1) and Department of Physical Sciences, The Wellcome Research Laboratories, Langley Court, Beckenham, Kent BR3 3BS U.K. (2)

INTRODUCTION

In recent years we have explored the application of high resolution proton nuclear magnetic resonance (PMR) spectroscopic analysis of blood, plasma, urine and other body fluids to investigate metabolic disorders, drug metabolism and toxicity states in man and animals (1). PMR studies on body fluids and intact cell systems can provide detailed information on the biochemical and toxicological effects of a wide range of xenobiotic compounds. Although conventional enzymatic and chromatographic methods may be more sensitive than PMR for detecting low levels of metabolites, significant advantages may be conferred by using PMR to follow biochemical responses of animals or cells to foreign compounds. These are best understood by considering a key question in mechanistic toxicology i.e. "What is the critical biochemical lesion in the cell and how does this relate mechanistically to the exhibited pathological condition?". To answer this question using a conventional bioanalytical approach normally requires the subjective selection of a battery of biochemical methods to be used in conjunction with histopathological techniques in both in vivo and selected in vitro systems. This is necessarily a complex and time consuming process and if an inappropriate range of biochemical methods or metabolic parameters is used, important metabolic disturbances may be overlooked. PMR spectroscopy is well suited to the study of toxicological events, as multi-component analyses on biological materials can be made simultaneously, without bias imposed by the experimenters' expectations of toxin-induced metabolic changes. For example, the PMR spectrum of a biofluid or tissue extract gives a characteristic (fingerprint) pattern of resonances for a range of important endogenous metabolites (1). Quantifiable changes in metabolite patterns often give information not only on the location and severity of a toxic lesion, but also insights into the underlying biochemical features of the toxic process (2-5). These patterns are often unique for different toxin types and hence can be used as a basis for their classification. PMR spectra of biological materials are very rich in information which is carried in the overall pattern of the metabolite resonances. However, the information contained in the PMR biofluid metabolite patterns is often extremely complex, and subtle biochemical alterations may be lost even in extensive conventional quantitative and statistical analysis of the spectral data. We have, therefore, used a computer-based pattern recognition (PR) approach to analyse the PMR urinalysis data obtained in various experimental nephrotoxicity states. The object being to uncover new relationships between urinary metabolites that may be relevant to the understanding of toxicological mechanisms, and to find combinations of novel diagnostic markers that may be useful in screening for toxic side-effects of experimental therapeutic agents.

METHODS

Experimental details pertaining to animals, doses etc. are described in Table 1. Any increase in urine flow rate caused by the toxins was corrected by lyophilisation of a calculated volume using the method described by Gartland et al. (4). PMR measurements were made at 400 MHz (9.4 Tesla). All other PMR experimental conditions are as described previously (4). Pattern recognition (PR) is a general term applied to methods of data analysis which can cope not only with fully quantitative data, but also with discrete or scored data, for example, that obtained from histological or behavioural studies or in this case semi-quantitative PMR studies. PMR spectra of urine (containing equal concentrations of 3-trimethylsilyl-[2,2,3,3-^{2}H$_4$]-1-pro-pionate (TSP)) from rats exposed to six nephrotoxins were compared with spectra obtained from untreated control animals at the same time-point plotted on the same vertical scale.

The following seven-level scoring system was employed relating to metabolite signal intensities and the added standard: +3, a major elevation in urinary concentration corresponding to 3 times control level; +2, a significant elevation corresponding to 2 to 3-times control; +1, a visually detectable, but minor elevation of <2-times control level; 0, not detectably different from control; -1, minor reduction (up to 50% of control); -2, moderate reduction (50-90% reduction from control); -3, signals from metabolite not detectable by PMR spectroscopy.

This procedure is rapid and easy to apply and generates a scaled matrix containing information on the changes in metabolite concentrations induced by various classes of toxin (Table 2).

The data set was analysed using a variety of pattern recognition methods including mainly non-linear mapping and principal components analysis (PCA) which form part of the software package ARTHUR running on a DEC VAX 11/750 computer. Non-linear mapping techniques were introduced to the chemical literature by Kowalski and Bender (6) based on the method published by Sammon (7). The methods work in the multi-dimensional parameter space where in this case each dimension is the concentration of one metabolite but can also provide dimension reduction techniques for display purposes. In simple terms the technique of non-linear mapping presents the data values as coordinates in n-dimensional space and then compresses this into a non-linear map (NLM) which is a 2-dimensional approximation to the true multidimensional interpoint distances. Two

Table 1. Doses, routes, and vehicles employed for the administration of the 6 nephrotoxins.

Treatment	Rat Strain (n)*	Dose	route	vehicle	Urine Collection Points		
					0-8	8-24	24-48h
Control	F344 (5)	—	i.p.	saline	+	+	+
PAP	F344 (3)	100 mg/kg	"	saline	+	+	+
Na$_2$CrO$_4$	" (5)	20 mg/kg	s.c	"	+	+	+
HgCl$_2$	" (4)	2 mg/kg	i.p.	"	+	+	+
HCBD	" (5)	200 mg/kg	"	corn oil	+	+	+
PI	" (5)	20 ul/kg	"	saline	+	+	+
BEA	" (5)	250 mg/kg	"	"	+	+	+

*number of rats. PAP: p-aminophenol; Na$_2$CrO$_4$: sodium chromate; HgCl$_2$: mercuric chloride; HCBD: hexachlorobutadiene; PI, propylene imine; BEA: bromoethanamine.

Table 2. Scored data for 16 metabolites obtained from PMR spectra of urine following exposure to 6 region-specific nephrotoxins[a].

	HgCl$_2$	PAP	Na$_2$CrO$_4$	HCBD	PI	BEA
acet	1	1	1	1	3	2
ala	1	2	1	2	1	1
HB	0	1	0	1	0	0
cn	-1	-1	-1	0	0	0
cit	-3	-2	0	0	1	-2
glc	2	3	3	3	1	1
gln	1	2	2	2	0	0
2-OG	-2	-1	-1	-1	-2	-3
hip	-1	-1	-2	-3	0	-1
lac	3	3	1	3	1	1
suc	-3	1	-1	1	3	2
TMAO	-2	0	0	0	-3	-3
val	1	2	0	2	0	0
DMA	-1	0	0	0	2	2
lys	1	2	1	2	0	0
DMG	0	0	0	0	3	3

See methods section for a description of the scoring system used. For key to metabolite abbreviations see legend to Figure 2.

points which are close on the map should be more similar in terms of input variables than two distant points. PCA is a well established statistical technique for dimension reduction (8,9). Principal components (PCs) are new variables created from linear combinations of the starting variables with appropriate weighting coefficients. The properties of these PCs are such that: (i) Each PC is orthogonal (uncorrelated) with all other PCs, (ii) The first PC contains the largest part of the variance (information content) of the data set with subsequent PCs containing correspondingly smaller amounts of variance. Thus a plot of the first and second PCs which may have negligible contributions from some of the input parameters gives a selective representation in terms of information content of the data.

RESULTS

The urinary excretion pattern of endogenous metabolites detected by PMR spectroscopy following toxic insult, depends strongly on the site

of action of the toxin and the perturbed biochemical processes that are involved. The PMR spectra obtained from rats following exposure to a variety of toxins are shown in Figure 1. The change in pattern of low molecular weight (MW) metabolites following proximal tubular insult consists of glycosuria, aminoaciduria and L-lactic aciduria, although the latter two changes are more marked following necrosis of the pars recta (induced by p-aminophenol) than the pars convoluta (induced by sodium chromate) (Figure 1). This pattern of perturbed urinary metabolites is distinct to that seen following toxicity to the renal papilla induced by propylene imine (PI) or bromoethanamine (BEA). Elevations in urinary dimethylamine (DMA), N,N-dimethylglycine (DMG), succinate and acetate can be seen in urine following exposure to these toxins. However, differences exist in the pattern of urinary metabolites following exposure to PI or BEA. PI causes a minor elevation in urinary L-lactate while BEA causes a hypocitraturia (Figure 1).

Non-linear maps (NLM) and principal component plots of toxins in metabolite space show clustering of toxins according to the site of toxicity (Figure 2A and B). PCA of metabolites in toxin space, the transposition of the dataset, shows clustering of markers of site-specific nephrotoxicity (Figure 2C). Amino acids, lactate and glucose are known markers of proximal tubular injury and cluster together, while succinate, TMAO, N,N-dimethylglycine and dimethylamine form another cluster of markers associated with renal papillary necrosis (Figure 2C). 3-D-Hydroxybutyrate (HB) is also associated with proximal tubular necrosis in particular that caused by PAP, HCBD and uranyl nitrate (4,5,10). A further cluster seen in Figure 2C comprising of citrate (cit), creatinine (cn), hippurate (hip) and 2-oxoglutarate (2-OG) represents a zone of activity of metabolites which can be described as non-specific renal markers, that is, they display altered excretion following both proximal tubular necrosis and RPN (Figure 2C).

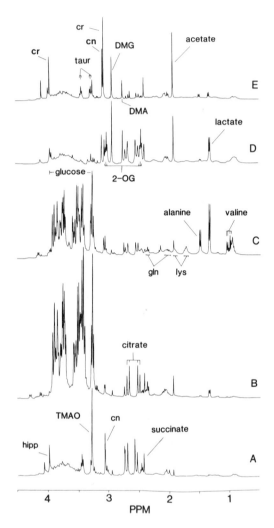

Figure 1. 400 MHzPMR spectra (region to low frequency of water) of 24 hr urines obtained from a control rat (A) and 24-48hr after dosing with 2 mg/k Na₂CrO (b) 10 mg/k PA (C) 2 μl/kg PI (D) and 250 mg/kg BEA. Abbreviations: cr, creatine; taur, taurine; other abbreviations are as in the legend to Figure 2.

DISCUSSION

PMR provides a simple and elegant method for detecting and monitoring toxicity through body fluid analysis. However, the complexity of biofluid PMR spectra requires that considerable care be taken in the interpretation and analysis steps in order to extract meaningful biological data and this approach to toxicological assessment is still at an early stage of development. The present studies show that PR provides an efficient means of reducing a large dataset to interpretable proportions and also classifies the toxins in terms of biochemical effects using a large number of metabolic dimensions. We have used 16 metabolic dimensions in the present study but many other metabolites (especially those present in lower concentrations) could also be used as input data for the PR routines, possibly giving increased discriminatory power.

PMR urinalysis has uncovered novel combination metabolic markers of organ-specific toxicity in the laboratory rat. For example, increased levels of acetate, DMA, DMG, succinate and TMAO may be indicative of damage to the renal papilla (4,5). In effect this means that the diagnosis of RPN can only be made with confidence if all of these metabolites appear in abnormal levels. This conclusion is supported by PR analysis (Figure 2). DMA, DMG and TMAO are chemically related to the trimethylamines that are known to be present in the inner medulla of the kidney at high concentrations where they function as osmolytes (11); the occurrence of elevated levels of these compounds in the urine following renal papillary damage may therefore also have mechanistic significance during the onset and progression of the disease process. At present there are no known biochemical markers for renal papillary damage in man, a condition that may occur in nephrogenic diabetes insipidus or in analgesic nephropathy (which has a poorly understood mechanism) following long term non-steroidal anti-inflammatory drug therapy. The novel combination markers for renal medullary damage detected by PMR with pattern recognition analysis may be clinically relevent and the detection of these substances in the urine may help in the early detection of analgesic nephropathy.

PMR based toxicological methods should at least for the present time be regarded as a novel means of supplementing conventional toxicity data. The technique shows consider-

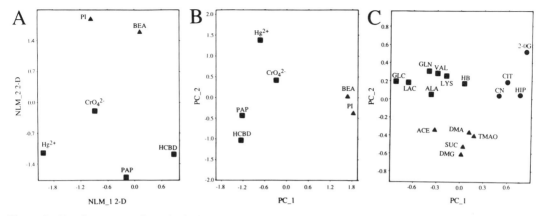

Figure 2. Non-linear map (A) and principal components plot (B) of toxins in metabolite space and metabolites in toxin space (C). Key to parts A and B: square represents toxicity to the proximal tubule; triangle represents toxicity to the renal papilla. BEA, bromoethanamine; CrO42-, sodium chromate; HCBD, hexachlorobutadiene; Hg2+, mercuric chloride; PAP, p-aminophenol; PI, propylene imine. Key to part C: square represents markers of proximal tubular toxicity; triangle represents markers of renal papillary toxicity; circle represents other less closely assigned markers. ac, acetate; ala, alanine; cit, citrate; cn, creatinine; DMA, dimethylamine; DMG, N,N-dimethylglycine; glc, glucose; gln, glutamine; hipp, hippurate; lac, lactate; lys, lysine; 2-OG, 2-oxoglutarate; succ, succinate; TMAO, trimethylamine N-oxide; val, valine.

able promise in toxicology and could be of great value in the early screening programme used for investigating the biochemical side-effects of drugs for acute side effects at an early stage of their development as therapeutic agents and hence contribute to the minimisation of the use of laboratory animals for toxicological testing. In addition, PMR methodology could be used to monitor the recovery phase from reversible toxic insult or disease states, and in the latter case, may represent a novel means of monitoring therapy.

ACKNOWLEDGEMENTS

We thank F.W. Bonner, J.A. Timbrell and E Rahr for their advice and technical assistance, S. Moncada FRS for encouragement and support, and The Wellcome Foundation and The National Kidney Research Fund, for financial support of this and related work. We thank the MRC for the use of central NMR facilities.

REFERENCES

1. Nicholson JK, Wilson ID: High resolution nuclear magnetic resonance spectroscopy of biological samples as an aid to drug development. Prog Drug Res 31:427-479, 1987.

2. Nicholson JK, Gartland KPR: A nuclear magnetic resonance approach to investigate the biochemical and molecular effects of nephrotoxins. In: Cells, Membranes and Disease (Methodological Surveys in Biochemistry and Analysis) (Ed Reid E, Cook GMW and Luzio JP) Plenum Press, New York pp 397-408, 1987.

3. Nicholson JK, Timbrell JA, Sadler PJ: Proton NMR spectra of urine as indicators of renal damage: Mercury-induced nephrotoxicity in rats. Mol Pharmacol 27:644-651, 1985.

4. Gartland KPR, Bonner FW, Nicholson JK: Investigations into the biochemical effects of region-specific nephrotoxins. Mol Pharmacol 35:242-250, 1989.

5. Gartland KPR, Bonner FW, Timbrell JA, et al.: The biochemical characterisation of p-aminophenol-induced nephrotoxic lesions in the F344 rat. Arch Toxicol 63:97-106, 1989.

6. Kowalski BR, Bender CFJ: Pattern recognition. A powerful approach to interpreting

chemical data. Am Chem Soc 94:5632-5639, 1972.

7. Sammon JW: A non-linear mapping for data structure analysis. IEEE Trans Comput, C-18, (5), 401-409, 1969.

8. Seal H, "Multivariate Statistical Analysis for Biologists", Methuen & Co. Ltd., London, 101-102, 1968.

9. Chatfield C, A J Collins. "Introduction to Multivariate Analysis" Chapman and Hall, London and New York, pp. 57-59, 1980.

10. Gartland KPR, Sweatman BC, Beddel CR et al.: PMR urinalysis studies on the biochemical effects of a nephrotoxic dose of uranyl nitrate in the fischer 344 rat. Proceedings of the Fourth International Symposium on Nephrotoxicity, eds. Bach PH, Delacruz L, Gregg NJ, Wilks MF. Marcel Decker, New York (in press).

11. Bagnasco S, Balaban R, Fales HM et al.: Predominant osmotically active organic solutes in rat and rabbit renal medullas. J Biol Chem 261:5872- 5877, 1986.

81

PROTON NUCLEAR MAGNETIC RESONANCE URINALYSIS STUDIES ON THE BIOCHEMICAL EFFECTS OF A NEPHROTOXIC DOSE OF URANYL NITRATE IN THE FISCHER 344 RAT

K.P.R. Gartland (1), B.C. Sweatman (2), C.R. Beddell (2), J.C. Lindon (2) and J.K. Nicholson (1)

Department of Chemistry, Birkbeck College, University of London, 29 Gordon Square, London WC1H 0PP U.K. (1) and Department of Physical Sciences, Wellcome Research Laboratories, Beckenham, Kent, BR3 3BS, UK (2)

INTRODUCTION

Small doses of uranyl nitrate (UN) and other uranyl compounds cause reproducible acute nephronal damage and have been employed as models of experimental acute renal failure (1-4). The site of the UN-induced lesion is the pars recta of the proximal tubule and is characterised by swelling, necrosis and shedding of epithelial cell cytoplasm into the tubular lumina (3). The functional changes observed following a single nephrotoxic dose of UN include increases in blood urea nitrogen, plasma renin activity, urine flow rate and urinary sodium with decreases in glomerular filtration rate, renal blood flow and urine osmolality (1-4). We have previously shown that proton nuclear magnetic resonance (PMR) urinalysis studies can provide novel information on the biochemical effects of nephrotoxins (5-7). In the present study we have chosen to examine UN-induced nephrotoxicity employing conventional clinical chemical and high resolution PMR spectroscopic urinalysis techniques in an attempt to evaluate the effects of this chemical on the profile of low molecular weight (MW) urine components and hence generate new information on its biochemical effects.

METHODS

Animals and Treatments.

Six male Fischer 344 rats were allocated to 2 groups (n=3) placed individually in plastic metabolism cages and allowed free access to food and tap water. Rats were housed in well ventilated animal rooms with regular light cycles (12 hour: 0700-1900 hr). Following an acclimatisation period of 3 days rats were dosed with either 0.9% NaCl (control) or a 13 mg/ml solution of $UO_2(NO_3)_2.6H_2O$ equivalent to a dose of 10 mg/kg $UO_2(NO_3)_2$.

Conventional Biochemical Urinalysis and Plasma Analysis.
Urine was collected over ice for 20 hr prior to dosing and at 8, 24 and 48 hr after dosing and tested for glucose by the hexokinase method, L-lactic acid and 3-D-hydroxybutyric acid (HB), and plasma was tested at 48 hr for urea nitrogen, HB and glucose employing commercially available enzymatic test kits. These methods were all based on the appearance or disappearance of NADH at 340 nm. Statistical analysis of data was carried out using unpaired Student's t-test. A probability of $p < 0.05$ was taken as the level of significance.

PMR Analysis.
Measurements were made on a Bruker WH400 spectrometer operating at a field strength of 9.4 Tesla at ambient probe temperature ($298 \pm 1°K$). Any increase in urine flow rate seen in the treated group was cor-

rected by lyophilisation as described previously (6). The lyophilisate was then redissolved in 0.45 ml ^2H_2O (field/frequency lock) and diluted with 0.05 ml ^2H_2O containing the internal chemical shift reference 3-trimethylsilyl-[2,2,3,3,-$^2H_4$]-1-propionate (TSP) in 5 mm tubes. For each sample 64 free induction decays were collected into 16,384 computer points using 40° (4 μs) pulses, a sweep width of 5000 Hz and an acquisition time of 1.7 seconds. A delay of 3.0 seconds between pulses was added to allow full T_1 relaxation. An exponential line broadening function of 0.6 Hz was applied prior to Fourier transformation. Water suppression was achieved by gated (decoupler off during acquisition) irradiation. Spin Echo spectra of lyophilised plasma in ^2H_2O were recorded using the Hahn sequence (90 - t - 180 - t - collect FID) (8) with a t value of 60 msec and a delay between cycles of 3 sec (8). Resonance assignments were made by chemical shift, spin-spin coupling patterns, pH-dependencies of chemical shifts and ultimately standard addition employing the procedure adapted by Bales et al (9).

RESULTS

Conventional Analyses

Urine. The effects of UN on urine flow rate, and the excretion of D-glucose, L-lactate and HB are shown in Table 1. Considerable increases in urine flow rate and the excretion of D-glucose and HB can be seen as early as 24 hr after dosing with UN, whereas only a minor increase in L-lactic acid excretion is seen.

Plasma. Plasma levels of urea nitrogen, glucose and HB from control and UN-treated animals are shown in Table 2. UN causes a 4-fold increase in plasma urea at 48 hr but only a minor increase in plasma HB levels at this time. UN has no effect on plasma glucose 48 hr after dosing.

PMR Analysis

Urine. Figures 1 and 2 show the high and low field portions respectively of the PMR spectra of urine before and after exposure to 10 mg/kg UN. A gradual decrease in citrate, creatinine and 2-oxoglutarate excretion can be seen in addition to aminoaciduria and glycosuria

Table 1. Urine flow rate and D-glucose, L-lactate and HB levels in urine from control and UN-treated (10 mg/kg) animals.

	0-8 hr	8-24 hr	24-48 hr
Urine Flow Rate			
Control	0.4±0.09	0.5±0.1	0.3±0.03
10 mg/kg UN	0.9±0.17	1.7±0.45	1.1±0.27*
Urine D-Glucose			
Control	1.8±0.3	3.1±0.08	4.5±0.5
10 mg/kg UN	20.2±10.9	144.7±42.1*	175.6±24.9+
Urine L-Lactate			
Control	3.3±0.6	6.7±0.9	5.9±0.3
10 mg/kg UN	7.3±0.6**	12.7±1.3*	14.2±2.2*
Urine HB			
Control	1.3±0.2	2.8±0.1	2.4±0.3
10 mg/kg UN	1.1±0.4	15.5±8.3	40.7±7.1**

(Values represent the mean ± standard error of the mean; n = 3 for both groups) Units: urine flow rate, ml/hr; D-Glucose, L-lactate, and 3-D-Hydroxybutyrate, μmol/hr/kg. HB, 3-D-hydroxybutyrate. Statistics: * p< 0.05; ** p< 0.01; − p< 0.001 when compared to control.

Table 2. Plasma urea, D-glucose and 3-D-hydroxybutyric acid levels 48 hr after 10 mg/kg UN.

	Urea mg/100 ml	D-Glucose mM	HB mM
Control	17.1±1.1	0.91±0.04	0.82±0.08
10 mg/kg UN	67.5±3.3*	1.02;0.95	1.08±0.12

Values represent mean ± standard error of the mean; n = 3 for both groups. For glucose in the treated group two values are shown. Statistics: * p<0.001 when compared to control.

throughout 8-24 hr and 24-48 hr after UN. Additionally, a minor L-lactic aciduria is apparent together with a progressive HB-aciduria (Figure 1). The glycosuria is confirmed in Figure 2 by the sugar α-anomeric proton. In addition, hippurate and allantoin both display a gradual decrease in excretion after UN (Figure 2).

Plasma. Hahn Spin-Echo PMR spectra of plasma UN-treated rats (Figure 3) also show differences from control. Increases in plasma creatinine and HB can be seen in addition to a decrease in the resonances P_1 and P_2 arising from mobile fatty acids.

DISCUSSION

PMR spectroscopy is well suited to the study of toxicological events. The combination of non-selectivity with high chemical specificity provided by this technique is potentially of great value in the field of toxicology since a variety of metabolic effects can be investigated simultaneously without prior knowledge of the nature of the toxic lesion. We have previously explored the potential of PMR urinalysis in uncovering novel low MW markers of region-specific nephrotoxicity (5-7). Indeed, this technique highlighted the link between L-lactic aciduria and proximal tubular necrosis, and in addition, the association between increased levels of urinary dimethylamine (DMA), trimethylamine N-oxide (TMAO), N,N-dimethylglycine (DMG) and succinate and experimentally induced renal papillary necrosis (6).

In the present study a dose of 10 mg/kg UN produced a reproducible pattern of changes in both the urine and plasma from treated rats. PMR urinalysis uncovered changes in recognised markers of renal injury such as amino acids, creatinine and glucose as well as changes in more novel low MW urine components like HB, citrate and L-lactate. The lactic aciduria seen following UN is modest in comparison to that seen following other toxins targeting the pars recta such as p-aminophenol, hexachlorobutadiene or $HgCl_2$ (5-7). The reason for this is unclear although sodium chromate, a toxin causing necrosis in the pars convoluta of the proximal tubule, has also been shown to produce a modest lactic aciduria (6). Thus it would appear that proximal tubular necrosis and lactic aciduria are only associated in certain types of nephrotoxic injury. The hypocitraturia displayed after UN is in common with that seen following exposure to 2 mg/kg $HgCl_2$ (5,6) but with a differing timecourse. Whereas citrate in urine was undetectable by PMR 8-24h after $HgCl_2$ (6) here this Krebs cycle intermediate is undetectable only at the ultimate time point i.e. 24-48 hr. Such an effect of UN on urine citrate indicates an effect on renal acid-base status. In fact, UN may be precipitating a renal tubular acidosis similar to that induced by $HgCl_2$ (5).

The most novel finding reported here following UN is the effect on urinary HB level - a 17-fold increase over control values during the last time point. Although urinary HB has previously been shown to be increased following hexachlorobutadiene and p-aminophenol (6,7) these changes were minor in comparison with those seen here. The HB-uria could arise from a number of causes including an effect of the toxin on food intake causing an appetite suppressant effect, overflow of increased plasma HB levels, or a biochemical effect within the kidney itself. The first of these possibilities can be eliminated immediately since in the fasting state plasma glucose is depressed (10) and in the present study UN produced no change in plasma glucose levels 48h after dosing (Table 2). The second possible explanation of this effect can also be eliminated since no such

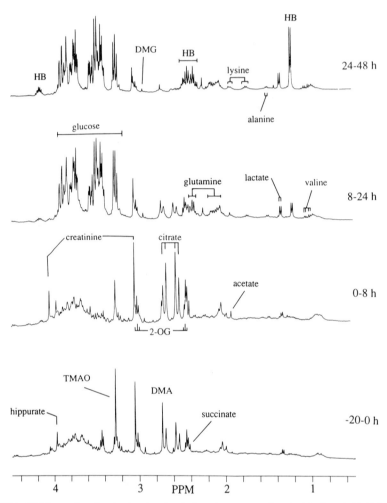

Figure 1. 400 MHz PMR spectra of rat urine (region to low frequency of water) before (-20-0h) and after 10 mg/kg uranyl nitrate. See text for experimental conditions. DMA, dimethylamine; DMG, N,N-dimethylglycine; HB, 3-D-hydroxybutyrate; TMAO, trimethylamine N-oxide

increase in plasma HB was seen (Table 2). More considerable increases in plasma HB were seen in fasting human subjects as well as in an insulin-dependent diabetic during insulin withdrawal (10). The lack of any increase in plasma HB levels following UN also rules out that the HB-uria arises from a systemic effect. Consequently, the data suggest that the HB-uria is due to a wholly renal effect, in particular, perturbed biochemistry such as incomplete oxidation of this ketone body by the cells of the proximal tubule. This finding combined with the disapppearance of resonances from plasma mobile fatty acids following UN (Figure 3) strongly suggests increased fatty acid catabolism. Disappearance of these resonances has been shown previously employing PMR spectroscopic analysis in plasma taken from normal fasting human subjects as well as in an insulin-dependent diabetic following insulin withdrawal (10). However, the situation seen following UN does not mimic either of these two examples

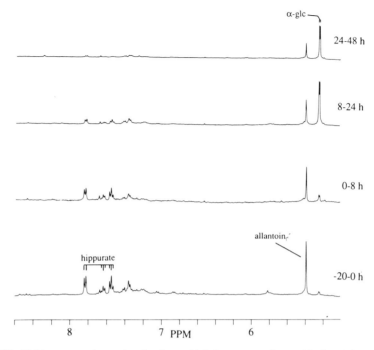

Figure 2. 400 MHz PMR spectra of rat urine (region to high frequency of water) before (-20-0 hr) and after 10 mg/kg uranyl nitrate. See text for experimental conditions. alpha-glc, alpha-anomeric proton of glucose.

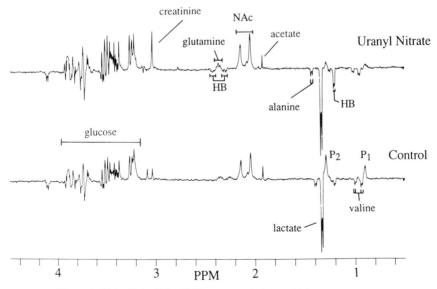

Figure 3. Hahn Spin-Echo PMR spectra of plasma UN-treated rats.

insofar as no changes in either plasma HB or glucose were observed here. The kidney is well known to use as energy sources not only fatty acids (11) but also ketone bodies (12). Indeed the highest activity of HB dehydrogenase in the kidney was recovered from the proximal and distal convoluted tubules (13). Further work is required in order to establish a dose-effect relationship, as well as experiments in which concentrations of UN are incubated with selected enymes of renal lipid metabolism such as HB dehydrogenase to test the hypothesis that UN is causing incomplete renal oxidation of HB. In the present study we have succeeded in characterising the biochemical effects of UN on the kidney including changes in the excretion of novel low MW urine components such as citrate, L-lactate and HB following toxic injury.

ACKNOWLEDGEMENTS

We thank The Wellcome Foundation and The National Kidney Research Fund, for financial support of this and related work. We thank the MRC for use of central NMR facilities.

REFERENCES

1. Flamenbaum W, McNeil JS, Kotchen TA, et al.: Experimental acute renal failure induced by uranyl nitrate in the dog. Circ Res 31: 682-698, 1972.

2. Flamenbaum W, Huddleston ML, McNeil JS, et al.: Uranyl nitrate-induced acute renal failure in the rat: Micropuncture and renal hemodynamic studies. Kidney Int 6: 408-418, 1974.

3. Stein JH, Gottschall J, Osgood RW et al.: Pathophysiology of a nephrotoxic model of acute renal failure. Kidney Int 8: 27-41, 1975. 4. Flamenbaum W, Hamburger RJ, Huddleston ML: The initiation phase of experimental acute renal failure: An evaluation of uranyl nitrate-in-duced acute renal failure in the rat. Kidney Int 10: S-115 - S-122, 1976.

5. Nicholson JK, Timbrell JA, Sadler PJ: Proton NMR spectra of urine as indicators of renal damage: Mercury-induced nephrotoxicity in rats. Mol Pharmacol 27: 644-651, 1985.

6. Gartland KPR, Bonner FW, Nicholson JK: Investigations into the biochemical effects of region-specific nephrotoxins. Mol Pharmacol 35: 242-250, 1989.

7. Gartland KPR, Bonner FW, Timbrell JA, et al.: The biochemical characterisation of p-aminophenol-induced nephrotoxic lesions in the F344 rat. Arch Toxicol 63: 97-106, 1989.

8. Hahn EL: Spin echoes. Physiol Rev 80: 580-594, 1950.

9. Bales JR, Higham DP, Howe I, et al.: Use of high resolution proton nuclear magnetic resonance spectroscopy for the rapid multicomponent analysis of urine. Clin Chem 30: 426-432, 1984.

10. Nicholson JK, O'Flynn MP, Sadler PJ, et al.: Proton nuclear magnetic resonance studies of serum, plasma and urine from fasting normal and diabetic subjects. Biochem J 217: 365-375, 1984.

11. Guder WG, Wirthensohn G. Renal turnover of substrates. In: Greger R, Lanf F, Silbernagl S (eds); Renal Transport of Organic Substances. Berlin, Heidelberg, Springer-Verlag, 1981.

12. Wirthensohn G, Guder WG. Renal lipid metabolism. Mineral Elect Metab 9: 203-211, 1983.

13. Guder WG, Purschel S, Wirthensohn G. Renal ketone body metabolism. Distribution of 3-oxoacid-CoA-transferase and 3-hydroxybu-tyrate dehydrogenase along the mouse nephron. Hoppe-Seyler's Z Physiol Chem 364: 1727-1737, 1983.

82

METALLOTHIONEIN AS A MARKER IN MERCURY NEPHROTOXICITY

B. Ribas, I. Bando, M.M. Martínez Trueba (1); J. Santamaría and M.A. Morcillo (2)

Institute of Biochemistry, CSIC-Complutense University, Faculty of Pharmacy (1) and Centro de Invest. Energéticas Medioambientales y Tecnológicas (CIEMAT) (2), Madrid, Spain

INTRODUCTION

Despite many attempts to control environmental mercury pollution, it is ubiquitous in both organic and inorganic forms which are toxic (1). More mercury is accumulated in the kidney (2) where it contributes to nephrotoxicity than in the liver or the gastrointestinal system. However, chronic systemic and degenerative diseases including effects on the nervous system (3) are also a frequent consequence of mercury toxicity. Metallothionein (MT) is induced after subchronic exposure to mercury (4). Copper and zinc levels were increased 8- and 1.5-times respectively in the kidneys of rats exposed to mercury, while the level of mercury increased up to 132 µg Hg/g wet tissue (5). These data show the inter-relationship between metals, their binding to MT and their great affinity to this low MW protein. The high renal accumulation of Hg after its chronic administration as $HgCl_2$ (6) relates to the induction of MT, which normally contains Cu^{2+} and Zn^{2+} (7). The anaemic condition in mammals predisposes to the absorption of heavy metals (8,9) and to the synthesis of MT (10,11).

The anaemic model rat was used in this study to observe the absorption of low doses of Hg^{2+}, and to find out if the MT levels are also detectable in their multiple molecular isoforms. The extrapolation of these results to humans will be proposed, focusing the interest on the population group of anaemic patients who may be susceptible to absorbing higher levels of environmental toxins, and developing pathological renal lesion.

METHODS

Male Sprague-Dawley rats of 200 ± 10 g distributed in control and pretreated groups were used. The treated rats were ferropenic and post-haemorrhagic anaemic animals and were administered 0.1 mg $HgCl_2$/kg/day po for 5 consecutive days. Anaemia was induced to the rats by ferropenic diet and by bleeding twice a week (11).

Kidneys were homogenized with Tris-HCl buffer 2.5×10^{-2}M pH 7.4 (1:2;w:v), ultracentrifuged to 40 000 rpm for 60 min. The supernatants were filtered and applied to a Sephadex G-50 (37x2.5 cm) column, and the elution profile established at the optical density of 262 nm. The mercury concentration at sub-ppm levels was analyzed and established for the collected fractions from the Sephadex G-50 column by atomic absorption spectrophotometry, and total protein was determined (13). In order to isolate and purify MT, the peak eluted from Sephadex G-50 containing this low MW protein, and 83 ppb Hg^{2+} was applied to a Glass Pack (TSK G 2 000 SW) column and the peak containing MT separated by high performance liquid chromatography (HPLC), and compared to the profile of MT obtained from rabbit liver (Sigma Nr: 5392).

HPLC was carried out using a Kontrol gradient former-425 Pump 420 and Ultra violet Unit at 220 nm (Knauer), Computer system (ACER500) and a CI-4000 integrator (Milton Roy). Separations were undertaken on column RP-18 5µ or MN-300-7C4, 25x0.3 cm column.

The gradient used was A:Tris-HCl buffer 2.5 x 10^{-2}M pH 7.4; and B:the same as A with 60% Acetonitrile (12,14).

RESULTS

The mercury administrated to the rats is mainly accumulated in the kidneys, its concentration is measured by atomic absorption spectrophotometry. The maximal concentration of mercury is found in fraction 19, eluted from Sephadex G-50 column, as shown in Figure figure 1. The peak of Hg^{2+} is composed by the fractions 18-20, and the higher concentration in fraction 19 is 83 ppb, belonging to the peak of MT as seen in Figure 1. The elution profile from the Glas Pac column of fraction 19 for kidneys of Hg^{2+} treated rats, established at 220 nm, is shown in Figure 2. For comparison, Figure 3 shows the elution profiles and retention times of the six metallothionein isoforms of rabbit liver induced by cadmium (Sigma Nr: 5392) used as control to establish the standard conditions for kidney of rats treated with HgCl2 (12).

DISCUSSION

There were significant differences between the protein concentration of kidneys of control and anaemic rats treated with 0.1 mg/kg HgCl2 during 5 consecutive days. This dose is equivalent to environmental doses of mercury, ingested or inhaled by some individuals or human groups (1). The results expressed here from the MT analysis, show the possibility of detecting environmental doses of mercury in rats. MT in 5 ml of urine or blood was not detected.

In non-anaemic (control) rats mercury is not detected if administered at the same low dose as in anaemic animals. This corroborates the tendency for anaemic animals to incorporate heavy metals.

The HPLC method for MT purification and for the separation and quantification in each individual isometallothionein used here (12) shows promise in assessing the effects of subclinical and environmental doses of mercury.

The pharmacological method used in this preliminary experiment, with an injection of 20 μg HgCl2 to the anaemic rats shows an increase of Hg^{2+} absorption compared to the controls. The detection of the peak of mercury of 83 ppb after relatively low oral doses corroborates the successful absorption and MT synthesis. The anaemic status alters the homeostatic regulatory mechanism for essential and heavy metals (15,16).

Ecological studies have shown the natural biotransformation of heavy metals, such as mercury. Comparison of results from different animal species, such as birds and mammals, shows that they have nephrotoxic lesions (of a similar type and severity) with comparable levels of metals (17). Microscopical and biochemical changes begin with doses presently considered subclinical for humans by the World Health Organization (17). The synthesis of MT could be one of the detoxification mechanisms established early in the evolution to minimise the presence of natural heavy metals in the body. The changes which occur at the molecular level before the physiological function of the kidney is affected need to be scientifically established. In addition, the early molecular modifications of isometallothioneins or which ones are the most affected also need to be determined.

These data suggest that isometallothionein 1 is induced during low levels of mercury exposure, before the physiological and morphological changes occur in the kidney. In spite of the difficulties in extrapolating between species, the morphologic nephrotoxic lesion caused by Hg^{2+} is similar for birds and mammals (17). The determination of the multiple molecular isoforms of the MT offers an early molecular marker for nephrotoxicity in several species. During mercury exposure, copper concentration are much greater in kidneys (8 times) compared to the controls, while zinc concentration is 1.5-times higher, and the MT contents are also increased markedly, a fact closely related to the association of Hg^{2+}, Cu^{2+} and Zn^{2+} to the MT (5). The increased levels of MT after Hg^{2+} exposure, are a result of metal

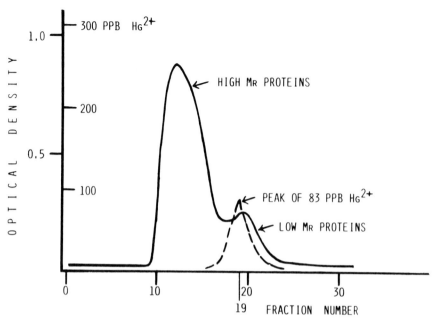

Figure 1. Elution profile from Sephadex G-50 at optical density of 262 nm and peak of Hg^{2+} from a kidney extract of anemic rats treated with Hg^{2+}, and control ones.

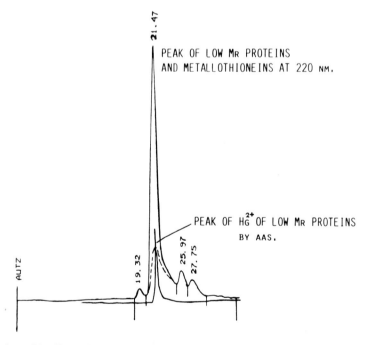

Figure 2. Profile from Glas Pac column of fraction 19 from Sephadex G-50 of kidney extract from anemic treated with Hg^{2+}, and control rats, detected at 220 nm.

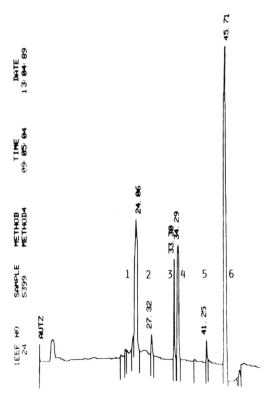

Figure 3. Elution profile and retention times of six isometallothionein isoforms of rabbit liver induced by cadmium (Sigma Nr: 5392) used as control to establish the standard conditions for comparison to rat kidney (12).

interaction, probably substituting Hg^{2+} for Zn^{2+}, in the native and synthesized de novo renal MT, with the consequent inactivation of MT.

The relatively low molecular mass and high percentage of cysteine residues present in the MT molecule, permits binding to heavy metals through mercaptide bonds (which are very stable), with heavy metals, making the use of MT as a low molecular weight marker for environmental pollution feasible. RIA is a method with several orders of magnitude lower sensitivity in its detection limit. Theoretically it would be possible to quantify each MT isoform more easily, rapidly and inexpensively.

The detection of MT after the doses of mercury used in this preliminary experiment shows that these low doses induce the accumulation of mercury and the synthesis of MT. Since mercury also induces a toxic response in the nervous system and degenerative diseases, the possibility arises of using MT detection to study diseases of the nervous system of unknown etiology.

REFERENCES

1. Mitra S: Mercury in the Ecosystem. Its Dispersion and Pollution Today. Trans Tech Publications, Switzerland, Germany, UK, USA, 1986.

2. Klonne DR, Johnson DR: Enzyme activity and sulphydryl status in rat renal cortex following mercuric chloride and dithiothreitol administration. Tox Lett 42: 199-205, 1988.

3. Clarkson TW: Metal toxicity in the central nervous system. Environm Health Perspect 75: 59-64, 1987.

4. Nolan CV, Shaikh ZA: Induction of metallothionein in rat tissues, following subchronic exposure to mercury shown by radioimmunoassay. Biol Trace Element 12: 419-428, 1987.

5. Skreblin M, Stegnar P, Kregar I: Effect of mercury on the subcellular distribution of endogenous copper and zinc and the presence of Hg-Cu-Zn-Metallothionein in the kidney of rats exposed to mercury vapor. Trace Element Anal Chem Med Biol, Walter de Gruyter Co, Berlin-New York, Vol 5, 1988, pp 570-575.

6. Piotrowski JK, Trojanowska B, Wisniewska-Knypl JM, Bolanowska W: Mercury binding in the kidney and liver of rats repeatedly exposed to mercury chloride: Induction of metallothionein by mercury and cadmium, Toxicol Appl Pharmacol 27: 11-19, 1974.

7. Stillman MJ, Law AYC, Cai W, Zelazowski AJ: Information on metal binding properties of metallothioneins from optical spectroscopy, In: Kagi JHR, Kojima Y (eds); Metallothionein II, 2nd Intern. Congress on Metallothionein, University of Zurich, August 1985, pp 203-211.

8. Hamilton DL, Valberg LS: Relationship between cadmium and iron absorption. Am J Physiol 227: 1033-1037, 1974.

9. Valberg LS, Sorbie J, Hamilton DL: Gastrointestinal metabolism of cadmium in experimental iron deficiency. Am J Physiol 231: 462-467, 1976.

10. Ribas B, Brenes MA, Basagoiti I, Sánchez Reus MI: Die Beteiligung des Gehirnmetallthioneins an der Eisenhomöstase. M. Anke, W. Baumann, H. Braunlich, Chr. Bruckner, B. Groppel (eds), Trace Elements 5:405-412, 1986.

11. Ribas B, Pelayo JF, Rodrígues NL: New data on the hypothesis of the brain participation in iron homeostasis. Trace Element Anal Chem Med Biol, Walter de Gruyter Co, Berlin-New York, Vol 5, 1988, pp 548-555.

12. Ribas B, Iniesta MP: Induction of metallothionein 1 with cadmium, by high pressure liquid chromatography. Anal Real Acad Farm 55:533-540, 1989.

13. Lowry OH, Rosebrough NJ, Farr AL, Randall RJ: Protein measurement with Folin phenol reagent. J Biol Chem 193: 265-275, 1951.

14. Hunziker PE, Kagi JHR: Human hepatic metallothioneins: Resolution of six isoforms. In: (Kagi JHR, Kojima Y (eds); Metallothionein II, Experientia Suppl Vol 52, Basel-Boston, Birkhauser Verlag, 1987, pp 257-264.

15. Ribas B, Pelayo JF: Isolation of brain metallothionein labelled with ^{59}Fe in anemic rats. Toxicol Environ Chem 23: 9-15, 1989.

16. Ribas B, Brenes MA, De Pascual FJ: Brain metallothionein labelled with [109]Cd and ^{59}Fe and its involvement in iron homeostasis. Toxicol Environ Chem 23: 33-40, 1989.

17. Nicholson JK, Kendall MD, Osborn D: Cadmium and Mercury Nephrotoxicity, Nature 304: 633-635, 1983.

83

THE CLEARANCE OF ENDOGENOUS N-1-METHYLNICOTINAMIDE: A NEW MARKER OF NEPHROTOXICITY?

J.-C. Cal, A. Maiza and P. T. Daley-Yates

Department of Pharmacy, University of Manchester, Manchester M13 9PL, United Kingdom

INTRODUCTION

In an attempt to assess the nephrotoxic side-effects of drugs, a wealth of indicators have been proposed and used to date. Among these, histopathological analysis of the kidneys is invaluable in describing the site and type of structural damage (1-3), but does not give an indication of functional loss. In addition, this procedure requires a surgical removal or biopsy of the kidneys. Traditional renal function measurements such as serum creatinine or urea and creatinine or inulin clearance are often insensitive to subtle renal damage (4-6). In order to find a more sensitive functional test of nephropathy, the clearance of p-aminohippurate (PAH) has been investigated but found to have drawbacks since its clearance falls in uraemia due to the accumulation of endogenous anions which compete for the same transport processes. The in vitro accumulation of PAH and of organic cations such as tetraethylammonium (TEA) or N-1- methylnicotinamide (NMN), by renal cortical slices have also been used (7-9), but are laborious and invasive techniques. In contrast, non-invasive tests based, according to Piperno (10), on the analysis of "generously donated liquid biopsy" represented by urine specimens have proved to be indicative of the concentrating ability of the nephron and even a quantitative and persistent reflection of the severity of renal damage when proteinuria is determined. However, these tests may lack sensitivity and specificity (6,10), except when some specific low molecular weight protein (e.g. retinol binding protein or beta-2-microglo-

bulin) are assayed (11). More recently, enzymuria has been reported as an early, non-invasive, sensitive and relatively site-specific marker (12-14), but drug interference with the assay of enzymes is always a potential problem and changes in enzymuria are often transient.

Against this background, this study was designed to determine the value of the clearance of the prototypic organic cation, N-1-methylnicotinamide (NMN), as an indicator of proximal tubular secretory function in renal injury. A major advantage of this cation is that it is endogenous as the main metabolite of tryptophan and niacin i.e. its clearance may be determined without infusion of exogenous substances. To evaluate the advantages and limitations, NMN clearance was measured along with other markers in the well-known model of renal failure induced by mercuric chloride. Its regional specificity was also tested in several models of renal injury involving different segments of the nephron.

METHODS

Animals. Male adult Sprague-Dawley rats (250-450 g) were used throughout this study. They were allowed free access to food and water and housed in groups of 4 or 5 in temperature-controlled (22 ± 1°C) rooms under a 12-hr light/dark cycle (0800/2000) during a standardization period of 10 days. The animals were weighed every day during the study.

Induction of Renal Failure. During the first series of experiments, proximal tubular necrosis was induced by a single i.p. injection of 1 mg Hg/kg of mercuric chloride. The 24-hr urine was collected immediately before intoxication and 24-hr after. Clearance experiments were performed 24-hr after dosing. During the second series of experiments, proximal tubular necrosis was produced by a single i.p. injection of 5 mg/kg of cisplatin and four days were allowed for the development of the lesion. Papillary necrosis was induced by injecting i.v. under light anaesthesia 150 mg/kg of 2-bromoethylamine hydrobromide (BEA) and clearances performed 24-hr after. Drug-mediated glomerulonephritis was involved by 6 weekly i.p. injections of 0.05 mg/kg of sodium aurothiomalate. Clearances were performed three weeks after the beginning of the treatment. Immunologically-mediated glomerulonephritis has been developed in rats by a single i.v. injection of rabbit antiserum (0.5 ml) anti-glomerular basement membrane (antiGBM) raised by repeated i.d. injection of fraction FX1A (extracted from rat kidneys). Clearances were performed one week after dosing.

Clearance Experiments. Rats were anaesthetised with 50 mg/kg of sodium pentobarbital. Inulin was infused for about 2 hr via the jugular vein at a constant rate of 1.2 ml/hr, after injection of a loading dose of 100 mg/kg. Forty five minutes after the beginning of the infusion, a series of three 20-min urine collections from the catheterised bladder were performed. At the middle of each collection period, blood samples (0.5 ml) were taken, using a heparinised syringe, from the carotid artery and immediately centrifuged for the separation of plasma.

Biochemical Analyses. Creatinine was determined in plasma and urine by the Jaffé's method and urea by an enzymatic colorimetric method. Inulin was measured using the anthrone method (17). NMN was determined fluorimetrically according to the method of Clark et al. (15), revised by Shim et al. (16). Gamma-glutamyl-transpeptidase (GGT), alkaline phosphatase (AlP) and N-acetyl-beta-D-gluco-

saminidase (NAG) were assayed using Boerhinger Mannheim kits.

Statistical Analysis. All data are reported as mean $\pm$ standard error. Analysis of variance followed by intergroup comparisons was used to estimate the effect of the treatment on the different parameters studied. When these tests were not applicable, a Friedman test was used. Wilcoxon's tests or paired Student's t-tests were performed for comparing pre-dose and post-dose parameters.

RESULTS AND DISCUSSION

A 6-fold decreased clearance of NMN (Fig. 1) was observed 24-hr after injection of mercuric chloride ($p < 0.0001$) in comparison to a 2-fold decreased glomerular filtration rate (GFR) (as assessed by the clearance of inulin) ($p > 0.02$). Similarly, the clearance of creatinine and urea were reduced 3-fold, 24-hr post dosing. The glomerular filtration rate was still falling 48-hr post dosing whereas the clearance of NMN remained at the same level, both being 5- to 6-fold below their control values (Fig. 1). Therefore, compared to the clearance of inulin, creatinine or urea, the clearance of NMN may be an earlier marker of renal injury, whilst remaining depressed as long as the GFR and not requiring the infusion of exogenous compounds.

Compared to enzymuria (Fig. 2), the clearance of NMN proved to be as early a marker but remaining more significantly impaired for a longer period. In agreement with previous reports (14,18), the excretion of GGT, NAG and AlP were greatly increased 24-hr post dosing, 7-, 13- and 95-fold respectively ($p < 0.0001$), but fell to normal levels (GGT) or considerably decreased levels (AlP and NAG) 48-hr after the injection of mercury.

In addition, a significant decrease in the 24-hr urinary excretion of NMN (Fig. 3) was noted 24-hr post dosing (2.5-fold, $p < 0.0001$) and even 48-hr after (4-fold, $p < 0.001$). These data were correlated very closely with those for the clearance of NMN (correlation coefficient: 0.99) which suggests that the 24-hr urinary excretion

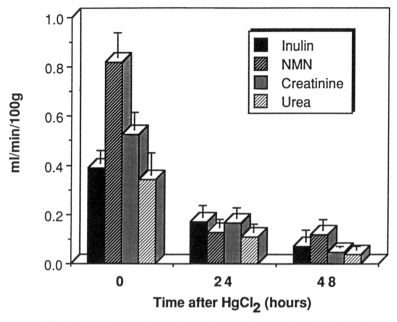

Figure 1. Clearances of inulin, NMN, creatinine and urea in control rats or in rats injected with 1 mg Hg/kg of mercuric chloride. Each bar depicts the mean ± SE of 3 measurements per rat, for 5 rats.

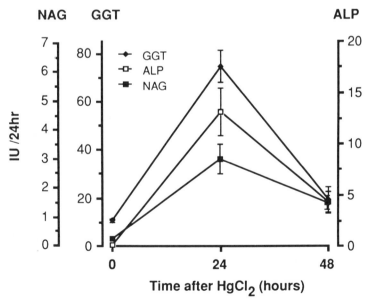

Figure 2. The 24-hr urinary activity of gamma-glutamyltranspeptidase (GGT), alkaline phosphatase (ALP) and N-acetyl-beta-D-glucosaminidase (NAG) before and after injection of 1 mg Hg/kg of mercuric chloride. Each point depicts the mean ± SE for 10 rats.

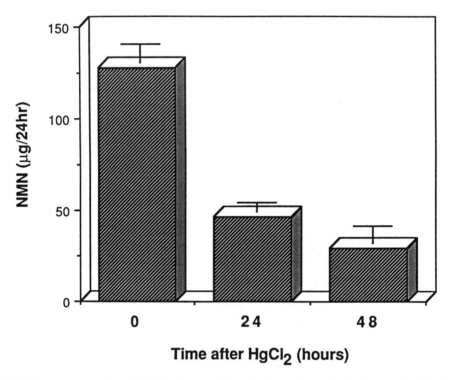

Figure 3. 24-hr urinary excretion of NMN before and after injection of 1 mg Hg/kg of mercuric chloride. Each bar depicts the mean ± SE for 10 rats.

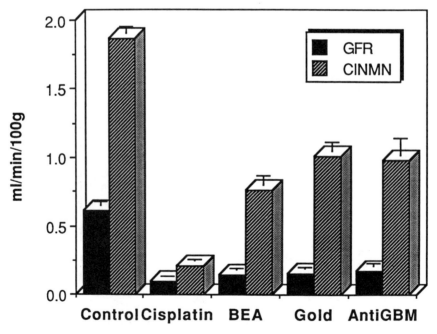

Figure 4. Clearances of inulin (glomerular filtration rate) and of NMN (CINMN) in control rats or in rats injected with several nephrotoxicants. Each bar depicts the mean ± SE of three measurements per rat for 5 rats.

of NMN may be used as an alternative to the clearance, providing an advantage in the experimental setting.

Figure 4 shows the regional specificity of the clearance of NMN as a marker of nephrotoxicity. Indeed, as NMN is excreted partly by filtration at the glomerular level, its clearance is reduced significantly (p<0.001) either in renal failure due to tubular necrosis (cisplatin) or to glomerulonephritis (gold, antiGBM) or even to papillary necrosis (BEA). However, as NMN is secreted at the proximal tubular level, the fall in its clearance is greater (9.1-fold) than the fall in GFR (6.7-fold) only in the model of renal tubular injury induced by cisplatin. These results are consistent with those described above in mercuric chloride-induced tubular necrosis indicating that the clearance of NMN is preferentially a marker for the proximal tubule.

Nevertheless, some questions remain unanswered, especially whether NMN only measures renal blood flow rather than the functional capacity of the proximal tubule. Although we have not directly addressed this point, if it is assumed that renal blood flow would be affected in a similar way to GFR in renal failure, it seems clear from our data (Fig. 4) that the clearance of NMN is more affected in cisplatin-induced renal injury (falling 9.1-fold compared to 6.7-fold for GFR) than in antiGBM-induced glomerulonephritis for example (falling 1.9-fold compared to 3.7-fold for GFR). Thus the clearance of NMN seems to reflect changes in the functional capacity of the nephron rather than changes in renal blood flow. These results are in agreement with findings from Shim et al. (16).

The other point to be made is that certain drugs or even endogenous compounds may compete for NMN tubular secretory processes due to their accumulation in the plasma during uraemia. Thus the fall in the clearance of NMN would not be a direct result of the fall in functional capacities of the nephron. This phenomenon has been observed for organic anions like PAH, but McNay et al. (19) have demonstrated that the extraction of TEA was independent of the degree of experimentally induced azotemia. In addition, Shim et al. (16)

have shown that, although the plasma concentration of NMN in various models of renal failure was much higher than that in the normal rats, it did not affect the urinary clearance of NMN. Thus it can be concluded that the clearance of NMN actually reflects the functional capabilities of the nephron.

Therefore, the clearance of NMN could be of value as a sensitive, site-specific and non-invasive marker of nephrotoxicity which may provide the clinician with a useful tool to monitor both the early and late stages of renal function impairment in contrast to the transient changes often observed in enzymuria.

ACKNOWLEDGEMENTS

J.C.C. has received a grant-in-aid fellowship from the European Science Foundation in support of the work described in this paper.

REFERENCES

1. Sharratt M, Frazer AC: The sensitivity of function tests in detecting renal damage in the rat. Toxicol Appl Pharmacol 5: 36-48, 1963.

2. McDowell EM, Nagle RB, Zalme RC, McNeil JS, Flamenbaum W, Trump BF: Studies on the pathophysiology of acute renal failure. I. Correlation of ultrastructure and function in the proximal tubule of the rat following administration of mercuric chloride. Virchows Archiv B 22: 173-196, 1976.

3. Daley-Yates PT, McBrien DCH: Cisplatin (cis-dichlorodiammine- platinum II) nephrotoxicty. In: Bach PH, Bonner FW, Bridges JW, Lock EA, (eds.); Nephrotoxicity, Assessment and Pathogenesis. Chichester, John Wiley & Sons, 1982, pp. 356-370.

4. Balazs T, Hatch A, Zawidzka Z, Grice HC: Renal tests in toxicity studies on rats. Toxicol Appl Pharmacol 5: 661-674, 1963.

5. Rosenbaum JL, Mikail M, Wiedmann F: Further correlation of renal function with kidney biopsy in chronic renal disease. Amer J Med Sci 254: 156-160, 1967.

6. Ansermet F, Mieville C, Diezi J: Urinary enzyme excretion and changes in renal functions induced by toxic substances or by renal ischemia in rats. Arch Toxicol Suppl 4: 201-207, 1980.

7. Hirsch GH: Differential effects of nephrotoxic agents on renal organic ion transport and metabolism. J Pharmacol Exp Ther 186: 593-599, 1973.

8. Berndt WO: Use of the renal slice technique for evaluation of renal transport processes. Environ Health Persp, 73-88, 1976.

9. Berndt WO: Use of renal function tests in the evaluation of nephrotoxic effects. In: Hook JB (ed.); Toxicology of the kidney. New York, Raven Press, 1981, pp. 1-29.

10. Piperno E: Detection of drug induced nephrotoxicity with urinalysis and enzymuria assessment. In: Hook JB (ed.); Toxicology of the Kidney. New York, Raven Press, 1981, pp. 31-55.

11. Bernard AM, Moreau D, Lauwerys R: Comparison of retinol-binding protein and beta-2-microglobulin determination in urine for the early detection of tubular proteinuria. Clin Chim Acta 126: 1-7, 1982.

12. Price RG: Urinary enzymes, nephrotoxicity and renal disease. Toxicology 23: 99-134, 1982.

13. Stonard MD, Gore CW, Oliver GJA, Smith IK: Urinary enzymes and protein patterns as indicators of injury to different regions of the kidney. Fund Appl Tox 9: 339-351, 1987.

14. Cal JC, Merlet D, Cambar J: In vitro and in vivo HgCl$_2$-induced nephrotoxicity assessed by tubular enzymes release. In: Bach PH, Lock EA (eds.); Nephrotoxicity, Extrapolation from in vitro to in vivo and from Animals to Man. London, Plenum Press, 1989, pp. 99-102.

15. Clark BR, Halpern RM, Smith RA: A fluorimetric method for quantitation in the picomole range of N-1-methylnicotinamide and nicotinamide in serum. Anal Biochem 68: 54-61, 1975.

16. Shim CK, Sawada Y, Iga T, Hanano M: Estimation of renal secretory function for organic cations by endogenous N-1-methylnicotinamide in rats with experimental renal failure. J Pharmacokin Biopharm 12: 23-42, 1984.

17. Greger R, Lang F, Knox FG, Lechene C: Analysis of tubule fluid. In: Martinez-Maldonado M (ed); Methods in Pharmacology. New York, Plenum Press, 1978, vol 4B, pp 105-140.

18. Stroo WE, Hook JB: Enzymes of renal origin in urine as indicators of nephrotoxicity. Toxicol Appl Pharmacol 39: 423-434, 1977.

19. McNay JL, Rosello S, Dayton PG: Effects of azotemia on renal extraction and clearance of PAH and TEA. Am J Physiol 230: 901-906, 1976.

84

DETERMINATION OF RAT URINARY KIDNEY-DERIVED ANTIGENS WITH MONOCLONAL ANTIBODIES – A NEW METHOD FOR THE DETECTION OF EXPERIMENTALLY INDUCED NEPHROTOXICITY

F.W. Falkenberg (1), B. Denecke (1) and E. Bomhard (2)

Abteilung für Medizinische Mikrobiologie und Immunologie, Medizinische Fakultät, Ruhr-Universität Bochum, 4630 Bochum, FRG (1) and Bayer AG, Institut für Toxikologie, Forschungszentrum Aprather Weg, 5600 Wuppertal, Germany (2)

INTRODUCTION

A variety of chemical and pharmaceutical compounds are known to cause nephrotoxicity. If profound morphological changes are induced by such substances they can be easily detected histologically, but subtle toxic effects need methods with high sensitivity. Chemically induced damage to the renal tubular cells will result in the release of cellular components which can then be determined in the urine. If the injury is limited and/or short-lived, the cells might recover and the process will be reversible. If, however, the toxic effect is pronounced or of long duration, epithelial cells, and other basic kidney tissue structures will be affected, and the process will become irreversible.

Under these conditions a variety of intracellular (e.g. enzymes) and extracellular components will be released into the urine. Some kidney-derived enzymes have been determined in urine, where the level of enzyme excretion has been used as an indicator for kidney damage. However, kidney-derived urinary enzymes represent only a small fraction of the large spectrum of macromolecular components released. Other biologically active or inactive components will be excreted in the urine. Such biological molecules - in this case termed "antigens" - can be determined with antibodies. If polyclonal or -

better - monoclonal antibodies to such kidney-derived urinary marker molecules were available, it would become possible to locate the site and extent of renal changes more precisely than with the present limited range of urinary enzymes.

We have, in the past, developed monoclonal antibodies to human kidney antigens (1) and used them for the determination of urinary kidney- derived antigens ("UA") in sandwich-ELISA tests. The results obtained with these tests indicated that the release of such antigens into the urine of patients suffering from renal diseases and of kidney transplant recipients permitted the location and extent of the damage occurring to the kidney to be identified (2). However, due to the complexity of the causes leading to phenotypical expression of kidney diseases it was not always possible to correlate antigen excretion patterns with the underlying primary processes.

Rats have been widely used for the study of nephrotoxicity of chemical and pharmaceutical compounds. The urine of rats treated with a substance with known nephrotoxic potential will contain all those cellular and extracellular components which are released from the cells/tissue as a consequence of the damage induced. Therefore, in contrast to the procedure applied in our previous work in which a membrane fraction prepared from human kidney tissue was used as a source of antigen (1), the urine of rats treated with toxic doses of mercuric chloride (HgCl2) was used as a source of antigens for the immunization of mice prior to hybridization of their lymphocytes. Applying this concept would give us a chance to obtain monoclonal antibodies to the kidney-derived antigens in the same form in which they are present and have to be determined in the urine. The results reported here show that it is possible to obtain such monoclonal antibodies with a variety of specificities for urinary antigens derived from cellular and extracellular compartments of the rat kidney. They have been applied to immunometric tests for the corresponding antigens in the urine.

MATERIALS AND METHODS

Preparation of antigen for immunization. Urine samples were collected from rats treated i.p. with 4.0 mg/kg body weight of HgCl2. The pooled urine samples were concentrated, dialyzed and fractionated on ConA-Sepharose into fractions differing in their glycoprotein content.

Immunization of mice and preparation of monoclonal antibodies. BALB/c mice were hyperimmunized by repeated injections over a period of several months with samples of the pooled fractions of the ConA-Sepharose elution peaks emulsified with CFA. Serum samples were tested for the presence of antibodies to rat kidney antigens in indirect immunofluorescence on rat kidney slices. Cell fusion and selection of hybridomas was done following standard procedures. Hybridomas secreting monoclonal antibodies of desired specificities were selected according to the staining pattern observed in indirect immunofluorescence on rat kidney tissue slices.

Purification and enzyme labelling of monoclonal antibodies. Monoclonal anti-bodies were purified from ascitic fluid by anion exchange chromatography on a DEAE-TSK column in a Pharmacia FPLC apparatus and labeled with horse radish peroxidase (HRP).

Sandwich ELISA. Following the same procedures as applied in previous work of our group (1,2) the purified monoclonal antibodies were adsorbed (1.0 µg per well) to the surface of micro ELISA plates. Rat urine samples were applied to the solid phase adsorbed "catcher" antibodies. After appropriate incubation and washing steps, the bound antigen was determined with the help of the HRP-labelled monoclonal "indicator" antibodies (1.0 µg per well). Antigen concentration was determined from the change in optical density at 405 nm in a SLT 8 channel ELISA Photometer. Since the rat urinary kidney-derived antigens were not available as standards in purified form, antigen concentration was given as arbitrary units (U/ml). One Unit of an antigen is defined as the amount of antigen contained in 1.0 ml of native urine when a 0.1 ml sample is applied under the conditions of the test and results in a change in optical density of 1.000 at 405 nm after 60 min of incubation at room temperature.

RESULTS

Antigens were characterised as shown in Table 1. In order to examine the usefulness of the tests, rats were treated with substances with known nephrotoxic potential. Urine was collected before, during and after the treatment as indicated and tested for the presence of rat urinary kidney-derived antigens ("RUA") in the five treatment groups.

1. Mercuric chloride. Urine collection started on day 1. On day 4, rats of group A (n=7) were injected with 2.0 ml 0.15 M NaCl i.p., group B (n=8) with 2.0 ml 0.3 M NaHCO3. On day 8, both groups received a single dose of 1.0 mg/kg HgCl2 i.p. The urine was collected daily until day 13.

The results of this experiment clearly showed that before treatment, low and stable baselines were observed for all the antigens. Only part of the rats ("Responders") showed enhanced urinary antigen levels. By contrast others ("Non-responders") had levels close to normal. Strongly enhanced excretion of RUA2 and moderately enhanced

Table 1: Designation and tissue localization of rat urinary kidney-derived antigens.

DESIGNATION OF ANTIGEN	TISSUE LOCALIZATION OF ANTIGEN	MOLECULAR SIZE OF ANTIGEN (kD)	MONOCLONAL ANTIBO-DIES USED IN TEST
RUA1	DISTAL TUBULUS	69	RaU I 17B3
RUA2	PROXIMAL TUBULUS	99	RaU I 2C8
RUA3	PROXIMAL TUBULUS	64, 77	RaU I 5C4
RUA4	DISTAL TUBULUS	16, 20, 24, 34	RaU I 6E9
RUA5	INTERSTICE	197	RaU II 1E8

excretion of RUAI and RUA5 is seen in the urine of animals of both groups after $HgCl_2$ treatment. Pretreatment with 2.0 ml of 0.30 M $NaHCO_3$ leads to a higher fraction of responders and higher antigen levels in the urine of responders.

2. Gentamycin Experiment Male Wistar rats (8 per group) received gentamycin daily for 7 consecutive days 0.0, 10.0, 50.0 or 250.0 mg/kg in saline i.p. Urine was collected on the day before, during the 7 days of treatment and during the 8 days after completion of the treatment. The results obtained showed that antigen release was observed only after application of the highest dose (250 mg/kg). Whereas the release of antigens RUA2, RUA3 and RUA5 was moderately enhanced, release of antigen RUA1 was strongly enhanced.

3. Methylated and chlorinated benzenes. Male Wistar rats (5 in each group) were gavaged with 500 mg/kg of monochlorobenzene, N,N-diethyl-toluamide (N-DET, Autan), 1,2-dichlorobenzene, 1,2-dimethylbenzene, 1,3-dichlorobenzene, 1,3-dimethylbenzene, 1,4-dichlorobenzene, 1,4-dimethylbenzene, 1,2,3-trichlorobenzene, 1,2,3-trimethylbenzene,1,2,4-trichlorobenzene, 1,2,4-trimethylbenzene, 1,3,5-trichlorobenzene, 1,3,5-trimethylbenzene, each dissolved in peanut oil daily for 7 consecutive days. Urine was collected on day 7 and tested for presence of rat urinary antigens and lactic dehydrogenase (LDH).

The results obtained showed that antigen excretion was within the normal range in untreated animals, but strongly enhanced excretion of most of the antigens was seen in part of the animals after dosing of 1,3,5-trichlorobenzene, 1,2-dimethylbenzene, 1,3-dimethylbenzene, 1,2,3-trimethylbenzene, 1,2,4-trimethylbenzene, 1,3,5-trimethylbenzene.

There was a slight to moderate enhancement of excretion of most of the antigens in animals dosed with the other aromatic compounds. Urinary level of all the antigens was within the normal range (RUA1, RUA2, RUA3) or slightly enhanced (RUA4, RUA5) in rats treated with N-DET (Autan).

In contrast, urinary level of LDH was in the normal range after application of all the other aromatic compounds, but was found significantly enhanced after application of N-DET (Autan).

Statistical analysis indicated that a correlation exists between the release of each of the 5 antigens. However, no correlation was found between release of the antigens and of LDH. Antigen excretion in female rats treated with the same aromatic compounds (results not shown) was only slightly enhanced. For better comparison the results of the experiments described above are compiled in the figure below.

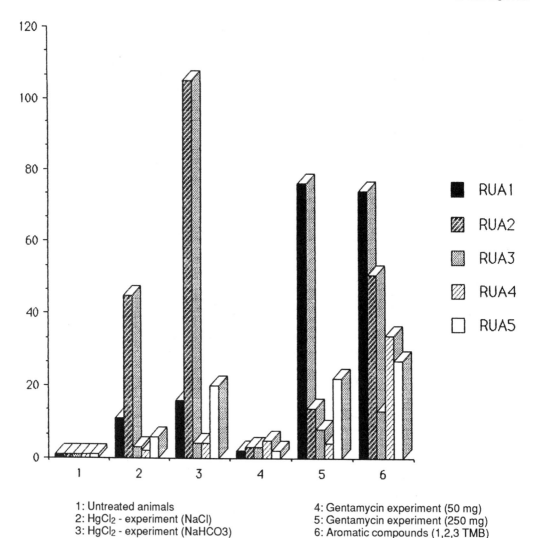

Figure 1. The relative numbers on the y-axis indicate the factor by which the mean value o f the highest peak of the mean excretion curve of a certain antigen is higher than the pretreatment value.

DISCUSSION

The results presented in this communication clearly show that it is possible to determine the levels of urinary antigens from different compartments of the cells/tissue of the kidney of rats under conditions of toxic damage. The monoclonal antibodies applied in these tests were produced by fusion of spleen lymphocytes of mice immunized with urinary antigen fractions obtained from rats treated with a toxic dose of $HgCl_2$. It was therefore expected that these antigens would be found in the urine of rats treated with this compound. However, this was not the case for all the antigens. A high urinary level was found only for the proximal tubular antigen RUA2, urinary levels of RUA1 and RUA5 were only moderately higher than in untreated animals (bar cluster 1). RUA3 and RUA4, however, remained very low indicating that these antigens obviously represent minor antigenic constituents in the urine of $HgCl_2$ treated rats. Nevertheless, hybridomas secreting antibodies specific to these antigens were obtained, and RUA3 and RUA4 were found in higher levels in the urine of rats treated with aromatic compounds.

Furthermore, practically all the animals of group B, which were pretreated with 2.0 ml of 0.3 M $NaHCO_3$ (bar cluster 3) responded to some extent to the application of $HgCl_2$ as compared to only 30-50% of the animals of group A (NaCl pretreatment, bar cluster 2). In this context gentamycin, the aromatic compounds and $HgCl_2$ considerably enhanced levels of some of the antigens. This is especially so in the experiment in which the effects of the various aromatic compounds were screened. Most of the antigens (RUAl, RUA2, RUA4 and RUA5) were found in very high levels in the urine of the animals (up to 700-fold above pretreatment level in some individual animals). In these animals the distal tubular RUA4 which was found low in the $HgCl_2$ and gentamycin experiments was released in high concentration as well. The fact that in the gentamycin experiment high antigen release was observed only after dosing of 250 mg/kg daily for 7 days (bar cluster 5 for the 250 mg dose, bar cluster 4 for the 50 mg dose) indicated that antigen release is not a very sensitive indication of kidney alteration/damage for this nephrotoxin. In contrast, the results of this experiment indicate that release of these antigens seems to be indicative only for very serious changes. Having this in mind, the observation that practically all the antigens are released in high concentrations after application of aromatic compounds (bar cluster 6) might indicate that the changes induced by these nephrotoxins are more serious than they were thought to be. From the results reported two major conclusions can be drawn:

The patterns of antigens released after application of $HgCl_2$, gentamycin and of the aromatic compounds are rather different. This indicates that the alteration/damage on the kidney epithelium is different and the fact that an antigenic component derived from the interstium (RUA5) is released indicates that the changes induced go far beyond the sensitive cells of the kidney epithelium and extend to the basic kidney tissue structures.

REFERENCES

1. Falkenberg FM, Müller E, Riffelmann H-D, Behrendt B, Waks T: The production of monoclonal antibodies against glomerular and other antigens of the human nephron. Renal Physiol. 4: 150-156, 1981.

2. Falkenberg FW, Mai U, Puppe C, Risse P, Herrmann G, Hecking E, Bremer K, Mondorf AM, Shapira Z: Kidney-derived urinary antigens assayed with monoclonal antibodies for the detection of renal damage. Proceedings of the 6th European Congress of Clinical Chemistry, Jerusalem/Israel, 1985. Clinica Chimica Acta 160, 171-182: 1986.

85

NEW MICROMOLECULAR MARKERS OF NEPHROTOXICITY: VILLIN AND TAMM-HORSFALL PROTEIN AS INDICATORS OF REGIONAL TUBULAR REGENERATION/DAMAGE AFTER RENAL TRANSPLANTATION

L.B. Zimmerhackl[1], G. Weber[1], D. Höfer[2], T. Fabricius[3], D.M. Scott[3], M. Brandis[1], D. Drenckhahn[2] and R. Kinne[3]

[1]Department of Pediatrics, Albert-Ludwigs-University, D-7800 Freiburg; [2]Department of Cell Biology Philipps-University, D-3550 Marburg; and [3]Max-Planck-Institut for Systemphysiology, D-4600 Dortmund, Germany

INTRODUCTION

Renal transplantation mimics the experimentally induced ischaemic renal failure induced by clamping of the renal artery or the infusion of nor-epinephrine (1). An anuric phase is followed by polyuria and thereafter the damaged cells of proximal and distal tubular origin regenerate. A regional differentiation of these processes is possible by invasive techniques, including renal biopsy (2). In order to assess, noninvasively, regional differences, we determined the renal excretion of a specific proximal tubular antigen, villin, and a specific distal tubular antigen, Tamm-Horsfall protein, by a newly developed enzyme-immuno-assay. The excretion of these proteins was compared to overall renal function.

METHODS

1: Villin Villin is a protein of the renal proximal tubular and intestinal cytoskeleton (3). Villin was isolated from chicken intestinum according to methods reported earlier (4). Polyclonal antibodies were raised in rabbit and one batch was labeled by the Biotin-Avidin system. Determination of villin was performed by polyclonal Sandwich-Enzyme-Immuno-Assay (Sandwich-ELISA) using rabbit anti-chicken villin antibodies. By histochemical staining of human kidney sections villin was found exclusively in the proximal tubular brushborder, not in the medullary tissue. After purification of villin the molecular weight, as determined by SDS-polyacrylamide-electrophoresis, was 95,000 Daltons. Western blotting of urine from children after transplantation showed villin could be determined as an intact protein and as two fragments with 70,000 and 45,000 Daltons. In urine of control patients, without renal insufficiency, villin could not be determined.

2: Tamm-Horsfall Protein (THP)

Tamm-Horsfall protein was prepared by salt precipitation with 0.58M NaCl overnight according to the original description by Tamm and Horsfall (5). Thereafter THP was purified by gel filtration (Sephadex) twice and finally freeze dried overnight. Antibodies against THP were raised in mice and monoclonals were separated according to standard procedures (6). A polyclonal antibody linked to horseradish peroxidase was purchased from SEROTEC, UK. THP was determined by monoclonal-polyclonal Sandwich-ELISA. The molecular weight of the glycoprotein was between 85-100,000 Daltons. Western blotting showed only intact protein could be determined in urine of children. No fragments were detectable. After histochemical staining of human kidney sections, activity was found in loops of Henle, initial distal tubule and within the lumen of the tubule (Figure 1a,b). Urine of pediatric patients and controls was

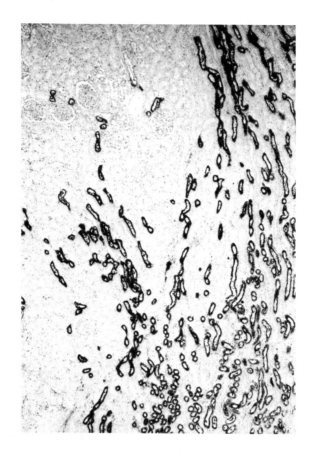

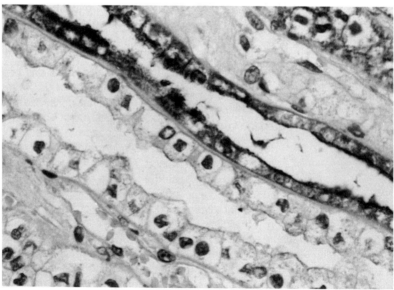

Figure 1. a: Histochemical image of Tamm-Horsfall protein in human kidney by polychlonal antibody as used in Sandwich ELISA. Note staining of the medullary region and lack of staining in the cortex. b: Higher magnification of medullary region. Note staining in loop of Henle and lack of staining in the collecting duct.

stored immediately after voiding and was determined after appropriate dilution to reach concentrations of THP of 0.1 to 1 mg/l to avoid precipitation of the protein. A dilution profile (1:2 to 1:512) of each urine was detected by ELISA and at least two concentrations had to be within 5%. Interassay variation was below 10% and coefficient of variation, within the range of concentrations given, was 5%.

Patients: Eight children, 2 female and 6 male, age 5-18 years, were studied after transplantation. Seven children received their first cadaver transplant, and 1 girl the second kidney. Immunosuppression was performed by cyclosporin (Sandimmun, Sandoz) and predisone. After initiation of diuresis furosemide was added in high dose (10mg/kg/day). Urine was collected every day for the first 3 weeks. Overall renal function was assessed by endogenous crea-

tinine clearance and fractional excretion of sodium (FE$_{Na}$).

RESULTS

Figure 2 depicts the excretion of antigens within the first 3 weeks after transplantation in a 12 year old male without a rejection period. After an initial rise, serum creatinine values decrease towards normal within three weeks after transplantation. FE$_{Na}$ decreases in parallel. Villin excretion is low the first days probably due to anuric renal failure and increases to maximal values around days 5-10. Thereafter the villin excretion falls. THP is not detectable the first two days, probably as a result of nonfunction of the transplant. Thereafter the excretion increases to normal values after two weeks.

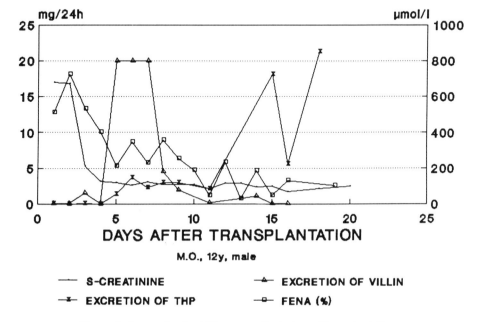

Figure 2. Curve of patient #1; uncomplicated renal transplantation.

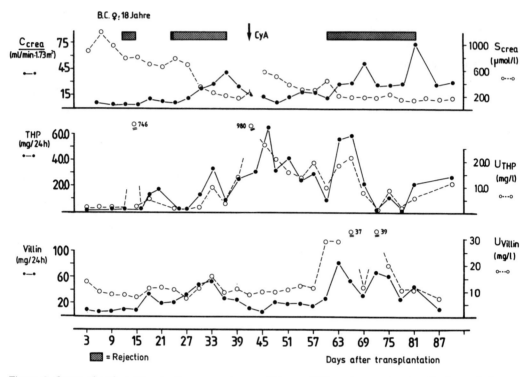

Figure 3. Curve of patient #2; rejection proven by renal biopsy. CYA and arrow denotes Cyclosporin A associated nephrotoxicity.

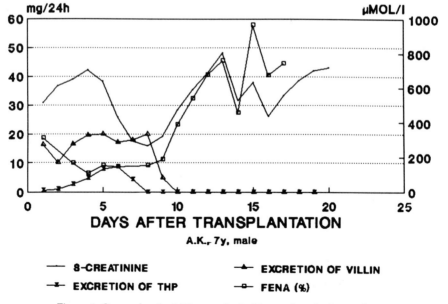

Figure 4. Curve of patient #3; complicated by nonfunctioning graft.

In Figure 3, a 7-year old male with non-functioning renal transplant is depicted. After a small rise in villin and THP excretion, both parameters fell to very low values after 10 days. On renal biopsy the graft was completely destroyed without signs of rejection.

In Table 1 the median of the parameters Villin and THP is given. During rejection (Figure 4) villin excretion increases to 5-10 fold over the initial values and falls after successful treatment. THP excretion falls before serum creatinine values rise as indicator of disturbed distal tubular function.

DISCUSSION

The results of this study demonstrate that renal antigen excretion is a new marker of tubular function and thus of damage or regeneration. Both markers, villin and Tamm-Horsfall protein are determined by novel ELISA-techniques. This technique is a new and simple tool with which to determine renal regional tubular damage on a structural but noninvasive level, and is easy to perform.

The microvillus is formed by actin filaments that are oriented towards the main axis of the villus. The filaments are anchored in the cell body by a complex network including "rootlets" and a "terminal web". The actin filaments are stabilized by bridging proteins which also anchor the membrane proteins to the cytosceleton

TABLE 1. URINARY ANTIGEN EXCRETION IN UNCOMPLICATED RENAL TRANSPLANTATION IN CHILDREN

DAYS AFTER TRANSPLANTATION	1-2	5-15	16-21
U_{VILLIN} (mg/l)	12.3	19.4	9.4
E_{VILLIN} (mg/24h/BSA)	20.2	55.1	32.5
U_{THP} (mg/l)	0.23	3.5	7.9
E_{THP} (mg/24h/BSA) (Median)	0.28	12.72	38.5

U = urinary concentration; E = urinary excretion; BSA = body surface area;(1.73 m2); THP = Tamm-Horsfall protein

(3). Villin is one of the bridging proteins necessary to maintain cell stability. After renal transplantation villin fragments and intact molecules are detectable in urine. Shedding of proteins (antigens) into urine can be caused by increased turnover brush border fragments or by direct damage to brushborders. At present we cannot differentiate between the two possible explanations. However, as indicated by patient #2 diminution of villin excretion can also be explained by complete death of the cell and, when no material is present, no antigen excretion of brush border fragments will occur. Thus decrease in shedding can be a sign of repair and of complete damage: This can be differentiated by other methods.

After its first description in 1950, THP has attracted attention with variable hypotheses (5). In particular the hypothesis that THP might represent the (furosemide inhibitable) ion transporter (Na-K-Cl) of the thick ascending loop of Henle, has been of interest to renal physiologists, although it was later shown that this was not the case (7). Despite further micromolecular clarification (8) its detailed function still remains speculative. At present it seems that THP is secreted in distinct portions of the tubule, the loop of Henle and the initial distal tubule and reflects the energy turnover of tubular cells. Ion reabsorption is linked to energy and solute supply and thus absorption of solutes and secretion of THP may be indirectly linked. In the present study excretion of THP was inversely related to sodium excretion (FE_{Na}) which supports this hypothesis. However, to clarify this issue further experiments are necessary.

THP secretion increases when kidney function improves. Thus, in contrast to shedded antigens, THP directly reflects renal tubular transporting ability. The rise in THP secretion within the first week after transplantation is a good parameter of initial graft response. Yet, its validity during and before rejection periods has to be clarified.

ACKNOWLEDGEMENTS

We thank Mrs. M. Kramer, R. Weller and Mrs. A. Brecht for excellent technical assistance.

We thank Dr. Neumann, Department of Pathology, Marburg for the help in histochemistry of THP and Prof. Vogt and Dr. S. Batsford, Department of Microbiology, Albert-Ludwigs-Universität, Freiburg for their help in Western blotting. This study is supported by the German Research Foundation (DFG-Zi 314).

REFERENCES

1. Steinhausen M, Parekh N, Zimmerhackl B: Pathophysiology of acute renal failure. In: Sybold G, Gessler U (eds); Acute Renal Failure, Basel, Karger, 1982, pp. 9-20.

2. Zimmerhackl B, Robertson CR, Jamison RL: The medullary microcirculation. Circ Res 57: 657-667, 1985.

3. Coudrier E, Kerjaschki D, Louvard D: Cytoskeleton organization and submembraneous interactions in intestinal and renal brush borders. Kidney Int 34: 309-320, 1988.

4. Drenckhahn D, Mannherz HG: Distribution of actin and the actin associated protein myosin, tropomyosin, alpha-actinin, vinculin and villin in rat and bovine exocrine glands. Eur J Cell Biol 30: 167-176, 1983.

5. Tamm I, Horsfall FL: A mucoprotein derived from normal urine which reacted with influenza, mumps and Newcastle disease viruses. J Exp Med 95: 71-97, 1952 .

6. Fabricius TH: Untersuchungen zur biochemischen und funktionellen Charakterisierung des Tamm-Horsfall Proteins vom Kaninchen. PhD thesis, University Münster, FRG, 1988.

7. Santoso AWB, Scott DW, Kinne R: Localization of Tamm-Horsfall protein in chloride transporting epithelia: lack of correlation with Na,K,Cl cotransporter. Eur J Cell Biology 43:104-109, 1987.

8. Pennica D, Kohr WJ, Kuang WJ, Glaister D, Aggarwal BB, Chen EY, Goeddel DV: Identification of human uromodulin as the Tamm-Horsfall urinary glycoprotein. Science 236: 83-88, 1987.

86

ENZYMURIA AS AN INDEX OF NEPHROTOXICITY OVER LONG-TERM EXPOSURE OF RATS TO GENTAMICIN

D.K. Obatomi, D.T. Plummer and J.D. Haslam

Department of Biochemistry and Physiology, King's College (KQC), University of London, Campden Hill Road, London, W8 7AH, UK

INTRODUCTION

Gentamicin is a powerful antibiotic used in the treatment of severe bacterial infections. However, it has been found by several workers to be nephrotoxic in man and laboratory animals. Quite often, evidence of nephrotoxicity is detected by histological and ultrastructural studies (1,2) and by the measurement of various renal function parameters (3,4). The former is tedious and time consuming while the latter is not very sensitive. There is a wealth of literature reporting an increase in urinary enzymes following renal injury induced by gentamicin in rats (5-7) and in man (8,9). Selection of enzymes for investigation in many cases appears to be almost random and only rarely are the reasons for a particular choice given. Previous investigations have also focussed more attention on the sensitivity of urinary enzyme measurement over other parameters with little or no attention given to the sequence of cellular injury involved. The present study therefore investigated the excretion of various enzymes which are markers of different regions of the cell so that the sequence of cell injury and the possible involvement of organelles in this process can be followed when the kidneys are damaged.

Alkaline phosphatase (ALP) is a membranous enzyme found at the brush border of the proximal convoluted tubule, glutamate dehydrogenase (GDH) is present in the mitochondria, lactate dehydrogenase (LDH), in the cytoplasm of the cell and N-acetyl-μ-glucosaminidase (NAG) is a lysosomal enzyme. The other enzyme assayed was muramidase (MUR) which readily passes through the glomerular membrane from the plasma and is reabsorbed from the renal tubules. The urinary muramidase activity therefore provides a useful index of the tubular reabsorptive capacity of the kidney. We also compared the excretion of these enzymes with other parameters of renal function. In addition, changes of these enzymes in serum were measured.

METHODS

Animals Adult male, Fischer 344 rats weighing 180-200g were used in the present study. Normal rat chow and water was provided ad libitum during the day while access to water alone was provided during overnight urine collection period.

Administration of Gentamicin Successive doses of 50 mg/kg gentamicin was administered to 18 rats for 10 days. The doses were given subcutaneously at 24 hr intervals. Control rats received saline solution.

Collection and Preparation of Urine Samples Urine was collected from groups of rats housed in perspex restraint cages overnight to avoid faecal contamination (10). Rats were kept in the cage for a 12 hr period. Urine samples were collected daily into test tubes maintained at 0°C in an ice-filled bucket. The volume of each sample was measured and time of collection noted. The pH was measured routinely and the presence of blood, glucose and ketone bodies was tested semi-quantitatively by Labstix (Ames Laboratories Ltd.; Stoke Poges, Buckinghamshire). The urine was centrifuged at 3000 g for 15 min and the supernatant removed. A suitable aliquot was diluted with an appropriate volume of buffer for the enzyme assay to eliminate the effects of inhibitors or activators (11).

Collection of Blood Unhaemolysed samples of blood were collected from the jugular veins of rats 12 hr after the last injection of gentamicin. The blood was allowed to clot at $37^{o}C$ and the serum separated by centrifugation. Enzyme assays were then carried out on appropriate aliquot of the serum.

Enzyme Assays and Protein Determination The activities of ALP, GDH, LDH, MUR were determined as described by Plummer & Ngaha (12) and NAG by the methods described Price et al (13) at $37^{o}C$ under optimal conditions.

The excretion of the enzymes into the urine was then expressed as mU excreted per hour and MUR as μg/ml/hr while the activities of enzymes in serum was expressed as μmoles/min/ml. Protein was estimated using a Biuret method (14).

Determination of Ions and Osmolality The concentration of Na^+ and K^+ in the urine was measured using a flame photometer (Radiometer, Copenhagen). The concentration of Cl^- was determined using a chloride meter (Corning-Eel, Halstead, Essex). The excretion of these ions was then calculated from the volume of urine passed and the weight of rat expressed as μmoles excreted/hr/100g weight of rat. The Wescor Inc. 5100B vapour pressure Osmometer was used to measure osmolality by the vapour pressure measurement. Osmolar excretion was calculated as μmoles excreted/hr/100g body weight.

Upper Limit of Normal Normal ranges were established for all measurements and the upper limit of normal determined. The upper limit of normal (ULN) was defined as the mean of control group rats ± twice the standard deviation of 200 rats.

RESULTS

Urinary enzyme excretion There appeared to be a biphasic pattern of excretion of LDH (Figure 1a) and NAG (Figure 1c). The rise in the first phase extended over 5 days for LDH and 4 days for NAG. However the 2nd phase extended over a longer period and the excretion of these enzymes were abnormal in both phases. Although the excretion of GDH was significantly higher than the control on days 1, 3 and 8 ($p<0.05$), it fell below the ULN (Figure 1b).

The excretion of MUR was normal until the 8th day when there was sharp increase in its excretion which reached a peak on the 11th day and then progressively returned to normal (Figure 2a). An initial increase in the excretion of ALP was obtained (Figure 2b), but rose above the ULN from the 12th day.

Serum Enzymes Serum enzymes measured after the 3rd and 10th injection of gentamicin did not show any significant increase compared to the control (Table 1).

Protein There was an increase in protein excretion from the 1st day of injection (Figure 3b). This increase was highly significant ($p<0.01$) when compared to the control. On the 4th day, the level returned to normal level. There was an increase in excretion on the 9th day and by the l5th day a peak value was obtained after which it finally returned to normal.

Osmolar Excretion This showed daily fluctuations and was only significantly elevated ($p<0.01$) above the control on days 11, 15, 17 and 18.

Electrolytes The excretion of Na^+ and Cl^- followed similar patterns (Figure 4a,b) significant excretion of these electrolytes was obtained on day 3 ($p<0.05$) and day 10 ($p<0.01$) but fall below the ULN. K^+ excretion shows daily fluctuations but remained within the normal range throughout the period of the experiments (Figure 4c).

Urinary pH and Abnormal Constituents The pH of the urine samples recorded were be-

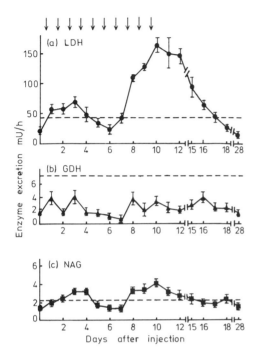

Figure 1. The effect of repeated injections of gentamicin (50mg/kg) on the excretion of LDH, GDH and NAG before (day 0), during (days 1-10) and after (days 11-28) treatment. (POINTING ARROWS indicate gentamicin administration while horizontal dotted lines indicate upper limit of normal.)

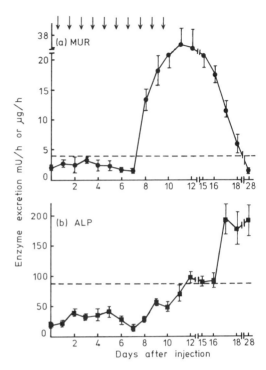

Figure 2. The effect of repeated injections of gentamicin (50mg/kg) on the excretion of Mur and ALP before (day 0), during (days 1-10) and after (days 11-28) treatment. (POINTING ARROWS indicate gentamicin administration while horizontal dotted lines indicate upper limit of normal.)

tween 5.3-8.3. Large amounts of glucose started appearing in the urine from the 9th day and remained until the 11th day. No glucose was detected afterwards.

DISCUSSION

The aim of this study was to determine, if possible, the sequence of cell injury when the kidneys are damaged by gentamicin. The gentamicin dosage employed in these rats was considerably higher than those used in man compared on a weight basis, but remained a standard toxic dose employed in a laboratory. The damage to the kidney was reflected in the changes seen in the excretion of some of the enzymes measured into urine. The pattern and

level of GDH excretion did not suggest any severe damage to the mitochondria. Studies by Plummer and Ngaha (12) indicated that this enzyme was only increased at a very high dose of cephaloridine (20mg/kg body weight) in Wistar rats. It therefore appears that mitochondria are not involved in the early damage to the kidney following the administration of this drug. In vitro studies conducted by Morin et al (15) indicate slight swelling of mitochondria when incubated with gentamicin but did not cause any leakage of enzymes into the medium. It is therefore possible that accumulation of gentamicin in mitochondria may be unrelated to the mechanism that produces cell damage.

Table 1. The activities of enzyme in serum before (day 0), during (day 1,3,10) and after (day 28) treatment of rats with gentamicin (50 mg/kg/day).

Enzyme	SERUM ACTIVITY (umoles/min/ml ± SD)				
	day 0	day 1	day 3	day 10	day 28
ALP	108.00±27.2	407.00±32.5**	158.00±887	102.00±15.4	110.00±35.6
GDH	29.80±11.0	95.20±47.5**	47.60±19.4	24.70±1.52	32.70±12.3
LDH	2775.00±1306	3036.00±1338	3353.00±1058	2176.00±885	2771.00±1126
MUR	118.00±51.4	273.00±123*	205.00±148	330.00±207*	212.00±60.2
NAG	5.05±0.74	4.03±1.12	4.36±1.02	7.45±3.06	5.62±1.25

*p<0.05; **p<0.01 compared to control; n = 6.

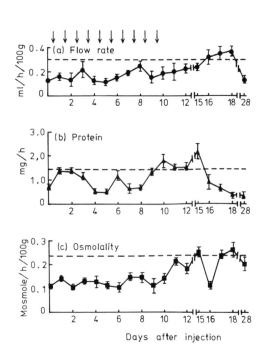

Figure 3.   The effect of repeated injections of gentamicin (50mg/kg) on the flow rate, protein and osmolar excretion before (day 0), during (days 1-10) and after treatment. (POINTING DOWN ARROWS indicate gentamicin administration while horizontal dotted lines indicate upper limit of normal.)

The pattern of excretion of ALP suggests that the brush border membrane is probably only affected when severe damage is inflicted upon the kidney.   An early observations made by Wellwood et al (16) showed that urinary ALP was highly elevated after injecting 100mg/kg gentamicin for 5 days into rats. Kempson et al (17) also reported a sharp increase in ALP caused by HgCl₂ and this was attributed to its primary effect on the proximal tubule causing a loss of brush border membrane thereby provoking a sharp increase in ALP. Price (18) in his recent review noted that the excretion of ALP normally occurs later when the membrane is damaged and is therefore indicative of a severe damage. This appears to be the case as obtained in this study. The appearance of MUR in significant amounts in urine after the 7th day of injection is an indication of tubular proteinuria and possible incomplete reabsorption in the proximal tubule. This also corresponds with the protein measurement and appeared to be a resultant effect of late damage to the kidney. From the results of Adelman et al (19), administration of 10mg/kg of gentamicin every 8 hr for 11 days leads to a significantly increased urinary muramidase at the later part of the experiments but for the first few days, the excretion was normal. Recently Cojocel and Hook (20) reported a decreased reabsorption

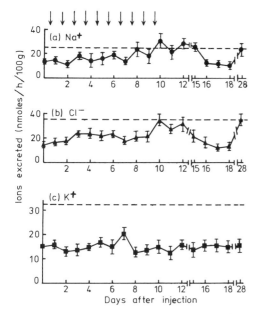

Figure 4. The effect of repeated injections of gentamicin (50mg/kg) on electrolyte excretion before (day 0), during (days 1-10) and after (days 11- 28) treatment. (POINTING DOWN ARROWS indicate gentamicin administration while horizontal dotted lines indicate upper limit of normal.)

of MUR after treatment with gentamicin (30mg/kg) for 14 days but recovery of tubular reabsorption capacity continued after the 14 days of treatment. Two phases of NAG and LDH excretions were obtained. Renal injury as determined by the measurement of these 2 enzymes showed that the first phase of damage was over a shorter period (1-4 days for LDH) than the second phase which extended over a longer period (Figure 1b). The trough between these phases may possibly represent regeneration of cells despite ongoing treatment with gentamicin, while the final return of excretion of these enzymes to normal level may indicate that the damage is reversible. The findings of Gilbert et al (7) using male Fischer rats given gentamicin (40mg/kg/day in 2 divided doses) over 14 days support our results. They observed a cyclical pattern of gentamicin nephrotoxicity based on morphological evi-

dence. In the first phase of damage, there was no observable tubular necrosis whereas this was evident by the 10th day when the peak renal gentamicin concentration was obtained. They also observed that tubular regenerating cells have lost their functional and metabolic vulnerability. Luft and Patel (6) have observed progressive excretion of some lysosomal enzymes on days 3, 5 and 10 and decreases on days 12 and 15 when a dose of 60mg/kg gentamicin was administered daily for 15 days. The peak excretion of the enzyme was obtained on day 10 which correlates with the observation made in this study. The significance of this cyclical pattern of damage to the cytoplasm and lysosomes is not well understood but has shown the vulnerability of these organelles to the dose of gentamicin given.

The various renal function parameters measured did not give any additional information to that obtained in measuring urinary enzymes. It is therefore concluded that these measurements are not as sensitive as urinary enzyme measurements and do not indicate the pattern of renal injury. In contrast to urinary enzymes, some of the serum enzymes were only significantly elevated on the first day after receiving gentamicin. However, there was a modest rise in serum MUR on day 10 (Table 1). In all, the serum enzymes were of little value in detecting renal damage and sequence of injury. From the results of our study, it appears that selection of appropriate enzymes can give information on the sequence of cell injury and the involvement of the organelles in this process. For instance GDH was not elevated above normal in the urine suggesting the absence of mitochondrial injury while the significant rise in MUR on days 8-17 is indicative of tubular damage. The increased urinary excretion of LDH and NAG at an early and late phase would support the idea that damage to the organelles and the kidney as whole is a gradual process and when this damage is severe, then the plasma membrane ALP is also released. Out of the enzymes examined, LDH and NAG appear to relate the sequence of injury and are recommended in the routine screening of renal injury.

ACKNOWLEDGEMENTS

DKO would like to thank May & Baker (Nigeria) Ltd for providing a Travelling Fellowship to enable him present this work.

REFERENCES

1. Kosek JC, Mazze RI, Cousins MJ: Nephrotoxicity of gentamicin. Lab Invest 30: 48-57, 1974.

2. Houghton DC, Houtnett M, Campbell-Boswell M, et al: A light and electron microscopic analysis of gentamicin nephrotoxicity in rats. Am J Path 82: 589-599, 1976.

3. Parker RA, Bennett WM, Porter GA: Animal models in the study of aminoglycoside nephrotoxicity. In: Whelton A, Neu HC (eds); The Aminoglycosides: Clinical use and Toxicology. New York, Marcel Dekker, 1982, pp. 235-267.

4. Luft FC, Block R, Sloan RS, et al: Comparative nephrotoxicity of aminoglycoside antibiotics in rats. J Infect Dis 138: 541-545, 1978.

5. Patel V, Luft FC, Yum MN, et al: Enzymuria in gentamicin induced kidney damage. Antimicrob Agents Chemother 7: 364-369, 1974.

6. Luft FC, Patel V: Lysosomal acid hydrolases as urinary markers of aminoglycoside nephrotoxicity in the rat. In: Fillastre JP (ed); Nephro toxicity: Interactions of drugs with membrane systems Mitochondria- lysosomes. New York, Massons Inc, 1978, pp. 127-141.

7. Gilbert DN, Houghton DC, Bennett WM, et al: Reversibility of gentamicin nephrotoxicity in rats: recovery during continuous drug administration. Proc Soc Exp Biol Med 160: 99-103, 1979.

8. Wellwood JM, Simpson PM, Tighe JR, Thompson AE: Evidence of gentamicin nephrotoxicity in patients with renal allografts. Br Med J 3: 278-281, 1975.

9. Wellwood JM, Price RG, Ellis BG, Thompson AE: A note on practical aspects of assay on N-acetyl-a-glucosaminidase in human urine. Clin Chim Acta 69: 85-91, 1976.

10. Leathwood PD, Plummer DT: Enzymes in rat urine: a metabolic cage for the complete separation of urine and faeces. Enzymologia 37: 240-250, 1969.

11. Plummer DT, Noorazar S, Obatomi DK, Haslam JD: The assessment of renal injury by urinary enzymes. Uraemia Invest 9: 97-102, 1986.

12. Plummer DT, Ngaha EO: Urinary enzyme as an index of kidney damage. In: Fillastre JP (ed); Nephrotoxicity: Interaction of drugs with membrane- systems Mitochondria-lysosomes. New York, Masson Inc, 1978, pp.175-191.

13. Price RG, Dance N, Richards B, Cattell WR: The excretion of N-acetyl-B- glucosaminidase following surgery to the kidney: Clin Chim Acta 27: 65-72, 1970.

14: Plummer DT: An Introduction to Practical Biochemistry, 3rd ed. London, McGraw-Hill Book Company, 1987, p.159.

15. Morin JP, Viotte G, Bendirdjian JP, et al: Aminoglycoside nephro toxicity: lysosomal and mitochondrial alterations in rat kidneys after aminoglycosides treatment. In Whelton A, Neu UC (eds); The Aminoglycosides: Clinical Use and Toxicology. New York, Marcel Dekker, 1982, pp 117-131.

16. Wellwood JM, Lovell D, Thompson AE, Tighe JR: Renal damage caused by gentamicin: a study of the effects on renal morphology and urinary enzyme secretion. J Pathol 118: 171-182, 1976.

17. Kempson SA, Ellis BG, Price RG: Changes in rat renal cortex, isolated plasma membrane and urinary enzymes following the injection of mercury chloride. Chem-Biol Int 18: 217-234, 1977.

18. Price RG: Urinary enzymes, nephrotoxicity and renal disease. Toxicol 23: 99-134, 1982.

19. Adelman RD, Conzelman G, Spangler W, Ishizaki G: Comparative nephro toxicity of gentamicin and netilmicin: Functional and morphological correlation with urinary enzyme activities. In: Dubach UC, Schmidt U (eds);

Diagnostic significance of enzymes and proteins in urine. Bern, Hans Huber Publisher, 1979, pp 166-182.

20. Cojocel C, Hooks JB: Aminoglycoside nephrotoxicity. Trends in Pharmacol Sci 4: 177-179, 1983.

87
URINARY TREHALASE AS A NEW MARKER FOR RENAL TUBULAR DAMAGES

M. Nakano (1) and K. Higuchi (2)

Institute for Medical Science of Aging (1), and Department of Obstetrics and Gynecology (2), Aichi Medical University, Nagakute-cho, Aichi-ken 480-11, Japan

INTRODUCTION

With any disease it is important to detect the disorder as early as possible. There are some indicators for renal failure such as glucosuria, proteinuria, enzymuria, and $beta_2$-microglobulin excretion. The enzyme trehalase [EC 3.2.1.28] hydrolyzes trehalose [1-alpha-D-glucopyranosyl- alpha-D-glucopyranoside] to two glucose moieties. It has been demonstrated biochemically (1) and histochemically (2) that trehalase is localized in brush borders of intestine and of proximal tubules. Urinary trehalase activity is elevated with mercuric chloride-induced acute tubular necrosis (3) and chronic cadmium poisoning (4) in experimental animals.

We have reported that Itai-Itai disease which is a serious case of chronic cadmium poisoning (5), and inhabitants in the Jinzu river basin (Toyama, Japan) show a significant increase in urinary trehalase activity (6). Urinary trehalase activity in Itai-Itai disease was inversely correlated with urinary glucose and urinary total protein (5). Urinary trehalase activity of inhabitants in the Jinzu river basin is increased and correlated statistically with other urinalysis components, such as $beta_2$-microglobulin, glucose, and total protein (6). In this paper, we describe a clinical role of urinary trehalase, and elucidate a severity of renal tubular lesions.

MATERIALS AND METHODS

The study populations: Pregnant women studied in this paper were inpatients and outpatients of the Aichi Medical University and Gamagohori City Hospital. The populations studied in this paper were female patients of Itai-Itai disease which are inpatients and outpatients of Hagino Hospital, and inhabitants of Jinzu river basin in Toyama prefecture (Japan), where there is one of the most severe cadmium polluted areas in the world. Patients with diabetes mellitus and inpatients and outpatients with other diseases were studied inpatients and outpatients at the Nagoya University Hospital and Aichi Medical University Hospital.

Collection of samples: Urine was collected as morning urine (7:00-9:00) in a poly-ethylene bottle, then divided into two portions and frozen at -80°C: One portion was used for the enzyme assay and the other for determination of $beta_2$-microglobulin, glucose, total protein, and creatinine contents. The urine for determination of $beta_2$-microglobulin was adjusted to pH ~ 6.0 by adding ammonia solution.

Assay methods for enzyme activity: The enzyme activity was assayed in the week after the collection of the urine. Pretreatment of urine and assay method of trehalase activity were based on the method described previously (3). Briefly, 5 ml of urine was dialyzed against distilled water and concentrated 10-fold (0.5 ml) by Minicon B-15 (Amicon Co.). The reaction mixture contained 20 alphamoles of phosphate buffer, pH 6.2, 40 alphamoles of trehalose and enzyme solution in a total volume of 0.25 ml. The reaction was stopped by the addition of

Tris-glucose oxidase-peroxidase reagent of Dahlqvist (7).

Assay for N-acetyl-alpha-D-glucosaminidase (NAG) was determined with an NAG Kit (Shionogi Co., Japan) using sodium m-cresolsulfonphthaleinyl N-acetyl-alpha-D-glucosaminide (MCP-NAG) as the substrate.

Analytical Procedures: Urinary beta$_2$-microglobulin was determined by radioimmunoassay Kit (Eiken Chemical Co.) or by enzyme immunoassay Kit (Imuzyne beta$_2$-M; Fujirebio Co.). Creatinine content was measured by the Foli-Wu method (8).

Statistical analysis: Differences between means were tested with the student's t-test.

RESULTS

Urinary trehalase is quite stable, and no significant loss of the activity was observed during storage at 4°C or at -80°C for at least 2 weeks. Satisfactory reproducibility was obtained with samples from both healthy and pathological individuals. Table 1 shows the urinary trehalase activity of various patients with diseases such as diabetes mellitus, acute nephritis, and toxaemia of pregnancy. Urinary trehalase activity of these patients was significantly higher than that of healthy individuals. As shown in Table 2, urinary beta$_2$-microglobulin and urinary trehalase activity in patients of Itai-Itai disease and of inhabitants in the Jinzu river basin were significantly elevated compared to the reference area. As shown in Figure 1, urinary trehalase activity was significantly increased in the early stages of the pregnancy (the first trimester). In this stage, no significant change was observed in urinary NAG activity and beta$_2$-microglobulin (Table 3). At the second and the third trimester, urinary trehalase activity, NAG activity and urinary beta$_2$-microglobulin were significantly higher than the level of non-pregnant women. After delivery, urinary trehalase activity became low level at the puerperal 30th day. Similar phenomena were observed with urinary NAG activity and beta$_2$-microglobulin.

Table 1. Urinary Trehalase Activity of Various Patients

	Trehalase activity (umole glucose/hr/g creatinine)
Healthy (n=51)	4.02 ± 0.58
Diabetes mellitus (n=21)	17.60 ± 2.38 **
Acute nephritis (n=6)	51.80 ± 16.00 **
Others (n=20)	5.20 ± 0.95
Non-pregnant women (n=17)	6.40 ± 1.50
Mild toxemia (n=22)	57.50 ± 10.30 **

Values show mean±S.E. Figure in parentheses show number of cases. Significant difference: ** $p<0.01$.

Table 2. Urinary Trehalase Activity of Itai-Itai Disease and Inhabitants of Cadmium Polluted Area

	Trehalase activity (umole/hr/g creatinine)
Control (n=53)	4.28 ± 0.78
Inhabitants (n=55)	15.20 ± 2.87 **
Itai-Itai disease (n=43)	25.70 ± 3.30 **

Values show mean±S.E. Figure in parentheses show number of cases. Significant difference: ** $p<0.01$.

As shown in Figure 2, urinary trehalase activity showed a parabolic curve against urinary beta$_2$-microglobulin. The maximum trehalase activity was observed in the group with 100-125 mg beta$_2$-microglobulin. In the case of relatively lower levels of beta$_2$-microglobulin (Figure 2B), urinary trehalase activity showed a maximum in the group with 0.0-0.15 mg beta$_2$-microglobulin, and the activity was significantly higher than that of the lowest group of beta$_2$-microglobulin (0-0.15 mg) (p<0.05).

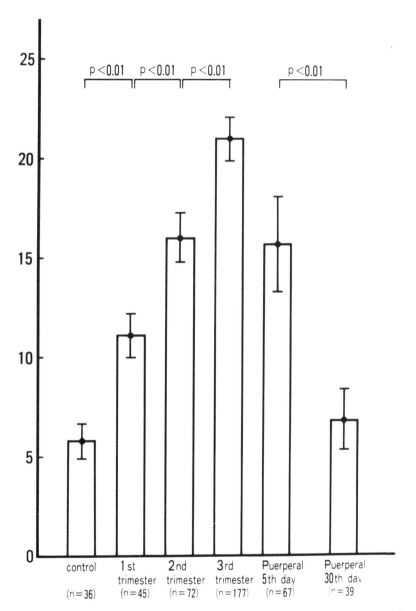

Figure 1. Urinary trehalase activity of pregnant women. Numbers in parentheses show number of cases.

Urinary trehalase activity in each group of total urinary protein was significantly increased compared with the group of 0-0.5 g protein (Figure 3). The activity showed an apparently parabolic curve against urinary total protein, and the maximum was observed at the group of 1.0-1.5 g protein.

DISCUSSION

Previously, we reported that acute tubular ne-

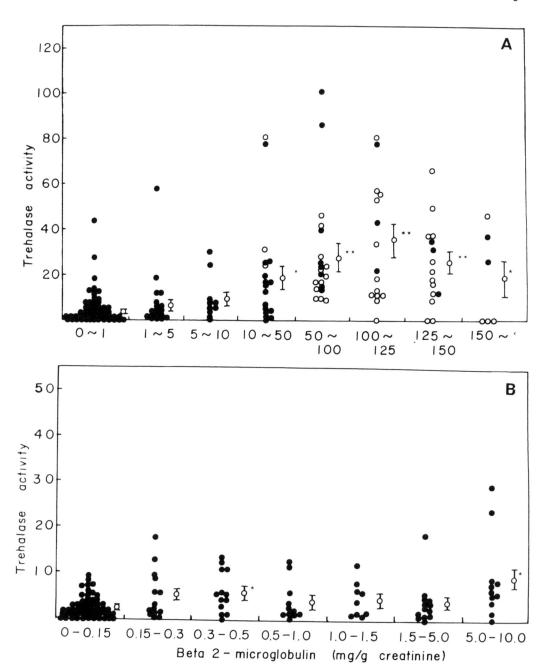

Figure 2. Urinary trehalase activity against urinary beta2-microglobulin in patients of Itai-Itai disease and inhabitants of cadmium polluted area. A: Relatively high urinary beta2-microglobulin, B:Relatively low urinary beta2- microglobulin . Open circle; Itai-Ita disease, closed circle; Inhabitants. Trehalase activity and beta2-microglobulin were expressed as umole/hr/g creatinine and mg/g creatinine. Significant difference: * p<0.05, ** p<0.01.

Table 3. Urinary Beta₂-microglobulin and NAG Activity in Normal Pregnancy

	Control	trimester			puerperal	
		1st	2nd	3rd	5th day	30th day
Beta₂-MG	88.7±24.7 (n=15)	120±22.2 (n=16)	175±15.9 (n=36)	380±53.3 (n=27)	115±25.5 (n=19)	68.9±6.3 (n=14)
NAG	2.7±0.6 (n=10)	3.0±0.5 (n=19)	4.8±0.6 (n=36)	5.0±0.6 (n=27)	3.2±0.5 (n=19)	1.8±0.2 (n=14)

Beta₂-microglobulin and NAG activity were expressed as ug/g creatinine and unit/g creatinine, respectively. Values show mean±S.E. Figure in parentheses shows number of cases. Significant difference: * p<0.05, ** p<0.01.

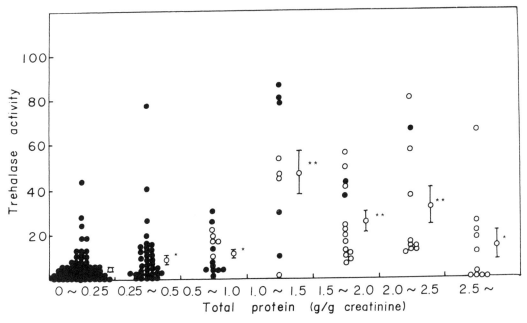

Figure 3. Urinary trehalase activity against urinary total protein in patients of Itai-Itai disease and the inhabitants of cadmium polluted area. Trehalase activity was expressed as in Figure 1, and total protein content was expressed as g/g creatinine. Open circle: Itai-Itai disease, closed circle; inhabitants. Significant difference: * p<0.05, ** P<0.01.

crosis with mercuric chloride (3) and chronic cadmium poisoning (4,5) showed the elevation of urinary trehalase activity, and that urinary trehalase had the same antigenicity as renal trehalase (3).

Urinary trehalase activity of various patients and of inhabitants in cadmium polluted area showed significantly higher values than that in controls (Tables 1 and 2). We reported that a statistically linear relationship was observed between urinary trehalase activity and urinary beta$_2$-microglobulin in the inhabitants in the Jinzu river basin (6), and in normal pregnancy (9). From these results, it is suggested that urinary trehalase is a good indicator for renal tubular damages. From the data of Figure 2, urinary trehalase showed parabolic relationship against urinary beta$_2$-microglobulin. In healthy individuals, small molecular substances such as beta$_2$-microglobulin, amino acid and glucose are freely filtered through the glomerulus and completely reabsorbed at the tubular site (10). Urinary excretion of beta$_2$-microglobulin seems to show a maximum level of about 150 mg per g creatinine (5) in Itai-Itai disease (11,12). This maximum level would be caused by no or little reabsorption at the tubular site. Namely, in these stages of disease severe damages should have occurred at tubular sites causing a severe loss of epithelial cells and/or brush borders. As a result, little brush border enzymes could be excreted in the urine at extremely high concentration of beta$_2$-microglobulin or glucose (5, 13).

It is interesting that urinary trehalase activity is rather low at extremely high beta$_2$-microglobulin, glucose or urinary total protein levels (Figures 2 and 3). Urinary trehalase and beta$_2$-microglobulin reveal different phenomena of tubular injury. The former shows a direct morphological injury of the tubular brush border, whereas the latter shows a dysfunction of reabsorption at tubular sites. Generally, urinary excretion of low molecular substances which pass freely through glomerulus and are reabsorbed at the tubular sites, are increased with progressive injury of renal tubules because of the dysfunction of reabsorption.

In summary, urinary trehalase activity was significantly elevated with normal pregnancy, diabetes mellitus, acute nephritis, and toxaemia of pregnancy, and correlated with beta$_2$-microglobulin. Activity of urinary trehalase was parabolically correlated with urinary beta$_2$-microglobulin and with urinary total protein. From these results, it is concluded that urinary trehalase activity is a good indicator for renal tubular injury, and that measuring both urinary trehalase and urinary beta$_2$-microglobulin can help to elucidate the degree of tubular injury.

REFERENCES

1. Berger SJ, Sacktor B: Isolation and biochemical characterization of brush borders from rabbit kidney. J Cell Biol 47: 637-645, 1970.

2. Nakano M: Localization of renal and intestinal trehalase with immunofuorescence- and enzyme-labeled antibody techniques. J Histochem Cytochem 30: 1243-1248, 1982.

3. Nakano M, Itoh G: Elevation of urinary trehalase in mercuric chloride- induced nephrotic rabbits: urinary trehalase as a specific indicator of renal brush border damage. Chem Biol Interact 45: 179-189, 1983.

4. Nishimura N, Ohshima H, Nakano M: Urinary trehalase as an early indicator of cadmium-induced renal tubular damage in rabbit. Arch Toxicol 59: 255-260, 1986.

5. Nakano M, Aoshima K, Katoh T, Teranishi H, Kasuya M: Elevation of urinary trehalase activity in patients of Itai-Itai disease. Arch Toxicol 60: 300-303, 1987.

6. Nakano M, Aoshima K, Katoh T, Teranishi, H, Kasuya M: Urinary trehalase activity and brush border damages of inhabitants in cadmium polluted area (The Jinzu river basin). Toxicol Lett 34: 159-166, 1986.

7. Dahlqvist A: Assay of intestinal disaccharidases. Anal Biochem 22: 99-107, 1968.

8. Bonsnes RW, Taussky HH: On the colo-

rimetric determination of creatinine by the Jaffe reaction. J Biol Chem 158: 581-591, 1945.

9. Higuchi K, Asai M, Suzuki M, Noguchi M, Ishihara M, Nakano M: Urinary trehalase activity in normal pregnancy: Renal tubular damages. Acta Obst Gynaec Jpn 38: 2045-2049, 1986.

10. Flynn FV, Platt HS: The origin of the proteins excreted in tubular proteinuria. Clin Chim Acta 21: 377-399, 1968.

11. Kjellstrom T, Piscator M: Beta2-microglobulin in urine induced by cadmium. In Padedoc No. 1, diagnostic communications. Pharmacia Diagnostics, Uppsala, Sweden.

12. Shiroishi K, Kjellstrom T, Kubota K, Evrin P-E, Anayama M, Vesterberg O, Shimada T, Piscator M, Iwata T, Nishino M: Urine analysis for detection of cadmium-induced renal changes, with special reference to beta2-microglobulin. Environ Res 13: 407-424, 1977.

13. Nakano M, Aoshima K, Katoh T, Teranishi H, Kasuya M, Katoh T: Severity of tubular brush border damage in cadmium-polluted area (Jinzu river basin): Clinical role of urinary trehalase. Environ Res 44: 161-168, 1987.

88

URINARY GLUTATHIONE S-TRANSFERASE IN SEVERAL MODELS OF PRIMARILY GLOMERULAR, DISTAL TUBULAR OR PAPILLARY DAMAGE

E. Bomhard (1), D. Maruhn (2) and H. Mager (3)

Institute of Industrial Toxicology (1), Institute of Clinical Research (2), Institute of Biometry (3), BAYER AG, D-5600 Wuppertal 1, Germany

INTRODUCTION

In the rat and the rabbit nephron the glutathione S-transferase (GST) is confined to the P_1 segment of the proximal convoluted and P_3 segment of the proximal straight tubule (1-3). A similar distribution has recently been confirmed for the human kidney (4). Injury to the proximal tubule leads to leakage of the cytosolic contents into the urinary space, which should make GST readily detectable in the urine. By contrast, lactate dehydrogenase (LDH) is distributed along most parts of the nephron (5) and measurement of both enzymes can be expected to provide information about the localisation of the nephron damage.

There are some published data on urinary GST measurements after acute and chronic toxic damage to the proximal tubule (6-13), but there is no data following treatment with model nephrotoxins that affect the glomeruli, distal tubules or papilla.

MATERIAL AND METHODS

Female Sprague-Dawley rats (average weight 250-350g) were housed individually in metabolic cages. Experimental group size was 10-12 animals per dose. Nephrotoxicity was induced by intraperitoneal injections twice daily on 3 consecutive days of 2.5 os 7.14 g/kg bovine serum albumin (BSA) or single intraperitoneal injections of puromycin aminonucleoside (PAN); 130 mg/kg, folic acid (FA; 125, 250 or 375 mg/kg) and ethyleneimine

(EI; 0.5, 2.0 or 5.0 ul/kg) respectively. The vehicles used were 0,9 % NaCl for BSA, H_2O for PAN and 0.3 m $NaHCO_3$ for FA, respectively. EI was administered undiluted. Urine was collected at 0°C immediately after the injections, in 24hr sampling periods for 4 days (all compounds) and days 7 to 10 (PAN). GST and LDH activity measurements (14,15) included a gel filtration step (16) to remove low molecular weight inhibitors. Enzyme excretion rates were calculated as mU/24hr and expressed as % control for that 24hr period. For the purpose of histopathological investigations the kidneys were fixed in formalin by in situ perfusion at the end of the urine sampling periods. Statistical analysis was performed by variance F-test or, if the F-test rejected, by the Dunnett-test.

RESULTS

BSA at a dose of 2.5 g/kg did not affect enzymuria. After 7.14 g/kg excretion rates were significantly increased for both enzymes on day 1 and 2 (Figure 1).

Glomerular damage with tubular involvement induced by PAN shows the typical delayed enzymuria (Figure 2). During the first 4 days enzyme excretion is normal, but it is significantly increased on days 7 through 10. A relative increase is more pronounced for LDH, but the GST profile parallels it.

Following administration of 375 mg FA/kg a very small transient increase in GST excretion could be measured on day 1 with median

571

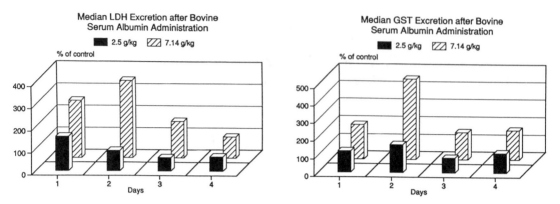

Figure 1. Effects of bovine serum albumin on lactate dehydrogenase (LDH) and glutathione S-transferase (GST) excretion.

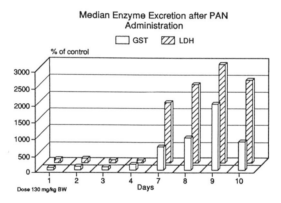

Figure 2. Effects of puromycin aminonucleoside on lactate dehydrogenase (LDH) and glutathione S-transferase (GST) excretion.

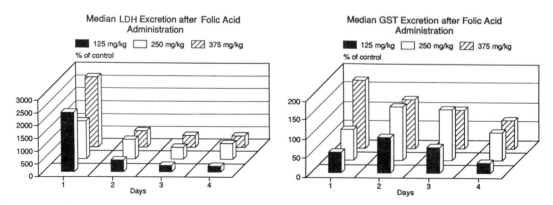

Figure 3. Effects of folic acid on lactate dehydrogenase (LDH) and glutathione S-transferase (GST) excretion.

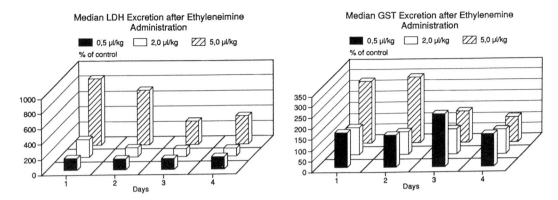

Figure 4. Effects of ethyleneimine on lactate dehydrogenase (LDH) and glutathione S-transferase (GST) excretion.

values of 177% of controls (Figure 3). LDH was elevated between about 1500 and 1700% of controls on day 1 with no clear-cut dose-dependency and remained significantly elevated from day 2 to 4.

Both enzymes were not affected after EI 0.5 µl/kg (Figure 4). Median LDH excretion was slightly elevated (220% of controls) the following 24hr after injection of 2.0 µl/kg but not subsequently. GST was unaffected in this group. Following EI 5.0 µl/kg, LDH increased 8.5-fold on day 1, 7-fold on day 2, and about 3-fold on day 3 and returned to control values on day 4. GST excretion was less, but was distinctly elevated 3- to 4-fold on day 1 and 2. Normal GST levels were measured on day 3 and 4.

Histopathological investigations revealed the well described lesions for each model compound, plus slight indications of proximal tubular involvement after high doses of BSA, FA and EI. In contrast, marked degenerative proximal tubular effects were seen after PAN corresponding to the highly elevated GST output.

CONCLUSIONS

The data suggest that the assay of urinary enzymes such as LDH and GST reflect slight alterations of renal cellular integrity. The simultaneous determination of LDH and GST proved to be valuable in identifying the site of damage due to their different distribution along the nephron. Continuous monitoring of enzymuria seems to be mandatory since enzyme excretion rates may return to normal levels even if morphological damage persists. Effects in the proximal tubule are qualitatively and quantitatively identified by GST determination. High doses of model substances that damage the glomeruli and distal nephron also cause secondary proximal tubule changes, thus interpretations of elevated GST excretions must be treated with caution.

ACKNOWLEDGEMENTS

We are grateful to Dr. O. Vogel for performing the histopathological investigations.

REFERENCES

1. Fine LG, Goldstein EG, Arias IM: Localization of glutathione transferase activity in the

rabbit nephron using isolated segments. Kidney Int 8: 474 (Abstr), 1975.

2. Fine LG, Goldstein EG, Trizna W, Rozmaryn L, Arias IM: Glutathione-S- transferase activity in the rabbit nephron: segmental localization in isolated tubules and formation of thiol adducts of ethacrynic acid. Proc Soc Exp Biol Med 157: 189-193, 1978.

3. Fleischner GM, Kamisaka K, Gatmaitan Z, Arias IM: Immunologic studies of rat and human ligandin. In: Arias IM, Jakoby WB (eds); Glutathione: Metabolism and function, Raven Press, New York, pp. 259-265, 1976.

4. Harrison DJ, Kharbanda R, Cunningham DS, McLellan LI, Hayes JD: Distribution of glutathione S-transferase isoenzymes in human kidney: basis for possible markers of renal injury. J Clin Pathol 42: 624-628, 1989.

5. Guder WG, Ross BD: Enzyme distribution along the nephron. Kidney Int 26: 101-111, 1984.

6. Bass IM, Kirsch RE, Tuff SA, Campbell JA, Saunders JS: Radioimmunoassay measurement of urinary ligandin excretion in nephrotoxin-treated rats. Clin Sci 56: 419-426, 1979.

7. Bomhard E, Maruhn D, Paar D, Wehling K: Urinary enzyme measurements as sensitive indicators of chronic cadmium nephropathy. In: Bianchi C, Bertelli A, Duarte E (eds); Kidney, Small Proteins and Drugs, Contributions to nephrology, Karger S, Basel, Vol. 42, pp. 142-147, 1986.

8. Bomhard E, Maruhn D, Vogel O: Comparative investigations on the effects of acute intraperitoneal cadmium, chromium and mercury exposure on the kidney. Uremia Invest 9: 131-136, 1986.

9. Feinfeld DA, Bourgoignie JJ, Fleischner G, Goldstein EJ, Biempica L, Arias IM: Ligandinuria in nephrotoxic acute tubular necrosis. Kidney Int 12: 387-392, 1977.

10. Feinfeld DA, Fleischner GM, Goldstein EJ, Levine RD, Levine SD, Avram MM, Arias IM: Ligandinuria: an indication of tubular cell necrosis. Curr Probl Clin Biochem 9: 273-278, 1979.

11. Feinfeld DA, Fleischner GM, Arias IM: Urinary ligandin and glutathione- S-transferase in gentamycin-induced nephrotoxicity in the rat. Clin Sci 61: 123-125, 1981.

12. Feinfeld DA, Sherman RA, Safirstein R, Ohmi N, Fuh VL, Arias IM, Levine SD: Urinary ligandin in renal tubular cell injury. In: Bianchi C, Bertelli A, Duarte E (eds); Kidney, Small Proteins and Drugs, Contributions to nephrology, Karger S, Basel, Vol. 42, pp. 111-117, 1984.

13. Feinfeld, DA, Safirstein R, Anderson H, Johnson R. Hardy M, Benvenisty A and D'Agati V: Urine glutathione S-transferase associated with nephrotoxic drugs. In: Bach PH, Lock EA (eds); Nephrotoxicity: Extrapolation from in vitro to in vivo and from animals to man. Plenum Press, London, pp. 705-710, 1989.

14. Goldstein EJ, Feinfeld EA, Fleischner GM, Elkien M: Enzymatic evidence of renal tubular damage following renal angiography. Radiology 121: 617-619, 1976.

15. Recommendations of the German Society of Clinical Chemistry (Empfehlungen der Deutschen Gesellschaft fr Klinische Chemie). Z Klin Chem Klin Biochem 10: 182-192, 1972.

16. Maruhn D: Preparation of urine for enzyme determinations by gel filtration. Curr Probl Clin Biochem 9: 22-30, 1979.

89

FUTURE MARKERS FOR THE DIAGNOSIS OF RENAL LESIONS

W.G. Guder and W. Hofmann

Institut für Klinische Chemie, Städtisches Krankenhaus München-Bogenhausen, Englschalkinger Strasse 77, D-8000 München 81, Germany

INTRODUCTION

The analysis of urine and blood for markers of renal diseases has a long tradition and is part of routine screening tests in the medical assessment of many patients. Compared to laboratory tests for liver and muscle integrity, however, the present routine programme to screen glomerular filtration rate (creatinine, urea in serum) and proteinuria (dipstick test) is neither sufficiently sensitive nor specific enough to detect renal functional defects at an early and possibly reversible stage. This holds especially for the detection of defects in tubular integrity, as caused by nephrotoxic agents and for minor impairments of glomerular filtration rate and quality.

A large battery of new techniques and possibly new parameters have been presented at this meeting, which might usefully be included into a future screening programme (Table 1). The clearance of Li^+, N- methylnicotinamide and free water have been proposed to monitor proximal and distal tubular function respectively (1-3). Metabolites which are either transported or synthesized by the tubule can be analyzed by chromatographic procedures. Microproteins, which are completely filtered are widely used as markers of reduced tubular protein reabsorption (4,5). In addition to tubular enzymes, a broad spectrum of tubular antigens are now being measured using monoclonal antibodies (6). These macromolecular markers can be measured with either the qualitative techniques of electrophoresis. Increasingly, however, the techniques of biotechnology are being applied to measure macromolecules in urine. This includes immunoblotting and immunotest strips, quantitating with homogeneous and heterogeneous immunoassays. DNA analysis in urine has just opened a new approach for possible future nephrotoxicity assessment (7). Using the technique of the polymerase chain reaction it is possible to analyse genes from single cells (8). Surface markers help to characterize cells in monitoring immunoligial processes (9). These high technology developments are also paralleled by better physiochemical techniques to image organs and even single atoms and molecules in the kidney in situ and in vitro with the aid of NMR and electron probe techniques (10,11).

When discussing the possible future implications of these analytical techniques one has to differentiate between projects which try to clarify the mechanisms of nephrotoxicity and those which will be used to monitor renal dysfunction in more or less defined animal and patient groups. This is the reason why most of the "new" parameters given above are widely used for mechanistic studies. The clinical biochemistry, however, has to analyze hundreds of samples per day from an unselected patient population. The application of most of these new methods is neither scientifically established nor are they currently cost-effective. The long experience which has already been accumulated for urinary enzymes, proteins and antigens will be the focus of this presentation.

Table 1 New parameters and techniques applicable to monitor nephrotoxicity

Parameters	Techniques
Clearance of Li^+, H_2O, and N-methylnicotinamide	
Metabolites	High pressure liquid chromatography
Enzymes and Antigens	Fluorimetric and luminometric Immunoassays
Microproteins	2-Dimensional electrophoresis Immunoblotting techniques Nephelometry, turbidimetry
DNA, mRNA	Southern blotting Pulse field electrophoresis Northern blotting Restricted fragment length analysis
In vivo imaging	Nuclear magnetic resonance spectroscopy
In vitro imaging	Electron probe analysis
Surface markers	Cell sorting

WHAT ARE THE CRITERIA FOR THE DIAGNOSTIC USE OF TUBULAR ENZYMES OR ANTIGENS?

Most diagnostic tests are introduced on the basis of empirical knowledge about their usefulness in diseased states.   As can be seen from Table 2, this knowledge can be divided into technical and biological criteria which together characterize the diagnostic quality of the parameter.

These criteria have been tested and proven to be acceptable for only a few parameters tested thus far.   Urinary N-acetyl-beta-D-glucosaminidase (NAG) may serve as an example. Intranephron localization in human nephron has recently been documented by Schmid et al. (12).   In contrast to previous studies in the kidney (13), highest activities were found in the S_3 segment of the proximal tubule and considerable activity resided in the final segments of the distal nephron. The lysosomal origin of this enzyme is also well known.   However, the mechanisms of enzyme release into the proximal and distal tubular urine is not well understood. Besides cell destruction, several other mechanisms have to be taken into consideration which may complicate interpretation of results obtained in an undefined urine (Table 3).

Thus the increased urinary NAG activity observed in early untreated diabetics may not be taken as a sign of tubular dysfunction, since tubular and glomerular hypertrophy may contribute to increased urinary enzyme excretion (13,14).   The observed increase of urinary NAG in hypertensive patients is likewise not yet explained (15).   Upon appropriate therapeutic treatment, hyperenzymuria in both diabetics and hypertensives seems to be reversible (14,15).

On the other hand the analytical criteria for the use of NAG as a marker have greatly improved. New substrates have become available which allow automation of tests in undiluted urines (16-18), and biological variation and other factors that influence the assay and interpretation have also been studied in detail (18,19). This allows the use of NAG in mass screening programmes, as proposed by Price 10 years ago (20).   When used in a screening profile, urinary

Table 2 Criteria for the diagnostic use of enzymes and antigens in urine

Technical	Biological
1. Precision.	1. Origin in the nephron and body
2. Standardization (accuracy)	2. Intracellular localization
3. Interferences	3. Mechanism(s) of release into urine
4. Technical performance (automation)	4. Stability in urine at 37°C
5. Costs	5. Influence factors (diet, blood pressure) (biological variation)
	6. Sampling conditions

NAG activity proves to be a very sensitive parameter to exclude nearly all kinds of tubular dysfunction, whereas its diagnostic power to differentiate between various types of renal diseases is poor (18) (see below).

WHAT PROTEINS SHOULD BE MEASURED IN URINE?

Albumin is well established as a sensitive marker for screening the quality of glomerular filtration in urine (5,18,21).   In contrast, less uniform opinions are found regarding the use of proteins to screen for tubular proteinurias based on technical and biological factors. As summarized in Table 4, several microproteins have been described which can be found in urine and may be useful to monitor tubular protein reabsorption.

Beta$_2$-Microglobulin has found the widest application, although it has poor stability in urine under physiological conditions (22).   Cystatin C, described to behave similarly in plasma to creatinine in renal insufficiency has not been well studied in urine yet (23).   On the other hand, retinol binding protein is easily measured in urine, it increases in renal tubular dysfunction, but major extrarenal factors affect plasma levels and filtration in a wide variety of clinical states (24). In addition to these limitations, the detection limits of the presently available assay systems hardly reach the levels needed to quantify at the upper level of normals. Alpha$_1$-microglobulin (the function of which is not understood) is only partially filtered, because its plasma level contains a free and covalently bound macromolecular fraction (25), but its plasma level is much less subject to extrarenal factors.   Furthermore, its urinary stability and low biological variance together with the availability of turbidimetric (18) and nephelometric (24) procedures make this parameter of tubular protein reabsorptive function one of great future potential. Studies in acute renal failure patients (26), diabetics (27) and patients on nephrotoxic drugs (26) look promising but require further validation.   This parameter may replace measuring urinary low molecular weight enzymes of plasma origin, which are markedly influenced by extrarenal diseases and can therefore only be interpreted when plasma activities are monitored simultaneously (28).

USE OF "NEW" MARKERS IN UNSELECTED HOSPITALIZED PATIENTS

In order to test the usefulness of urinary NAG, albumin and alpha$_1$- microglobulin as markers for glomerular and tubular function we measured these parameters in an automated version (18) in 409 urines sent to the laboratory for screening purposes.   The results were compared with the usual test strip procedure (pH, protein, leucocytes, blood, glucose). Whereas 191 urines were positive in at least one of the test strip fields, 255 urines exhibited at least one result outside the normal range with the quantitative parameters.   Together only 127 urines proved to be negative in both test profiles. Urines found to be positive in either NAG or albumin, but not in the test strip, were

Table 3 Possible mechanisms of enzyme (antigen) release into urine

Glomerular filtration

Inhibition of tubular reabsorption

Tubular or postrenal secretion

Induction by drugs and/or hormones

Change in cell and organelle turnover

Cell lesion and destruction

SUGGESTIONS FOR A FUTURE SCREENING PROFILE

In conclusion, the following profile is suggested to exclude glomerular and tubular diseases as well as postrenal and malfunction in hospitalized patients:- albumin, N-acetyl-beta-D-glucosaminidase activity, haemoglobin peroxidase and leucocyte esterase.

In addition, a quantitative test for total protein in urine is performed to detect all kinds of prerenal proteinuria (Bence-Jones, haemoglobin- and myo-lobinuria).   Only if one or more of

Table 4 Criteria for the use of microproteins as markers for tubular proteinuria.

Protein	Mol. weight kD	Analytical procedure	Stability in urine	Disturbing influence factors
Beta$_2$-Microglobulin	11.8	RIA, EIA	Not	+
Cystatin C	13.3	RIA, EIA	Unknown	?
Retinol binding protein	21	RID, nephel. turbid.	Yes	++
Alpha$_1$-Microglobulin	33	RID, nephel. EIA	Yes	(+)
Lysozyme	17	turbidimetry	Yes	+
Amylase	50	photometry	Yes	++

+ blood concentration changed by diseases, ++ blood concentration heavily changed by various diseases, (+) blood concentration little changed, ? no data available.

tubular and selective glomerular proteinurias. On the other hand most of those urines, which were negative with the quantitative procedure (but had a positive test strip result) had micro-haematuria or leucocyturia (18).   This experience led to the preliminary recommendation that haemoglobin peroxidase and leucocyte esterase should be included in a screening profile in spite of the increased sensitivity of the quantitative parameters. On the other hand, alpha$_1$-microglobulin excretion was rarely increased without simultaneous increase in urinary NAG activity (18).

these parameters is outside the normal range, quantitative measurements of alpha$_1$-microglobulin, IgG and other tests are performed to differentiate the various forms of renal proteinurias (29). It is hoped that the application of this profile will increase our capability in early detection of nephrotoxic and other renal diseases.

REFERENCES

1. Koomans HA, Boer WH, Dourhout Mees EJ: Evaluation of lithium clearance as a marker of proximal tubular sodium handling. Kidney Int 36: 2-12, 1989.

2. Holper K, Struck E, Sebening F: Die freie Wasser-Clearance zur frühen Diagnose akuter Niereninsuffizienz nach Operationen am offenen Herzen mit extracorporaler Zirkulation. Herz 2: 217-223, 1977.

3. Daley-Yates PT, Cal JC, Maiza A: Endogenous N-1-methylniconinamide as a marker of proximal tubular injury in animals and man. In: Bach PH, Delacruz L, Gregg NJ, Wilks MF (eds); Proceedings of the Fourth International Symposium on Nephrotoxicity. New York, Marcel Dekker, 1990, this volume.

4. Piscator M: Clinical and epidemiological validity of markers of tubular dysfunction. Tox Let 46: 197-204, 1989.

5. Yu H, Yanagisawa Y, Forbes MA, Cooper EH, Crockson RA, MacLennan ICM. Alpha-1-microglobulin: an indicator protein for renal tubular function. J Clin Pathol 36: 253-259.

6. Falkenberg FW, Denecke B, Bomhard B: Determination of rat urinary kidney-derived antigens with monoclonal antibodies - a new method for the detection of experimentally induced nephrotoxicity. In: Bach PH, Delacruz L, Gregg NJ, Wilks MF (eds); Proceedings of the Fourth International Symposium on Nephrotoxicity. New York, Marcel Dekker, 1990, this volume.

7. Bret L, Lul J, Pourrat JP, Fourni GJ: Extracellular DNA in blood and urine as a new marker of cytotoxicity. Technical aspects and pilot study on gentamycin nephrotoxicity in the mouse. Renal Failure, in press, 1990.

8. Saiki RK, Gelfand DH, Stoffel S, Scharf SJ, Higuchi R, Horn GT, Mullis KB, Ehrlich H: Primer-directed enzymatic amplification of DNA with a thermostable DNA polymerase. Science 239: 487-491, 1988.

9. Neumeier D, Pauls R, Wifling I, Fateh-Moghadam A, Knedel M: Immunophenotyping of lymphocyte subsets by the use of monoclonal antibodies and analytical flow cytometry: Evaluation of the method and reference values. J Clin Chem Clin Biochem 23: 765-775, 1985.

10. Gartland KPR, Sweatman BC, Beddell CR, Lindon JC, Nicholson JK: The application of high resolution proton nuclear magnetic resonance spectroscopy to the investigation of nephrotoxic lesions. In: Bach PH, Delacruz L, Gregg NJ, Wilks MF (eds); Proceedings of the Fourth International Symposium on Nephrotoxicity. New York, Marcel Dekker, 1990, this volume.

11. Mandel LJ, LeFurgey A, Ingram P: Quantitative elemental analysis of subcellular organelles in proximal renal tubules: Effects of alterations in active transport and metabolism. Presented at the 3rd Biannual meeting of the Am. Soc. Renal Biochem. Metabolism, jointly with the 9th Intern. Symp. "Biochemical Aspects of Kidney Function", Salamanca, 1989, p. 47 (abstr.).

12. Schmid H, Mall A, Bockhorn H: Catalytic activities of alkaline phosphatase and N-acetyl-beta-D-glucosaminidase in human cortical nephron segments: heterogenous changes in acute renal failure and acute rejection following kidney allotransplantation. J Clin Chem Clin Biochem 24: 961-970, 1986.

13. LeHir M, Dubach UC, Guder WG: Distribution of acid hydrolases in the nephron of normal and diabetic rats. Int J Biochem 12: 41-46, 1980.

14. Hofmann W, Guder WG: Urinary proteins of patients with diabetes mellitus. Klin Wochenschr 67 (Suppl 17): 37-39, 1989.

15. Alderman MH, Melcher L, Drayer DE, Reidenberg MM: Increased excretion of urinary N-acetyl-beta-D-glucosaminidase in essential hypertension and its decline with antihypertensive therapy. New Engl J Med 309: 1213-1217, 1983.

16. Noto A, Ogawa Y, Mori S, Yoshioko M, Kitahaze T, Hori T, Nakamura M, Miyake T: Simple rapid spectrophotometry of urinary N-acetyl-beta- d-glucosaminidase with use of a new chromogenic substrate. Clin Chem 29: 1713-1716, 1983.

17. Yuen C-T, Kind PRN, Price RG, Praill

PFG, Richardson AC: Colorimetric assay for N-acetyl-beta-D-glucosaminidase in pathological urine using the omega-nitrostyryl substrate:the development of a kit and the comparison of manual procedure with the automated fluorometric method. Ann Clin Biochem 21: 295-300, 1984.

18. Hofmann W, Guder WG: A diagnostic programme for quantitative analysis of proteinuria. J Clin Chem Clin Biochem 27: 589-600, 1989.

19. Schulze G, Goebel H: Harnenzymdiagnostik - ein Vorschlag zur Definition der pranalytischen Bedingungen. Z med Lab Diag 29: 381- 386,1988.

20. Price RG: Urinary-N-acetyl-beta-D-glucosaminidase as an indicator of renal disease. In: Dubach UC, Schmidt U (eds); Diagnostic significance of enzymes and proteins in urine. Bern, Hans Huber Publishers, 1979, pp. 150-163.

21. Mogensen CE: Hyperfiltration, microalbuminuria and hypertension in diabetic involvement and nephropathy. Akt Endokr Stoffw 10: 47-54, 1989.

22. Evrin PE, Wibell L: Serum levels and urinary excretion of beta-2- microglobulin in apparently healthy subjects. Scand J Clin Lab Invest 26: 69, 1972.

23. Simonsen O, Grubb A, Thysell H: The blood serum concentration of cystatin C (gamma-trace) as a measure of glomerular filtration rate. Scand J Clin Lab Invest 45: 97-101, 1985.

24. Hofmann W: Erste Erfahrungen mit der nephelometrischen Bestimmung von Einzelproteinen im Urin und ihrer diagnostischen Anwendung an ausgewhlten Beispielen. In: Fateh-Moghadam A (ed); Nephelometrie- Symposium. Marburg, Verlag Deutsches Grnes Kreuz, 1989, pp. 89-105.

25. Vincent C, Bouic P, Revillartd JP, Bataile R: Complexes of alpha- 1-microglobulin and monomeric IgA in multiple myeloma and normal human sera. Molecular Immunology 22: 663-673, 1985.

26. Kristof O: Harnproteine und Harnenzyme beim akuten Nierenversagen, Dissertation, Mnchen, 1990.

27. Hofmann W, Guder WG: Harnproteine bei Patienten mit Diabetes mellitus. Klin Wochschr 67 (Suppl XVII): 37-39, 1989.

28. Jung K, Pergande P, Schimke E, Ratzmann KP: Harnenzyme und niedermolekulare Proteine als Indikatoren der diabetischen Nephropathie. Klin Wochschr 67 (Suppl XVII): 27-30, 1989.

29. Hofmann W, Guder WG: Modern methods for differentiation of urinary proteins. Lab Med 13: 336-344, 1989.

INDEX

ABOUT THE EDITORS

PETER H. BACH is Head of the School of Science at the Polytechnic of East London and Head of the Nephrotoxicity Research Group at the Robens Institute of Health and Safety, University of Surrey, Guildford, Surrey, England. A member of the British Toxicological Society, Royal Microscopial Society, Renal Association of the United Kingdom, and Society of Toxicologic Pathologists, among others, Dr. Bach serves on the editorial boards of *Toxicologic Pathology, Toxicology,* and *Renal Failure* (Marcel Dekker, Inc.). Dr. Bach received the B.Sc. (1969) and M.Sc. (1972) degrees from the University of Natal, South Africa, and Ph.D. (1982) degree from the University of Surrey, England.

NEILL J. GREGG is a Toxicologist at the Boots Company PLC, Thurgarton, Nottingham, England. A member of the British Toxicological Society and Royal Microscopial Society, Dr. Gregg received the B.Sc. degree (1984) in anatomy and cell biology from the University of Sheffield, and Ph.D. degree (1990) in toxicology from the University of Surrey, both in England.

MARTIN F. WILKS is a clinical Toxicologist with ICI Central Toxicology Laboratory in Alderly Park, Macclesfield, Cheshire, England. A member of the British Toxicological Society, Federal Medical Chamber (Germany), and British Medical Association, Dr. Wilks received the M.D. degree (1986) from the Medical School in Hannover, Germany, and Ph.D. degree (1990) in toxicology from the University of Surrey, England.

LIGIA DELACRUZ is a Research Fellow in the Nephrotoxicity Research Group at the University of Surrey, Guildford, Surrey, England. A member of the British Toxicological Society, she received the B.Sc. degree (1971) in pharmaceutical chemistry from the University of Antioquia, Colombia; M.S. degree (1981) in animal nutrition from the National University of Colombia, Bogotá; and M.Sc. (1984) and Ph.D. (1988) degrees, both in toxicology, from the University of Surrey, England.